Musculoskeletal Ultrasound in Rheumatology Review

Minna J. Kohler
Editor

Musculoskeletal Ultrasound in Rheumatology Review

Second Edition

Springer

Editor
Minna J. Kohler
Massachusetts General Hospital
Harvard Medical School
Boston, MA
USA

ISBN 978-3-030-73554-8 ISBN 978-3-030-73555-5 (eBook)
https://doi.org/10.1007/978-3-030-73555-5

This Springer imprint is published by the registered company Springer Nature Switzerland AG
The registered company address is: Gewerbestrasse 11, 6330 Cham, Switzerland

I would like to dedicate this book to my parents Kahp and Michelle So, my husband Ed, and daughter Evelyn; thank you for your unconditional love and support.

Foreword

More than 20 years ago now, the first report of the use of ultrasound to guide the diagnosis of giant cell arteritis appeared, serving as my own introduction to the idea that this imaging modality could be useful in the rheumatic diseases [1]. The report was met with both excitement and skepticism at the time, and it was unclear which emotion to believe more. The ensuing years have confirmed, fortunately, that the excitement was in fact appropriate and well founded. The techniques of musculoskeletal ultrasound (MSK) have continued to evolve and progress, growing now to play important and sometimes critical roles in the diagnosis not only of giant cell arteritis, but also inflammatory arthritis, other joint conditions, and dozens of soft-tissue rheumatologic syndromes. In my own practice, I have often found the input of MSK crucial to the diagnosis and management of difficult patients, often obviating the need for additional, more invasive procedures.

Broad education and rigorous training have been essential to these advances. I have no doubt that this second edition will contribute substantially to these important developments in our field and am pleased to recommend it to all trainees and practitioners of our craft.

1. Schmidt WA, Kraft HE, Vorpahl K, et al. Color duplex ultrasonography in the diagnosis of temporal arteritis. N Engl J Med. 1997;337(19):1336–42.

John H. Stone, MD, MPH
Professor of Medicine, Harvard Medical School
The Edward A. Fox Chair in Medicine
Massachusetts General Hospital
Boston, MA, USA

Preface

Point-of-care ultrasound, or ultrasound performed and interpreted by the clinician in the clinic/office or at the bedside, has been rapidly expanding in use among multiple medical specialties. Musculoskeletal ultrasound has added value to clinical care to expedite diagnoses by visualizing mechanical versus inflammatory features and correlating these findings with patient's symptoms. The use of power Doppler to assess for subclinical inflammation or active hyperemia has been a distinguishing use of ultrasound for rheumatologists. Accurate needle guidance with ultrasound for joint and tendon procedures has allowed expansion of procedures in the clinic and has been associated with less pain and precise targeting of affected structures. Musculoskeletal ultrasound education is now offered in nearly all rheumatology fellowship training programs in the United States and is also included in residency training in other specialties (e.g., physical medicine and rehabilitation, orthopedics, podiatry, emergency medicine, and family medicine). Since the publication of the first edition of *Musculoskeletal Ultrasound in Rheumatology Review*, I have been excited to see the growth of musculoskeletal ultrasound in the field of rheumatology as well as other musculoskeletal specialties. This concise review book is designed for rheumatologists and other musculoskeletal providers learning and practicing the valuable skill of point-of-care musculoskeletal ultrasound. It is intended to serve as a practical guide for learning the fundamentals of normal sonographic anatomy and understanding how ultrasound can be incorporated into clinical care to assist in the diagnosis and management of common rheumatologic and musculoskeletal problems. Review questions are presented at the end of each chapter designed to highlight the essential concepts the reader should learn. These questions also serve as a self-evaluation and may be helpful for exam preparation.

Organization

This book begins with an introduction to musculoskeletal ultrasound use in rheumatologic disease, basic physics, and a "how-to" approach on learning about ultrasound equipment, image acquisition techniques, and common artifacts.

The next chapter, "Basic Sonopathology and Implementing Musculoskeletal Ultrasound into Clinical Practice," reviews the general sonographic appearance of normal anatomy in contrast to commonly encountered rheumatologic abnormalities with an updated review of the supporting literature. This chapter is newly organized to include practical aspects of adding musculoskeletal ultrasound into a clinical practice, including maintenance of equipment and cleaning guidelines.

Chapters 3 to 18 review the normal sonoanatomy of the upper and lower extremity joint regions (hand/wrist, elbow, shoulder, hip, knee, ankle /foot) and image acquisition of these areas using standardized scanning protocols. Commonly encountered sonopathology in rheumatologic and musculoskeletal conditions is reviewed, with updated case examples.

Musculoskeletal providers are well versed in joint aspiration and injections. Supporting literature review for ultrasound-guided injections and description of commonly used injection techniques with image examples are reviewed in Chap. 9, "Ultrasound-Guided Injections."

The state of pediatric ultrasound in rheumatology continues to grow. Chap. 10, "Pediatric Musculoskeletal Ultrasonography," reviews important sonographic differences to consider between adults and children with particular focus on careful interpretation of normal versus pathologic ultrasound images in rheumatologic patients. Due to the scope of this book, emphasis on fractures, dislocations, and other musculoskeletal issues that may be seen in emergency settings is not provided.

New to this second edition are chapters dedicated to rheumatologic disease, which provide a more in-depth review of the growing information we are learning through the power of ultrasound and how it may be applicable in the clinical setting. Chapters 11 to 15 include the use of ultrasound in the following diseases: rheumatoid arthritis, psoriatic arthritis, crystalline arthritis, osteoarthritis, systemic sclerosis, and systemic lupus erythematosus.

The final chapters of this book (Beyond Musculoskeletal Ultrasound, Chaps. 16 to 19) showcase the evolution of ultrasound use for non-musculoskeletal indications including vascular ultrasound for large vessel vasculitis, salivary gland ultrasound for Sjogrens and other mimickers, lung ultrasound for rheumatic interstitial lung disease, and a new advanced ultrasound technology chapter on the potential of ultrasound elastography and contrast-enhanced ultrasound in rheumatologic diseases.

It is incredible to see the expansion of ultrasonography within the field of rheumatology since the publication of the first book. This second edition strives to provide the fundamentals, as well as the latest updates, on how advancing ultrasound technology has changed our approach to everyday clinical practice by enhancing our clinical skills, in both diagnostic and procedural aspects. I hope this book fills a continued educational need for providing a comprehensive, practical guide to point-of-care musculoskeletal ultrasound for rheumatologic and musculoskeletal diseases.

Boston, MA, USA Minna J. Kohler, MD, RhMSUS

Acknowledgments

I would like to thank all the authors and contributors who have made this second edition book come to fruition. Their time, energy, expertise, and commitment to this project have made this concise, up-to-date review book for musculoskeletal ultrasound in rheumatology a valuable resource for clinicians incorporating musculoskeletal into their clinical care. I sincerely appreciate all their hard work, dedication, forward-thinking, and enthusiasm in bringing the latest updates in rheumatologic ultrasound to a wide audience. I feel blessed to have them as my rheumatology ultrasound colleagues. Without them, this book would not have been possible.

I would like to give special thanks to:

Dr. Joseph Craft is a Paul B. Beeson Professor of Medicine (rheumatology) and professor of immunobiology; former section chief, rheumatology section; and program director of investigative medicine at Yale University School of Medicine. His guidance and advice in my academic career have profoundly influenced my efforts. I am forever grateful for his encouragement to choose academic rheumatology as a career, where I have been able to pursue innovation to enhance clinical care as well as continue my passion for teaching.

Dr. Liana Fraenkel is former professor of medicine (rheumatology) at Yale University School of Medicine, now director of Patient Center Population Health Research at Berkshire Medical Center, and adjunct professor of medicine at Yale University School of Medicine. Dr. Fraenkel has inspired me by being an amazing role model and mentor. She has provided unconditional mentoring, support, and encouragement throughout my career and research endeavors.

Dr. John S. Reach is an associate professor of orthopaedics and rehabilitation and director of the foot and ankle section at Yale University School of Medicine. Dr. Reach first introduced me to point-of-care musculoskeletal ultrasound, and I am grateful for the unique, dedicated opportunity I had to learn from him.

Dr. John H. Stone is the Edward A. Fox Professor of Medicine at Harvard Medical School and director of clinical trials at Massachusetts General Hospital, Division of Rheumatology, Allergy, and Immunology. I thank Dr. Stone for his guidance, support, and encouragement for my academic career.

Dr. Andrew D. Luster is the Persis, Cyrus, and Marlow B. Harrison Professor of Medicine at Harvard Medical School; chief of the Division of Rheumatology, Allergy, and Immunology at the Massachusetts General Hospital; and director of the Center for Immunology and Inflammatory Diseases. I greatly appreciate and treasure the amazing opportunities and continuous support Dr. Luster has given me to start and grow the Massachusetts General Hospital Rheumatology Musculoskeletal Ultrasound Program.

I would also like to express my gratitude for Janakiraman Ganesan, project coordinator, Sydney Keen, and the entire Springer team in assembling, editing, and publishing this beloved project. It has been a pleasure working with all of you on this second edition!

Contents

Contributors

Catherine J. Bakewell, MD, FACR, RhMSUS Rheumatology, Intermountain Medical Group, Salt Lake Clinic, Salt Lake City, UT, USA

Arnold Ceponis, MD, PhD, FACR, RhMSUS Division of Rheumatology, Allergy and Immunology, University of California San Diego School of Medicine, La Jolla, CA, USA

Paul J. DeMarco, MD, FACP, FACR, RhMSUS Arthritis & Rheumatism Associates PC, Center for Rheumatology and Bone Research, Wheaton, MD, USA

Andreas P. Diamantopoulos, MD, PhD Department of Rheumatology, Martina Hansens Hospital, Bærum, Norway

Department of Rheumatology, Akershus University Hospital, Lørenskog, Norway

Amy Evangelisto, MD, FACR, RhMSUS Arthritis, Rheumatic and Back Disease Associates, Voorhees, NJ, USA

Robert M. Fairchild, MD, PhD, FACR, RhMSUS Division of Immunology and Rheumatology, Stanford University School of Medicine, Palo Alto, CA, USA

Hilde Berner Hammer, MD, PhD Department of Rheumatology, Diakonhjemmet Hospital, Oslo, Norway

Jay B. Higgs, MD, FACP, FACR, RhMSUS Brooke Army Medical Center, Rheumatology SVC, MCHE-MDR, Houston, TX, USA

Gurjit Singh Kaeley, MBBS, MRCP, FACR, RhMSUS Division of Rheumatology, University of Florida College of Medicine, Jacksonville, FL, USA

Eugene Y. Kissin, MD, FACR, RhMSUS Division of Rheumatology, Department of Medicine, Boston University Medical Center, Boston, MA, USA

Minna J. Kohler, MD, FACR, RhMSUS Division of Rheumatology, Allergy, and Immunology, Department of Medicine, Massachusetts General Hospital, Harvard Medical School, Boston, MA, USA

Gary A. Kunkel, MD, FACR, RhMSUS Division of Rheumatology, University of Utah, Salt Lake City, UT, USA

Anna M. Lafian, DO Division of Rheumatology, Department of Medicine, Loma Linda University School of Medicine, Loma Linda, CA, USA

Mark A. Matza, MD, FACR, RhMSUS Division of Rheumatology, Allergy, and Immunology, Department of Medicine, Massachusetts General Hospital, Harvard Medical School, Boston, MA, USA

Amanda E. Nelson, MD, MSCR, FACR, RhMSUS Thurston Arthritis Research Center and Division of Rheumatology, Allergy, and Immunology, University of North Carolina at Chapel Hill, Chapel Hill, NC, USA

Midori Jane Nishio, MD, FACR, RhMSUS Rheumatology, Walnut Creek, CA, USA

Naina Rastalsky, MD, FACR, RhMSUS SQZ Biotechnologies, Watertown, MA, USA

Johannes Roth, MD, PhD, FRCPC, RhMSUS Division of Pediatric Dermatology and Rheumatology, Children's Hospital of Eastern Ontario, Ottawa, ON, Canada

University of Ottawa, Ottawa, ON, Canada

Jonathan Samuels, MD, FACR, RhMSUS Division of Rheumatology, Department of Medicine, Center for Musculoskeletal Care, NYU Langone Hospital for Joint Diseases, New York, NY, USA

Vaneet K. Sandhu, MD, FACR, RhMSUS Division of Rheumatology, Department of Medicine, Loma Linda University School of Medicine, Loma Linda, CA, USA

Wolfgang A. Schmidt, MD Medical Center for Rheumatology Berlin-Buch, Immanuel Krankenhaus Berlin, Berlin, Germany

Veronika Sharp, MD, FACR, RhMSUS Division of Rheumatology, Department of Medicine, Santa Clara Valley Medical Center, San Jose, CA, USA

Wilmer L. Sibbitt Jr, MD, FACR Division of Rheumatology, Department of Internal Medicine, University of New Mexico Health Sciences Center, University of New Mexico, Albuquerque, NM, USA

Lene Terslev, MD, PhD Center for Rheumatology and Spine Diseases, Rigshospitalet-Glostrup, Copenhagen, Denmark

Ralf G. Thiele, MD, FACR, RhMSUS Division of Allergy/Immunology & Rheumatology, Department of Medicine, University of Rochester School of Medicine and Dentistry, Rochester, NY, USA

Karina D. Torralba, MD, MACM, FACR, RhMSUS Division of Rheumatology, Department of Medicine, Loma Linda University School of Medicine, Loma Linda, CA, USA

Janeth Yinh, MD, FACR, RhMSUS Division of Rheumatology, Allergy, and Immunology, Department of Medicine, Massachusetts General Hospital, Harvard Medical School, Boston, MA, USA

Introduction: Musculoskeletal Ultrasound Indications and Fundamentals

1

Wolfgang A. Schmidt

Key Points

- Point-of-care ultrasound can be performed and interpreted by the rheumatologist in the clinic or at the bedside as part of the clinical examination for clearly distinguishing between normal and abnormal conditions and for differentiation of pathology.
- An increasing number of indications are emerging for performing ultrasound in daily rheumatology practice, as well as other musculoskeletal care clinics.
- Musculoskeletal ultrasound is performed with linear transducers with frequencies of around 10 MHz (3–22 MHz). Higher frequencies provide better resolution but decreased depth.
- Anatomic structures are distinguished by different levels of echogenicity. For instance, bone is hyperechoic, fat tissue is isoechoic, synovium is hypoechoic, and fluid is anechoic.
- The sonographer should be aware of artifacts and can use them to help identify anatomic structures (i.e., anisotropy can help to find tendons).

W. A. Schmidt (✉)
Medical Center for Rheumatology Berlin-Buch, Immanuel Krankenhaus Berlin, Berlin, Germany
e-mail: w.schmidt@immanuel.de

M. J. Kohler (ed.), *Musculoskeletal Ultrasound in Rheumatology Review*,
https://doi.org/10.1007/978-3-030-73555-5_1

Introduction

Rheumatology is a fascinating specialty. Diagnosis strongly relies on history and clinical examination. Once a diagnosis is established, promising treatment options are available for the majority of rheumatologic conditions. Can ultrasound improve our clinical skills to examine a patient with suspected rheumatic disease? Yes, it definitely can! Combining history and clinical examination with ultrasound enables the rheumatologist to clearly define rheumatic disease entities. Ultrasound can be performed and interpreted by the rheumatologist at the point of care while interviewing and examining the patient. The added benefit of ultrasound with clinical correlation allows for expedited diagnosis and management and targeted treatment (e.g., ultrasound-guided injections) of rheumatologic conditions with the potential for improved clinical outcomes and decreased healthcare costs.

Indications for Ultrasound in Rheumatology

As rheumatology includes a wide range of diseases, ultrasound can be used for an increasing number of indications. The American College of Rheumatology has published a report of reasonable use of musculoskeletal ultrasonography in rheumatology clinical practice which provides a summary of clinical scenarios achieving positive evidence-based recommendations based on the current literature (Table 1.1) [1]. Additional recommendations have been published by EULAR for adults [2] and in pediatric rheumatology [3]. The following questions should be considered for the use of ultrasound in clinical practice:

- *Does my patient have articular pathology?* Clinical findings are often ambiguous particularly in large joints or in obese patients, which may only reveal painful impairment of the range of movement. It is also sometimes difficult to examine smaller joints, like the MTP joints. An examiner experienced in both sonography, and the clinical examination can clearly distinguish normal from abnormal conditions.
- *If pathology is present, which structure is affected?* Ultrasound can easily distinguish synovitis, effusion, tenosynovitis, tendinitis, paratenonitis, enthesitis, bursitis, and fasciitis. The respective pathologies are explicitly described in Chap. 2.
- *Does the abnormality represent inflammation?* Color or power Doppler ultrasound allows visualization of the vascularity in synovial tissue, tendon sheaths, and tendons. Increased vascularity correlates with inflammation [4]. An inflamed joint is treated differently than a swollen uninflamed joint.
- *Has pathology already lead to structural damage?* If joint swelling is already obvious, ultrasound is more sensitive than X-ray for detecting erosive disease. It takes only seconds to screen the MCP 2, MCP 5, and MTP 5 joints for the presence of erosions [5].
- *Is it rheumatoid arthritis (RA) or osteoarthritis (OA)?* Ultrasound is particularly sensitive for detecting osteophytes. OA of MCP joints may mimic RA. Ultrasound

Table 1.1 Summary of clinical scenarios for reasonable use of musculoskeletal ultrasound (MSUS) [1]

Indications for evaluation	Joints to evaluate	Level of evidence
Joint pain, swelling, or mechanical symptoms without definitive diagnosis	Glenohumeral, acromioclavicular, sternoclavicular, elbow, wrist, metacarpophalangeal, interphalangeal, hip, knee, ankle, midfoot, and metatarsophalangeal	B
Monoarthralgia or oligoarthralgia without definitive diagnosis (consider subclinical inflammatory arthritis or enthesitis)	Glenohumeral, acromioclavicular, sternoclavicular, elbow, wrist, metacarpophalangeal, interphalangeal, hip, knee, ankle, midfoot, and metatarsophalangeal	B
New or ongoing symptoms of inflammatory arthritis without definitive diagnosis on clinical examination (assess inflammatory disease activity, structural activity, or other causes)	Glenohumeral, acromioclavicular, elbow, wrist, metacarpophalangeal, interphalangeal, hip, knee, ankle, midfoot and metatarsophalangeal, and entheseal	B
Hip pain or mechanical symptoms without definitive diagnosis	Intra-articular and periarticular lesions and adjacent regional soft tissue structures of the hip	B
Periarticular pain without definitive diagnosis (consider tendon and soft tissue pathologies)	Shoulder, elbow, hand, hip, knee, ankle, and forefoot	B
Inflammatory-sounding entheseal, sacroiliac, or spine pain (enthesopathy)	Entheses	B
Shoulder pain or mechanical symptoms, without definitive diagnosis (consider underlying structural disorders)	Glenohumeral, acromioclavicular, rotator cuff	B
Inflammation, tendon, and soft tissue pathologies with regional mechanical symptoms, without definitive diagnosis	Shoulder, elbow, hand, wrist, hip, knee, ankle, and foot	B
Parotid and submandibular gland (consider Sjögren's disease)	Parotid and submandibular glands	B
Difficult to evaluate symptomatic joints due to fat or other soft tissue	Glenohumeral, acromioclavicular, elbow, wrist, hand, metacarpophalangeal, interphalangeal, hip, knee, ankle/foot, and metatarsophalangeal	C
Regional neuropathic pain without definitive diagnosis (e.g., median nerve entrapment)	Carpal tunnel, ulnar nerve at the cubital tunnel, and posterior tibial nerve at the tarsal tunnel	B
Guidance for articular and periarticular aspiration or injection	Synovial, tenosynovial, bursal, peritendinous, and perientheseal areas	A
Guidance for synovial biopsy procedures	Synovial areas	C
Monitoring disease activity and structural progression of joints in patients with inflammatory polyarthritis	Glenohumeral, acromioclavicular, elbow, wrist, hand, metacarpophalangeal, interphalangeal, hip, knee, ankle, foot, and metatarsophalangeal sites	B

can clearly differentiate between erosions and osteophytes in order to distinguish the two diseases [6].

- *Is it RA or psoriatic arthritis?* Psoriatic arthritis is characterized by multiple small erosions and proliferations different when compared to RA with larger erosions and less osteophytes [7]. Extra-articular manifestations of dactylitis and enthesitis can be differentiated.
- *Is it a pain syndrome, enthesitis, or tear?* Particularly the lateral humeral epicondyles, but also other anatomic areas like the medial femoral condyles and greater trochanter regions, are often painful either in the context of a musculoskeletal pain syndrome or because of inflamed anatomic structures. Tendons are hypoechoic and with increased hyperemia in enthesitis. Chronic inflammation leads to erosions, osteophytes, and calcifications [8]. Degenerative tendon tears can be visualized as a potential pain generator.
- *Is it trauma or inflammation?* In addition to tendon and ligament tears, ultrasound can visualize bony irregularities or disruptions together with hyperperfused edema along the bone in fractures. Stress fractures of the metatarsal bones can be easily distinguished from primary inflammatory conditions [9].
- *Is there nerve pathology?* Nerves are well visualized with ultrasound. Abnormal nerves are thickened and hypoechoic proximal or distal to a compression [10]. The median nerve is most commonly examined for carpal tunnel syndrome. In addition to nerve pathology, ultrasound can detect causes for compression such as tenosynovitis, synovitis, ganglion cysts, and soft tissue masses.
- *Does my patient have gout?* Urate crystal deposits on the articular cartilage generate a hyperechoic, often irregular, band known as a "double-contour sign;" its appearance and diameter can be similar to bone [11]. Intra-articular and extra-articular tophi have a hyperechoic "snowstorm" appearance. In addition, small hyperechoic spots, called "aggregates," or a "sugar in water clump" appearance, are often reported. Ultrasound is particularly valuable if there is no joint effusion amenable to aspiration and in patients with hyperuricemia without previous gout attacks in order to verify crystal deposition. Ultrasound is now included in the imaging domain for the ACR/EULAR gout classification criteria [12].
- *What about calcium pyrophosphate disease (CPPD)?* CPPD is often misdiagnosed as RA, gout, or OA. Ultrasound shows characteristic hyperechoic rounded and linear densities in fibrocartilage [menisci, discus triangularis carpi aka triangular fibrocartilage complex (TFCC)] and in the hyaline cartilage, particularly in the intercondylar cartilage of the knee [13].
- *What is the reason for acute swelling of the lower leg?* Ruptured Baker's cysts are common due to arthritis of the knee. Ultrasound can easily and quickly show the pathology and differentiate swelling from peripheral edema, abscess formation, soft tissue masses, and deep vein thrombosis.
- *How can I correctly place a needle for aspiration and injection?* Ultrasound guidance increases accuracy and particularly allows for identification of small amounts of abnormal fluid or synovitis that may have been missed with standard palpation-guided methods (see Chap. 9).
- *Does my patient have polymyalgia rheumatica (PMR)?* Most untreated patients exhibit inflammation in the shoulder and hip region, such as subdeltoid and

trochanteric bursitis, biceps tenosynovitis, and joint effusions. The specificity of classification criteria increases when incorporating ultrasound and hip ultrasound [14]. CPPD and calcific tendinitis may also be differentiated, which can be a mimicker for PMR.

- *Does the patient with PMR or with headache have giant cell arteritis (GCA)?* Even small arteries like the temporal arteries can be visualized due to the excellent spatial resolution of ultrasound [15]. Arterial walls exhibit concentric, noncompressible wall thickening, known as the "halo sign" in cases of acute vasculitis. The EULAR recommendations on imaging in large vessel vasculitis recommend ultrasound of temporal and axillary arteries as the first imaging modality particularly in cranial GCA [16] (see Chap. 16).
- *Is this primary or secondary Raynaud's phenomenon?* Likewise, ulnar, radial, and digital arteries are well visualized with ultrasound. Narrowing, stenoses, and occlusions are common in several rheumatic diseases such as systemic sclerosis, dermatomyositis, systemic lupus erythematosus, antiphospholipid syndrome, or vasculitis [17].
- *Is this Sjögren's syndrome?* Salivary gland ultrasound has become a specific, noninvasive tool in the diagnosis of Sjögren's syndrome. The parotid glands become inhomogeneous with characteristic hypoechoic areas representing dilated glandular ducts and lymph nodes [18] (see Chap. 17).
- *Can we assess the lungs with ultrasound?* Yes, we can. Pleural effusions occur in many rheumatic diseases. An inflamed pleura becomes thickened and irregular. B lines ("comet tails") represent several pathologies, but they are particularly common in pulmonary fibrosis. Ultrasound allows to see pneumothorax, peripheral tumors, and infiltrates. Infiltrates may have a triangular shape in pulmonary embolism (see Chap. 18).

Technical Fundamentals of Ultrasound

Ultrasound Waves

Ultrasound waves are generated by a transducer which represents the core of the ultrasound probe. The transducer consists of a disc with crystals of lead zirconate titanate. These crystals show a marked piezoelectric effect. They transform electrical potentials into mechanical vibrations and vice versa. When an electrical current passes through the crystals, the disc generates an ultrasound pulse. Conversely, when the disc receives an ultrasound wave that returns from the tissue, it will deform, and a voltage is generated on the transducer surface. Subsequently, the electronic potential is converted by a computer into an ultrasound image. The transducer functions as a receiver of returning ultrasound echoes for about 99.9% of the time. In the remaining 0.1% of time, it acts as an emitter of sound waves. Newer technology different from the standard piezoelectric crystals has also been developed to allow a single silicon chip with artificial intelligence capability to provide ultrasound images in frequencies between 1 and 10 MHz [19].

The term "ultrasound" refers to sound which is above the acoustic spectrum that can be heard by a human being. Humans can hear sound frequencies between 20 hertz (Hz) and 20,000 Hz. 1,000,000 Hz equate to 1 megahertz (MHz). Medical diagnostic ultrasound applies frequencies between 1 and 70 MHz [20].

Sound is a vibration that spreads as mechanical waves of compression and decompression. Sound waves travel with a velocity of 1540 m/s through air. They reach a distance of 10 cm after 0.000065 s. Within 1 second, about 1000 ultrasound waves can be emitted and received from an object at a distance of 10 cm from the ultrasound probe. Frequency (f) and wavelength (λ) are inversely proportional to each other, i.e., $f = 1/\lambda$. A higher frequency of the sound wave leads to a lesser penetration but to a higher resolution of structures. A lower frequency with longer wavelength leads to a greater penetration in the body, but resolution decreases.

The emitted waves are subject to transmission and reflection. Transmission occurs when a pulse passes through tissues. Reflection back to the source of the pulse occurs when an ultrasound pulse is reflected at an interface. The more two tissues differ in density from each other, the higher the amount of reflection; the more they are similar, the higher the amount of transmission. The boundary between two different tissues is called an acoustic interface. A marked interface exists between air and the skin. If one places the transducer on the skin surface without using a coupling medium, i.e., ultrasound gel, only 0.1% of the ultrasound pulse would be transmitted into the skin tissue, and 99.9% would be reflected by the skin surface. Therefore, with the use of ultrasound gel or water, a much higher amount of the ultrasound pulse penetrates into the tissue that will be examined. Liquids, like blood, urine, or synovial fluid, do not reflect sound waves. When the surface of an object is flat and no air is present between the source and the object, almost all of the ultrasound waves will be reflected from the object at right angles [21, 22].

Ultrasound Energy

Ultrasound loses its energy as it propagates through the tissue. This loss of energy is called "attenuation." There are three causes of attenuation: diffraction, scattering, and absorption. Diffraction refers to the bending of waves when they interact with obstacles in their path. Scattering means that waves are forced to deviate by nonuniformities of the tissue such as density fluctuations in fluids and inhomogeneous organs. Absorption means that acoustic energy is converted into heat energy. This implies warmth in body tissue. This phenomenon is applied for therapeutic ultrasound. Diagnostic ultrasound uses lower energies with a much lower effect on tissue temperature. A material or surface that absorbs sound waves does not reflect them. Absorption of a given material is frequency-dependent. Attenuation results in echoes from deep body tissues being displayed less intense than those returning from superficial structures. A function of the ultrasound system, called time-gain control, corrects the attenuation and technically intensifies the echoes returning from deeper structures.

Ultrasound Modes

A-mode is the simplest mode of ultrasound. A single transducer scans a line through the body. Along this line, the echoes are displayed on the screen as a function of depth. This mode is still sometimes used in ophthalmology to determine distances in the eye. The term B-mode stands for "brightness"-mode. This is the most commonly used mode in musculoskeletal ultrasound. It is also called gray-scale ultrasound. An array of transducers simultaneously scans a plane through the body. The information is displayed as a two-dimensional image on the monitor. M-mode stands for "motion"-mode. This mode is most commonly used in echocardiography for determining the movement of cardiac structures. It can also show the pulsation of an artery. M-mode displays the depth of echo-producing interfaces along one axis and time along the second axis, recording motion of the interfaces toward and away from the transducer. Doppler modes are explained in Chap. 11.

Ultrasound Equipment

An ultrasound machine consists of a computer, a monitor, a keyboard, and probes. Newer technology also includes probes with downloadable software or app to connect directly into a tablet or mobile phone device. Linear probes are capable of covering all indications for musculoskeletal ultrasound and most indications for vascular ultrasound. Abdominal ultrasound is mainly performed with curved array probes. Echocardiography is performed with sector array probes. Most linear probes are 4–5 cm long. Short probes with a length of about 2 cm are often called "hockey stick" or "footprint" probes because of their shape. They mainly serve to examine small superficial structures or for assessing regions that are difficult to reach, such as to determine MCP joint pathologies in hammertoes.

To date, most probes offer a range of frequencies, e.g., 10–22 MHz, 6–18 MHz, or 3–13 MHz. Therefore, only one or two probes are needed to cover most of the indications that are relevant in rheumatology. Low frequencies of about 5 MHz are needed for examining deep structures such as hip joints or glenohumeral joints. Higher frequencies are needed for examining superficial structures such as finger joints (>10 MHz) or temporal arteries (≥15 MHz).

The size of ultrasound machines differs considerably. Larger stationary equipment may provide higher image quality; however, with improving technology, smaller, portable ultrasound equipment has allowed wide expansion of ultrasound use by the clinician, varying in size from a laptop computer to pocket-sized equipment. Portable ultrasound machines are useful for orientation of office/bedside procedures, guided aspirations, and injections and allow the use of ultrasound in multiple clinical locations.

How to Use Ultrasound Equipment: "Knobology"

When starting to use the ultrasound machine, the diversity of possible functions may be overwhelming. However, the sonographer needs to particularly know a few specific knobs. Figure 1.1 shows a panel of a stationary ultrasound machine. The arrangement of the operating components differs between different ultrasound machines.

- *Power button (1)*: To date, most ultrasound machines have it clearly visible in the front. In older machines, the power button or a second power button may be located in the back.
- *Starting a new examination (2)*: After completing the last examination, data needs to be saved. For examining a new patient, this button leads to a menu for entering the new patient data.
- *Select probe (3)*: If you have more than one probe, pressing these buttons allows selecting the probe that is needed for the examination. In this machine, this function is found on the touch screen (16).
- *Preset (4)*: This button provides a variety of musculoskeletal, vascular, small parts (or thyroid) and other presets. Subgroups can exist [e.g., specific preset for shoulder/large joint v. hand (small joints)]. The sonographer can create or modify presets according to his or her preferences. Some smaller ultrasound equipment may already have defined presets that cannot be changed. In this machine, this function is found on the touch screen.
- *Frequency (5)*: Most transducers allow a choice between three and five frequencies. Some ultrasound machines indicate "resolution" for high frequencies and "penetration" for low frequencies. The sonographer should choose a higher frequency in order to receive a good resolution. If the image is too dark at the bottom of the image, the frequency needs to be lowered in order to increase the penetration. Some machines automatically adjust frequency.

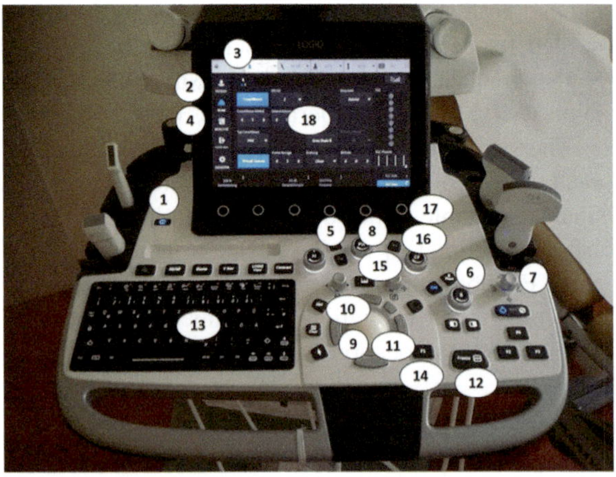

Fig. 1.1 Panel of an ultrasound machine showing important operating components. (*1*) Power button, (*2*) button for starting a new examination, (*3*) select probe, (*4*) preset, (*5*) frequency, (*6*) gain, (*7*) image depth, (*8*) focus, (*9*) track ball, (*10*) select, (*11*) set, (*12*) freeze, (*13*) keyboard/annotation, (*14*) save or print, (*15*) measure, (*16*) color and power Doppler, (*17*) PRF, (*18*) touch screen

- *Gain (6)*: This button adjusts the acoustic power of the transmitted signals. When increasing the power, the ultrasound image becomes brighter. The brightness may be also changed in a specific image depth by the sliders on the right side, also called "time-gain compensation controls." The sonographer needs to avoid too bright or too dark images ("over-gain" and "under-gain").
- *Image depth (7)*: It changes the field of view. The depth should be adjusted according to the size and depth of the examined structures.
- *Focus (8)*: The focus needs to be localized close to the anatomic area of interest. Two or more foci may be applied. The frame rate (the number of images produced within 1 s) may decrease with increasing number of foci. The frame rate should be at least 12 images per second for achieving an adequate image quality. The ultrasound equipment shown in the figure has an autofocus. In many machines, the focus button is localized at the bottom of the touch screen. In other machines, the focus position is adjusted with the track ball (9).
- *Track ball (9)*: The track ball may have several functions, e.g., placing a caliper or an arrow or adjusting the focus. When the freeze button is activated, scrolling the track ball allows review of the last sequences of the ultrasound examination (cine loop function, also known as "movie clip").
- *Select (10)*: Hitting this button leads to the different functions of the track ball.
- *Set (11)*: This button serves as the enter button for confirming an action. It may be located on the left or on the right side of the track ball. This button is labeled as "enter" on some machines.
- *Freeze (12)*: The button is pressed for acquiring a still image ("freeze"), e.g., for measurement or documentation and for starting the examination again ("unfreeze").
- *Keyboard/Annotation (13)*: By pressing a key on the keyboard, text can be written to label the ultrasound images, which is required for appropriate report documentation.
- *Save or print (14)*: These buttons allow saving still images and videos electronically or printing out images.
- *Measure (15)*: The sonographer can measure distances when using this button. Calipers appear ("+" at Fig. 1.4) that can be moved to an area of interest with the track ball.
- *Color Doppler and Power Doppler gain (16)*: By hitting these buttons, color or power Doppler mode will be activated. The color intensity (gain) increases or decreases by turning the button clockwise or anticlockwise, respectively. On some machines, the gray-scale gain is a knob that automatically will adjust color or power Doppler gain when a Doppler setting is activated.
- *Pulse repetition frequency (PRF, 17)*: This button increases or decreases the PRF for high- or low-flow velocities. It is often called "scale" button.
- *Touch screen (18)*: Many machines provide additional functions that can be managed with a touch screen.

How to Sit and Hold the Probe: Ultrasound Ergonomics

Ultrasound is a safe imaging technique for the patient, but the sonographer may develop medical problems because of inappropriate posture when performing ultrasound on a regular basis. The sonographer should sit comfortably on a chair. Preferably, the chair should revolve. The monitor should be at or below eye level. If space and patient positioning allows, the monitor can be adjusted in a way that both the sonographer and the patient can see the ultrasound image. The sonographer's hand that is holding the probe should rest comfortably on the patient. It is important to hold the probe firmly with the first three or four fingers and place the fifth or the fourth and the fifth finger and the ulnar part of the hand on the patient for probe stability. The sonographer should be aware of holding the arm comfortably to avoid rotator cuff problems of his/her own shoulders. Figure 1.2 shows an example ultrasound workplace.

The sonographer performs longitudinal (long axis) and transverse (short axis) views in relation to the body axis. Some views are oblique, e.g., for examining the sternoclavicular joints. The probe can be moved in different ways (Fig. 1.3).

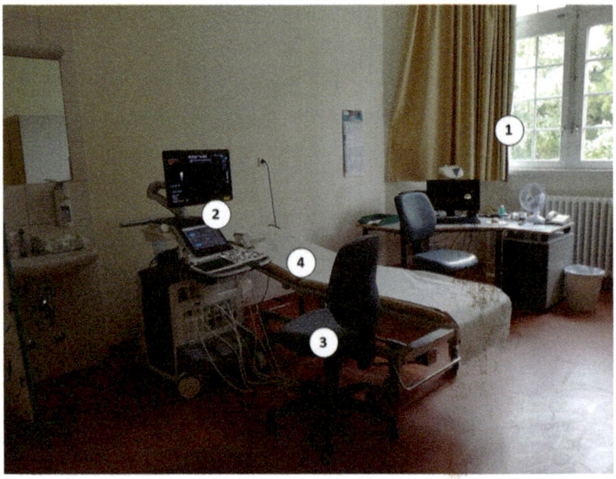

Fig. 1.2 Ultrasound workplace with (*1*) availability for dimming the daylight (*2*) ultrasound machine with monitor adjusted to the level of the sonographer's eyes, (*3*) revolving chair, (*4*) height-adjustable examination bed

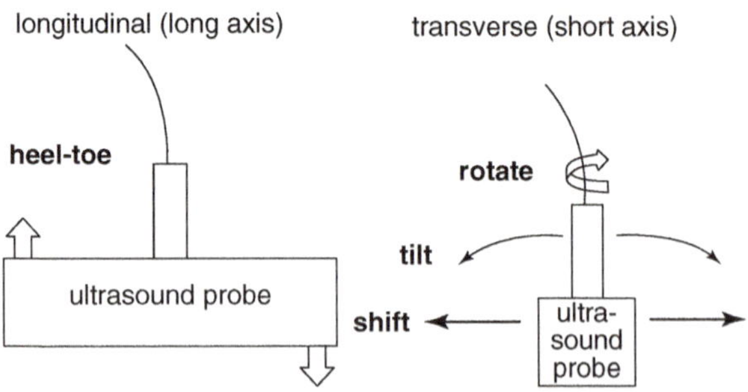

Fig. 1.3 How to move the ultrasound probe. Heel-toe, rotate, tilt, shift (axis change)

- Heel-toe: Angling the probe in a longitudinal plane, e.g., for avoiding anisotropy of the biceps tendon
- Shift or slide (or change the axis): Moving the probe side-to-side, e.g., for examining the full length of the biceps tendon
- Tilt (or rock): Angling the probe in a transverse plane, e.g., for adjusting the probe parallel to an anatomic structure
- Rotate: Change direction around the axis of the probe, e.g., for adjusting the probe parallel to a structure, e.g., a needle

How Anatomic Structures Appear on an Ultrasound Image

Structures can be isoechoic to soft tissue or deeply localized fat tissue, hyperechoic (brighter), hypoechoic (darker), or anechoic (black) (Fig. 1.4). Fat and connective tissue are heterogeneous. The skin is isoechoic or slightly hyperechoic. Tendons show a fibrillar pattern in longitudinal views. They are hyperechoic if located parallel to the probe and hypoechoic when insonation is not perpendicular because the reflected waves divert and miss the transducer. This phenomenon is called "anisotropy" (see below). Nerves are hypoechoic with a more dotted appearance than tendons (Figs. 1.5 and 1.6). The epineurium and fascicles of the nerve are typically hyperechoic in a honeycomb-like pattern. Fluid is anechoic or hypoechoic. Ultrasound may display physiologic amounts of fluid in normal joints or pathologic amounts of fluid (effusions) in inflamed joints. Synovium and synovial proliferations are hypoechoic. Cartilage is hypoechoic or anechoic. The bone surface is hyperechoic. Ultrasound waves cannot penetrate through the bone, and therefore,

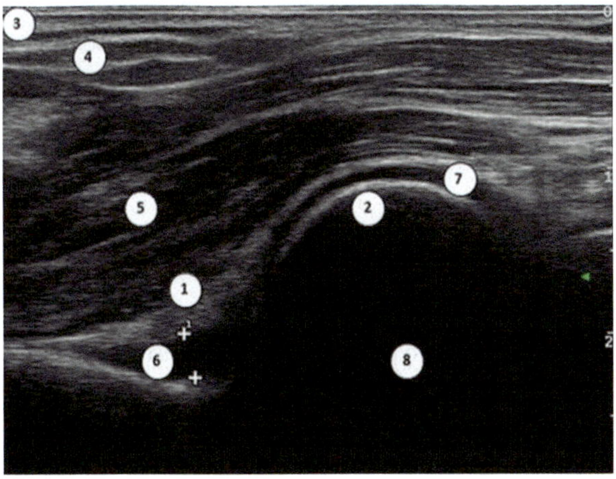

Fig. 1.4 Anterior longitudinal ultrasound image of an elbow with different types of echogenicity: (*1*) Soft tissue (fat pad)—isoechoic. (*2*) Bone—hyperechoic. (*3*) Skin—isoechoic. (*4*) Fat tissue—hypoechoic with hyperechoic septae. (*5*) Muscle—hypoechoic with hyperechoic septae. (*6*) Small amount of intra-articular fluid—anechoic, compressible. (*7*) Cartilage—anechoic. (*8*) Area under bone surface—anechoic

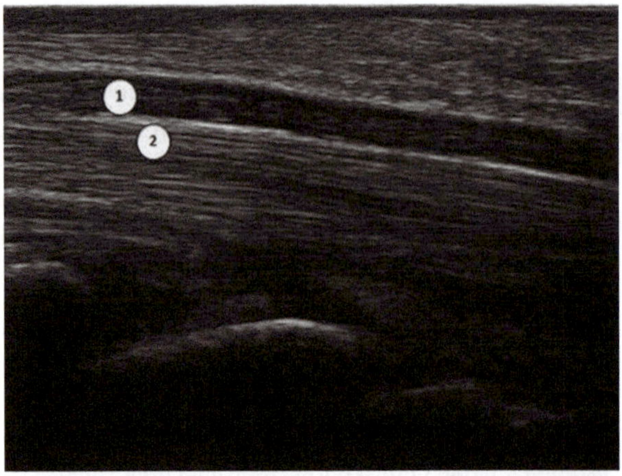

Fig. 1.5 Longitudinal palmar view of a wrist with (*1*) median nerve (hypoechoic) and (*2*) flexor digitorum tendons (fibrillar pattern)

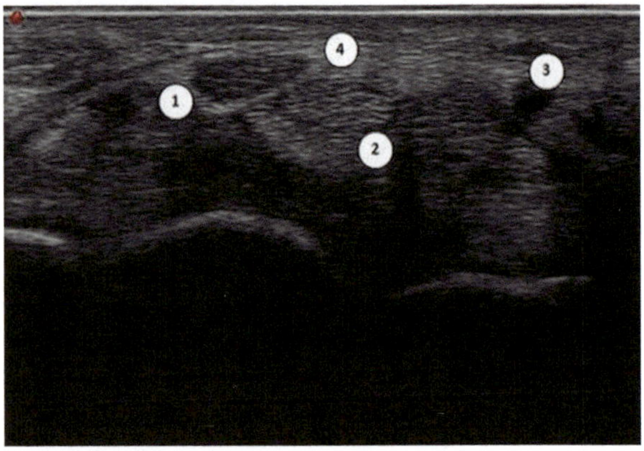

Fig. 1.6 Transverse palmar view of the wrist showing the different appearance of (*1*) median nerve, (*2*) flexor tendons, (*3*) radial artery, and (*4*) flexor retinaculum (anechoic)

musculoskeletal ultrasound cannot depict structures underneath the bone surface. Figure 1.4 shows different types of echogenicity.

1. Soft tissue (fat pad)—isoechoic
2. Bone—hyperechoic
3. Skin—isoechoic
4. Fat tissue—hypoechoic with hyperechoic septae
5. Muscle—hypoechoic with hyperechoic septae (fibrillar pattern in longitudinal view, "starry night" pattern in transverse view)
6. Small amount of intra-articular fluid—anechoic, compressible
7. Cartilage—anechoic
8. Area under bone surface—anechoic

Common Artifacts

When beginning to perform ultrasound, artifacts may cause some confusion because nonexisting structures or pathology may be suspected on ultrasound images [21]. With increasing ultrasound experience, artifacts may become helpful, for instance, in distinguishing a tendon from another structure by anisotropy.

Anisotropy

Tendons are strongly reflecting the sound waves. If tendons are not parallel to the probe, the reflected waves are not traveling back to the transducer (Fig. 1.7). The tendon appears hypoechoic. The proximal part of the biceps tendon is located more anteriorly than the distal part of the biceps tendon. By heel-toeing the probe, i.e., by pressing the distal end of the probe down, the probe becomes parallel to the tendon with increasing echogenicity of the tendon (Fig. 1.8).

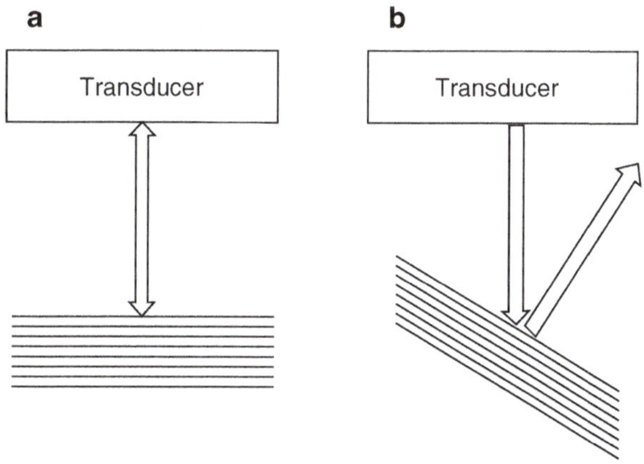

Fig. 1.7 (**a**) The tendon is parallel to the probe. The sound waves are reflected toward the probe. The tendon appears bright (hyperechoic). (**b**) The tendon is not parallel to the probe. The sound waves are reflected away from the probe. The tendon would appear dark (hypoechoic)

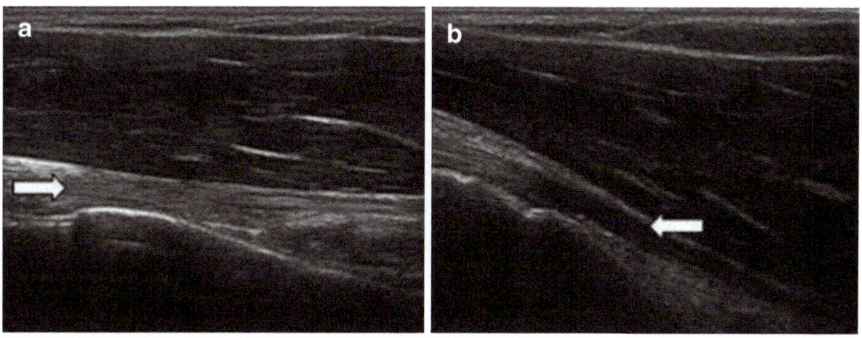

Fig. 1.8 Ultrasound image of a biceps tendon (*arrows*) (**a**) without and (**b**) with anisotropy

Posterior Acoustic Shadowing (Attenuation Artifact)

Sound waves are totally reflected or absorbed by bone or calcifications. The area below is anechoic. It is impossible to visualize structures below bone or calcifications (Fig. 1.9).

Posterior Acoustic Enhancement

Anechoic or hypoechoic lesions, such as fluid collections, cause reduced attenuation, i.e., transmission is increased with increased brightness of structures below the lesion (Fig. 1.10).

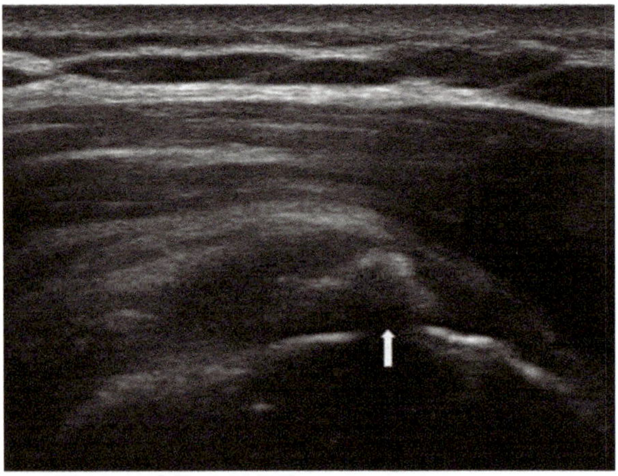

Fig. 1.9 A calcification of the supraspinatus tendon causes posterior acoustic shadowing mimicking a cortical break of the humeral head (*arrow*). The humeral head itself causes acoustic shadowing. The area below the bone is anechoic

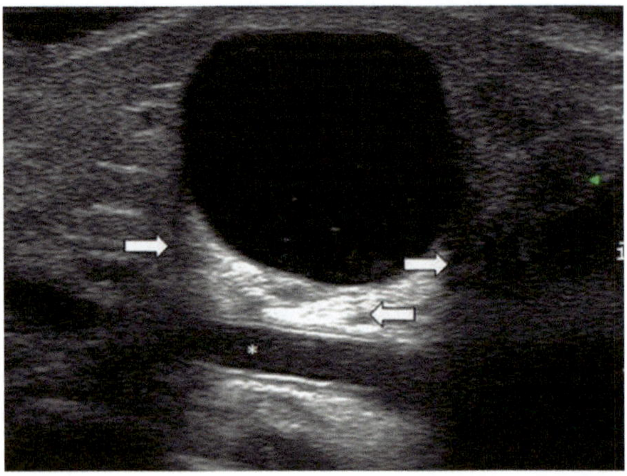

Fig. 1.10 Longitudinal image of a ganglion cyst at the volar side of a wrist. The echogenicity is increased below the anechoic ganglion (←). The radial artery (*) is much better visualized in this region. The two hypoechoic lines on both sides of the posterior acoustic enhancement represent lateral edge shadowing (→)

Lateral Edge Shadowing

This artifact is a thin acoustic shadow that appears behind edges of anechoic, hypoechoic, or curved structures, often tendons, but also fluid collections (Fig. 1.10). Sound waves encountering a curved surface at a tangential angle are scattered and refracted. Due to loss of energy, hypoechoic shadows appear.

Posterior Reverberation

When ultrasound encounters two parallel highly reflective surfaces, the sound waves are bounced back and forth between the two layers before returning back. The transducer detects a prolonged traveling time and displays additional images in deeper layers. Figure 1.11 shows reverberation by an injection needle. The sound waves bounce back and forth between the two sides of the needle with additional layers below the needle.

If the reverberation artifact appears more continuously below a metal surface, it is called a "ring-down artifact" (Fig. 1.12). If these artifacts are very thin with a marked difference in acoustic impedance to the surrounding tissue, they are also called "comet tail artifacts" (Fig. 1.13). These artifacts appear below metal nails and screws as well as below air. They are common in pulmonary fibrosis and may help diagnose pulmonary involvement in systemic sclerosis.

Mirror Image

This artifact is relevant both in gray-scale and color Doppler ultrasound. If a structure is located adjacent to a strong reflector, it may be duplicated on the other side of the reflector. The reflector causes additional sound waves that bend toward the neighboring anatomy, from where they are bounced back toward the strong reflector and return to the transducer (Fig. 1.14).

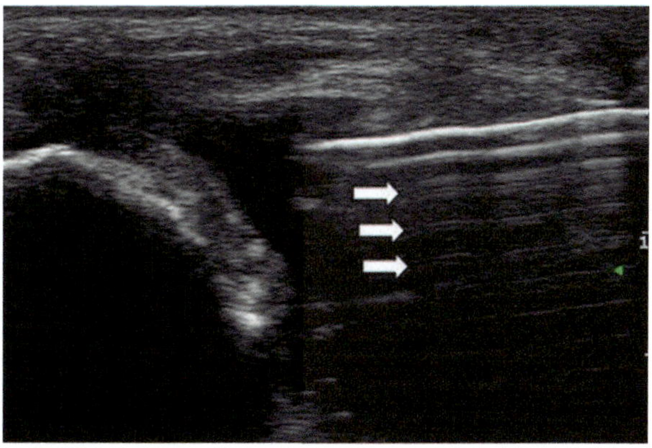

Fig. 1.11 Reverberation artifacts (→) below an injection needle

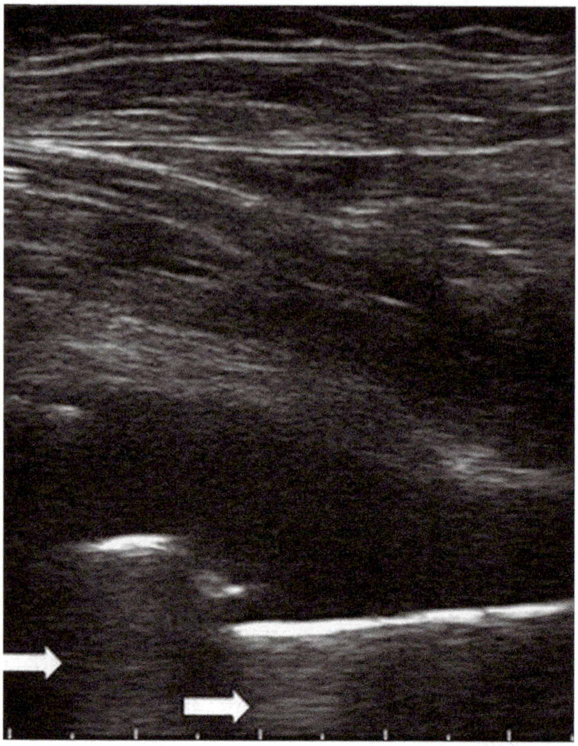

Fig. 1.12 Ring-down artifacts below a hip joint prosthesis (→)

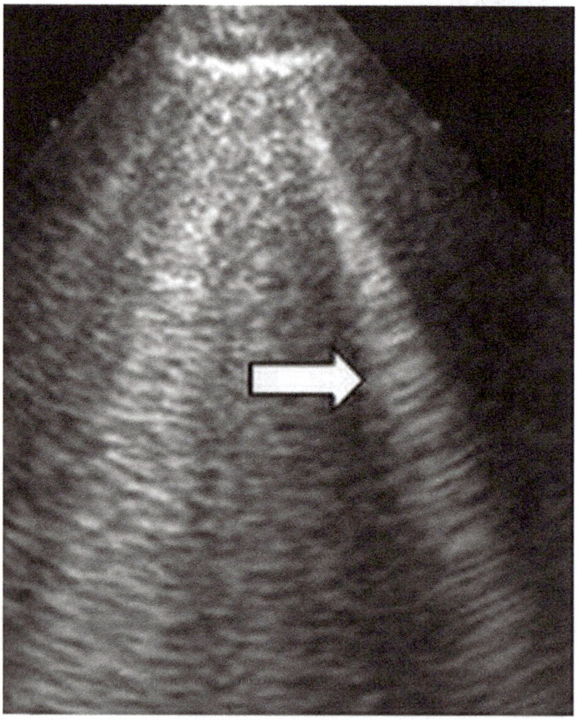

Fig. 1.13 Comet tail artifact in pulmonary fibrosis (→)

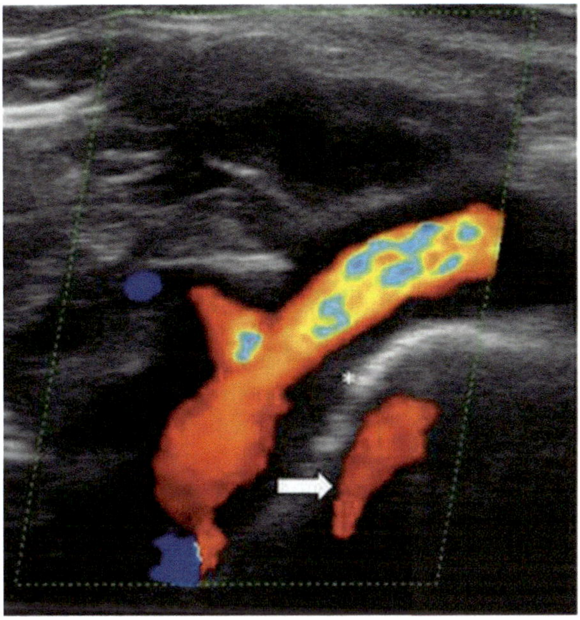

Fig. 1.14 Proximal left subclavian artery in large vessel giant cell arteritis (see Chap. 16). The clavicle (*) serves as strong reflector. The color signal of the subclavian artery is mirrored on the other side of the clavicle

Further artifacts with power Doppler and color Doppler ultrasound are covered in Chaps. 11 and 16.

Conclusion

Point-of-care ultrasound allows the clinicians to use their history and exam skills correlating with an ultrasound examination of specific joint regions to help identify pathology and/or confirm disease activity for better evaluation and management of musculoskeletal and rheumatologic conditions. Techniques to improve image acquisition and recognition of artifacts are important to the accurate interpretation of the ultrasound examination.

Review Questions

1. Which of the following is *not* a typical indication for ultrasound in rheumatology?
   (a) Search for erosions at MCP 2 and 5 and MTP 5 joints in early arthritis.
   (b) Detect bone marrow edema of sacroiliac joints in spondyloarthritis.
   (c) Estimate the inflammatory activity in the synovium of a swollen joint.
   (d) Distinguish osteoarthritis from rheumatoid arthritis lesions in finger joints.
   (e) Distinguish stress fracture from synovitis of MTP joints.
2. Which rheumatic disease has *no specific ultrasound finding*?
   (a) Sjögren's syndrome
   (b) Carpal tunnel syndrome

   (c) Small vessel vasculitis
   (d) Large vessel giant cell arteritis
   (e) Chondrocalcinosis (CPPD)
3. Which of the following statements is true?
   (a) Medical ultrasound refers to sound frequencies only between 10 and 20 Hz.
   (b) Higher ultrasound frequencies lead to better penetration.
   (c) The transducer functions as an emitter of sound waves for most of the time.
   (d) The loss of energy of ultrasound when traveling through tissue is called "attenuation."
   (e) Diagnostic ultrasound implies more heat in the body tissue than therapeutic ultrasound.
4. Which of the following statements about ultrasound modes is true?
   (a) A-mode is the ideal mode for examining joints.
   (b) B-mode stands for "brightness" mode.
   (c) M-mode is used for static structures.
   (d) 3D mode is essential for musculoskeletal ultrasound.
   (e) Doppler mode is useless for vascular imaging.
5. Which of these frequencies is most adequate for the respective anatomic region?
   (a) 1 MHz for ankle joint
   (b) 2 MHz for elbow joint
   (c) 10 MHz for wrist joint
   (d) 100 MHz for MCP joint
   (e) 200 MHz for DIP joint
6. Which of the following statements on ultrasound equipment is true?
   (a) The preset button serves for raising and lowering of the monitor.
   (b) The gain adjusts the acoustic power of transmitted signals.
   (c) The frequency can be adjusted by the time-gain compensation controls.
   (d) More foci increase the image frame rate.
   (e) Decreasing the frequency allows for higher image resolution.
7. How should the sonographer hold and move the probe?
   (a) The sonographer's fingers should not touch the patient's skin.
   (b) The monitor should be above the sonographer's eye level.
   (c) The sonographer's arm should be elevated while performing the examination.
   (d) For performing the heel-toe maneuver, the probe is angled along the transverse axis.
   (e) Tilting the probe helps adjust it parallel to an anatomic structure.
8. Which echogenicity corresponds correctly to a tissue?
   (a) Fluid is hyperechoic.
   (b) Soft tissue is anechoic.
   (c) Bone is isoechoic.
   (d) Synovitis is hypoechoic.
   (e) Hyaline cartilage is hyperechoic.
9. Which statement about anisotropy is true?
   (a) Anisotropy is due to reverberation.

(b) Anisotropy is typically found in vessels.
(c) The anatomic structure becomes dark when being parallel to the transducer.
(d) Anisotropy may be avoided by rotating the probe.
(e) Anisotropy may lead to misdiagnosis of fluid collections.

10. Which statement on other artifacts is true?
    (a) Posterior acoustic enhancement leads to increased echogenicity below a cyst.
    (b) Mirror images only occur in gray-scale images.
    (c) Due to lateral edge shadowing, the lateral areas of an ultrasound image are darker.
    (d) The area below bone is anechoic because of posterior reverberation.
    (e) A comet tail usually appears in fluid.

Answers

1. (b) Detect bone marrow edema of sacroiliac joints in spondyloarthritis.
2. (c) Small vessel vasculitis
3. (d) The loss of energy of ultrasound when traveling through tissue is called "attenuation."
4. (b) B-mode stands for "brightness" mode.
5. (c) 10 MHz for wrist joint.
6. (b) The gain adjusts the acoustic power of transmitted signals.
7. (e) Tilting the probe helps adjust it parallel to an anatomic structure.
8. (d) Synovitis is hypoechoic.
9. (e) Anisotropy may lead to misdiagnosis of fluid collections.
10. (a) Posterior acoustic enhancement leads to increased echogenicity below a cyst.

References

1. McAlindon T, Kissin E, Nazarian L, Ranganath V, Prakash S, Taylor M, et al. American College of Rheumatology report on reasonable use of musculoskeletal ultrasonography in rheumatology clinical practice. Arthritis Care Res. 2012;64:1625–40.
2. Möller I, Janta I, Backhaus M, Ohrdorf S, Bong DA, Marinoli C, et al. The 2017 EULAR standardised procedures for ultrasound imaging in rheumatology. Ann Rheum Dis. 2017;76:1974–9.
3. Colebatch-Bourn AN, Edwards CJ, Collado P, D'Agostino MA, Hemke R, Jousse-Joulin S, et al. EULAR-PReS points to consider for the use of imaging in the diagnosis and management of juvenile idiopathic arthritis in clinical practice. Ann Rheum Dis. 2015;74:1946–57.
4. Larché MJ, Seymour M, Lim A, Eckersley RJ, Pétavi F, Chiesa F, et al. Quantitative power Doppler ultrasonography is a sensitive measure of metacarpophalangeal joint synovial vascularity in rheumatoid arthritis and declines significantly following a 2-week course of oral low-dose corticosteroids. J Rheumatol. 2012;37:2493–501.
5. Wakefield RJ, Gibbon WW, Conaghan PG, O'Connor P, McGonagle D, Pease C, et al. The value of sonography in the detection of bone erosions in patients with rheumatoid arthritis: a comparison with conventional radiography. Arthritis Rheum. 2000;43:2762–70.
6. Iagnocco A, Naredo E. Ultrasound of the osteoarthritic joint. Clin Exp Rheumatol. 2017;35:527–34.

7. Riente L, Carli L, Delle SA. Ultrasound imaging in psoriatic arthritis and ankylosing spondylitis. Clin Exp Rheumatol. 2014;32(1 Suppl 80):S26–33.
8. Terslev L, Naredo E, Iagnocco A, Balint PV, Wakefield RJ, Aegerter P, et al. Defining enthesitis in spondyloarthritis by ultrasound: results of a Delphi process and of a reliability reading exercise. Arthritis Care Res (Hoboken). 2014;66:741–8.
9. Banal F, Gandjbakhch F, Foltz V, Goldcher A, Etchepare F, Rozenburg S, et al. Sensitivity and specificity of ultrasonography in early diagnosis of metatarsal bone stress fractures: a pilot study of 37 patients. J Rheumatol. 2009;36:1715–9.
10. Cartwright MS, Walker FO. Neuromuscular ultrasound in common entrapment neuropathies. Muscle Nerve. 2013;48:696–704.
11. Gutierrez M, Schmidt WA, Thiele RG, Keen HI, Kaeley GS, Naredo E, et al. International Consensus for ultrasound lesions in gout: results of Delphi process and web-reliability exercise. Rheumatology (Oxford). 2015;54:1797–805.
12. Neogi T, Jansen TL, Dalbeth N, Fransen J, Schumacher HR, Berendsen D, et al. 2015 Gout Classification Criteria: an American College of Rheumatology/European League Against Rheumatism collaborative initiative. Arthritis Rheumatol. 2015;67:2557–68.
13. Filippou G, Scirè CA, Adinolfi A, Damjanov NS, Carrara G, Bruyn GAW, et al. Identification of calcium pyrophosphate deposition disease (CPPD) by ultrasound: reliability of the OMERACT definitions in an extended set of joints-an international multiobserver study by the OMERACT Calcium Pyrophosphate Deposition Disease Ultrasound Subtask Force. Ann Rheum Dis. 2018;77:1194–9.
14. Macchioni P, Boiardi L, Catanoso M, Pazola G, Salvarani C. Performance of the new 2012 EULAR/ACR classification criteria for polymyalgia rheumatica: comparison with the previous criteria in a single-centre study. Ann Rheum Dis. 2014;73:1190–3.
15. Schmidt WA. Ultrasound in the diagnosis and management of giant cell arteritis. Rheumatology (Oxford). 2018;57(suppl_2):ii22–31.
16. Dejaco C, Ramiro S, Duftner C, Besson FL, Bley TA, Blockmans D, et al. EULAR recommendations for the use of imaging in large vessel vasculitis in clinical practice. Ann Rheum Dis. 2018;77:636–43.
17. Schmidt WA, Krause A, Schicke B, Wernicke D. Color Doppler ultrasonography of hand and finger arteries to differentiate primary from secondary forms of Raynaud's phenomenon. J Rheumatol. 2008;35(8):1591–8.
18. Wernicke D, Hess H, Gromnica-Ihle E, Krause A, Schmidt WA. Ultrasonography of salivary glands – a highly specific imaging procedure for diagnosis of Sjögren's syndrome. J Rheumatol. 2008;35:285–93.
19. European Society for Radiology (ESR). ESR statement on portable ultrasound devices. Insights Imaging. 2019;10:89.
20. Schmidt WA, Backhaus M. What the practising rheumatologist needs to know about the technical fundamentals of ultrasonography. Best Pract Res Clin Rheumatol. 2008;22:981–99.
21. Bruyn GA, Schmidt WA. Introductory guide to musculoskeletal ultrasound for the rheumatologist. Bohn Stafleu van Loghum/Springer: Houten; 2011. ISBN 978-90-313-9206-3.
22. Taljanovic MS, Melville DM, Scalcione LR, Gimber LH, Lorenz EJ, Witte RS. Artifacts in musculoskeletal ultrasonography. Semin Musculoskelet Radiol. 2014;18:3–11.

Basic Sonopathology and Implementing Musculoskeletal Ultrasound into Clinical Practice

2

Jonathan Samuels, Karina D. Torralba, and Minna J. Kohler

Key Points

- The Outcomes in Measures of Rheumatology (OMERACT) Ultrasound Task Force has developed consensus-based, standardized definitions for ultrasound pathology in rheumatology.
- Synovial thickening, synovial effusions, and cortical erosions can be seen in inflammatory arthritis; numerous studies in rheumatoid arthritis have focused on semiquantitative scoring/grading systems.
- Seronegative spondyloarthropathies, including psoriatic arthritis, may have differing ultrasound pathology compared to that of rheumatoid arthritis, such as enthesitis and/or dactylitis.
- Crystal arthropathies, such as gout and pseudogout, may be visualized by ultrasound, which can be important for diagnosis particularly when synovial fluid is unavailable for aspiration.

J. Samuels (✉)
Division of Rheumatology, Department of Medicine, Center for Musculoskeletal Care, NYU Langone Hospital for Joint Diseases, New York, NY, USA
e-mail: jonathan.samuels@nyumc.org

K. D. Torralba
Division of Rheumatology, Department of Medicine, Loma Linda University School of Medicine, Loma Linda, CA, USA
e-mail: ktorralba@llu.edu

M. J. Kohler
Division of Rheumatology, Allergy, and Immunology, Department of Medicine, Massachusetts General Hospital, Harvard Medical School, Boston, MA, USA
e-mail: mkohler@mgh.harvard.edu

M. J. Kohler (ed.), *Musculoskeletal Ultrasound in Rheumatology Review*,
https://doi.org/10.1007/978-3-030-73555-5_2

- Clinical guidelines for cleaning and preparing the use of ultrasound transducers, equipment, and between patients as well as safe handling of the use of ultrasound coupling gel have been created by the AIUM (American Institute of Ultrasound in Medicine).
- Adequate electronic medical record documentation of ultrasound examinations is required for billing.

Introduction

The use of musculoskeletal ultrasound has greatly enhanced our diagnostic capabilities within rheumatology. Before delving into the detailed anatomy and diverse sonopathology of specific joints, we would like to introduce some definitions of general sonographic findings that correspond to various pathologies that are frequently encountered. Such sonopathology spans across anatomic locations and often in multiple rheumatic/musculoskeletal disease processes. In this chapter, we present an overview of the breadth of sonographic pathology and describe the hallmark pathologic findings in a handful of the more common rheumatic diseases. We additionally provide logistical tips to start incorporating your new skill set into your daily clinical practice. We hope this foundation will serve as a stepping stone for the joint-specific chapters throughout the rest of the book.

Definitions

In 2005, the OMERACT ultrasound task force, a group of international rheumatology ultrasound experts, developed standardized, consensus-based sonographic pathology definitions for use in rheumatology ultrasound research and clinical practice [1]. These definitions, particularly for evaluation of inflammatory arthritis, have become the gold standard for reporting of rheumatologic ultrasonography findings.

Bone Erosion An intra-articular discontinuity of the bone surface that is visible in two perpendicular planes (see Fig. 2.1)

Synovial Effusion Abnormal hypoechoic or anechoic (relative to subdermal fat, but sometimes may be isoechoic or hyperechoic) intra-articular material that is displaceable and compressible, but does not exhibit Doppler signal (see Fig. 2.2)

Synovial Hypertrophy Abnormal hypoechoic (relative to subdermal fat, but sometimes may be isoechoic or hyperechoic) intra-articular tissue that is nondisplaceable and poorly compressible and which may exhibit Doppler signal (see Fig. 2.3; see Chap. 11 “Ultrasound in Rheumatoid Arthritis” for further details on synovitis)

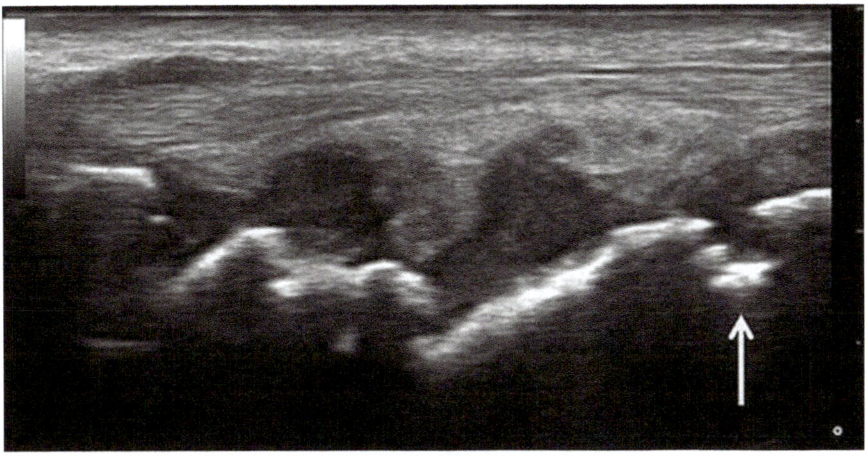

Fig. 2.1 Erosion. Wrist dorsal longitudinal view (*arrow* pointing to capitate)

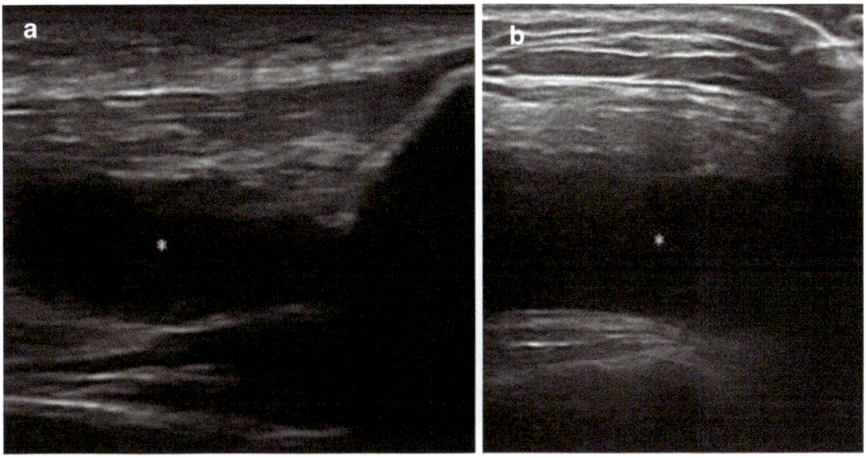

Fig. 2.2 Synovial effusion. (**a**) Knee, suprapatellar longitudinal view. (**b**) Knee, suprapatellar transverse view

Tenosynovitis Hypoechoic or anechoic thickened tissue with or without fluid within the tendon sheath, which is seen in two perpendicular planes and which may exhibit Doppler signal (see Fig. 2.4; see Chap. 11 "Ultrasound in Rheumatoid Arthritis" for further details on tenosynovitis)

Enthesopathy Abnormally hypoechoic (loss of normal fibrillar architecture) and/or thickened tendon or ligament at its bony attachment (may occasionally contain hyperechoic foci consistent with calcification), seen in two perpendicular planes that may exhibit Doppler signal and/or bony changes including enthesophytes, erosions, or irregularity.

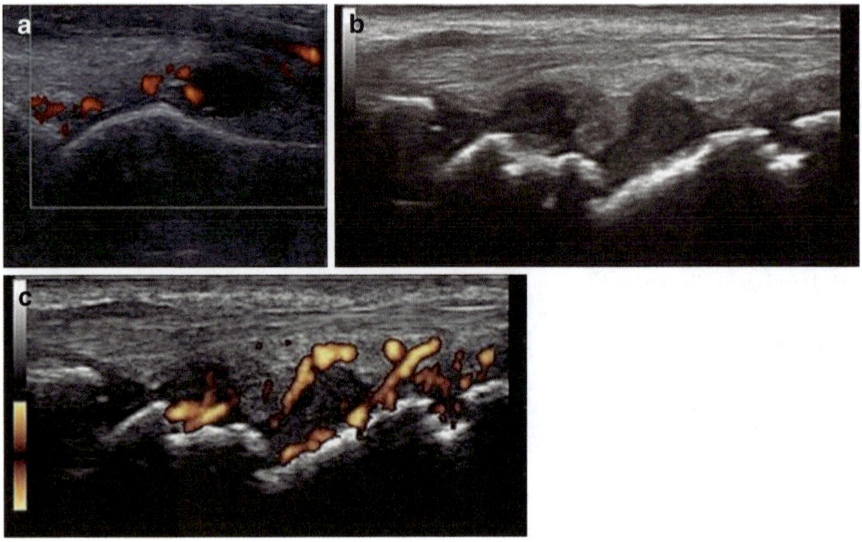

Fig. 2.3 Synovial hypertrophy. (**a**) First MTP, dorsal longitudinal view with power Doppler. (**b**) Wrist, dorsal longitudinal view in gray scale and (**c**) with power Doppler

Fig. 2.4 Tenosynovitis. (**a**) Ankle, dorsal longitudinal view. (**b**) Ankle, dorsal transverse view. (Courtesy of Jay Higgs, MD). The views expressed herein are those of the author(s) and do not reflect the official policy or position of Brooke Army Medical Center, the US Army Medical Department, the US Army Office of the Surgeon General, the Department of the Army, and the Department of Defense or the US Government

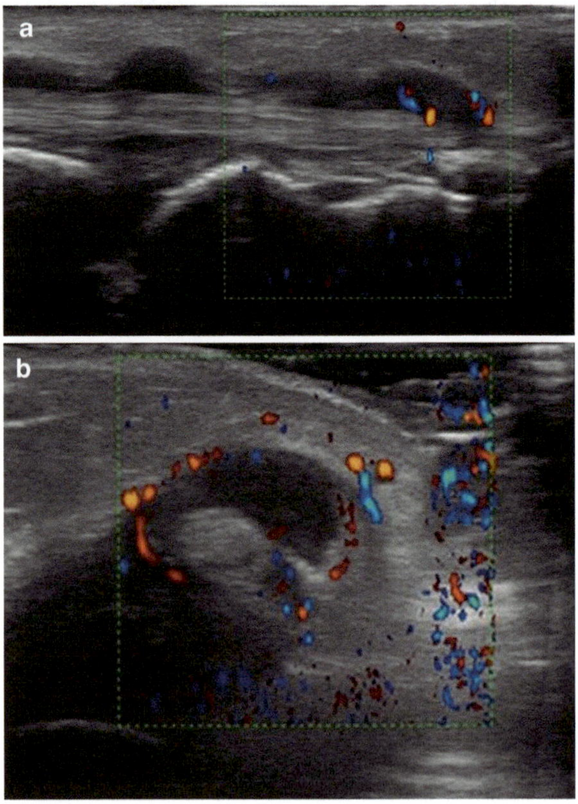

While OMERACT initially focused on these key findings in inflammatory arthritis such as rheumatoid arthritis (RA) and psoriatic arthritis (PsA), the utility of ultrasound in rheumatology has become apparent in other diseases as we have gained more experience. See Chap. 12 "Ultrasound in Psoriatic Arthritis" for further details of key findings in PsA. Thus, it is important to include other basic pathologic findings that have been described in the inflammatory arthritides and in other rheumatic and musculoskeletal diseases. The following definitions are compiled from a review of the literature reported from the OMERACT 10 Ultrasound Task Force in 2011 [2]:

Articular Cartilage Damage Focal increase in echogenicity, focal decreased thickness or loss of sharp contour, or punctate/linear hyperechoic spots on the surface or inside the anechoic structure (i.e., crystal disease) (see Fig. 2.5)

Bone Productive Change Hyperechoic elevated or "step-up" bony prominence in two perpendicular planes close to the joint space (whether osteophytes in primary or secondary osteoarthritis (OA) or new formation in a spondyloarthropathy) rarely showing Doppler signal (see Fig. 2.6)

Bursitis Abnormal anechoic or hypoechoic extra-articular collection between tissue layers that may be compressible depending on location and may exhibit some Doppler signal or hyperechoic material depending on the etiology

Dactylitis Heterogeneous and variable changes in a digit affecting different tissue compartments (i.e., tendons/sheaths, ligaments, joints, soft tissue)

Calcifications Hyperechoic areas of variable size and tissue location, not demonstrating power Doppler signal, although these densities can be adjacent to such areas

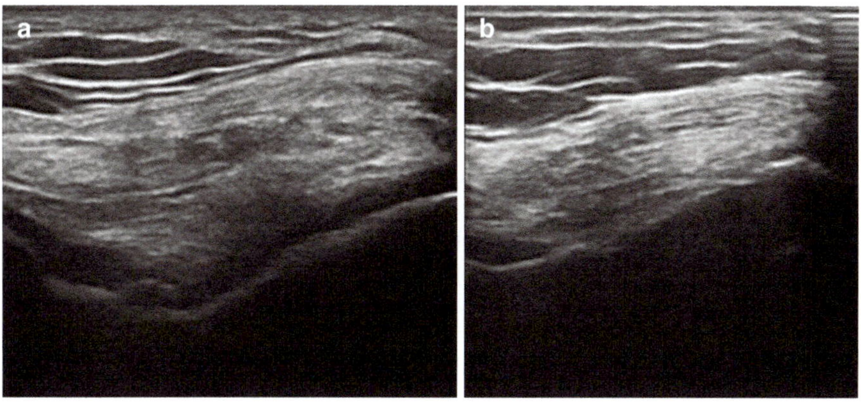

Fig. 2.5 Articular cartilage damage. Femoral hyaline articular cartilage wear, suprapatellar transverse knee in flexion (two different knees with different degrees of cartilage wear, (**a**) mild/moderate and (**b**) severe))

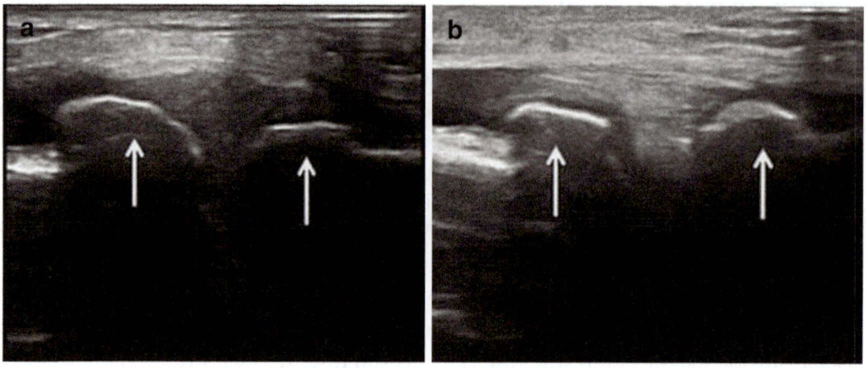

Fig. 2.6 Bone productive change. (**a**) Osteophytes, medial longitudinal knee. (**b**) Osteophytes, lateral longitudinal knee

Many of these pathologic elements appear in a number of diseases discussed in the following sections.

Rheumatoid Arthritis

Ultrasound (US) has clinical utility in both acute and chronic stages of RA, for diagnosis, prognosis, and assessment of response to treatment. The key findings of synovitis and tenosynovitis (by both gray scale and Doppler signal), effusions, and bony erosions are easily identifiable at the clinic visit and are useful in both clinical practice and research studies. They can help confirm a diagnosis of RA in an ambiguous case or shed light on disease activity when the physical exam or plain radiographs are not sufficient [3].

Synovitis and Tenosynovitis

Numerous studies have validated sonographic evaluation of synovitis in RA at multiple anatomic sites such as the shoulders [4], wrists and small joints of the hands [5, 6], knees [7], and feet [8], while others have found it to be reliable across anatomic sites with respect to both intraobserver and interobserver concordance [9, 10].

Rheumatoid synovitis, or pannus, appears on ultrasound as synovial hypertrophy that is hypoechoic or isoechoic on the screen, with or without an anechoic (black) effusion [1] (Fig. 2.3). In these gray-scale images, readers can quantify synovial pathology by measuring the synovial thickness or the size of the effusion. However, gray-scale imaging for synovial hypertrophy cannot accurately differentiate between chronically and acutely inflamed synovial membranes, which retain thickness over time. Color power Doppler assessment can detect the amount of microvascular flow within pathologic synovial membranes with hypervascularity. Color power Doppler is more sensitive than gray-scale ultrasound alone for the detection of early disease and can more accurately differentiate chronic and acute disease in the thickened synovium, thus helping assess response to treatment [11].

Assessment of vascularity using color power Doppler has been shown to correlate with the histopathologic features of synovitis. A study evaluating patients who had total knee replacements revealed a high correlation between preoperative Doppler scores for the synovium and postoperative histologic analysis of the tissue by qualitative and quantitative vessel density ($p < 0.01$) [12]. The same group subsequently looked at hip arthritis and found similar results, suggesting that Doppler reliably estimates vascularity of synovial tissue [13].

In assessment for synovitis, US has proven better than both conventional radiography and clinical examination by many investigators [5, 8, 14]. In fact, many studies have shown US to be on par with MRI in detecting synovitis [15], while one found US superior to MRI in detecting this tissue thickening [16].

With tenosynovitis, US is overall better in diagnosis than MRI. The anechoic (black) fluid inside the tendon sheath (in both longitudinal and transverse views) and hypoechoic (gray) synovial tissue displacing other structures are easily seen with the sonographic images (Fig. 2.4). The hand and wrist are common locations for RA involvement of tendons, including the flexor digitorum, extensor digitorum, extensor carpi ulnaris, and extensor carpi radialis [17]. One recent study found US to be more sensitive [18], while another comparison of ultrasound with MRI in an early RA cohort found US has a better specificity and positive predictive value for tenosynovitis, with good intra- and inter-reader reliability of tendon assessment in RA [19, 20]. The reliability with acceptable intraobserver and interobserver concordance has been perpetuated in recent studies looking at evaluation of tenosynovitis using US [20, 21].

Effusions

While plain radiographs can suggest the presence of effusions, US is able to directly visualize and quantify the amount of fluid versus synovial thickening present; US guidance allows localization of fluid to assist with diagnostic and therapeutic arthrocentesis. Anechoic, compressible synovial fluid (without Doppler signal) can be found by US in many diseases, including OA. But in RA, these pathologic collections are more common and are often seen in any active, inflammatory joint—from the small interphalangeal joints to the larger shoulders and hips (Fig. 2.2).

Erosions

US has also had a great impact on diagnosing and prognosticating cases of RA because it vividly showcases bone erosions—one of the hallmark signs of focal joint damage. While erosive changes are not pathognomonic for RA, these lesions in the right setting can help to establish a diagnosis as well as predict more aggressive disease and worse clinical outcomes to support the use of more aggressive therapy. Identification of the erosions also facilitates enrollment into many research studies and contributes to outcome measures.

Erosions are visible with US in a host of areas, with the highest yield including the ulnar styloid process, the radial aspect of the second MCP joint, and the ulnar aspect of the fifth MCP [22]. Due to limitations in probe positioning and anatomy that decrease acoustic windows, US is less useful in evaluation of the carpal bones. In significant erosions, the hyperechoic articular or periarticular bony cortex appears to have a "dip" or break of at least 2 mm deep and must be visualized in orthogonal planes to ensure that it is not an artifact (Fig. 2.1).

While conventional radiography had long been considered the test of choice to look for the presence or worsening of erosions, with biannual imaging as a standard of care to assess progression and treatment efficacy, US has in fact become a common alternative. Numerous studies have shown that US identifies erosions missed by conventional radiography in early RA [5, 15, 23–25], at times justifying immunosuppressive treatment at an earlier time to protect the patient from further joint damage. Plain X-rays can also miss erosions that are obscured by superimposed secondary degenerative changes, while US is able to detect such erosions [11, 25, 26]. As early as the year 2000, one group reported 6.5-fold more erosions by US vs. plain radiography in an early RA cohort (disease duration more than 12 months), while 3.4-fold more erosions were visualized by US in a late RA cohort (disease duration less than 12 months), using MRI as the gold standard [25]. Many studies suggest US performs nearly as well, or as well, as MRI in identifying such erosions [5, 27, 28] and also effectively detects erosions when CT is used as the gold standard [27].

Questions of reproducibility and operator dependence continue to surface when evaluating the role of US, though studies suggest a high interobserver reliability in the detection of bone erosions, including one with the two participants being a rheumatologist and an experienced radiologist [29]. A similar study with a US-naïve rheumatologist (after a 4-week training course) and one experienced in US found high interobserver rates for detecting bone erosions [30].

RA Synovitis Scoring Systems

While US can identify disease activity in RA at the joint level, many groups have devised scoring methods at the "patient" level for use in both research and patient care. These systems aid in measuring clinical trial outcomes, help the clinician evaluate patient improvement (or worsening), and often provide important prognostic information—even in the cases of subclinical inflammation. No clinicians and few researchers have time to scan all joints of the hands and feet, though too few joints may sacrifice sensitivity.

The proposed number of joints to scan for studies and clinical care has ranged from 78 to 6 [31, 32]. One of the first proposals for a global patient "score" encompassing various joints reported that a comprehensive 78-joint assessment was highly sensitive to change after biologic therapy. Not surprisingly, other investigators have proposed scoring systems requiring fewer joints but retaining sensitivity or specificity—which would be more feasible for clinicians in the hurried outpatient setting and even in research. Options have included a 44-joint system taking more than an hour [33], a 28-joint count that the authors boasted "can be performed in 15 min" [5], and both 12- and 6-joint (bilateral wrists, second MCPs, and knees) versions by another group (excluding erosions), reporting significant correlations with DAS-28 that were sensitive to improvement over 3 months [32]. A comparison of the 44 and 12 joints (bilateral elbow, wrist, second and third MCP, knee, and ankle) [34] found highly correlative improvements with biologic therapy.

In creating what may be the most widely used system (at least in research studies), Backhaus and her colleagues validated a seven-joint exam (dominant wrist, second and third MCPs and PIPs, and second and fifth MTPs). They incorporate both semiquantitative grading for synovitis/tenosynovitis and the presence/absence of erosions, and they estimate the exam takes up to 20 min to complete. The system results in scores that correlate well with DAS-28, both at baseline and with medication-induced clinical improvement over the course of a year [35, 36]. The OMERACT Ultrasound Task Force, which aims to improve the role of ultrasound in arthritis clinical trials, subsequently endorsed a synovitis-specific score to assess disease activity and response to biologic therapy [37]. Their US Global Synovitis Score (US-GLOSS) combines synovial hypertrophy and power Doppler signal levels. Recently, Ben-Artzi et al. developed a synovitis grading system and atlas to attempt to provide more objective, reproducible, clinically relevant information than what current systems used [38]. Still, there is no overall consensus regarding the optimal number of joints that should be scanned for either research studies or in clinical practice. Further details on scoring systems for rheumatoid arthritis are discussed in Chap. 11 "Ultrasound in Rheumatoid Arthritis".

Prognosis

What do these sonopathologic findings mean for the early RA patient? While erosions indicate damage and help justify more aggressive treatment, synovitis and color power Doppler signal have been shown to predict future damage. One group found that MCP joints in RA patients displaying an increased power Doppler signal at baseline assessment were 12 times more likely to develop radiographic damage at 1 year than those without such hyperemia [39]. Other studies have documented that US findings, particularly power Doppler signal, are predictive of erosive disease over time [40–42]. Another group found that wrist synovitis by US at baseline is significantly more predictive than marrow edema on MRI of future erosions in 12 months [43].

In fact, older studies suggested that many RA patients who appear to be in clinical remission actually have persistent subclinical synovitis on US [44]. A more recent study estimated that more than one-third of patients considered to be in clinical remission by the DAS-28 and ACR/EULAR criteria showed significant gray-scale synovitis ($p = 0.01$ and 0.0002, respectively) and power Doppler activity ($p = 0.005$ and 0.0005, respectively) [45].

Still, pending further follow-up studies, it is not yet clear if such inflammation leads to future erosions when more aggressive treatment is withheld from seemingly well-controlled patients. While longitudinal studies will ultimately answer these treatment questions, the present data does suggest that clinical and biochemical assessments are less sensitive than US in detecting low or early disease activity [46].

Osteoarthritis

US can play a role in the diagnosis of OA and has been shown more recently to provide prognostic information as well. There are a number of classic findings, many of which are specific to OA, most often in the knee and hip joints (the two joints most often affected by OA) but also in the upper extremities. XR is often ordered to evaluate joint space narrowing and osteophytes; however, US, despite its limitations with acoustic windows (unable to penetrate bone), can still potentially identify OA changes earlier with findings of osteophytes, cartilage damage, and synovitis/effusions [47, 48]. Patients can see evidence of their degenerative joint disease in the exam room before ever going for an X-ray. While one group recently proposed a comprehensive knee OA ultrasound scoring system to complement and correlate with global scores by radiography and patient symptoms [49], other research has focused on the importance of the specific sonographic findings in OA as described below. See Chap. 14 "Ultrasound in Osteoarthritis" for further details on sonographic findings in OA.

Osteophytes

These bone spurs that are found in most osteoarthritic joints are clearly visible by their raised or elevated hyperechoic segments along the bony contour (not sporadically found as in calcium deposits). Many have described a sonographically identified osteophyte as the "inverse" of an erosion, which is seen as a focal depression in the bony contour.

In the knees, osteophytes are usually found along the medial and lateral joint lines from the distal femur and proximal tibia. Longitudinal views can reveal an elevation of the edges of the hyperechoic triangle in which the meniscus resides and are easily measured for later comparison or scored by a semiquantitative scale [47, 48] (Fig. 2.6).

The hip joint is another common location to find raised osteophytes, on both the acetabulum and the femoral head—and these should be confirmed with the orthogonal view as well. Many authors have also reported that US detects more hand osteophytes compared with X-rays [50], with one author finding twice as many osteophytes by ultrasound (448 vs. 228 in the PIPs DIPs and MCPs in 37 patients) [51].

Articular Cartilage Damage

Articular cartilage manifestations of OA are seen with changes to the thick anechoic (water-filled) layer usually seen in healthy joints. With injury or wear to the cartilage that overlies the bony cortex, there is often focal, or more diffuse, disease seen in the cartilage that is revealed with patient positioning. For instance, in the knee, the femoral articular cartilage is exposed with knee flexion that moves the patella out of the way. Patients with focal disease (i.e., medial vs. lateral) have blurring of the clear demarcation and eventually thinning of the anechoic layer with isoechoic infiltration. This provides more information beyond what X-rays can provide—a defined loss of joint space that is acceptable as a surrogate for cartilage damage.

While seen most easily in larger joints like the knee (Fig. 2.5), this cartilage damage is also apparent in hand OA, where damage and loss of joint space are detected more readily by US. One study of 37 patients found that US detected nearly twice as many narrowed individual joints in the fingers [52].

Effusions and Baker's Cysts

While effusions have been detected clinically and aspirated for years in OA patients, US has dramatically allowed more rapid and comprehensive diagnosis of the effusions—seen as compressible, displaceable anechoic collections without Doppler signal. US has also improved the ability to diagnose Baker's cysts (see Fig. 2.7) that

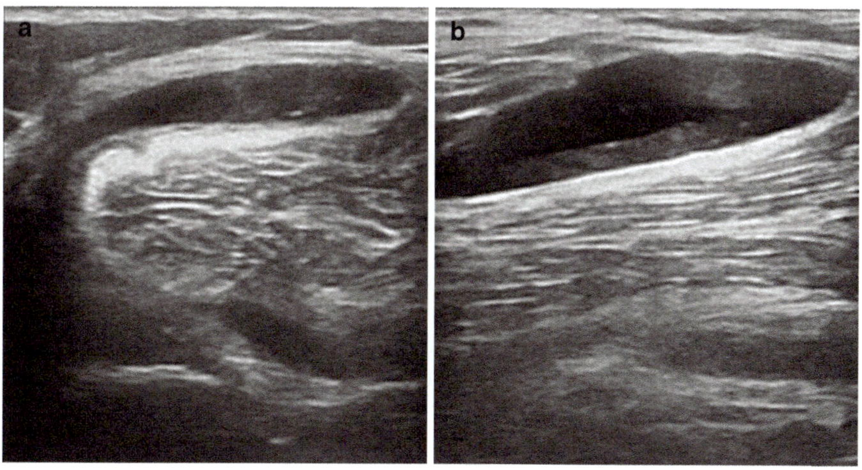

Fig. 2.7 Popliteal (Baker's) cyst. (**a**) Posterior knee transverse. (**b**) Posterior knee longitudinal

are present in up to 25% of patients with knee OA yet usually missed by the physical exam [52]. This is especially helpful in patients with obesity or bulky knees where the physical exam lacks sensitivity and specificity [53]. Furthermore, as most clinicians will attest, the anechoic, compressible effusions are at times hard to aspirate blindly without image guidance; most clinicians have refrained from aspirating popliteal cysts without image guidance given the proximity and potential for inadvertent trauma to the popliteal vessels.

There is also emerging evidence that sonographic identification of large effusions is important prognostically. A prospective multicenter European study of 531 patients with painful knee OA found those with knee effusions measuring greater than 4 mm in size were 2.6 times as likely to need total joint replacement within 4 years ($p < 0.0001$), while effusions found by physical exam alone were not similarly predictive [54].

Synovitis

While OA has long been heralded as a noninflammatory, degenerative disease, more recent US research supports other clinical, biochemical, and imaging evidence that synovitis is a characteristic feature of OA. Beyond identifying osteophyte effusions and articular cartilage damage, sonographers now describe synovitis by both gray scale and Doppler in a variety of joints including the knee [55, 56]. As with synovitis seen in other inflammatory arthritis syndromes, it can be seen as isoechoic or hypoechoic synovial thickening—but in the suprapatellar recess of the knee, it can appear frond-like. At times, it can also demonstrate some mild power Doppler signal.

One European study of 600 patients with knee OA identified 17% with synovial thickening (and 44% with anechoic effusions)—but without power Doppler assessment because the Doppler data at that time was "highly machine-dependent." Even so, they suggested that gray-scale synovitis identified by US correlated statistically with clinical signs and symptoms of increased pain and swelling or "flares" [57].

This diagnostic ability of US can be very helpful in patient care as well as in OA research, as X-rays do not detect synovial inflammation, while most MRIs (without the use of specific windows or using gadolinium) are not as sensitive. Thus, when there is a discrepancy in early OA between X-ray severity and a patient's symptoms, sonographic evaluation could be an important modality to diagnose the patient's disease earlier.

Sonographic features of OA may also provide important prognostic information to potentially guide treatment. In a prospective, randomized controlled trial of steroid injections for hip OA, those patients with US-proven synovitis predicted a better response to the injection at weeks 4 and 8 ($p < 0.05$) [58].

In hand OA, there have been many studies to suggest that US can detect statistically significant synovitis in the small joints [51, 59, 60]. While one author found 46% of the patients' joints with gray-scale synovitis and 7% with Doppler signal ($p < 0.001$ for both when compared with controls) [50], a more recent study suggested a higher burden of synovitis in erosive hand OA [61].

Spondyloarthropathies

Significant progress in the use of US imaging for spondyloarthropathies (SpA) including psoriatic arthritis (PsA) have been made, particularly with the role of US in identifying enthesitis in ankylosing spondylitis (AS) and undifferentiated SpA. Minimal effort has been placed on the arthritides associated with inflammatory bowel diseases and reactive arthritis.

Tendon/Enthesis

US has been used to study pathogenesis of structural tendon and entheseal abnormalities in SpA. US is reliable and sensitive to noting changes in erosions related to the Achilles enthesitis. A 12-month-long study noted improvement of these erosions and development of new ones [62]. Entheseal fibrocartilage (EF) derangement has been thought to contribute to enthesopathy, and EF at the Achilles tendon (AT) insertion can be visualized well [63]. Relating to bovine hindfeet and SpA AT insertions in patients, EF in the former is described as a thin, uncompressible, well-defined, anechoic layer between the hyperechoic bone and the hyperechoic fibrils of the enthesis both in longitudinal and transverse scans, and these correlated with histological examination; discontinuities of the anechoic layer around the erosions and enthesophytes were observed in SpA patients [63]. Furthermore, the Achilles enthesis bursa in early SpA can be visualized in 67.4% of SpA patients vs. 58.7% of controls and 21.7% in RA controls; bursal thickening and Doppler signal were increased in the SpA group vs. controls and appears to correlate with CRP levels and disease activity scores [64].

In the evaluation of enthesitis, specifically in AS, power Doppler use is helpful and complementary to the physical examination [65]. US appears to be able to distinguish signs of chronic enthesitis [66]. Local etanercept injection under US guidance for Achilles enthesitis in AS was effective and safe in a study involving 12 patients followed over 3 months [67]. Subclinical Achilles enthesitis was noted to improve after 2 months of therapy with anti-TNF therapy [68].

Ankylosing Spondylitis

There are a number of studies specifically dealing with US findings in AS, and many of the findings for PsA apply here as well. Changes on hip appear to correlate with C-reactive protein and pain scores; CRP elevations were even noted to correlate with sonographic abnormalities in the hip in patients without hip tenderness on exam [69]. Color Doppler ultrasound (CDUS) has been established as a useful tool in evaluating disease activity in AS, with a sensitivity of 82% (95% CI, 68–91%) and a specificity of 92% (95% CI, 85–96%) [70]. Vascularity in the sacroiliac joint (SIJ) in AS appears to involve two or more different flow patterns, but in general increased vascularity and venous flow in active cases are particularly noted [71]. In another study using CDUS, a lower resistive index value and vascularization in the SIJ correlated with AS activity [72]. CDUS was more sensitive (92%) in detecting active sacroiliitis than enthesitis (52.2%) and correlates with Bath Ankylosing Spondylitis Disease Activity Index (BASDAI) scores [73]. Power Doppler US evaluation of sacroiliitis is useful in following response to infliximab [74].

Psoriatic Arthritis

The key sonographic features of psoriatic arthritis and nail psoriasis are described in the following subsections and summarized below in Table 2.1. Further details can be found in Chap. 12.

Table 2.1 Sonographic changes in patients with psoriatic arthritis: synovitis, enthesitis, psoriasis nail changes, and dactylitis

Synovitis
Power Doppler changes
Effusion
Synovial proliferation or hypertrophy
Joint effusion
Enthesitis (MASEI, Leeds systems)
Thickening and structural changes of the tendon insertion
Calcification at the tendon insertion
Bone erosions
Enthesophyte formation
Perientheseal soft tissue edema
Entheseal thickening
Bursitis
Power Doppler changes at site of enthesis
Nail changes
Power Doppler signal in nail bed
Increase in ventral plate—osseous margin distance
Adjacent distal interphalangeal joint extensor tendon enthesopathy
Wortsman psoriasis nail classification
Wortsman type I: focal hyperechogenicity of the ventral plate without involvement of the dorsal plate
Wortsman type II: loosening of the borders of the ventral plate
Dactylitis
Flexor tenosynovitis
Small joint soft tissue edema including involvement of the palmar plate and collateral ligament

MASEI (Madrid Sonographic Enthesitis Index) sites: patella at insertions of the quadriceps femoris and patellar tendons, Achilles tendon and plantar fascia insertions in the calcaneus, triceps tendon insertion to the olecranon process

Leeds Enthesitis Index sites: lateral epicondyles of the humerus, medial condyles of the femur; Achilles tendon insertions

Early PsA may have findings of subclinical synovitis by US especially in the wrist, knee, and metatarsophalangeal and metacarpophalangeal joints resulting in a change of assessment of number and symmetry of joint involvement, especially with 81.8% of oligoarthritis patients being reclassified as having polyarthritis [74]. However, the prevalence of subclinical enthesitis noted by sonography in early PsA is low [75]. Occult enthesitis in PsA, evaluated using the Glasgow Ultrasound Enthesitis Scoring System (GUESS), appears to be independent of clinical features and psoriasis severity, with many patients having a positive power Doppler US signal in 40% of cases, and clinical examination noting tenderness in only about 29% [76].

About 15–20% of cases of PsA may precede psoriasis, and up to 70% of patients develop PsA after the onset of their psoriasis even by about 10 years [77]. Psoriasis patients may have features of subclinical arthritis and enthesitis [78, 79]. Patients with no known arthritic involvement can have structural changes in the fingers and toes, up to 11% by conventional radiography and 69% by US [78]. There is significantly more frequent synovitis and enthesopathy in patients with psoriasis than in controls with psoriasis being the only significant predictive variable of synovitis and enthesopathy by US [79]. Tendon thickness and entheseal abnormalities were useful in identifying psoriasis patients who are most likely to develop psoriatic arthritis [80, 81]. These studies underscore the importance of early evaluation of psoriasis patients for PsA. Baseline power Doppler and gray-scale scores of ≥2, enthesitis, higher score, onychopathy, and persistent synovitis and enthesitis at 6 months were all associated with progressive early PsA [82]. Despite clinical remission, joint inflammation can still persist in up to 62% of 25 patients after 1 year of anti-TNFα treatment when evaluated using contrast-enhanced US 1 year later [83]. Further study is needed using a larger population of patients.

In PsA, hip US assessment is useful and subclinical effusions have been noted [84]. Disease activity scores correlate with and findings of synovitis or enthesitis on US. Power Doppler ultrasound can detect extensive entheseal abnormalities in PsA [85]. Composite scores (*d*isease *a*ctivity in *ps*oriatic *a*rthritis (DAPSA) and Boolean's remission definition) correlated with US findings of remission or minimal disease activity [85]. GRAPPA (Group for Research and Assessment of Psoriasis and PsA) has developed a Diagnostic Ultrasound Enthesitis Tool (DUET) to identify PsA at earlier stages to optimize early diagnosis and treatment and seeks to validate a sonographic enthesitis scoring system [86].

Dactylitis

Dactylitis, commonly known as "sausage digit," appears to be inflammation related to multiple tissue compartments [87, 88]. A number of studies have looked at the sources of inflammation in dactylitis, beginning with the concept that it involved mainly a flexor tenosynovitis; however, a number of US and MRI studies have concluded that in addition to tenosynovitis, there is small joint soft tissue edema including involvement of the palmar plate and collateral ligament [89–94].

Psoriasis of the Nails

Nails are considered an extension of the enthesis. US can evaluate nail diseases in psoriasis [95–99]. A transducer with a frequency of 6–18 MHz and Doppler frequency 7–14 MHz can be used. Wortsman [98] devised a classification system (Table 2.1). Changes of both Wortsman types have been noted in 50% of patients with cutaneous psoriasis and also 50% in those with PsA [96, 98]. A significant difference was also noted in the mean distance between ventral plate and osseous margins of the distal phalanx. Power Doppler US detected in the DIP joints and nail beds were also noted in a significant number of PsA patients [98]. DIP joint extensor tendon enthesopathy appears relevant to the pathogenesis of nail disease in both psoriasis and clinically evident and subclinical PsA patients [99].

Scoring Systems for SpA

The Maastricht Ankylosing Spondylitis Enthesitis Score (MASES) was developed to evaluate the predictive value of US to detect enthesitis and has been studied in correlation with history and clinical examination; the sensitivity of selected MASES points was 66.7–86.4% for history and 71.4–87% for clinical examination, and the specificity was 85–91.7% for history and 47.4–75% for clinical examination ($p < 0.05$ for each) [100]. The Madrid Sonographic Enthesitis Index (MASEI) can be used to classify patients as having PsA, with the severity of sonographic entheseal abnormalities highest in patients with PsA [101] with a sensitivity of 30% and a specificity of 95% [101]. Using the Leeds enthesitis index, a study involving RA and PsA showed that these scores by US alone did not distinguish these two populations of patients [102].

Ultrasound scoring systems for both large and smaller joints have been used in SpAs. The SOLAR (*so*nography of *la*rge joints in *r*heumatology) score, a large joint assessment scoring system validated initially for RA, was found to be useful in the evaluation of PsA and AS [103]. Other studies looking at large joint involvement have noted significantly higher frequency of acromioclavicular synovitis (66% vs. 5%, $p < 0.0001$) and unilateral involvement (64% vs. 26%, $p < 0.0001$) in SpA patients over RA patients [104]. Power Doppler US to evaluate hyperemia of joints is also useful in SpAs [105]. Scoring for peripheral joint, tendon, and entheseal sites of inflammation was useful in detecting responsiveness to treatment in SpA [106].

Crystal Arthropathies: Gout and CPPD/Pseudogout

Demonstration of crystals on synovial fluid analysis has been the gold standard in the diagnosis of crystalline-related arthritides [107]. However, fluid is not always present to aspirate, and advances in imaging are changing the way that crystalline disease can be diagnosed. Ultrasonography can identify crystalline deposition that may not always be seen on radiographs. Distinctive features to differentiate gout and pseudogout have been described. The high reflectivity of crystalline particles and the sensitivity of US to detect even small amounts make US ideal as an imaging modality for the evaluation of crystalline arthritides [108]. The development of scanning protocols and scoring systems and further validation of techniques including the use of power Doppler sonography warrant further study [109]. US, along with XR and DECT, is now included in the imaging domain of the 2015 ACR/EULAR classification criteria for gout [110]. A similar collaborative ACR/EULAR initiative is working to develop classification criteria for CPPD, including an imaging domain to include US. See Chap. 13 "Ultrasound in Crystalline Diseases" for further details.

Gout

Gout classically starts in the foot or other lower extremity involvement. Numerous studies have shown that US is useful in diagnosing and evaluating gout. The sonographic features of monosodium urate (MSU) crystal deposition in gout described in the literature to date include the presence of hyperechoic irregular band overlying the superficial margin of the articular cartilage (see Fig. 2.8) also known as a double-contour sign (DCS), hyperechoic stippled foci, and hyperechoic cloudy areas (HCA); tophi are depicted by the presence of hypoechoic to hyperechoic inhomogeneous material surrounded by an anechoic rim; and erosive bone changes [111] (Table 2.2). Terminology describing urate crystals in a "snowstorm" pattern and "sugar clumps in water" appearance has also been reported.

On radiographs, the classic features of gout are punched out periarticular erosions with overhanging edges. However, these findings are not evident until about 6–12 years after the onset of gout [107, 112]. Assessment of foot joints in gout patients reveal a higher detection rate of inflamed foot joints by sonography when compared with physical examination and X-ray [113], with the talonavicular and first metatarsophalangeal joints having the highest prevalence of sonographic signs of MSU crystal aggregates [114]. A study looking at first metatarsophalangeal joint

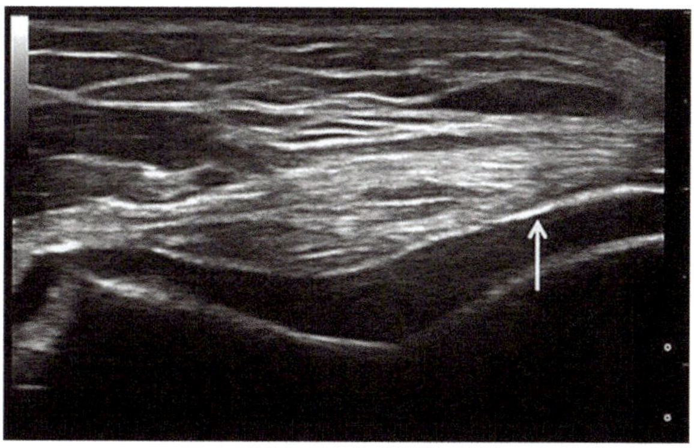

Fig. 2.8 Gout. "Double-contour" sign of the femoral articular cartilage

Table 2.2 Ultrasonographic features of acute and chronic gout

Acute	Chronic
"Snowstorm"—free monosodium urate crystals within synovial fluid	Erosions adjacent to tophaceous material
Synovial hypertrophy	Tophi: hyperechoic, inhomogeneous material with anechoic rim within joints, tendons, ligaments, bursae; can invade into bone
Power Doppler findings indicating hypervascularity	Double-contour sign (DCS)—hyperechoic, irregular band over the superficial margin of the articular cartilage
Hyperechoic spots in synovium, hyperechoic cloudy areas (HCAs)	

Table 2.3 Sonographic features of calcium pyrophosphate deposition disease

Principal sonographic features of CPPD
Crystal deposition within articular cartilage
Calcification of fibrocartilage
Focal crystal deposition within tendons
Patterns of CPPD calcification
Thin hyperechoic bands parallel to the surface of the hyaline cartilage
Punctate pattern—more common in fibrous cartilage and tendons
Homogeneous hyperechoic nodular or oval depositions—in bursae and articular recesses

examination by sonography and X-ray noted a higher detection of erosions by US; and similarly, DCS and tophi were also noted by US [115].

In a retrospective study involving 37 joints of 23 patients with MSU crystal-proven gout and 33 joints from 23 control patients, 92% of all gouty joints were noted to have DCS, 100% of MCP joints were noted to have tophi, and 65% of MTP and 25% of MCP joints were noted to have erosive changes adjacent to tophi [115]. In contrast, calcium pyrophosphate crystals tend to aggregate in the center of both hyaline and fibrous cartilage (Table 2.3).

Additionally, ultrasonography has been helpful based on some reports in diagnosing [116] and distinguishing gout from its mimics including cellulitis [117], psoriatic arthritis [118], and infectious tenosynovitis [119].

Asymptomatic Hyperuricemia and Early Gout

Some investigators have noted sonographic changes of gout in patients with asymptomatic hyperuricemia [120–122] and early gout not requiring urate-lowering therapy (ULT) [123]. Tophi and inflammatory changes were noted in 34% and 23%, respectively, in patients with a known duration of asymptomatic hyperuricemia of 5 years [120]. In a controlled study, 25% of first MTP joints were found to be affected vs. none in the control group [122]. Enthesopathy of the patellar (12% vs. 2.9%) and Achilles (15% vs. 1.9%) tendons was found, including tophi in both tendons and intra-articularly [122]. A prospective study on patients not yet requiring ULT noted articular MSU deposit in 60% of cases, with DCS noted in 40–47% and tophi in 27% of knees and MTP joints; they also noted that uric acid levels correlated with the presence of DCS but not with tophi [123].

Gout Vs. Calcium Pyrophosphate Dihydrate Deposition (Pseudogout)

US findings of MSU and calcium pyrophosphate dihydrate deposition at the knee cartilage had a high specificity, low sensitivity, and accuracy [124]. Knees in 32 gout patents and 48 calcium pyrophosphate arthropathy patients were evaluated with 52 rheumatoid arthritis, osteoarthritis, and psoriatic arthritis patients being disease controls. DCS was found in at least 1 knee of 14 of the gout patients (43.7%), giving a specificity of 99%; most of these were found on parapatellar views (51.1%) compared with 32.6% in the suprapatellar and 16.3% on posterior views. Hyperechoic spots within the cartilage layer were found in at least 1 knee of 33 pseudogout patients (68.7%) and in 1 patient with OA and another with RA giving a specificity of 97.6%; much of these findings were found on suprapatellar views (48.8%) vs. 34.9% on parapatellar and 16.3% on posterior views. Interobserver agreement between two sonographers was seen in 92.7% of 180 scans with regard to hyperechoic enhancement of the chondrosynovial interface and in 90% with regard to hyperechoic spots within the cartilage layer. Degree of concordance is 99–100% between readers of images for individual subjects, total joints, femoral articular cartilage, and first metatarsophalangeal joints [125].

Ultrasound Vs. Other Imaging Modalities for Diagnosis of Gout

When comparing US with other imaging modalities, US has comparable usefulness in detecting MSU deposits. When compared to X-rays, US has a sensitivity of 96% and a specificity of 73%, whereas X-rays have a sensitivity of 31% and a specificity of 93%, suggesting that US can be useful in cases where clinical suspicion of gout is high but laboratory findings and X-ray results are less than useful [126].

A number of studies have looked at the use of dual-energy computed tomography (DECT). DECT allows direct visualization of MSU crystal deposits and bone structures at the same time. US and DECT have comparable sensitivity [127]. A study involving four men with chronic tophaceous gout aimed to compare the usefulness of MRI, US, and CT in providing specific images of gouty tophi; it showed that CT images could clearly show MSU crystal deposits with a density of 160 Hounsfield units, whereas MRI and color Doppler US images showing masses surrounded by a hypervascular area was not thought to be specific enough [128]. MRI findings of bone edema can also be found in tophaceous gout, but this is much more mild compared to more severe findings in osteomyelitis which can also occur concomitantly with gout [129]. MRI appeared to be more sensitive than ultrasound in detecting destructive changes of synovial pannus, bone marrow edema, and soft tissue edema and erosions; in this study, none of these changes were noted by US in the asymptomatic joint, and on the index joint, ultrasound detected single cases of synovial pannus, soft tissue tophi, and erosion [128]. However, these findings are disputed by other authors who note that up to 2/3 of patients with clinical gout with normal conventional radiographs will have erosions by sonography [114, 115]. Bongartz et al. noted that DECT and US do not provide the same quantification of urate burden in feet and knees. The two techniques were discordant for assessing tophi volume, with DECT generally underestimating the volume compared to US. The agreement was improved when considering localized tophi in the feet, but small tophi of the first MTP often did not demonstrate any tophi via DECT. DECT tends to visualize tophi limited to crystals, whereas US provides an assessment of the overall tophaceous structure, soft tissue included [129].

Chronic Tophaceous Gout

Tophi can be generally described as hyperechoic, heterogeneous structures with poorly defined borders surrounded by an anechoic halo [130]. Tophi can be multiple and grouped or can be solitary or individual. In a prospective study looking at US features of tophi at the olecranon bursa, the most frequent feature was hyperechogenicity which was noted in 91.7% of a study of 35 involved sites, followed by poorly defined contours (88.6%), multiple grouped nodules (85.6%), and heterogeneity (68.6%) [131].

In the interest of measuring gout as part of outcome assessment in clinical therapeutic drug trials for gout, ultrasonography including other various methods of tophi measurement has been described [132]. US can be useful in distinguishing tophi located at unusual sites. It has been used to distinguish tophi involving extensor tendon from an abscess [133]. It has also been used to distinguish tophi from osteomyelitis, highlighting the increased value of US over MRI in these cases [134].

Calcium Pyrophosphate Deposition Disease

The principal findings of calcium pyrophosphate deposition disease (CPPD) by sonography are crystal deposits within cartilage and tendons, fibrocartilage calcification [109, 135] (Table 2.3). CPPD calcifications can further be described based on various patterns (Table 2.2) and noted that US had a sensitivity and specificity comparable to that of CR in identifying these calcifications. Gutierrez [135] and Sofka [136] notes the usefulness of US to detect calcifications in patients with negative radiographs, citing the limitations of the latter based on acquisition techniques and patient-dependent factors such as concomitant osteoarthritis with severe joint space narrowing. US is noted to have a high specificity (96.4%), sensitivity (86.7%),

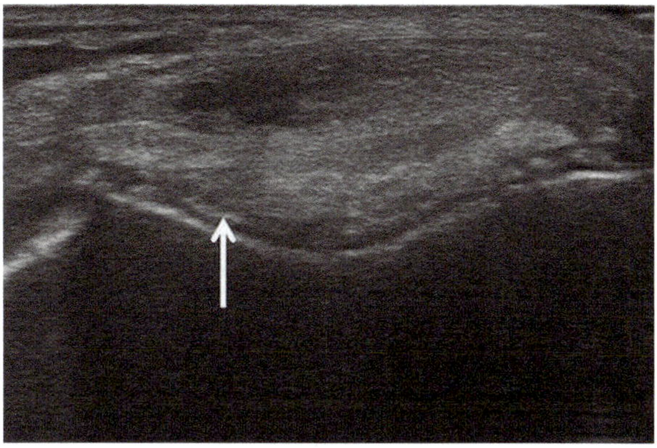

Fig. 2.9 Chondrocalcinosis. Femoral hyaline articular cartilage, suprapatellar transverse knee in flexion. (Courtesy of Jay Higgs, MD). The view(s) expressed herein are those of the author(s) and do not reflect the official policy or position of Brooke Army Medical Center, the US Army Medical Department, the US Army Office of the Surgeon General, the Department of the Army, and Department of Defense or the US Government

positive predictive value (92%), and negative predictive value (93%) [137]. In order to understand the extent of involvement of joints affected by CPPD, Filippou et al. [138] studied 42 consecutive patients and noted a mean involvement of 4.7 ± 1.7 sites affected, with the knee most affected followed by the wrist, Achilles tendons, plantar fascia, and metacarpophalangeal joints; the highest extent of deposition was reported in the menisci, followed by hyaline cartilage of the femoral condyles (see Fig. 2.9) and the entheses. Further studies looking at CPPD deposits in the Achilles tendon and plantar fascia noted calcification in 57% and 15.8%, respectively. Other changes were also noted including enthesophytes, increased vascularity, and cortical bone irregularity [139].

Interestingly, a case of an elderly patient with a mix of gout and CPPD findings by US has been described. Due to the deposition of MSU and CPPD crystals in the superficial surface of the cartilage and in the intra-articular deposition of hyperechoic dots resembling "rosary beads" due to chondrocalcinosis, respectively, a "triple-contour"-like appearance was described [140].

Systemic Sclerosis/Systemic Lupus Erythematosus

See Chap. 15.

Sjögren's Syndrome

See Chap. 17.

Large Vessel Vasculitis and Polymyalgia Rheumatica

See Chap. 16.

Implementing Ultrasound into Clinical Practice

Adding US into your existing clinical practice can initially feel daunting. When first starting, many are challenged by the additional time it takes to set up equipment for diagnostic scanning or US-guided procedure. A stepwise approach can be taken such as adding one diagnostic US exam or ultrasound-guided procedure for the last patient in your clinic day. An initial workflow to set aside a clinic session with increased time to add a few diagnostic ultrasound exams or procedure only visits can be helpful until there is more comfort level, experience, and speed in using your new skill set. Scheduling more time initially can avoid feeling rushed and can allow you to adequately and accurately scan the region of interest and interpret the findings. As you gain more experience, you may be able to return to your usual appointment time scheduling or feel comfortable adding an exam or procedure to your existing evaluation and management visit if preferred.

Maintenance of Equipment

Minimizing the impact of your US unit or probe being down for repairs is important to the reliability and performance for your equipment being used for clinical care. Before starting the examination, always check that connections to the US unit and make sure that probes are properly plugged in. Check your transducers and cords for any damage. It is important to maintain your equipment properly to ensure functional use for clinical safety and longevity of your equipment. Routine assessment of your US machine may also be required at your institution/practice with biomedical support.

Cleaning Guidelines

The AIUM (American Institute of Ultrasound in Medicine) has developed guidelines for cleaning and preparing US tranducers and equipment between patients as well as safe handling and use of coupling gel [141]. Recent changes due to COVID-19 outbreak have affected the level of disinfection needed. The no touch technique had previously been acceptable for musculoskeletal US-guided injection procedures; however, now with special attention to COVID-19 and other respiratory infection cases requiring aerosolization procedures, a transducer cover is recommended for interventional procedures breaking the skin barrier. Cleaning of the entire equipment from top to bottom (not just the tranducer and cord) is recommended. Following manufacturer guidance and institutional guidelines for proper cleaning of your equipment is also recommended.

Non-sterile, multiple-use ultrasound gel bottles have frequently been used for diagnostic ultrasound examinations; however, if there is concern for infection, single-pack US gel may be the preferred use. If you have a gel warmer, this also needs to be cleaned and disinfected according to the manufacturer's and infectious disease policy at your institution/clinic.

For interventional/percutaneous ultrasound-guided procedures, single-use probe cover or sterile probe cover is recommended with the use of sterile gel. After procedure has been completed, the cover should be discarded, not reused, and the probe and equipment should be cleaned. Varying degrees of disinfection are required depending on the sterility of a procedure. For example, an endocavitary procedure using an internal transducer may require a high level of disinfection or sterilization, whereas a joint injection procedure would require the use of a probe cover and low-level disinfection.

Documentation and Billing

Documentation in the form of a report and saving/archiving your images are required to be able to bill. The AIUM has developed general guidelines for documentation of US examination [142] and selected US-guided procedures [143]. Reimbursement for procedures varies by insurer and location.

Conclusion

US is an invaluable imaging modality in the evaluation and management of rheumatic diseases. It can identify key pathology in many diseases. While it is helpful diagnostically in many cases, it can also provide prognostic information that may change management and help guide treatment. Once you have learned the basics, steps to incorporating US into your clinical practice can be made to enhance your diagnostic and procedural capabilities.

Review Questions

1. Which of the following best defines the sonographic appearance of synovial hypertrophy?
   (a) Hypoechoic, compressible, and displaceable, exhibits Doppler signal
   (b) Hypoechoic, noncompressible, and nondisplaceable, exhibits Doppler signal
   (c) Anechoic, noncompressible, and nondisplaceable, exhibits Doppler signal
   (d) Hypoechoic, noncompressible, and nondisplaceable, does not exhibit Doppler signal

2. What is assessed in the US7 score for rheumatoid arthritis?
   (a) Erosions
   (b) Synovitis
   (c) Tenosynovitis
   (d) All of the above

3. How many ultrasound views/images are necessary to confirm the presence of an erosion in rheumatoid arthritis?
   (a) 1
   (b) 2
   (c) 3
   (d) 4
4. Which of the following is the best option to identify osteophytes of the knee?
   (a) Lateral tibiofemoral joint, transverse view
   (b) Medial tibiofemoral joint, longitudinal view
   (c) Suprapatellar longitudinal view
   (d) Posterior knee transverse view at the popliteal space
5. What is the best sonographic description of an osteophyte?
   (a) Hypoechoic area within the bony cortex
   (b) Raised hyperechoic area arising from the bony cortex, without any echogenicity below
   (c) Compressible anechoic accumulation near the joint space
   (d) Isoechoic noncompressible tissue
6. For lowering infection risk, it is recommended for a musculoskeletal ultrasound-guided injection procedure to use:
   (a) Sterile probe cover and sterile gel, followed by low-level disinfection
   (b) One-time use non-sterile probe cover and sterile gel, followed by low-level disinfection
   (c) Sterile probe cover and sterile gel, followed by high-level disinfection
   (d) a and b
7. Which of the following is a sonographic feature of acute gout?
   (a) Hyperechoic irregular band over the superficial margin of the articular cartilage
   (b) Hyperechoic, inhomogeneous material with anechoic rim within a joint
   (c) Hyperechoic cloudy areas and spots in thickened synovium
   (d) Erosions adjacent to inhomogeneous material with anechoic rim
8. Which of the following sonographic findings is suggestive of calcium pyrophosphate deposition disease?
   (a) Heterogeneous hypoechoic oval depositions in articular recesses
   (b) Thin hyperechoic bands parallel to the surface of the hyaline cartilage
   (c) Hyperechoic irregular band over the superficial margin of the articular cartilage
   (d) Hyperechoic cloudy areas
9. What percentage of psoriasis patients without any arthritic complaints can have subclinical sonographic findings of structural changes in their digits?
   (a) 40%
   (b) 55%
   (c) 69%
   (d) 75%

10. What is the most common sonographic feature of tophi at the olecranon bursa?
    (a) Heterogeneity
    (b) Multiple grouped nodules
    (c) Poorly defined contours
    (d) Hyperechogenicity

Answers

1. (b) Hypoechoic, noncompressible, and nondisplaceable, exhibits Doppler signal
2. (d) All of the above
3. (b) 2
4. (b) Medial tibiofemoral joint, longitudinal view
5. (b) Raised hyperechoic area arising from the bony cortex, without any echogenicity below
6. (d) a and b. Can use sterile probe cover and/or one-time use probe cover, with sterile gel, followed by low-level disinfection
7. (c) Hyperechoic cloudy areas and spots in thickened synovium
8. (b) Thin hyperechoic bands parallel to the surface of the hyaline cartilage
9. (c) 69%
10. (d) Hyperechogenicity

References

1. Wakefield RJ, Balint PV, Szkudlarek M, et al. Musculoskeletal ultrasound including definitions for ultrasonographic pathology. J Rheumatol. 2005;32:2485–7.
2. Naredo E, Wakefield RJ, Iagnocco A, et al. The OMERACT ultrasound task force – status and perspectives. J Rheumatol. 2011;38:2063–7.
3. Dalvi SR, Moser DW, Samuels J. Ultrasound and treatment algorithms of RA and JIA. Rheum Dis Clin N Am. 2013;39:669–88.
4. Bruyn GA, Pineda C, Hernandez-Diaz C, et al. Validity of ultrasonography and measures of adult shoulder function and reliability of ultrasonography in detecting shoulder synovitis in patients with rheumatoid arthritis using magnetic resonance imaging as a gold standard. Arthritis Care Res. 2010;62:1079–86.
5. Szkudlarek M, Klarlund M, Narvestad E, et al. Ultrasonography of the metacarpophalangeal and proximal interphalangeal joints in rheumatoid arthritis: a comparison with magnetic resonance imaging, conventional radiography and clinical examination. Arthritis Res Ther. 2006;8:R52.
6. Terslev L, Torp-Pedersen S, Savnik A, et al. Doppler ultrasound and magnetic resonance imaging of synovial inflammation of the hand in rheumatoid arthritis: a comparative study. Arthritis Rheum. 2003;48:2434–41.
7. Karim Z, Wakefield RJ, Quinn M, et al. Validation and reproducibility of ultrasonography in the detection of synovitis in the knee: a comparison with arthroscopy and clinical examination. Arthritis Rheum. 2004;50:387–94.
8. Wakefield RJ, Freeston JE, O'Connor P, et al. The optimal assessment of the rheumatoid arthritis hindfoot: a comparative study of clinical examination, ultrasound and high field MRI. Ann Rheum Dis. 2008;67:1678–82.

9. Naredo E, Moller I, Moragues C, et al. Interobserver reliability in musculoskeletal ultrasonography: results from a "Teach the Teachers" rheumatologist course. Ann Rheum Dis. 2006;65:14–9.
10. Cheung PP, Dougados M, Gossec L. Reliability of ultrasonography to detect synovitis in rheumatoid arthritis: a systematic literature review of 35 studies (1,415 patients). Arthritis Care Res. 2010;62:323–34.
11. Brown AK. Using ultrasonography to facilitate best practice in diagnosis and management of RA. Nat Rev Rheumatol. 2009;5:698–706.
12. Walther M, Harms H, Krenn V, et al. Correlation of power Doppler sonography with vascularity of the synovial tissue of the knee joint in patients with osteoarthritis and rheumatoid arthritis. Arthritis Rheum. 2001;44:331–8.
13. Walther M, Harms H, Krenn V, et al. Synovial tissue of the hip at power Doppler US: correlation between vascularity and power Doppler US signal. Radiology. 2002;225:225–31.
14. Naredo E, Bonilla G, Gamero F, et al. Assessment of inflammatory activity in rheumatoid arthritis: a comparative study of clinical evaluation with grey scale and power Doppler ultrasonography. Ann Rheum Dis. 2005;64:375–81.
15. Backhaus M, Burmester GR, Sandrock D, et al. Prospective two year follow up study comparing novel and conventional imaging procedures in patients with arthritic finger joints. Ann Rheum Dis. 2002;61:895–904.
16. Freeston JE, Brown AK, Hensor EM, et al. Extremity magnetic resonance imaging assessment of synovitis (without contrast) in rheumatoid arthritis may be less accurate than power Doppler ultrasound. Ann Rheum Dis. 2008;67:1351.
17. Boutry N, Lardé A, Lapègue F, et al. Magnetic resonance imaging appearance of the hands and feet in patients with early rheumatoid arthritis. J Rheumatol. 2003;30:671–9.
18. Schmidt WA, Schicke B, Ostendorf B, et al. Low-field MRI versus ultrasound: which is more sensitive in detecting inflammation and bone damage in MCP and MTP joints in mild or moderate rheumatoid arthritis? Clin Exp Rheumatol. 2013;31:91–6.
19. Grassi W, Filippucci E, Farina A, Cervini C. Sonographic imaging of tendons. Arthritis Rheum. 2000;43:969–76.
20. Micu MC, Serra S, Fodor D, et al. Inter-observer reliability of ultrasound detection of tendon abnormalities at the wrist and ankle in patients with rheumatoid arthritis. Rheumatology (Oxford). 2011;50:1120–4.
21. Bruyn GA, Möller I, Garrido J, et al. Reliability testing of tendon disease using two different scanning methods in patients with rheumatoid arthritis. Rheumatology. 2012;51:1655–61.
22. Boutry N, Morel M, Flipo RM, et al. Early rheumatoid arthritis: a review of MRI and sonographic findings. AJR Am J Roentgenol. 2007;189:1502–9.
23. Funck-Brentano T, Etchepare F, Joulin SJ, et al. Benefits of ultrasonography in the management of early arthritis: a cross-sectional study of baseline data from the ESPOIR cohort. Rheumatology (Oxford). 2009;48:1515–9.
24. Scheel AK, Hermann KG, Ohrndorf S, et al. Prospective 7 year follow up imaging study comparing radiography, ultrasonography, and magnetic resonance imaging in rheumatoid arthritis finger joints. Ann Rheum Dis. 2006;65:595–600.
25. Wakefield RJ, Gibbon WW, Conaghan PG, et al. The value of sonography in the detection of bone erosions in patients with rheumatoid arthritis: a comparison with conventional radiography. Arthritis Rheum. 2000;43:2762–70.
26. Lopez-Ben R, Bernreuter WK, Moreland LW, Alarcon GS. Ultrasound detection of bone erosions in rheumatoid arthritis: a comparison to routine radiographs of the hands and feet. Skelet Radiol. 2004;33:80–4.
27. Dohn UM, Ejbjerg BJ, Court-Payen M, et al. Are bone erosions detected by magnetic resonance imaging and ultrasonography true erosions? A comparison with computed tomography in rheumatoid arthritis metacarpophalangeal joints. Arthritis Res Ther. 2006;8:R110.
28. Ostergaard M, Szkudlarek M. Imaging in rheumatoid arthritis – why MRI and ultrasonography can no longer be ignored. Scandinavian J Rheumatol. 2003;32:63–73.

29. Szkudlarek M, Court-Payen M, Jacobsen S, et al. Interobserver agreement in ultrasonography of the finger and toe joints in rheumatoid arthritis. Arthritis Rheum. 2003;48:955–62.
30. Gutierrez M, Filippucci E, Ruta S, et al. Inter-observer reliability of high-resolution ultrasonography in the assessment of bone erosions in patients with rheumatoid arthritis: experience of an intensive dedicated training programme. Rheumatology (Oxford). 2011;50:373–80.
31. Hammer HB, Sveinsson M, Kongtorp AK, Kvien TK. A 78-joints ultrasonographic assessment is associated with clinical assessments and is highly responsive to improvement in a longitudinal study of patients with rheumatoid arthritis starting adalimumab treatment. Ann Rheum Dis. 2010;69:1349–51.
32. Perricone C, Ceccarelli F, Modesti M, et al. The 6-joint ultrasonographic assessment: a valid, sensitive-to-change and feasible method for evaluating joint inflammation in RA. Rheumatology (Oxford). 2012;51:866–73.
33. Scire CA, Montecucco C, Codullo V, et al. Ultrasonographic evaluation of joint involvement in early rheumatoid arthritis in clinical remission: power Doppler signal predicts short-term relapse. Rheumatology (Oxford). 2009;48:1092–7.
34. Naredo E, Rodriguez M, Campos C, et al. Validity, reproducibility, and responsiveness of a twelve-joint simplified power doppler ultrasonographic assessment of joint inflammation in rheumatoid arthritis. Arthritis Rheum. 2008;59:515–22.
35. Backhaus TM, Ohrndorf S, Kellner H, et al. The US7 score is sensitive to change in a large cohort of patients with rheumatoid arthritis over 12 months of therapy. Ann Rheum Dis. 2013;72(7):1163–9. Epub 2012 Sep 6.
36. Backhaus M, Ohrndorf S, Kellner H, et al. Evaluation of a novel 7-joint ultrasound score in daily rheumatologic practice: a pilot project. Arthritis Rheum. 2009;61:1194–201.
37. Iagnocco A, Naredo E, Wakefield R, et al. Responsiveness in rheumatoid arthritis. A report from the OMERACT 11 ultrasound workshop. J Rheumatol. 2014;41:379–82.
38. Ben-Artzi A, Kaeley GS, Ranganath VK. Ultrasound scoring of joint synovitis. Springer; 2021.
39. Brown AK, Conaghan PG, Karim Z, et al. An explanation for the apparent dissociation between clinical remission and continued structural deterioration in rheumatoid arthritis. Arthritis Rheum. 2008;58:2958–67.
40. Naredo E, Collado P, Cruz A, et al. Longitudinal power Doppler ultrasonographic assessment of joint inflammatory activity in early rheumatoid arthritis: predictive value in disease activity and radiologic progression. Arthritis Rheum. 2007;57:116–24.
41. Naredo E, Moller I, Cruz A, et al. Power Doppler ultrasonographic monitoring of response to anti-tumor necrosis factor therapy in patients with rheumatoid arthritis. Arthritis Rheum. 2008;58:2248–56.
42. Taylor PC, Steuer A, Gruber J, et al. Comparison of ultrasonographic assessment of synovitis and joint vascularity with radiographic evaluation in a randomized, placebo-controlled study of infliximab therapy in early rheumatoid arthritis. Arthritis Rheum. 2004;50:1107–16.
43. Boyesen P, Haavardsholm EA, van der Heijde D, et al. Prediction of MRI erosive progression: a comparison of modern imaging modalities in early rheumatoid arthritis patients. Ann Rheum Dis. 2011;70:176–9.
44. Brown AK, Quinn MA, Karim Z, et al. Presence of significant synovitis in rheumatoid arthritis patients with disease-modifying antirheumatic drug-induced clinical remission: evidence from an imaging study may explain structural progression. Arthritis Rheum. 2006;54:3761–73.
45. Zufferey P, Moller B, Brulhart L, et al. Persistence of ultrasound synovitis in patients with rheumatoid arthritis fulfilling the DAS28 and/or the new ACR/EULAR RA remission definitions: results of an observational cohort study. Joint Bone Spine. 2014;81:426–32.
46. Saleem B, Brown AK, Keen H, et al. Should imaging be a component of rheumatoid arthritis remission criteria? A comparison between traditional and modified composite remission scores and imaging assessments. Ann Rheum Dis. 2011;70:792–8.
47. Meenagh G, Filippucci E, Iagnocco A, et al. Ultrasound imaging for the rheumatologist VIII. Ultrasound imaging in osteoarthritis. Clin Exp Rheumatol. 2007;25:172–5.

48. Keen HI, Wakefield RJ, Conaghan PG. A systematic review of ultrasonography in osteoarthritis. Ann Rheum Dis. 2009;68:611–9.
49. Riecke BF, Christensen R, Torp-Pedersen S, et al. An ultrasound score for knee osteoarthritis: a cross-sectional validation study. Osteoarthr Cartil. 2014;22:1675–91.
50. Keen HI, Lavie F, Wakefield RJ, et al. The development of a preliminary ultrasonographic scoring system for features of hand osteoarthritis. Ann Rheum Dis. 2008;67:651–5.
51. Keen HI, Wakefield RJ, Grainger AJ, et al. Can ultrasonography improve on radiographic assessment in osteoarthritis of the hands? A comparison between radiographic and ultrasonographic detected pathology. Ann Rheum Dis. 2008;67:1116–20.
52. Picerno V, Filippou G, Bertoldi I, et al. Prevalence of Baker's cyst in patients with knee pain: an ultrasonographic study. Reumatismo. 2013;65:264–70.
53. Artul S, Khazin F, Hakim J, Habib G. Ultrasonographic findings in a large series of patients with knee pain. J Clin Imaging Sci. 2014;4:45.
54. Conaghan PG, D'Agostino MA, Le Bars M, et al. Clinical and ultrasonographic predictors of joint replacement for knee osteoarthritis: results from a large, 3-year, prospective EULAR study. Ann Rheum Dis. 2010;69:644–7.
55. Kristoffersen H, Torp-Pedersen S, Terslev L, et al. Indications of inflammation visualized by ultrasound in osteoarthritis of the knee. Acta Radiol. 2006;47:281–6.
56. Moller I, Bong D, Naredo E, et al. Ultrasound in the study and monitoring of osteoarthritis. Osteoarthr Cartil. 2008;16(Suppl 3):S4–7.
57. D'Agostino MA, Conaghan P, Le Bars M, et al. EULAR report on the use of ultrasonography in painful knee osteoarthritis. Part 1: prevalence of inflammation in osteoarthritis. Ann Rheum Dis. 2005;64:1703–9.
58. Atchia I, Kane D, Reed MR, Isaacs JD, Birrell F. Efficacy of a single ultrasound-guided injection for the treatment of hip osteoarthritis. Ann Rheum Dis. 2011;70:110–6.
59. Maheu E, Berenbaum F. Time for new outcome measures in hand osteoarthritis? Nat Clin Pract Rheumatol. 2009;5:136–8.
60. Keen HI, Wakefield RJ, Grainger AJ, et al. An ultrasonographic study of osteoarthritis of the hand: synovitis and its relationship to structural pathology and symptoms. Arthritis Rheum. 2008;59:1756–63.
61. Kortekaas MC, Kwok WY, Reijnierse M, et al. In erosive hand osteoarthritis more inflammatory signs on ultrasound are found than in the rest of hand osteoarthritis. Ann Rheum Dis. 2013;72:930–4.
62. De Miguel E, Falcao S, Castillo C, et al. Enthesis erosion in spondyloarthritis is not a persistent structural lesion. Ann Rheum Dis. 2011;70(11):2008–10.
63. Aydin SZ, Bas E, Basi O, et al. Validation of ultrasound imaging for Achilles entheseal fibrocartilage in bovines and description of changes in humans with spondyloarthritis. Ann Rheum Dis. 2010;69(12):2165–8.
64. Falcao S, De Miguel E, Castillo-Gallego C, et al. Achilles enthesis ultrasound: the importance of the bursa in spondyloarthritis. Clin Exp Rheumatol. 2013;31(3):422–7.
65. Spadaro A, Iagnocco A, Perrotta FM, et al. Clinical and ultrasonography assessment of peripheral enthesitis in ankylosing spondylitis. Rheumatology (Oxford). 2011;50:2080–6.
66. Hamdi W, Chelli MB, Ghannouchi MM, et al. Performance of ultrasounds compared with radiographs to detect chronic enthesitis signs in patients with ankylosing spondylitis. Rheumatol Int. 2013;33:497–9.
67. Huang Z, Cao J, Li T, et al. Efficacy and safety of ultrasound-guided local injections of etanercept into entheses of ankylosing spondylitis patients with refractory Achilles enthesitis. Clin Exp Rheumatol. 2011;29(4):642–9.
68. Aydin SZ, Karadag O, Filippucci E, et al. Monitoring Achilles enthesitis in ankylosing spondylitis during TNF-α antagonist therapy: an ultrasound study. Rheumatology (Oxford). 2010;49:578–82.
69. Sakellariou G, Iagnocco A, Meenagh G, et al. Ultrasound imaging for the rheumatologist XXXVII. Sonographic assessment of the hip in ankylosing spondylitis patients. Clin Exp Rheumatol. 2012;30(1):1–5.

70. Mohammedi A, Ghasemi-rad M, Aghdashi M, et al. Evaluation of disease activity in ankylosing spondylitis; diagnostic value of color Doppler ultrasonography. Skelet Radiol. 2013;42:219–24.
71. Zhu J, Xing C, Jiang Y, et al. Evaluation of complex appearance in vascularity of sacroiliac joint in ankylosing spondylitis by color Doppler ultrasonography. Rheumatol Int. 2012;32:69–72.
72. Hu Y, Zhu J, Xue Q, et al. Scanning of the sacroiliac joint and enthesis by color Doppler ultrasonography in patients with ankylosing spondylitis. J Rheumatol. 2011;38:1651–5.
73. Jiang Y, Chen L, Zhu J, et al. Power Doppler ultrasonography in the evaluation of infliximab treatment for sacroiliitis in patients with ankylosing spondylitis. Rheumatol Int. 2013;33:2025–9.
74. Freeston JE, Coates LC, Nam JL, et al. Is there subclinical synovitis in early psoriatic arthritis? A clinical comparison with gray-scale and power Doppler ultrasound. Arthritis Care Res. 2014;66(3):432–9.
75. Freeston JE, Coates LC, Helliwell PS, et al. Is there subclinical enthesitis in early psoriatic arthritis? A clinical comparison with power Doppler ultrasound. Arthritis Care Res. 2012;64(10):1617–21.
76. Bandinelli F, Prignano F, Bonciani D, et al. Ultrasound detects occult entheseal involvement in early psoriatic arthritis independently of clinical features and psoriasis severity. Clin Exp Rheumatol. 2013;31(2):219–4.
77. Gladman DD, Shuckett R, Russell MI. Psoriatic arthritis (PSA) – an analysis of 220 patients. Q J Med. 1987;62(238):127–41.
78. De Simone C, Caldarola G, D'Agostino M, et al. Usefulness of ultrasound imaging in detecting psoriatic arthritis of fingers and toes in patients with psoriasis. Clin Dev Immunol. 2011;2011:390726.
79. Naredo E, Moller I, De Miguel E, et al. High prevalence of ultrasonographic synovitis and enthesopathy in patients with psoriasis without psoriatic arthritis: a prospective case-control study. Rheumatology (Oxford). 2011;50:1838–48.
80. Tinazzi I, McGonagle D, Biasi D, et al. Preliminary evidence that subclinical enthesopathy may predict psoriatic arthritis in patients with psoriasis. J Rheumatol. 2011;38(12):2691–2.
81. Gutierrez M, Filippucci E, De Angelis R, et al. Subclinical entheseal involvement in patients with psoriasis: an ultrasound study. Semin Arthritis Rheum. 2011;40:407–12.
82. El Miedany Y, El Gaafary M, Youssef S, et al. Tailored approach to early psoriatic arthritis patients: clinical and ultrasonographic predictors for structural joint damage. Clin Rheumatol. 2015;34(2):307–13.
83. Bonifati C, Elia F, Graceffa D, et al. Clinical and contrast-enhanced ultrasound echography outcomes in psoriatic arthritis patients after one year of continuous therapy with anti-TNF drugs. ISRN Dermatol. 2014;2014:932721. eCollection 2014.
84. Riente L, Delle Sedie A, Sakellariou G, et al. Ultrasound imaging for the rheumatologist XXXVIII. Sonographic assessment of the hip in psoriatic arthritis patients. Clin Exp Rheumatol. 2012;30(2):152–5.
85. Iagnocco A, Spadaro A, Marchesoni A, et al. Power Doppler ultrasonographic evaluation of enthesitis in psoriatic arthritis. A multi-center study. Joint Bone Spine. 2012;79:323–34.
86. Eder L, Kaeley GS, Aydin SZ. Development and validation of a sonographic enthesitis instrument in psoriatic arthritis: the GRAPPA diagnostic ultrasound Enthesitis tool (DUET) project. J Rheumatol. 2020;96:50–2.
87. Husic R, Gretler J, Felber A, et al. Disparity between ultrasound and clinical findings in psoriatic arthritis. Ann Rheum Dis. 2014;73(8):1529–36.
88. Kaeley GS. Ultrasound imaging module: report from the GRAPPA 2012 annual meeting. J Rheumatol. 2013;40:1450–2.
89. Bakewell CJ, Olivieri I, Aydin SZ, et al. Ultrasound and magnetic resonance imaging in the evaluation of psoriatic dactylitis: status and perspectives. J Rheumatol. 2013;40:1951–7.
90. Healy PJ, Groves C, Chandramohan M, Helliwell PS. MRI changes in psoriatic dactylitis – extent of pathology, relationship to tenderness and correlation with clinical indices. Rheumatology. 2008;47:92–5.

91. Olivieri I, Scarano E, Padula A, et al. Fast spin echo-T2-weighted sequences with fat saturation in toe dactylitis of spondyloarthritis. Clin Rheumatol. 2008;27:1141–5.
92. Olivieri I, Barozzi L, Favaro L, et al. Dactylitis in patients with seronegative spondyloarthropathy. Assessment by ultrasonography and magnetic resonance imaging. Arthritis Rheum. 1995;39:1524–8.
93. Kane D, Greaney T, Bresnihan B, et al. Ultrasonography in the diagnosis and management of psoriatic dactylitis. J Rheumatol. 1999;26:1746–51.
94. Jevtic V, Watt I, Rozman B, et al. Distinctive radiological features of small hand joints in rheumatoid arthritis and seronegative spondyloarthritis demonstrated by contrast-enhanced (Gd-DTPA) magnetic resonance imaging. Skelet Radiol. 1995;24:351–5.
95. Fournie B, Margarit Coll N, Champetier De Ribes TL, et al. Extrasynovial ultrasound abnormalities in the psoriatic finger. Prospective comparative power-doppler study versus rheumatoid arthritis. Joint Bone Spine. 2006;73:527–31.
96. Gutierrez M, Wortsman X, Filippucci E, et al. High frequency sonography in the evaluation of psoriasis: nail and skin involvement. J Ultrasound Med. 2009;28(11):1569–74.
97. Wortsman X, Jemec G. Common inflammatory diseases of the skin: from the skin to the screen. Adv Psoriasis Inflamm Skin Dis. 2010;2:9–15.
98. Sandobal C, Carbo E, Iribas J, et al. Ultrasound nail imaging on patients with psoriasis and psoriatic arthritis compared with rheumatoid arthritis and control subjects. J Clin Rheumatol. 2014;20(1):21–4.
99. Aydin SB, Castillo-Gallego C, Ash ZR, et al. Ultrasonographic assessment of nail in psoriatic disease shows a link between onychopathy and distal interphalangeal joint extensor tendon enthesopathy. Dermatology. 2012;225:231–5.
100. Klauser AS, Wipfler E, Dejaco C, et al. Diagnostic values of history and clinical examination to predict ultrasound signs of chronic and acute enthesitis. Clin Exp Rheumatol. 2008;26(4):548–53.
101. Eder L, Jayaker J, Thavaneswaran A, et al. Is the Madrid Sonographic Enthesitis Index useful for differentiating psoriatic arthritis from psoriasis alone and healthy controls. J Rheumatol. 2014;41:466–72.
102. Ibrahim G, Groves C, Chandramohan M, et al. Clinical and ultrasound examination of the Leeds Enthesitis Index in PSoriatic arthritis and rheumatoid arthritis. ISRN Rheumatol. 2011;2011:731917.
103. Schafer VS, Fleck M, Kellner H, et al. Evaluation of the novel ultrasound score for large joints in psoriatic arthritis and ankylosing spondylitis: six month experience in daily clinical practice. BMC Musculoskelet Disord. 2013;14:358.
104. Ottaviani S, Gill G, Palazzo E, et al. Ultrasonography of shoulders in spondyloarthritis and rheumatoid arthritis: a case-control study. Joint Bone Spine. 2014;81:247–9.
105. Toprak H, Kilic E, Serter A, et al. Doppler US in rheumatic diseases with special emphasis on rheumatoid arthritis and spondyloarthritis. Diagn Interv Radiol. 2014;20:72–7.
106. Ruta S, Felquer MLA, Rosa J, et al. Responsiveness to therapy change of a global ultrasound assessment in spondyloarthritis patients. Clin Rheumatol. 2015;34(1):125–32.
107. McCarty DJ, Hollander JL. Identification of urate crystals in gouty synovial fluid. Ann Intern Med. 1961;54:452–60.
108. Filippucci E, Di Geso L, Girolimetti R, Grassi W. Ultrasound in crystal-related arthritis. Clin Exp Rheumatol. 2014;32(1 Suppl 80):S42–7.
109. Delle Sedie A, Riente L, Iagnocco A, et al. Ultrasound imaging for the rheumatologist X. Ultrasound imaging in crystal-related arthropathies. Clin Exp Rheumatol. 2007;25(4):513–7.
110. Neogi T, Jansen TLTA, Dalbeth N, et al. 2015 Gout classification criteria: an American College of Rheumatology/European League Against Rheumatism collaborative initiative. Ann Rheum Dis. 2015;74:1789–98.
111. Grassi W, Meenagh G, Pascual E, Filippucci E. "Crystal clear" – sonographic assessment of gout and calcium pyrophosphate deposition disease. Semin Arthritis Rheum. 2006;36:197–202.

112. Chen LX, Schumacher HR. Gout: can we create an evidence-based systematic approach to diagnosis and management? Best Pract Res Clin Rheumatol. 2006;20:673–84.
113. Filippucci E, Meenagh G, Delle Sedie A, et al. Ultrasound imaging for the rheumatologist XXXVI. Sonographic assessment of the foot in gout patients. Clin Exp Rheumatol. 2011;29(6):901–5.
114. Wright SA, Filippucci E, McVeigh C, et al. High-resolution ultrasonography of the first metatarsal phalangeal joint in gout: a controlled study. Ann Rheum Dis. 2007;66:859–64.
115. Thiele RG, Schlesinger N. Diagnosis of gout by ultrasound. Rheumatology. 2007;46:1116–21.
116. Daboiko JC, Ouali B, Ouattara B. Use of ultrasound guidance in an inaugural acute gout of the hip joint; apropos of a west African case. J Clin Rheumatol. 2011;17(2):94–5.
117. Wakefield R, Emery P, Pease C. Gout related upper limb cellulitis: an ultrasound study. J Rheumatol. 2003;30(2):417–9.
118. Le Goff B, Berthelot MJ, Andre V, Guillot P, Maugars Y. Ultrasonography for diagnosing atypical gout. Two case reports. Joint Bone Spine. 2008;75:610–2.
119. Aslam N, Lo S, McNab I. Gouty flexor tenosynovitis mimicking infection: a case report emphasizing the value of ultrasound in diagnosis. Acta Orthop Belg. 2004;70:368–70.
120. Puig JG, de Miguel E, Castillo MC, et al. Asymptomatic hyperuricemia: impact of ultrasonography. Nuclosides Nucleotides Nucleic Acids. 2008;27(6–7):592–5.
121. De Miguel E, Puig JG, Castillo C, et al. Diagnosis of gout in patients with asymptomatic hyperuricaemia: a pilot ultrasound study. Ann Rheum Dis. 2012;71(1):157–8.
122. Pineda C, Amezcua-Guerra LM, Solano C, et al. Joint and tendon subclinical involvement suggestive of gouty arthritis in asymptomatic hyperuricemia: an ultrasound controlled study. Arthritis Res Ther. 2011;13:R4.
123. Ottaviani S, Allard A, Bardin T, Richette P. An exploratory ultrasound study of early gout. Clin Exp Rheumatol. 2011;29(5):816–32.
124. Filippucci E, Gutierrez M, Georgescu D, et al. Hyaline cartilage involvement in patients with gout and calcium pyrophosphate deposition disease. An ultrasound study. Osteoarthr Cartil. 2009;17(2):178–81.
125. Howard RG, Pillinger MH, Gyftopoulos S, et al. Reproducibility of musculoskeletal ultrasound for determining monosodium urate deposition: concordance between readers. Arthritis Care Res. 2011;63(10):1456–62.
126. Rettenbecher T, Ennemoser S, Welrich H, et al. Diagnostic imaging of gout: comparison of high-resolution US versus conventional X-ray. Eur Radiol. 2008;18:621–30.
127. Gruber M, Bodner G, Rath E, et al. Dual-energy computed tomography compared with ultrasound in the diagnosis of gout. Rheumatology (Oxford). 2014;53(1):173–9. Epub 2013 Oct 17.
128. Gerster JC, Landry M, Dufresne L, Meuwly JY. Imaging of tophaceous gout: computed tomography provides specific images compared with magnetic resonance imaging and ultrasonography. Ann Rheum Dis. 2001;61:52–4.
129. Bongartz T, Glazebrook KN, Kavros SJ, et al. Dual-energy CT for the diagnosis of gout: an accuracy and diagnostic yield study. Ann Rheum Dis. 2015;74:1072–7.
130. De Avila FE, Kubota ES, Sandim GB, et al. Ultrasound features of tophi in chronic tophaceous gout. Skelet Radiol. 2011;40:309–15.
131. De Avila FE, Lopes MG, Mitraud SAV, et al. Ultrasound characteristics of gouty tophi in the olecranon bursa and evaluation of their reproducibility. Eur J Radiol. 2012;81:317–23.
132. Dalbeth N, Schauer C, MacDonald P, et al. Methods of tophus assessment in clinical trials of gout: a systematic literature review and pictorial reference guide. Ann Rheum Dis. 2011;70(4):597–604. Epub 2011 Jan 7
133. Balbir Gurman A, Nahir AM, Braun-Moscovici Y, Soudack M. Sonographic features of a tophaceous nodule. Isr Med Assoc J. 2005;7:746–7.
134. Kunkel G. Tophaceous gout mimicking osteomyelitis; the value of musculoskeletal ultrasound in establishing the diagnosis. J Clin Rheumatol. 2010;16(6):295–7.
135. Gutierrez M, Di Geso L, Filippucci E, Grassi W. Calcium pyrophosphate crystals detected by ultrasound in patients without radiographic evidence of cartilage calcifications. J Rheumatol. 2010;37(2):2602–3.

136. Sofka CM, Adler RS, Cordasco FA. Ultrasound diagnosis of chondrocalcinosis in the knee. Skelet Radiol. 2002;31:43–5.
137. Filippou G, Frediani B, Gallo A, et al. A "new" technique for the diagnosis of chondrocalcinosis of the knee: sensitivity and specificity of high-frequency ultrasonography. Ann Rheum Dis. 2007;66:1126–8.
138. Filippou G, Filippucci E, Tardella M, et al. Extent and distribution of CPP deposits in patients affected by calcium pyrophosphate dehydrate deposition disease: an ultrasonographic study. Ann Rheum Dis. 2013;72:1836–9.
139. Ellaban AS, Kamel SR, Abo Omar HAS, et al. Ultrasonographic findings of Achilles tendon and plantar fascia in patients with calcium pyrophosphate deposition disease. Clin Rheumatol. 2012;31:697–704.
140. Checa A, Wong H, Chun W. Sonographic characterization of mixed crystal arthropathy due to monosodium urate and calcium pyrophosphate dehydrate: the triple-contour sign. J Ultrasound Med. 2011;30:859–67.
141. American Institute of Ultrasound in Medicine. AIUM practice guidelines for cleaning and preparing external- and internal-use ultrasound transducers and equipment between patients as well as safe handling and use of ultrasound coupling gel. Reapproved 2020. aium.org/officialstatements/57.
142. American Institute of Ultrasound in Medicine. AIUM practice guideline for documentation of an ultrasound examination. J Ultrasound Med. 2014;33:1098–102.
143. American Institute of Ultrasound in Medicine. AIUM practice guidelines for selected ultrasound-guided procedures. 2014. aium.org/resources/guidelines/usguidedprocedures.pdf.

3 Ultrasound of the Hand and Wrist

Arnold Ceponis and Eugene Y. Kissin

Key Points

- Hand and wrist ultrasound can help in both identifying the source of symptoms and establishing the diagnoses in patients with hand and wrist pain.
- The most common pathologies that can be identified by ultrasound in hand and wrist region include synovitis and tenosynovitis, bony erosions, osteophytes, chondrocalcinosis, gouty tophi, ligamentous injury, tendinitis, retinacular pathology (e.g., DeQuervain's), and nerve impingement (e.g., median nerve).
- Hand and wrist ultrasound can be used in rheumatology practice to aid in the assessment of subclinical synovitis and treatment response.
- Hand and wrist ultrasound has been shown to increase both physician and patient confidence in therapeutic decision-making in rheumatoid arthritis.
- The use of ultrasound for procedural purposes can help with diagnostic synovial fluid aspiration and targeted corticosteroid injections.

A. Ceponis (✉)
Division of Rheumatology, Allergy and Immunology, University of California San Diego School of Medicine, La Jolla, CA, USA
e-mail: aceponis@health.ucsd.edu

E. Y. Kissin
Division of Rheumatology, Department of Medicine, Boston University Medical Center, Boston, MA, USA
e-mail: eukissin@bu.edu

M. J. Kohler (ed.), *Musculoskeletal Ultrasound in Rheumatology Review*,
https://doi.org/10.1007/978-3-030-73555-5_3

General Principles

Ultrasound evaluation of the hand and wrist is the most commonly performed ultrasound in rheumatology practice. It is especially valuable for the rheumatologist to better characterize structural damage caused by inflammation and can increase confidence in clinical decision-making [1]. Gray-scale and power Doppler ultrasound modalities, when used in conjunction, provide very sensitive and specific means to identify subclinical synovial abnormalities, assess disease activity, localize inflammation or other types of pathology to a particular tissue compartment, and determine the degree of damage that has been done to the soft tissues and to the underlying bone.

Proper scanning techniques and patient positioning are the key for accurate and reliable image acquisition. The following are hand and wrist ultrasound scanning tips.

Begin scanning by placing the hand, wrist, and forearm on a supportive surface between the examiner and the ultrasound screen. To avoid motion-related artifacts, the extremity should be relaxed and fully rested on the supporting surface.

The wrist should be kept in neutral position for scanning, as flexion or extension of the wrist will affect the appearance of the synovium—more prominent dorsally with wrist extension, less prominent with wrist flexion.

Lister's tubercle is a key anatomical landmark for obtaining standard proximal transverse view and identifying and scanning extensor tendon compartments and the distal radioulnar joint.

The pisiform and scaphoid tuberosity are the anatomical landmarks that help to identify the carpal tunnel on a volar transverse view of the wrist.

Synovial reflections should be evaluated fully by following them proximally or distally to the joint cleft depending on the joint being scanned. This is particularly important in scanning MCPs (metacarpophalangeal joints) because the dorsal synovial recesses of the MCPs continue far proximal to the joint cleft.

Localizing Doppler signal to synovial tissue identified during gray-scale scanning will help avoid mistaking feeding vessels for synovial hyperemia (or active inflammation).

Ligamentous structures such as the triangular fibrocartilage complex can be assessed for hyperechoic densities of calcium deposition such as chondrocalcinosis.

Soft tissue nodules can be differentiated based on their location and their echotexture: anechoic vs. isoechoic and homogeneous vs. isoechoic to hyperechoic and heterogeneous.

All pathology should be imaged in orthogonal planes for confirmation of abnormality.

The diagnosis of nerve impingement can be established by whether the nerve is swollen just proximal to the point of impingement in comparison to the nerve caliber further proximally.

Transducer "rocking" maneuver can be used to avoid artifacts caused by tendon and nerve anisotropy, which makes structures appear dark (hypoechoic or even anechoic), mimicking effusion.

One should avoid excessive compression of the tissues with the transducer (especially of the dorsal wrist and MCPs); otherwise, effusions and power Doppler signal could be missed. "Floating the transducer" by keeping a 1–3-mm layer of the gel between the transducer and the skin will prevent unintended tissue compression.

It is essential to perform scanning in a logical and routine progression to avoid missing/forgetting to scan any relevant structures. Slide the transducer from one view to the next, rather than picking up the transducer and setting it down in a different location. Doing the latter could result in missing pathology in the interval tissues. Table 3.1 shows recommended standard scans and corresponding common pathology that can be seen with hand and wrist ultrasound.

Table 3.1 Standard scans, indications, and key features

View	Structures and pathology	Key features
Dorsal wrist	Wrist joint synovitis Effusion Erosion Osteophytes Extensor tendinitis Tenosynovitis Ligament tears and calcifications	Use Lister's tubercle for orientation to the extensor tendons in transverse view Use radius, lunate, and capitate bones for orientation to the radiocarpal and intercarpal synovium in longitudinal view
Radial wrist	DeQuervain's tendinitis Tenosynovitis	Assess first compartment retinaculum at the level of the distal radius
Ulnar wrist	Extensor carpi ulnaris tenosynovitis ulnar erosions Triangular fibrocartilage calcification	Assess extensor carpi ulnaris at the level of the ulnar sulcus. Radially deviate the wrist to maximally expose the triangular fibrocartilage complex
Volar wrist	Wrist joint synovitis Effusion Erosion Flexor tendinitis Tenosynovitis Median nerve impingement Ulnar nerve impingement	Use the pisiform and scaphoid tuberosity for landmarks to the carpal tunnel. Angle the transducer slightly toward the elbow to make the tendons maximally bright in transverse
Dorsal finger	Dorsal synovitis and erosion Effusion Extensor tendinitis	Don't mistake the normal curvature just proximal to the metacarpal for an erosion. Float transducer to optimize visualization
Radial/ ulnar finger	Marginal erosions Collateral ligament damage	Assess collateral ligament origin for cortical erosions
Volar finger	Volar synovitis and erosions Flexor tendinitis and tenosynovitis volar plate damage	Pay particular attention to the synovial reflection just proximal to the palmar plate

Dorsal Wrist

Figure 3.1 shows schematic representation of extensor tendon compartments of the dorsal wrist.

Lister's tubercle, the bony prominence on the distal radius, is the key to scanning the dorsal wrist (Figs. 3.1 and 3.2). The extensor pollicis longus tendon can be followed proximally to this prominence and uses it as a pulley. All of the extensor tendon compartments of the wrist can be identified relative to Lister's tubercle. The extensor pollicis longus (third compartment) is just ulnar to the tubercle at the distal radius, and just radial to the tubercle is the extensor carpi radialis brevis and the extensor carpi radialis longus (both in the second compartment) and then the extensor pollicis brevis and the abductor pollicis longus (both in the first compartment). So, the progression from ulnar to radial is longus, brevis, longus, brevis, longus. Ulnar to the extensor pollicis longus is the fourth compartment containing the extensor indicis and the extensor digitorum. Further ulnar, in the space between the radius and ulnar, is the extensor digiti minimi (fifth compartment). These tendons can best be identified and evaluated in the transverse/short axis view. This view is also useful for evaluation of the distal radioulnar joint in a plane just deep to the extensor digiti minimi. Take care not to misidentify the extensor digiti minimi as radioulnar synovium due to anisotropic artifact making the tendon hypoechoic.

Sliding the transducer distally to Lister's tubercle will result in imaging the scaphoid bone and the scapholunate ligament (Fig. 3.2b). The radiocarpal joint capsule and synovium will fold distally over this region, while sliding slightly further distally will bring the capitate bone and the overlying intercarpal synovium into view (Fig. 3.2c). Note that the head of the capitate is more rounded than the lunate in the dorsal transverse view. In addition, notice that there is a dorsal feeding vessel

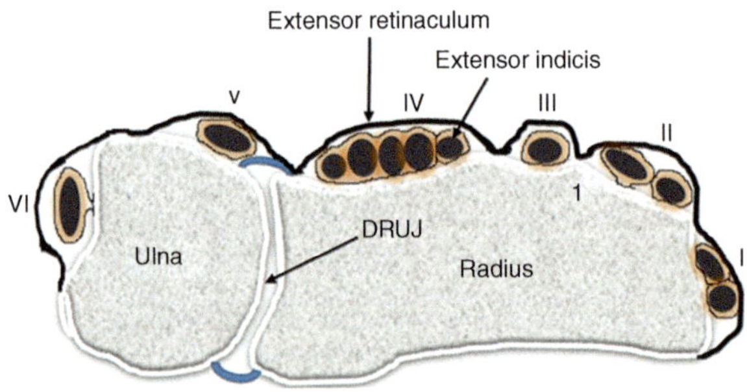

Fig. 3.1 Schematic representation of the anatomical landmarks and extensor tendon compartments of the proximal dorsal wrist. (1) Lister's tubercle, (DRUJ) distal radioulnar joint. Extensor compartments are numbered by roman numerals: (I) first extensor compartment contains abductor pollicis longus and extensor pollicis brevis; (II) second extensor compartment contains extensor carpi radialis longus and brevis; (III) third extensor compartment contains extensor pollicis longus; (IV) fourth extensor compartment contains extensor indices and extensor digitorum tendons; (V) fifth extensor compartment contains extensor digiti minimi; (VI) sixth extensor compartment contains extensor carpi ulnaris tendon

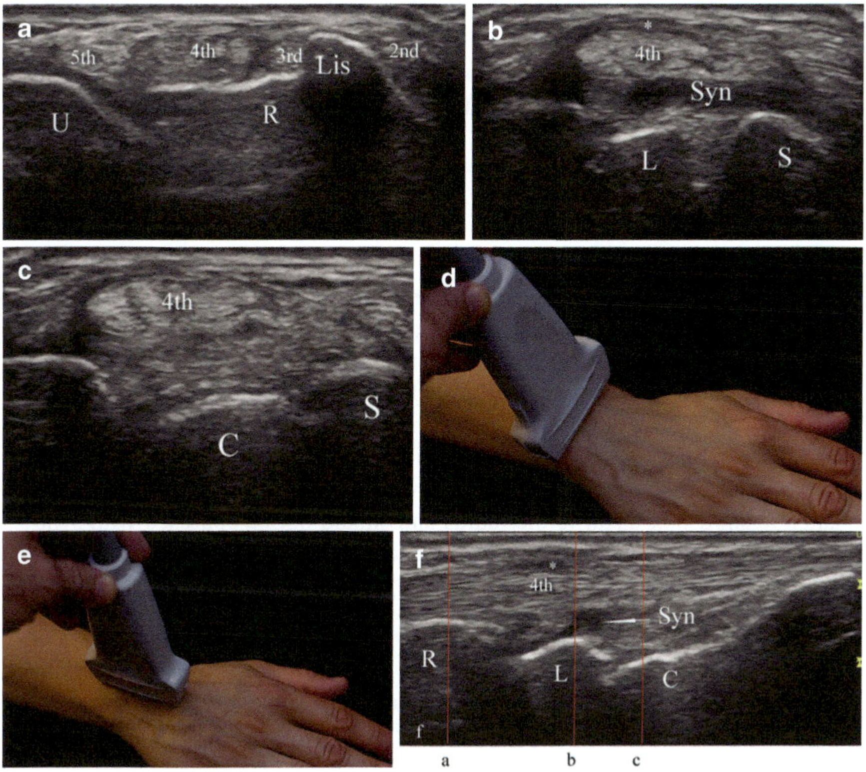

Fig. 3.2 Dorsal wrist. (**a**) shows a transverse ultrasound image through the radius (R) and ulna (U). Second, third, fourth, and fifth refer to the extensor compartments. Lister's tubercle (Lis) is the most important landmark used for orientation in this view. (**b**) shows a transverse view through the scaphoid (S) and lunate (L). The hyperechoic ligament connecting these two bones is clearly visible, and the hypoechoic radiocarpal synovium (Syn) is just superficial to the ligament. Note the normal retinaculum (*asterisk*) over the fourth compartment extensors at this level. (**c**) shows a transverse view at the level of the capitate (C). (**d**) is a photographic depiction of the transducer scanning position required to obtain images (**a**–**c**). (**e**) shows the transducer scanning position that should be used to obtain the wrist dorsal longitudinal view. (**f**) is a longitudinal view of the wrist with the transducer positioned over the radius (R), lunate (L), and capitates (C). The *orange lines* show where the transverse images were obtained relative to the longitudinal view. Radiocarpal synovium fold (Syn) and extensor retinaculum (*asterisk*) can also be appreciated on this image

that emerges from the lunate [2], which could be confused with a small erosion and synovial hyperemia.

The longitudinal view to the wrist can be obtained in the midline by positioning the proximal edge of the transducer just ulnar to Lister's tubercle and the distal end pointed at the third MCP (Figs. 3.2e, f). With this transducer position, the radius, lunate, and capitate bones should be visible, as well as the folds of the radiocarpal and intercarpal synovium. The normal extensor tendon retinaculum should be identified to avoid mistaking it for swollen tenosynovium. Sliding radially will bring the scaphoid into view. Note the effect that wrist flexion and extension have on the appearance of the synovium: extension of the wrist will make the synovial folds appear more prominent and could be mistaken for synovial hypertrophy. Power Doppler views in this plane will normally show signal from the dorsal carpal arch, superficial to the capitate, and should not be mistaken for acute synovitis/hyperemia.

Radial Wrist

The most common reason to scan the radial wrist is to evaluate for DeQuervain's tendinitis—retinacular thickening of the first compartment tendons (Fig. 3.3). The term DeQuervain's tenosynovitis, while classically used, is a misnomer as the flexor retinaculum (not tenosynovium) is the anatomic structure found surrounding the first compartment tendons at the distal radius. Normally this retinaculum is barely visible at less than a millimeter of thickness. Retinacular abnormalities are most easily appreciated in transverse view, while structural abnormalities of the tendon fibers are more easily seen in longitudinal view. The radial artery passes through the anatomic snuff box distal to the radius and should not be confused with synovial hyperemia. Slightly more distally, the first carpal-metacarpal joint can be seen, just deep to the abductor pollicis longus tendon.

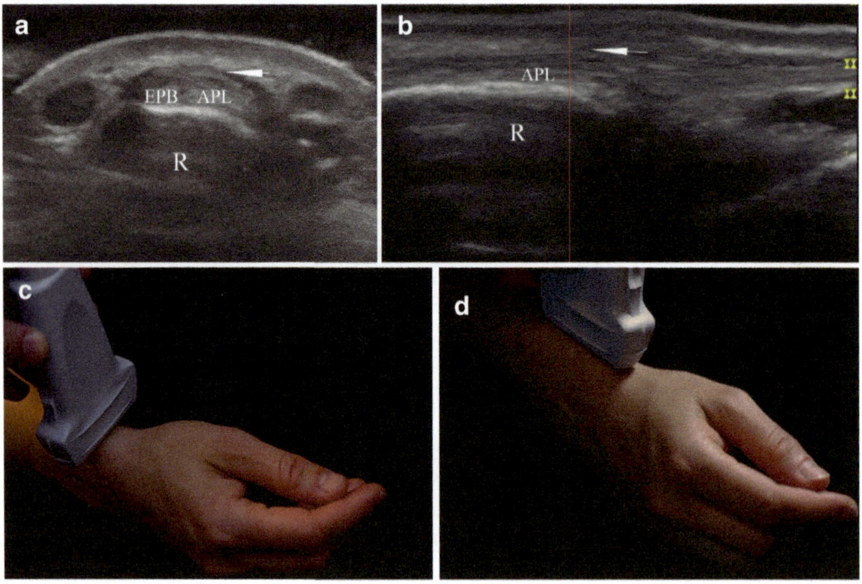

Fig. 3.3 Radial wrist. (**a**) is a transverse ultrasound image through the distal radius at the level of the orange line in (**b**), the longitudinal view through the radial wrist. The *arrows* point to the thin retinaculum normally seen over the first compartment tendons. (**c**, **d**) depict transducer scanning position over the radial wrist to obtain images (**a**, **b**). (EPB) extensor pollicis brevis, (APL) abductor pollicis longus, (R) radius

Scanning the radial wrist in longitudinal view can sometimes result in mistakenly positioning the transducer over the second compartment instead of the first. Avoid this mistake by first identifying the first and second compartments in transverse section and then scanning the intended tendons in longitudinal plane.

Ulnar Wrist

The ulnar wrist scan is performed to evaluate the extensor carpi ulnaris (ECU), the distal ulna, and the triangular fibrocartilage complex (TFCC) (Fig. 3.4). This view is especially important to the rheumatologist, given the frequency of ECU involvement in rheumatoid arthritis (RA) and the specificity of ulnar styloid erosions to RA [3]. Additionally, calcifications in the TFCC can help to evaluate for calcium pyrophosphate dihydrate (CPPD) arthropathy. In fact, ultrasound was shown to be highly specific and slightly superior to conventional X-rays in detecting chondrocalcinosis of TFCC [4]. Degenerative tears of the TFCC can also be found and commonly seen in people over 50.

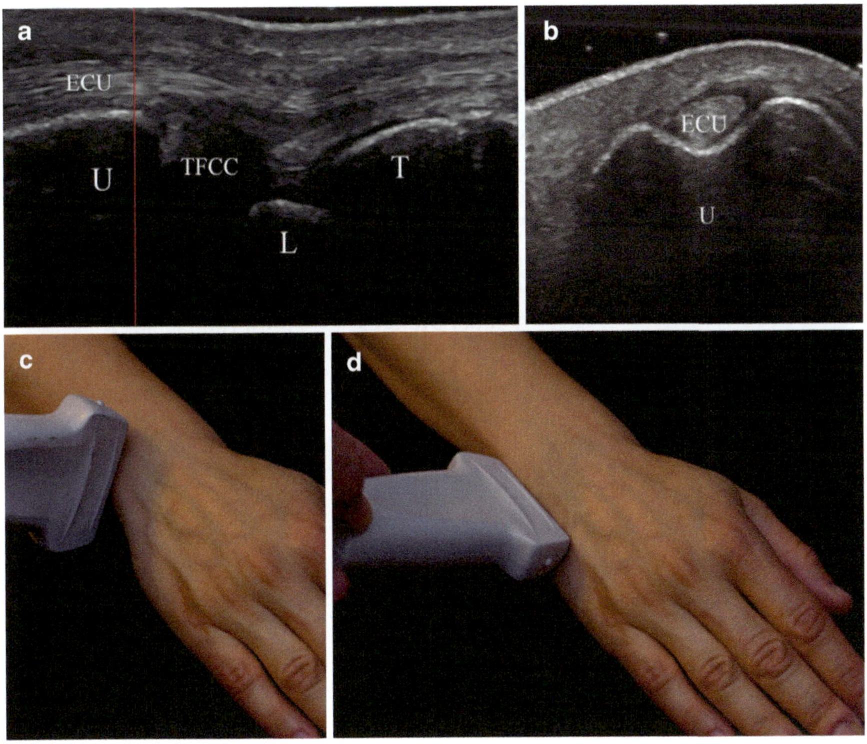

Fig. 3.4 Ulnar wrist. (**a**) shows a longitudinal ultrasound image for the ulnar wrist, with a focus on the extensor carpi ulnaris (ECU), and triangular fibrocartilage complex (TFCC). (**b**) shows the transverse view through the ECU and ulna (U) taken at the level of the orange line in (**a**). (**c**, **d**) show the transducer scanning position needed to achieve the images in (**a**, **b**). (U) ulna, (L) lunate, (T) triquetrum, (ECU) extensor carpi ulnaris, (TFCC) triangular fibrocartilage complex

To make the examination comfortable for the patient, have the patient sit across from the examiner, and bend the elbow to 90°, which will expose the ulnar wrist to the examiner. In finding proper transducer positioning, it will be helpful to remember that the ECU is dorsolateral to the styloid, rather than just lateral. Slight radial deviation of the wrist will help pull the ECU tight and reduce anisotropic artifact due to tendon curvature in a relaxed position.

Volar/Palmar Wrist

The volar view is most often used to assess for median nerve compression/carpal tunnel syndrome and flexor tendon "tenosynovitis" or retinaculitis. Schematic representation of the carpal tunnel at the level of scaphoid and pisiform is shown in Fig. 3.5. Flexor carpi radialis, palmaris longus, and flexor carpi ulnaris lay outside of the carpal tunnel, which is enclosed by the flexor retinaculum (Fig. 3.5). Ulnar artery and ulnar nerve lay within Guyon's canal, a separate compartment.

The volar view is also used for the assessment of the radiocarpal and intercarpal joints. For proper transducer placement, find the pisiform bone and the scaphoid tuberosity (Fig. 3.6)—each should be visible at the edge of the ultrasound image as these bones mark the carpal tunnel inlet with the flexor retinaculum stretching between them and the median nerve usually abuts the retinaculum and is surrounded by flexor tendons that are encased in thin tendon sheaths.

Typically in obtaining this view, the tendons in the tunnel are very anisotropic and can be made bright by rocking the transducer—pointing it more toward the elbow. As a more proximal slice of the wrist is obtained with this transducer

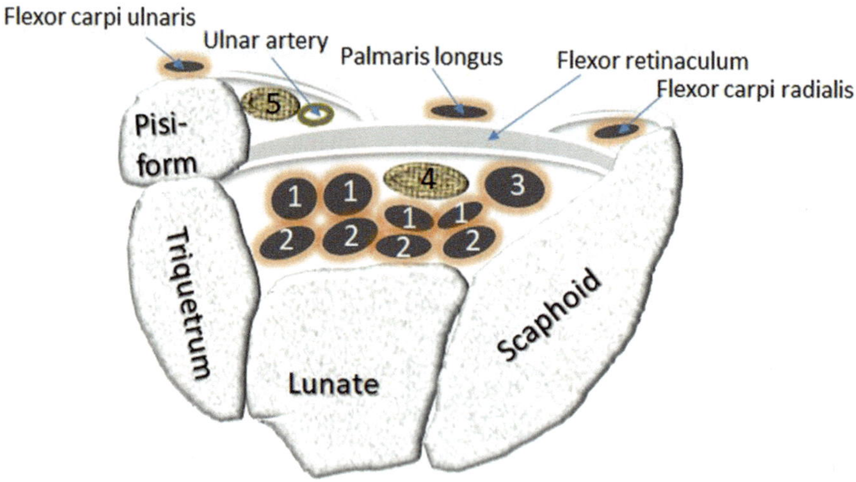

Fig. 3.5 Schematic representation of the volar wrist and carpal tunnel at the level of scaphoid-pisiform. (1) superficial flexor tendons, (2) deep flexor tendons, (3) flexor pollicis longus, (4) median nerve, (5) ulnar nerve

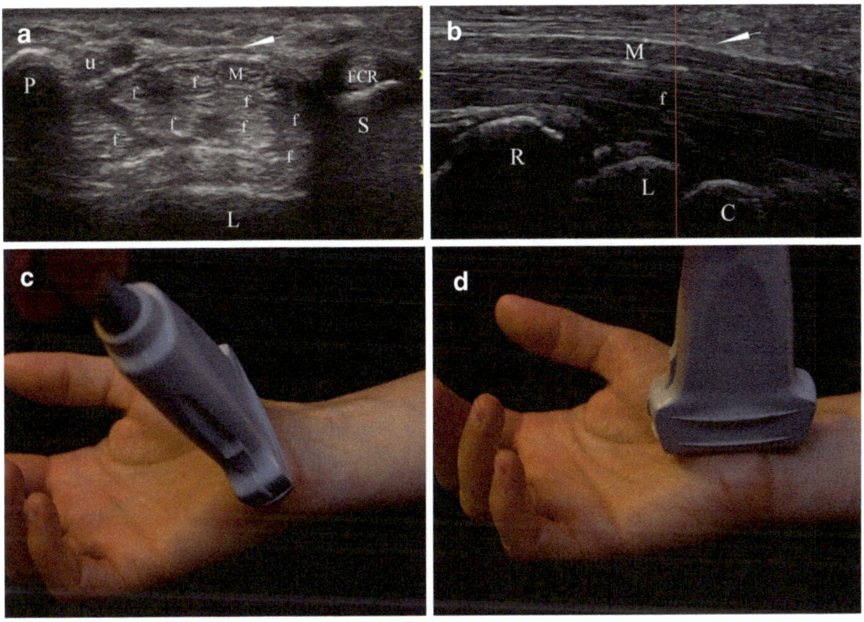

Fig. 3.6 Volar wrist. (**a**) shows a transverse view through the inlet to the carpal tunnel taken at the level of the *orange line* on the longitudinal view shown in (**b**). The pisiform (P) and scaphoid tuberosity (S) create the sides of the carpal tunnel, the lunate (L) is the bottom, and the retinaculum (*arrow*) is the top. The median nerve has a coarser, slightly more hypoechoic internal architecture than the surrounding tendons, and has a bright epineurium that the tendons lack. The probe scanning position necessary to achieve the images in (**a**, **b**) are illustrated in (**c**, **d**). (P) pisiform, (L) lunate, (S) scaphoid, (f) flexor tendon, (M) median nerve, (FCR) flexor carpi radialis, (u) ulnar nerve, (*arrow*) retinaculum, (R) radius, (C) capitate

position, the transducer should be slid distally at this new angle until the proper bone landmarks are once again visible. Making the tendons bright will help assess for tenosynovitis and synovitis deep to the palmar radiocarpal ligaments. Both synovitis and palmar carpal erosions are more easily identified on longitudinal views of the palmar wrist (Fig. 3.6b, d). The median nerve can be distinguished from the tendons by the bright epineurium surrounding it, which appears as hyperechoic "tram-track" lines on both sides of the nerve on longitudinal view and as a bright oval on transverse view. The fibers of the nerve itself are slightly hypoechoic relative to the tendons and do not have the fibrillar pattern typical for tendons, but rather a coarser pattern resembling a honeycomb. Nerves are also less anisotropic than tendons. Thus, in transverse view, when the tendons are very dark due to anisotropy, the nerve will be brighter than the tendons, but when the tendons are made maximally bright, the nerve will be slightly darker than the tendons. This technique can be useful to help identify the nerve. In longitudinal view, the tissues typically become anisotropic in the distal part of the carpal tunnel due to the wrist naturally assuming an extended position when it is supinated. By placing a rolled-up towel under the metacarpals, the wrist can be positioned closer to neutral, thus allowing better visualization of the distal carpal tunnel.

Finger Joints

Dorsal views of the metacarpal-phalangeal (MCP) joints require floating the transducer on a layer of gel to optimize the image. There is a natural dip in the contour of the bone between the articular portion of the metacarpal and the metacarpal neck, most prominently in the second MCP (Fig. 3.7). This dip can mimic an erosion, especially as this is a region that tends to get erosions. However, the bony groove will not have any irregularities in transverse views, thus differentiating normal anatomy from an erosion. Transverse views will also show synovium which has been pushed away from the midline by the extensor tendon. This highlights the importance of orthogonal views to confirm sonographic pathology.

Ulnar views of the fifth MCP joint and the radial views of the second MCP joint are critical for assessment of bone erosions and synovitis at the capsular attachment. In fact, ultrasound sensitivity for MCP joint erosions approaches that of MRI in the second and fifth MCP joints but is significantly less in the third and fourth MCP joints due to the lack of access for medial and lateral views. As one scans from a lateral to a dorsolateral view, the metacarpal part of the joint transitions from a curved to a flat, "ski slope"-shaped contour.

Volar views of the MCP joint need to extend proximally enough to visualize the full extent of the synovial capsule which stretches back beyond the palmar plate (Fig. 3.8). This reflection is normally a flat hypoechoic line which swells like a balloon when inflamed and with effusion. The flexor tendon lies superficial to the palmar plate over the metacarpal and is directly over the phalanx in the distal part of the joint. The A1 pulley is superficial to the flexor tendon at the level of the MCP joint and is normally very thin and hard to visualize, especially in longitudinal view. Thickening of the A1 pulley can contribute to mechanical "trigger finger."

The dorsal view of the proximal interphalangeal (PIP) joint shows the extensor hood, which can be inflamed and distended in cases of synovitis, but joint effusion is more likely to be visualized on the volar aspect of the joint where the capsule reflects proximally over the phalangeal bone surface (Fig. 3.8). Dorsal views of the distal interphalangeal (DIP) joint also allow visualization of the nail bed where lesions of psoriatic arthritis (PsA) might be found, while the volar views allow visualization of the flexor tendon insertion.

Pathology

Synovitis

Synovial tissue is intra-articular, typically hypoechoic, and poorly compressible. Power Doppler signal may be present depending on the degree of hyperemia. In the finger joints, the synovium reflects proximally from the joint cleft. In the dorsal wrist, the synovial tissue reflects distally for the radiocarpal and intercarpal joints, but the radioulnar synovium reflects proximally (Fig. 3.9). In the volar wrist, the radiocarpal synovium also reflects proximally. In evaluating Doppler signal, ensure

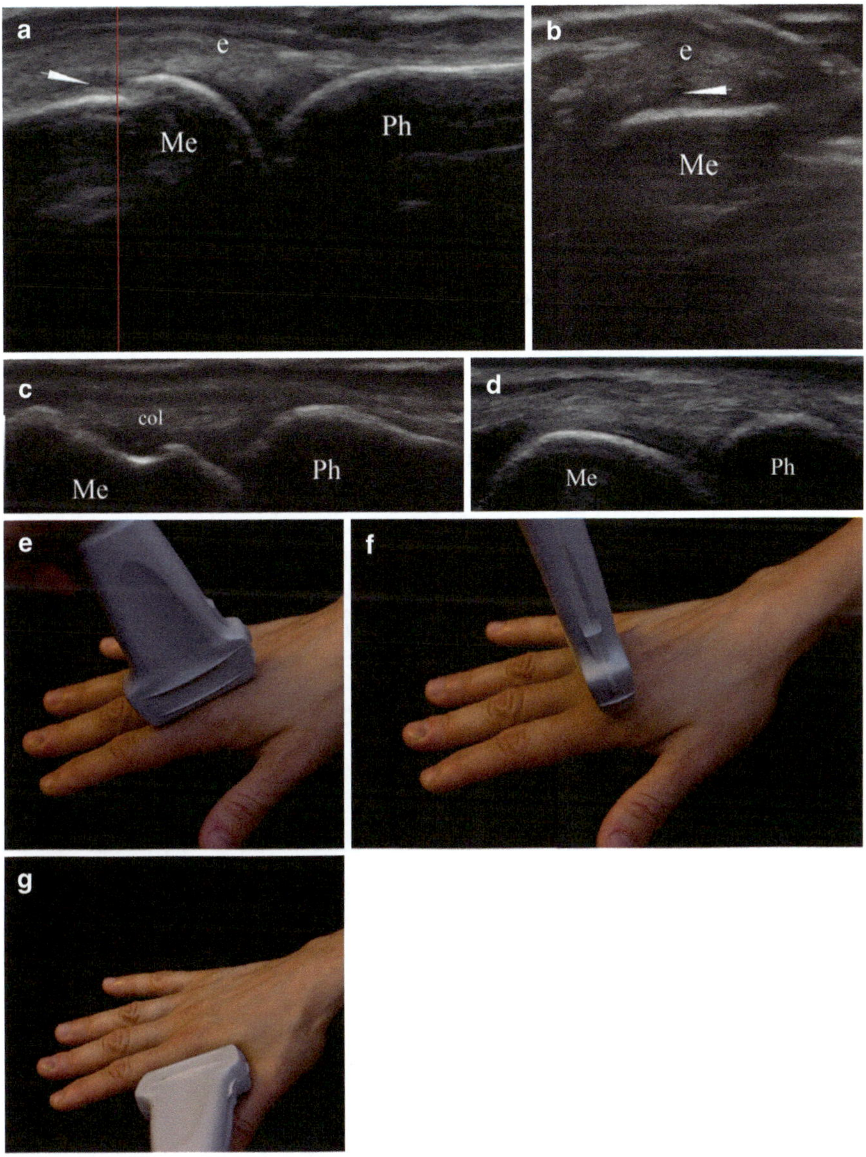

Fig. 3.7 Dorsal and lateral metacarpal–phalangeal joint. (**a**) shows a dorsal longitudinal view of a metacarpal-phalangeal joint (MCP). The transverse section through the *orange line* is shown in (**b**). The *arrow* points to the thin synovial reflection, normally seen proximal to the joint cleft. (**c**, **d**) are both lateral longitudinal views through the MCP, with **c** being more dorsal and 1d being more volar. The lateral collateral ligament is best seen in (**c**). (**e**–**g**) show transducer scanning position required to obtain the ultrasound images. (Me) metacarpal, (Ph) phalange, (e) extensor tendon, (col) collateral ligament

that you do not mistake normal vascular flow for synovitis by first identifying the synovium in gray scale and then looking specifically in that tissue for Doppler signal. The capsular attachment points are also worth evaluating for Doppler signal especially as these are the spots where erosions are most likely to occur in erosive arthritis.

The ultrasound assessment for wrist synovitis is comparable to MRI [5]. Semiquantitative assessment of power Doppler signal can be established based on previously established criteria: *grade 0* no signal, *grade 1* single dot of Doppler, *grade 2* less than half of the synovial tissue is filled with Doppler, *grade 3* more than half of the synovial tissue is filled with Doppler [6].

Erosions

Erosions are defined as intra-articular breaks in the cortical margin which can be seen in perpendicular planes. Sometimes, it is impossible to tell whether the image

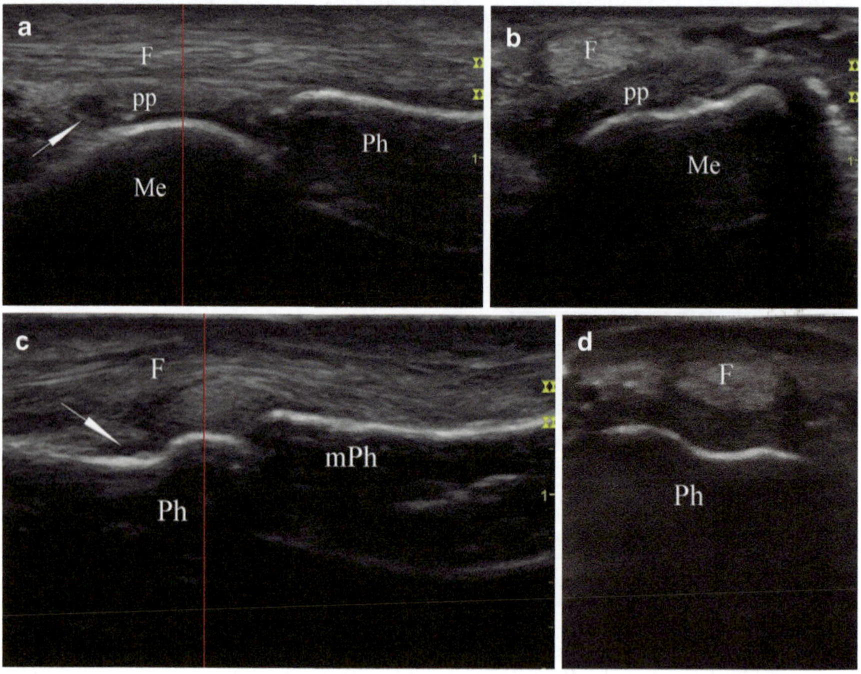

Fig. 3.8 Volar MCP and PIP joints. (**a**) shows the volar longitudinal view of the MCP joint with the *orange line* on the section where the transverse in (**b**) was taken. The *arrow* shows the small synovial reflection proximal to the MCP joint cleft and to the palmar plate (pp). Note that the palmar plate is between the flexor tendon and the metacarpal bone on the metacarpal side of the MCP joint. (**c**) shows the volar longitudinal view through the proximal interphalangeal joint, with the *orange line* indicating the level at which (**d**), the PIP volar transverse view, was taken. The *arrow* again points to the synovial reflection. Photographs (**e–h**) show transducer scanning position required to obtain images (**a–d**). (Me) metacarpal, (Ph) phalanx, (pp) palmar plate, (F) flexor tendon, (mPh) middle phalanx

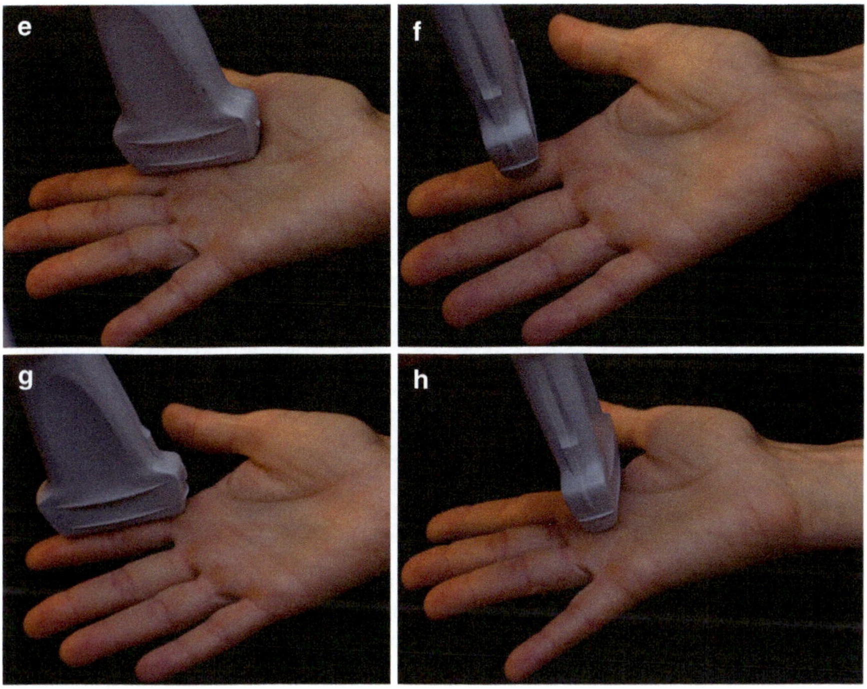

Fig. 3.8 (continued)

represents an erosion or an osteophyte in a single plane of view; however, on the orthogonal view, an erosion will still look like a "pot hole" in the cortex, while an osteophyte will be a hyperechoic lesion superficial to the surface of the cortex (Figs. 3.10 and 3.11). Ultrasound has been found to be more sensitive for erosive changes in the finger joints than radiographs [7]. The sides of the MCP and PIP joints are particularly important to evaluate for erosions. In the wrist, the lunate bone presents a challenge to the sonographer as there is normally a feeding vessel that enters the lunate. The spot where the vessel enters the lunate can appear as an erosion (Fig. 3.12) and sometimes as an erosion with Doppler signal! To complicate this issue further, real lunate erosions tend to occur in this same location. True pathologic erosions are generally larger, have more irregular cortical borders, and frequently cause reverberation artifacts deep to the surface of the erosion. Erosions that are larger than 2.5 mm are more specific to inflammatory erosive forms of arthritis like RA (specificity of 68%) [3]. Erosions smaller than 2 mm can be seen in osteoarthritis, and erosions of <1 mm can be seen in people without arthritis. The location of the erosion can also suggest its cause: erosions at the ulnar styloid, second MCP, and fifth MCP are more specific to RA (87% when greater than 2.5 mm). Sensitivity of ultrasound of MCP erosions is 42% compared to multidetector CT, with specificity of 91%. By comparison, MRI sensitivity is 68%, and specificity is 96% [8]. However, due to the availability of the lateral acoustic window in the

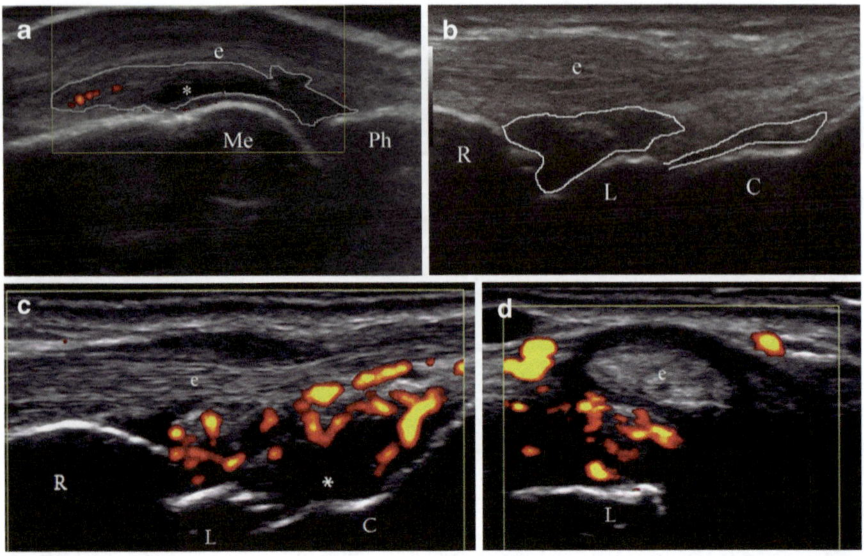

Fig. 3.9 Synovial hypertrophy, effusion, and power Doppler synovitis. (**a**) demonstrates a dorsal longitudinal view of an MCP joint with synovial hypertrophy outlined, extending far proximal to the joint cleft. This image also shows synovial hyperemia (grade 2—more than one vessel but less than half of the volume of the synovium) and synovial effusion (*asterisk*). (**b**) demonstrates a dorsal longitudinal view of the wrist with synovial hypertrophy outlined, extending distal to the joint cleft of the radiocarpal joint and to that of the intercarpal joint. (**c**) demonstrates a dorsal longitudinal view, while (**d**) demonstrates orthogonal (dorsal transverse) view of the same wrist. Note that there is synovial hypertrophy and grade 3 (radiocarpal) and grade 2 (midcarpal) power Doppler signal/synovitis. There is a small radiocarpal effusion (*asterisk*). (R) radius, (L) lunate, (C) capitate, (e) extensor tendons (fourth compartment)

second MCP, ultrasound sensitivity for erosion in these joint increases to 92%, compared to only 25% in the fourth MCP [8].

In addition to the location of erosion, other ultrasound findings may help differentiate RA from similarly erosive forms of arthritis such as psoriatic arthritis. The distance between the ventral side of the nail and the dorsal aspect of the distal phalanx may be increased in PsA compared to patients with RA [9]. Furthermore, Gutierrez M et al. have found that paratenon Doppler signal over the extensor tendons at the level of the MCP joints is found in 50/82 fingers studies in 20 patients with PsA, compared to only 4/83 fingers studies in 18 patients with RA [10] (Fig. 3.13).

Tendon and Ligament Pathology

Tenosynovitis can be the initial presentation of RA. In 90 consecutive patients with RA, half had tenosynovitis in at least one wrist tendon [11]. Tenosynovial effusions will appear as anechoic halos around tendons in transverse view. Very hypoechoic

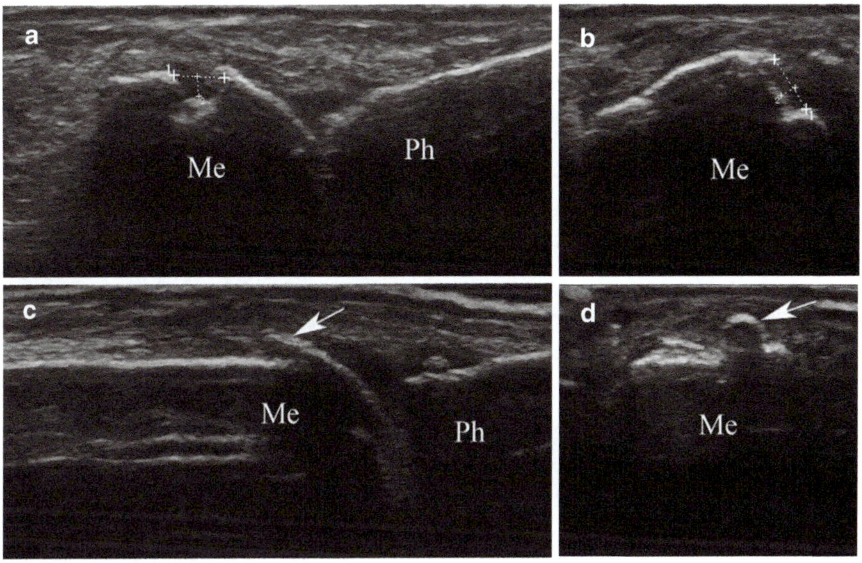

Fig. 3.10 Erosion vs. osteophyte. (**a**, **b**) demonstrate longitudinal and transverse views of a cortical erosion (*dashed measurement lines*) on the dorsal side of a metacarpal (Me), with a normal-appearing phalanx (Ph). In contrast, (**c**, **d**) show orthogonal views through an osteophyte (*arrows*) on the dorsal surface of an MCP joint. The erosion is a "pothole" in the cortical surface, while the osteophyte is a jagged protuberance from the bone surface which results in a cortical defect that is sometimes called "step-off" lesion

muscle fibers can be mistaken for a tenosynovial effusion as they transition into tendon fibers. These two are most easily differentiated by scanning proximally toward larger and more obvious parts of the muscle belly. Tenosynovial effusion can also be confused with thickened retinaculum on the dorsal wrist (especially first and fourth compartments) and with thickened pulleys on the volar MCP joints. Careful imaging will show that the retinaculum is outside of the tendon sheath and is hypoechoic rather than anechoic as long as no anisotropic artifact is present. Furthermore, both retinaculum and pulley lesions are very focal, while tenosynovial effusions tend to spread down tendon sheath (Fig. 3.14). On the dorsal side of the fingers, the extensor tendon lacks a tenosynovium; thus, a tendinitis and/or paratenonitis is possible but not a true tenosynovitis.

In stenosing tenosynovitis, the A1 pulley is thickened causing pinching of the flexor tendon as it tries to squeeze through the narrowed tunnel between the A1 pulley and the volar plate. The tendon thus becomes thickened distal to the A1 pulley, and with a dynamic exam, one can see the tendon fibers stop moving as the thickened tendon reaches the A1 pulley. In Dupuytren's contracture, the primary abnormality is thickened and disorganized fascia fibers superficial to the flexor tendon, which exerts a downward force on the tendon resulting in finger contracture.

The pathophysiology of DeQuervain's disease is similar to that of the trigger finger; due to microtrauma, the retinaculum at the distal radius becomes thickened

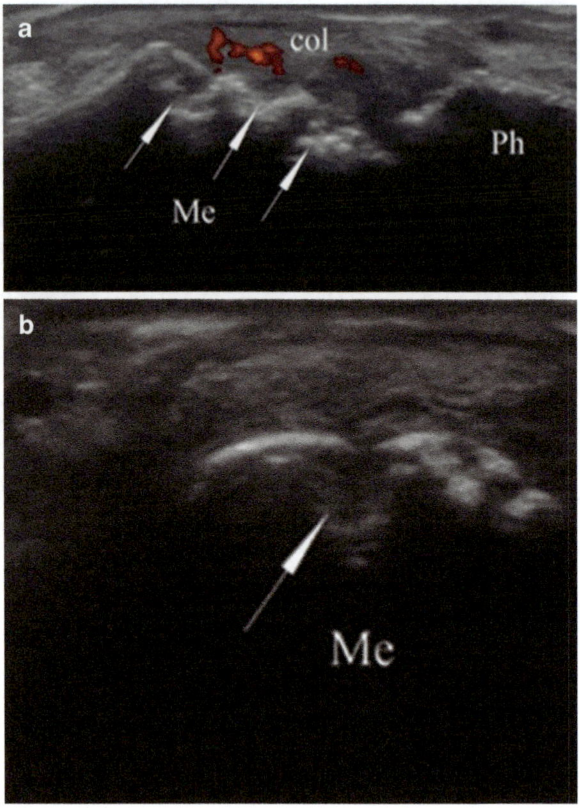

Fig. 3.11 Metacarpal radial side erosions. (**a**) demonstrates numerous small erosions (arrows) on the radial longitudinal view of the metacarpal (Me), just deep to the collateral ligament (col) and proximal to the phalanx (Ph). Doppler signal suggests that further damage is occurring. (**b**) demonstrates the transverse radial view of the metacarpal, confirming that the breaks in the cortical margin can be seen in perpendicular plains

and hypoechoic (Fig. 3.15). Thus, when providing an injection for treating this condition, the needle should be passed as quickly as possible through the sensitive retinaculum, and aspiration should not be attempted. In addition, some patients develop a true tenosynovitis which can be diagnosed by using power Doppler. Tenosynovitis of this compartment can occur due to microtrauma but also can be seen in scleroderma, crystal-induced, and inflammatory arthritis.

Medially, the extensor carpi ulnaris tendon sheath can be inflamed in RA and other inflammatory conditions (Fig. 3.16). There can also be associated erosions of the distal ulna which would be suggestive of RA. Distal to the ulna is the TFCC. Ultrasound has not been found to be a sensitive technique for evaluation of TFCC tears as these tears typically are in the deep part of the TFCC which is hidden from the ultrasound waves. However, calcification of the TFCC due to CPPD is better visualized by ultrasound than by radiography [4, 12]. The hyperechoic stippling that occurs in the ligaments and meniscal homologue due to CPPD is as dense as bone. Turning the gray-scale gain down until all the soft tissues become anechoic will highlight the bone and CPPD deposits (Fig. 3.16). Chondrocalcinosis deposits can also be seen in the scapholunate ligament. This ligament can be ruptured due to

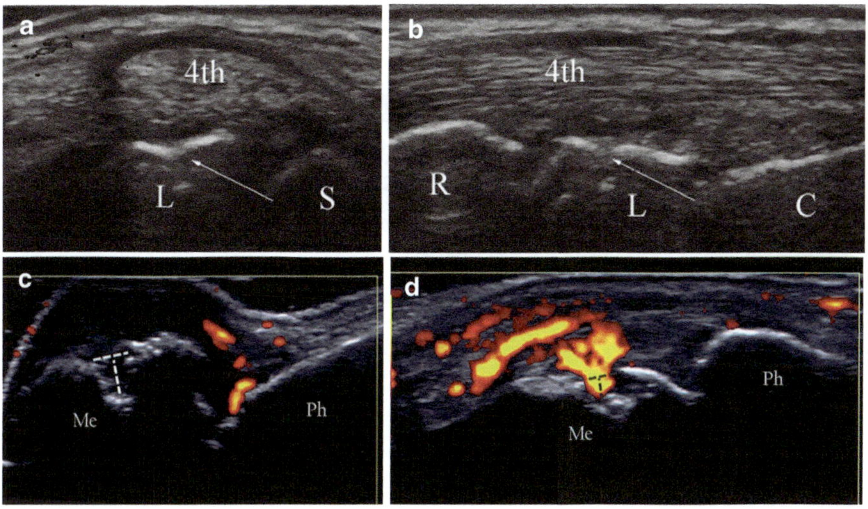

Fig. 3.12 Lunate vascular channel vs. quiescent erosion vs. active erosion. (**a**) is a transverse view through the first carpal row, and (**b**) is the longitudinal view through the midline of the wrist. The *arrows* point to the vascular channel in the lunate. (**c**) demonstrates quiescent erosion (i.e., doesn't contain power Doppler signal) (*dashed measurement lines*) in the dorsal aspect of the metacarpal head in advanced rheumatoid arthritis; please note that there is active power Doppler synovitis in the cleft of metacarpal joint, and the joint shows subluxation. (**d**) demonstrates active erosion (i.e., one that contains power Doppler signal indicative of active rheumatoid pannus) on the radial side of the second metacarpal in rheumatoid arthritis. (L) lunate, (S) scaphoid, (R) radius, (C) capitate, (4th) fourth compartment tendons, (Me) metacarpal, (Ph) phalanx

mechanical trauma and also due to severe inflammation from crystalline or erosive arthritis. Ligamentous tear presents as absence of the typical hyperechoic fibrils between the scaphoid and lunate, increased distance between the bones statically [13], or widening of the distance between the bones dynamically as the patient squeezes a ball in the palm of their hand (Fig. 3.17). The normal scapholunate interval has been reported to be 2.9–4.5 mm [14].

Ultrasound can aid in detection of subclinical tenosynovitis in scleroderma patients (27% with the use of ultrasound vs. 6% on clinical examination) [15]. The same study compared hand involvement between scleroderma and rheumatoid arthritis and showed that the frequency of ultrasound detected tenosynovitis was comparable between both conditions (27% of scleroderma vs. 25% of rheumatoid cases). While "inflammatory tenosynovitis" was seen in both scleroderma and rheumatoid patients, the so-called mixed and fibrosing tenosynovitis (described as hyperechoic tendon sheath thickening) were the unique sonographic patterns seen only in scleroderma patients. In addition, sclerosing tenosynovitis was typically localized to extensor tendons. It is not known, however, how these different sonographic patterns relate to different disease activities or different stages of the tendon and tenosynovial involvement in scleroderma patients (Fig. 3.18).

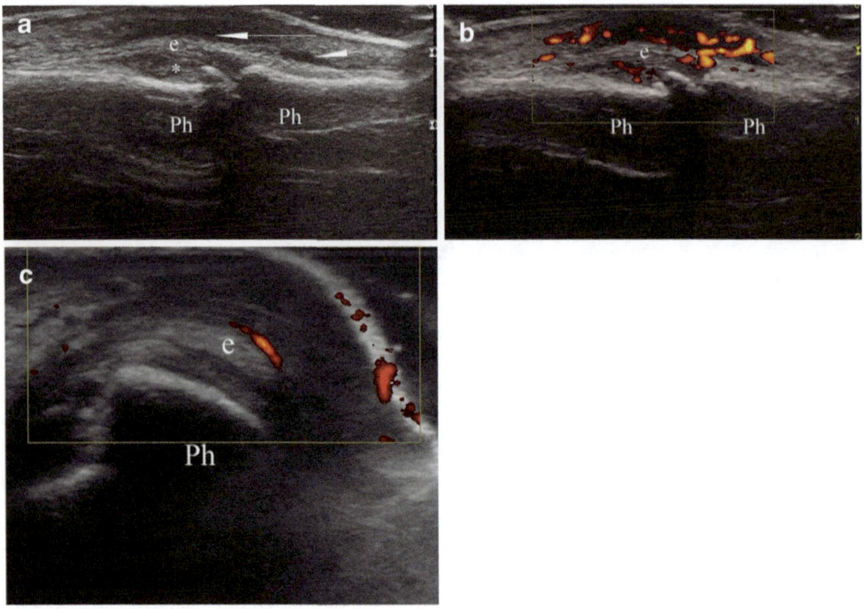

Fig. 3.13 Extensor tendinitis. (**a**) shows a dorsal longitudinal view of the interphalangeal joint. The *asterisk* indicates synovial proliferation, while the *arrows* indicate swelling around the extensor tendon (e). The Doppler view in (**b**) shows hyperemia in the synovium but more so in the paratenon region around the extensor tendon. This is also shown in transverse in (**c**)

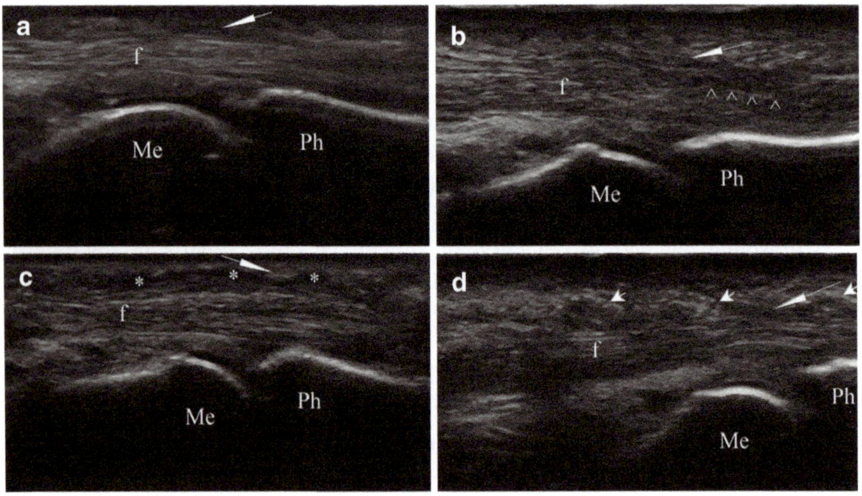

Fig. 3.14 Flexor tendon pathologies. (**a**) demonstrates a normal flexor tendon (f), with a normal A1 pulley (*arrow*). (**b**) shows the loss of normal fibrillar fibers of the flexor tendon (^) just distal to the A1 pulley (*arrow*) in a patient with a trigger finger. There is a subtle indentation of the A1 pulley on the flexor tendon. (**c**) shows a finger with flexor tenosynovitis (*asterisk*). Notice that the tenosynovium is swollen all along the flexor tendon, rather than focally, and is compressed at the level of the A1 pulley (*arrow*). (**d**) shows a mild case of Dupuytren's contracture, with the thick arrow pointing to the thickened and disorganized fascia, while the thin arrow points to the A1 pulley. The thickened fascia causes some artifactual hypoechoic signal from the tendon deep to it

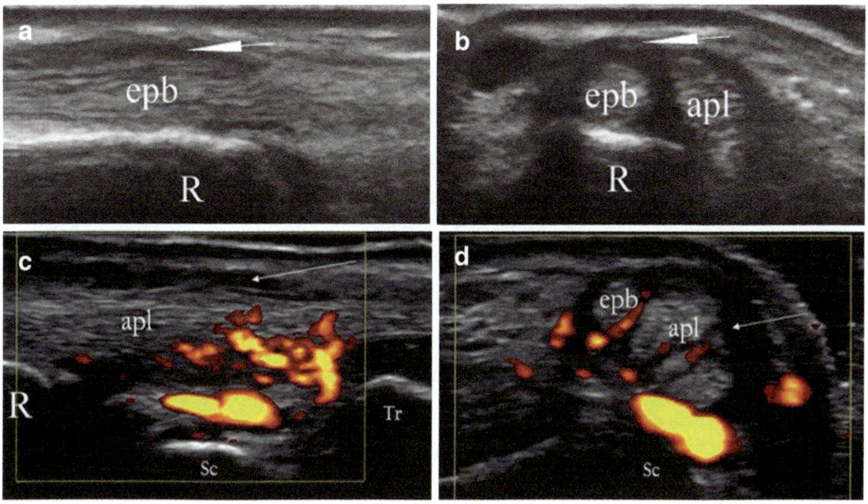

Fig. 3.15 DeQuervain's tenosynovitis. (**a**) shows a longitudinal view of the first extensor compartment: the extensor pollicis brevis (epb) tendon, with the thickened retinaculum (*arrow*) above, and the radial styloid below (R). (**b**) shows the first compartment in transverse. The retinaculum is thickened primarily around the extensor pollicis brevis (epb), and there is a septum between the epb and the abductor pollicis longus (apl). In such a case, ultrasound can help direct the injection to the most affected retinaculum. (**c**) demonstrates longitudinal while (**d**) demonstrated transverse view of the distal first extensor compartment with tenosynovial thickening (*arrows*), *apl* tendon thickening, and intrasubstance splitting indicative of chronic tendinosis. Active tenosynovitis and tendinitis distal to the extensor retinaculum are suggested by the presence of power Doppler signal within tenosynovium and the tendon proper, respectively. (R) radial styloid, (Sc) scaphoid, (Tr) trapezium

Nodules

Ligamentous tears can lead to ganglion cyst formation; cysts on the dorsal wrist are typically superficial to the scapholunate ligament (70%), while 13% are volar, arising from the flexor tendon sheath, and another 12% are volar but not from the flexor tendons [7]. These cysts tend to have well-defined margins, anechoic internal appearance, and produce acoustic enhancement (Fig. 3.19). Despite being fluid-filled, they are frequently non-compressible due to a tight surrounding capsule. In addition, large ganglia may contain some hyperechoic speckles within the anechoic gel-like material due to suspended air bubbles. These air bubbles are a clue to the hyperviscosity of the cyst contents, as air bubbles will not be found in regular synovial fluid. Most ganglia are multiloculated, while only 12% have surrounding Doppler signal [16]. Clinically, ganglion cysts may mimic giant cell tumors. By ultrasound, giant cell tumors are located near flexor tendons; are hypoechoic and homogeneous, as opposed to anechoic cysts; and almost all have either peripheral or central vascularity [17].

Gouty nodules in the wrist are quite different in appearance from ganglia, with heterogeneous internal echogenicity, no acoustic enhancement, and occasionally

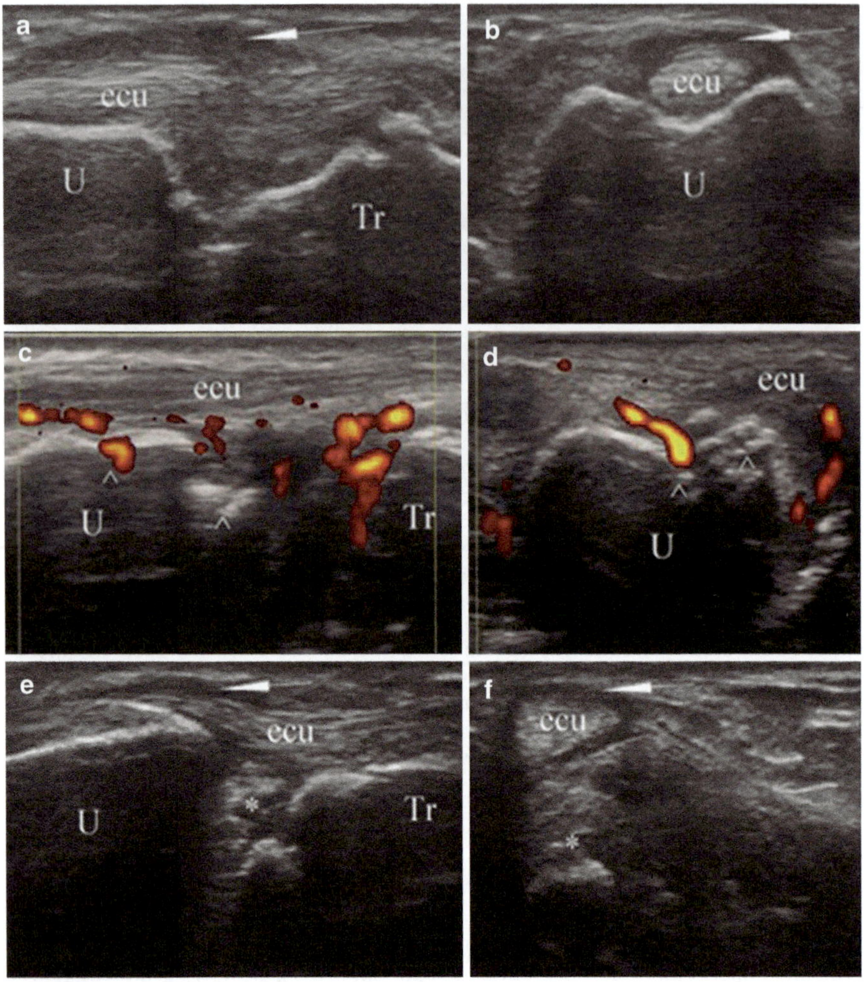

Fig. 3.16 Ulnar pathology. (**a**) demonstrates tenosynovitis of the extensor carpi ulnaris tendon (ecu) superficial to the ulna (U) sulcus and trapezium (Tr), with the *arrow* pointing to distended tenosynovium. (**b**) is the corollary transverse view of ECU tenosynovitis. (**c**) shows a longitudinal view of ECU tendinitis with hypogenic tendon fibers and Doppler signal along the tendon and along erosions (^) in the distal ulna. (**d**) shows the transverse view of the same region of erosion and clarifies that the ECU tendon is subluxed out of the ulnar sulcus. (**e**, **f**) exemplify hyperechoic changes of the triangular fibrocartilage complex (*asterisk*) typical for calcium pyrophosphate deposition disease in longitudinal and transverse views

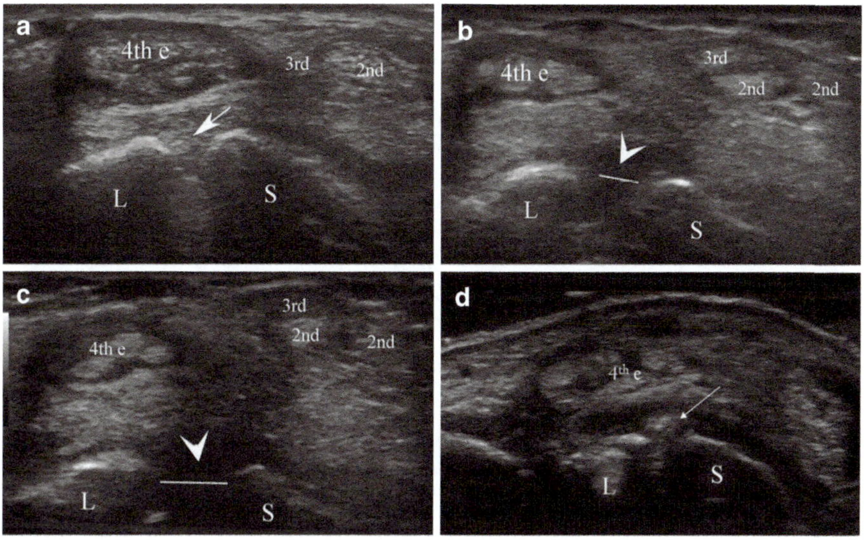

Fig. 3.17 Scapholunate ligament pathology. (**a**) demonstrates an intact scapholunate ligament (*arrow*) between the scaphoid (S) and lunate (L) and below the extensor tendons of the 4th, 3rd, and 2nd compartments. (**b**) depicts a torn scapholunate ligament (*arrowhead*) in a relaxed wrist—the hyperechoic ligament fibers are missing, and the distance between the scaphoid and lunate is slightly increased. (**c**) depicts the same wrist while squeezing a ball, resulting in widening of the distance between the scaphoid and lunate due to the torn ligament. (**d**) demonstrates calcification of the scapholunate ligament (*arrow*). Lunate osteophytes can also be readily appreciated

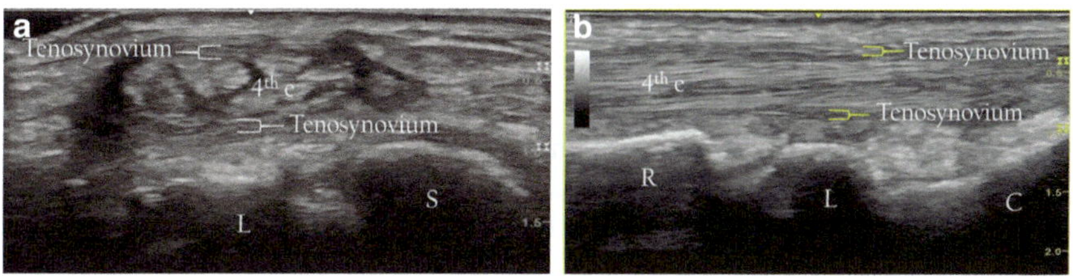

Fig. 3.18 Extensor tenosynovitis in scleroderma. (**a**) demonstrates dorsal transverse view, while (**b**) demonstrates dorsal longitudinal view of the distal wrist. Note the thickening and the fibrotic appearance of the tenosynovium of the fourth extensor compartment tendons. (R) radius, (L) lunate, (C) capitate, (S) scaphoid, (4th e) fourth extensor compartment tendons

cast shadows on the underlying tissues when the tophi are calcified [18, 19]. Gouty nodules are associated with other ultrasound findings typical for gout such as the double-contour sign, where monosodium urate crystals precipitate on the surface of hyaline cartilage and reflect ultrasound waves (Fig. 3.20). This produces a thick, irregular line parallel to the contour of the bone (double contour) that is visible

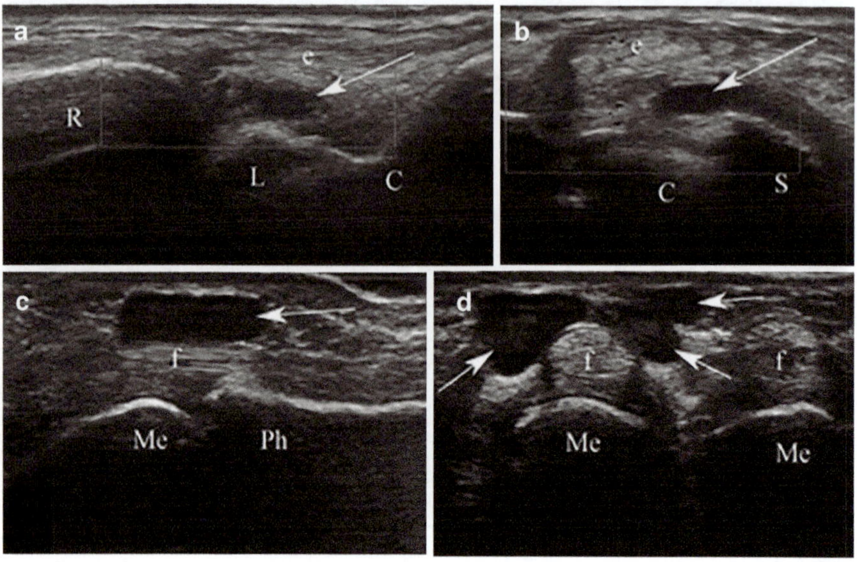

Fig. 3.19 Ganglion cyst. (**a**) shows a longitudinal view of a ganglion cyst (*arrow*) distal to the radius (R), superficial to the lunate (L) and capitate (C), and below the extensor tendons. The ganglion has very defined borders and an anechoic center. (**b**) shows the same cyst in transverse, between the scaphoid (S) and capitate (C). (**c**) demonstrates a ganglion cyst associated with a flexor tendon (f) over the metacarpophalangeal joint in longitudinal view. Notice that the flexor tendon is more hyperechoic deep to the cyst than to either side of the cyst due to "acoustic enhancement" artifact. The transverse view in (**d**) shows the characteristic multiloculated ganglion structure

independent of the angle with which the sound waves strike the monosodium urate lined surface [18]. Rheumatoid nodules can also be seen in the hands. In contrast to gouty nodules, these are most commonly homogeneous with a hypoechoic center [19]. Another distinguishing feature is that RA nodules are usually single, while tophaceous nodules tend to deposit in clusters [20].

Nerve Impingement

Ultrasonography is helpful in the evaluation of nerve impingement in the wrist, particularly median nerve impingement (Fig. 3.21). Numerous studies have shown that nerve impingement results in nerve swelling proximal to the impingement point and that the degree of nerve swelling correlates with the degree of nerve dysfunction as assessed by EMG/NCV studies [21]. Maximal median

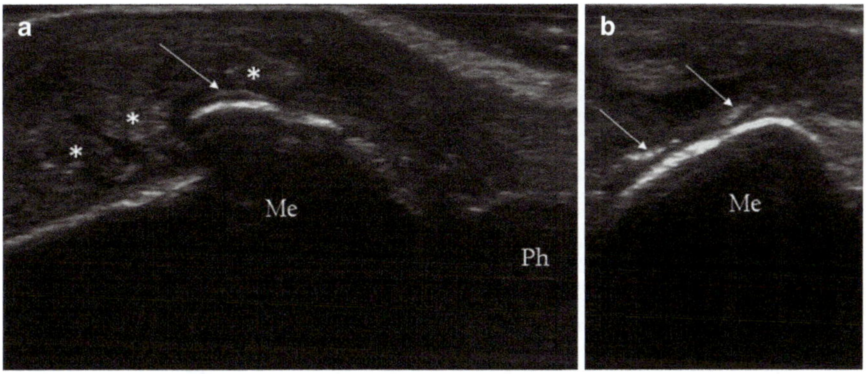

Fig. 3.20 Gouty nodules (tophi) and double-contour sign. (**a**) demonstrates dorsal longitudinal view of a metacarpophalangeal joint and (**b**) demonstrates an orthogonal view of the same joint through metacarpal head. Several clustered tophi (*asterisks*) and double-contour sign (*arrows*) can be readily identified. Double-contour sign is reproduced in both orthogonal views and has irregular and "bulky" appearance which distinguishes it from interface sign sometimes seen in joints with small effusion. (Me) metacarpal, (Ph) phalanx

nerve cross-sectional area measurement has emerged as the most validated ultrasound criteria for diagnosing median nerve impingement [22]. Median nerve size less than 8 mm^2 has a negative likelihood ratio for carpal tunnel syndrome of 0.13, while a size of equal to or greater than 12 mm^2 has a positive likelihood ratio of 19.9 [23]. For median nerve sizes between these limits, comparison to the asymptomatic side or comparison to the size of the same nerve 12 cm proximal to the carpal tunnel is useful: a distal to proximal ratio of greater than 1.4 has been shown to be both sensitive and specific for median nerve impingement [24]. In cases where the median nerve is bifid, the two portions of the median nerve can be measured separately, and then their surface areas are combined [25, 26]. In addition to establishing median nerve impingement, ultrasound can help detect causes for the impingement such as synovial or tenosynovial swelling or mass lesions (from crystal deposition, ganglion cysts, etc.). Furthermore, ultrasound can help detect anatomic abnormalities such as flexor digitorum muscle that extends further distally than normal into the carpal tunnel. Similarly, for questions of ulnar nerve impingement in Guyon's canal, the maximal nerve caliber can be compared to ulnar nerve caliber more proximally in the forearm.

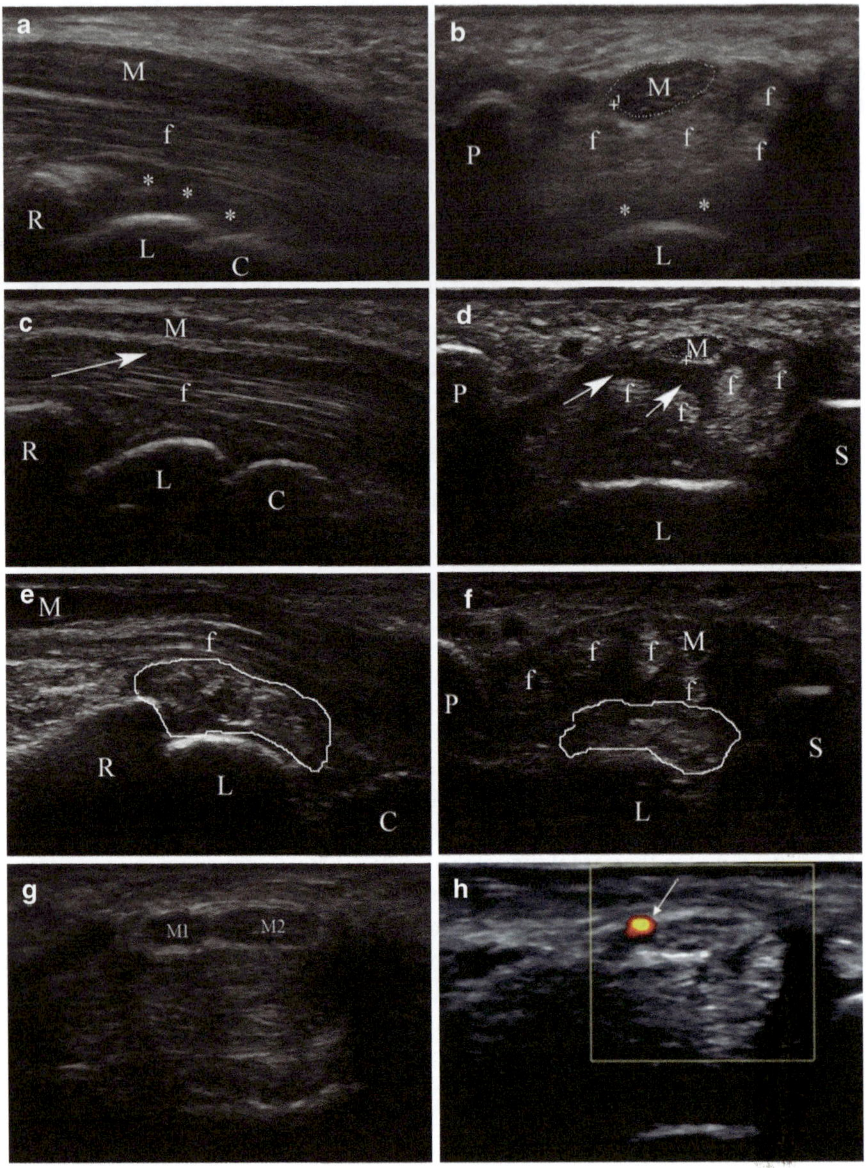

Fig. 3.21 Carpal tunnel pathology. (**a**) demonstrates, in longitudinal section, effusion and synovium (*asterisk*) from the joints between the radius (R), lunate (L), and capitate (C) exerting upward pressure on the flexor tendons (f) and the median nerve (M). This results in constriction of the nerve and swelling proximal to the retinaculum. (**b**) confirms the findings in transverse view of the carpal tunnel, with the pisiform (P) in view medially. (**c, d**) show tenosynovial hypertrophy and effusion (*arrows*) of the flexor (f) tendons surrounding the median nerve (M) and potentially causing nerve impingement. The scaphoid tuberosity (S) makes the lateral border of the carpal tunnel. (**e, f**) depict hyperechoic material (*outlined*) in the radiocarpal joint due to CPPD deposition disease causing constriction of the median nerve. (**g**) demonstrates transverse view of the carpal tunnel showing bifid median nerve (*M1, M2*), which is considered a normal variant but can be associated with median nerve dysfunction and predisposition to carpal tunnel syndrome. (**h**) demonstrates transverse view of the carpal tunnel showing bifid median nerve with patent median artery (*arrow*)

Conclusion

Ultrasound examination of the hand and wrist can be extremely useful in the evaluation of patients with tendon, joint, or nerve pathology. Evaluation and management of common rheumatologic conditions involving the hand and wrist, such as inflammatory arthritis and crystal-induced arthritis, as well as mechanical conditions such as DeQuervain's tendinitis or carpal tunnel syndrome, can be enhanced by the use of musculoskeletal ultrasound.

Review Questions

1. On a dorsal transverse image of a wrist, the radioulnar joint synovium can best be identified in which of the following locations?
   (a) Deep to the extensor digiti minimi tendon
   (b) Radial to Lister's tubercle
   (c) Distal to the radius
   (d) Distal to the lunate
2. On ultrasound imaging, DeQuervain's tendinitis is most commonly manifested by which of the following?
   (a) Anechoic, compressible material surrounding the first extensor compartment at the distal radius
   (b) Hypoechoic, non-compressible material surrounding the first extensor compartment at the distal radius
   (c) Loss of fibrillar architecture of the extensor pollicis longus tendon
   (d) Disruption of the cortical margin at the distal radius seen in orthogonal planes
3. Ulnar imaging of the wrist reveals a 2.5-mm cortical disruption of the ulna cortical surface and anechoic material surrounding the extensor carpi ulnaris tendon as well as Doppler signal surrounding the extensor carpi ulnaris. These findings most suggest which of the following?
   (a) Osteoarthritis
   (b) Gout
   (c) Rheumatoid arthritis
   (d) Psoriatic arthritis
4. Which of the following can help distinguish the median nerve from the surrounding tendons?
   (a) The nerve is more anisotropic.
   (b) The nerve has a finer echotexture.
   (c) The nerve slides more with finger flexion.
   (d) The nerve is surrounded by a bright epineurium.

5. This longitudinal view of the dorsal wrist clearly demonstrates which of the following?

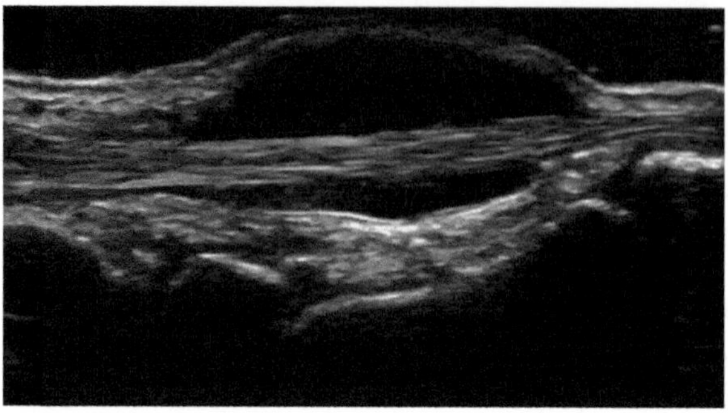

(a) Extensor tenosynovitis
(b) Radiocarpal synovitis
(c) Intercarpal synovitis
(d) Dorsal ganglion cyst

6. These orthogonal views of the volar metacarpal-phalangeal joint demonstrate which of the following?

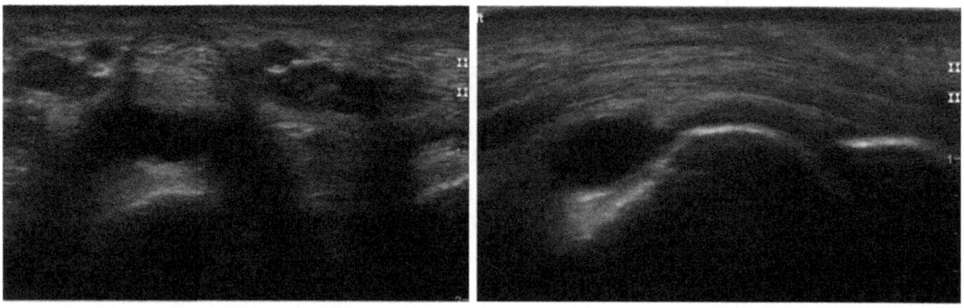

(a) Synovial effusion
(b) Tenosynovial effusion
(c) Gouty nodule
(d) Ruptured palmar plate

7. This longitudinal view of the volar wrist demonstrates which of the following?

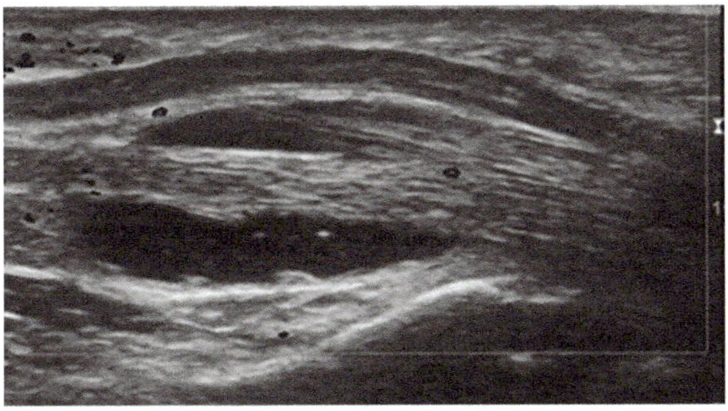

   (a) Muscle belly surrounding a flexor tendon, impinging the median nerve
   (b) Tenosynovial effusion impinging the median nerve
   (c) Median nerve with neuroma
   (d) Gouty tophus impinging on median nerve
8. This transverse power Doppler scan of the volar wrist demonstrates which of the following?

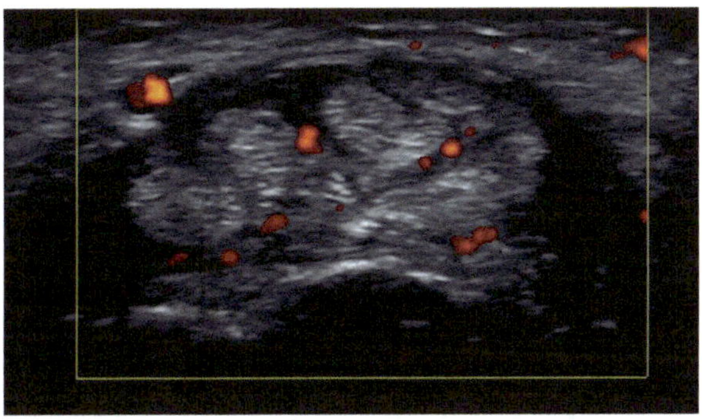

   (a) Wrist effusion
   (b) Neuroma of the median nerve
   (c) Flexor tenosynovitis
   (d) Thickening of the flexor retinaculum

9. Which of the following most accurately describe sonographic findings in this dorsal longitudinal power Doppler image of the wrist?

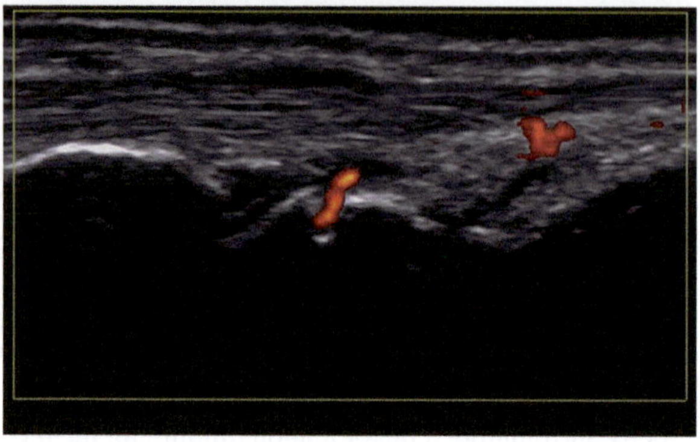

   (a) Lunate erosion, radiocarpal power Doppler synovitis, and blood flow in the dorsal carpal arch
   (b) Radiocarpal synovial hypertrophy, lunate erosion, and radiocarpal power Doppler synovitis
   (c) Dorsal fat pad hyperemia and cortical vascular channel of the lunate
   (d) Cortical vascular channel of the lunate and blood flow in the dorsal carpal arch

10. Which of the following findings are seen on this ulnar longitudinal view of the wrist?

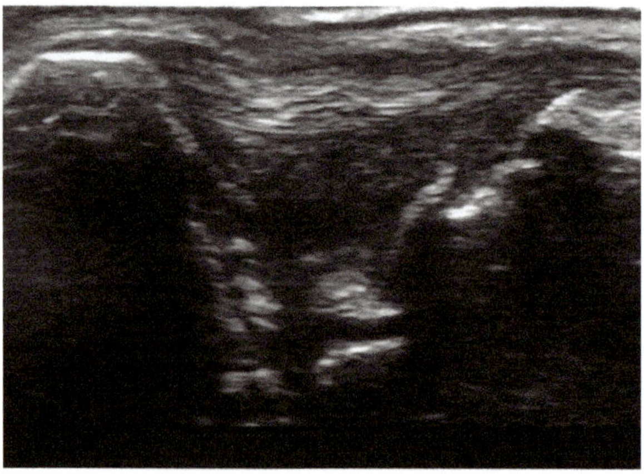

   (a) Tenosynovial thickening of ECU tendon, calcification of triangular fibrocartilage, and ulnar styloid erosion
   (b) Tenosynovial thickening of ECU tendon, calcification of triangular fibrocartilage, and ulnar styloid osteophytes
   (c) Calcification of triangular fibrocartilage and triquetrum erosion
   (d) Calcification of triangular fibrocartilage and triquetrum osteophytes

Answers

1. (a) Deep to the extensor digiti minimi tendon
2. (b) Hypoechoic, non-compressible material surrounding the first extensor compartment at the distal radius
3. (c) Rheumatoid arthritis
4. (d) The nerve is surrounded by a bright epineurium.
5. (a) Extensor tenosynovitis
6. (a) Synovial effusion
7. (b) Tenosynovial effusion impinging the median nerve
8. (c) Flexor tenosynovitis
9. (d) Cortical vascular channel of the lunate and blood flow in the dorsal carpal arch
10. (d) Calcification of triangular fibrocartilage and triquetrum osteophytes

References

1. Ceponis A, Onishi M, Bluestein HG, et al. Utility of the ultrasound examination of the hand and wrist joints in the management of established rheumatoid arthritis. Arthritis Care Res (Hoboken). 2014;66(2):236–44.
2. Lamas C, Carrera A, Proubasta I, et al. The anatomy and vascularity of the lunate: considerations applied to Kienbock's disease. Chir Main. 2007;26:13–20.
3. Zayat AS, Ellegaard K, Conaghan PG, et al. The specificity of ultrasound-detected bone erosions for rheumatoid arthritis. Ann Rheum Dis. 2015;74(5):897–903. Epub 2014 Jan 20.
4. Frediani B, Filippou G, Falsetti P, et al. Diagnosis of calcium pyrophosphate dihydrate crystal deposition disease: ultrasonographic criteria proposed. Ann Rheum Dis. 2005;64(4):638–40.
5. Terslev L, Torp-Pedersen S, Savnik A, et al. Doppler ultrasound and magnetic resonance imaging of synovial inflammation of the hand in rheumatoid arthritis: a comparative study. Arthritis Rheum. 2003;48:2434–41.
6. Szkudlarek M, Court-Payen M, Jacobsen S, et al. Interobserver agreement in ultrasonography of the finger and toe joints in rheumatoid arthritis. Arthritis Rheum. 2003;48:955–62.
7. Wakefield RJ, Gibbon WW, Conaghan PG, et al. The value of sonography in the detection of bone erosions in patients with rheumatoid arthritis: a comparison with conventional radiography. Arthritis Rheum. 2000;43:2762–70.
8. Dohn UM, Ejbjerg BJ, Court-Payen M, et al. Are bone erosions detected by magnetic resonance imaging and ultrasonography true erosions? A comparison with computed tomography in rheumatoid arthritis metacarpophalangeal joints. Arthritis Res Ther. 2006;8:R110.
9. Sandobal C, Carbo E, Iribas J, et al. Ultrasound nail imaging on patients with psoriasis and psoriatic arthritis compared with rheumatoid arthritis and control subjects. J Clin Rheumatol. 2014;20:21–4.
10. Gutierrez M, Filippucci E, Salaffi F, et al. Differential diagnosis between rheumatoid arthritis and psoriatic arthritis: the value of ultrasound findings at metacarpophalangeal joints level. Ann Rheum Dis. 2011;70:1111–4.
11. Filippucci E, Gabba A, Di Geso L, et al. Hand tendon involvement in rheumatoid arthritis: an ultrasound study. Semin Arthritis Rheum. 2012;41:752–60.
12. Ellabban AS, Kamel SR, Omar HA, et al. Ultrasonographic diagnosis of articular chondrocalcinosis. Rheumatol Int. 2012;32:3863–8.
13. Jacobson JA, Oh E, Propeck T, et al. Sonography of the scapholunate ligament in four cadaveric wrists: correlation with MR arthrography and anatomy. AJR Am J Roentgenol. 2002;179:523–7.

14. Kendi AT, Gudemez E. Sonographic evaluation of scapholunate ligament: value of tissue harmonic imaging. J Clin Ultrasound. 2006;34:109–12.
15. Avouac J, Freire V, Drapé JL, et al. Ultrasonographic hand features in systemic sclerosis and correlates with clinical, biologic, and radiographic findings. Arthritis Care Res (Hoboken). 2012;64(8):1244–9.
16. Teefy SA, Dahiya N, Middleton WD, et al. Ganglia of the hand and wrist: a sonographic analysis. AJR Am J Roentgenol. 2008;191:716–20.
17. Middleton WD, Patel V, Teefey SA, Boyer MI. Giant cell tumors of the tendon sheath: analysis of sonographic findings. AJR Am J Roentgenol. 2004;183:337–9.
18. Thiele RG, Schlesinger N. Diagnosis of gout by ultrasound. Rheumatology (Oxford). 2007;46:1116–21.
19. Nalbant S, Corominas H, Hsu B, et al. Ultrasonography for assessment of subcutaneous nodules. J Rheumatol. 2003;30:1191–5.
20. de Avila FE, Kubota ES, Sandim GB, et al. Ultrasound features of tophi in chronic tophaceous gout. Skelet Radiol. 2011;40:309–15.
21. El Miedany YM, Aty SA, Ashour S. Ultrasonography versus nerve conduction study in patients with carpal tunnel syndrome: substantive or complementary tests? Rheumatology (Oxford). 2004;43:887–95.
22. Roll SC, Case-Smith J, Evans KD. Diagnostic accuracy of ultrasonography vs. electromyography in carpal tunnel syndrome: a systematic review of literature. Ultrasound Med Biol. 2011;37:1539–53.
23. Ziswiler HR, Reichenbach S, Vogelin E, et al. Diagnostic value of sonography in patients with suspected carpal tunnel syndrome: a prospective study. Arthritis Rheum. 2005;52:304–11.
24. Hobson-Webb LD, Massey JM, Juel VC, Sanders DB. The ultrasonographic wrist-to-forearm median nerve area ratio in carpal tunnel syndrome. Clin Neurophysiol. 2008;119:1353–7.
25. Klauser AS, Halpern EJ, Faschingbauer R, et al. Bifid median nerve in carpal tunnel syndrome: assessment with US cross-sectional area measurement. Radiology. 2011;259:808–15.
26. Bayrak IK, Bayrak AO, Kale M, et al. Bifid median nerve in patients with carpal tunnel syndrome. J Ultrasound Med. 2008;27:1129–36.

Ultrasound of the Elbow

4

Janeth Yinh, Amy Evangelisto, and Minna J. Kohler

Key Points

- Ultrasound can be helpful in evaluating commonly encountered rheumatologic conditions involving the elbow, such as rheumatoid arthritis, psoriatic arthritis, and crystal-induced arthritis.
- Ultrasound investigation of the tendons can characterize structural abnormalities in the tendon to help differentiate from inflammatory vs. mechanical conditions.
- Ultrasound aids in the characterization of nodules in the elbow (e.g., heterogeneous echogenicity in gouty tophi vs. homogeneous echogenicity with hypoechoic center seen in rheumatoid nodules).
- Dynamic ultrasound of the elbow can enhance visualization of sonographic pathology affecting structures in motion (e.g., ulnar nerve subluxation, snapping tendon, confirmation of intra-articular loose bodies within the joint, ligament, and tendon disruption).

J. Yinh (✉) · M. J. Kohler
Division of Rheumatology, Allergy, and Immunology, Department of Medicine, Massachusetts General Hospital, Harvard Medical School, Boston, MA, USA
e-mail: janeth.yinh@mgh.harvard.edu; mkohler@mgh.harvard.edu

A. Evangelisto
Arthritis, Rheumatic and Back Disease Associates, Voorhees, NJ, USA

M. J. Kohler (ed.), *Musculoskeletal Ultrasound in Rheumatology Review*,
https://doi.org/10.1007/978-3-030-73555-5_4

Introduction

Ultrasound of the elbow is useful in evaluating the elbow for commonly encountered pathology in rheumatology and other musculoskeletal clinics. The articulations and synovium of the elbow joint and surrounding soft tissue structures such as tendons, ligaments, muscles, nerves, and bursa are easy to examine using musculoskeletal ultrasound. Synovitis, tendinitis, enthesitis, effusions, tendon, and ligament pathology can be characterized when physical exam findings are equivocal.

Elbow ultrasound of the joint recess can help distinguish the presence of synovial tissue vs. fluid and increase the likelihood of a successful aspiration. Evaluation of tendons with elbow sonography may complement in visualizing the extent of tendon derangement and on occasions help provide characteristic features that may help distinguish mechanical vs. inflammatory pathology.

Ultrasound Examination Technique

The ideal position to begin scanning the elbow is with the patient seated or supine with the elbow extended and the hand supinated. Positioning a pillow to support the extremity stabilizes the elbow in position to avoid motion artifact and provides comfort for the patient. In cases where elbow pathology does not allow full extension of the elbow, a generous amount of gel may assist in providing full contact of the probe for better visualization of anterior structures viewed longitudinally. Positioning the arm abducted with the elbow extended or semiflexed facilitates scanning of the medial elbow.

The use of a high-frequency linear array probe ranging from 5 to 12 MHz seeking the highest frequency that permits the best penetration of the structures of interest is recommended. The choice of probe and ideal frequency may be affected by the patient's body habitus. Adjustments in the depth can then be applied for more conspicuous visualization of deeper structures.

An organized scanning protocol (see Table 4.1) can visualize normal anatomy and allow the sonographer to focus on particular pathology related to the regional structures. Figure 4.1 provides a useful guide of the relevant bony landmarks of the elbow to keep in mind when scanning the elbow. Upon identifying the view or structure of interest, it is important to slide the transducer from side to side as well as proximally and distally to capture boundaries of structures and not miss any possible abnormalities.

Anterior Elbow

Scan of the anterior elbow can evaluate the humeroradial and humeroulnar joints with their corresponding radial and coronoid fossa: the articular cartilage, brachialis muscle, biceps brachii tendon, and median nerve.

Table 4.1 Elbow scanning protocol: structures of interest with indications and key features

View	Structures of interest	Indications/key features
Anterior	Anterior elbow recess (humeroradial/humeroulnar) Brachialis muscle Median nerve Biceps muscle/tendon insertion Femoral cartilage	Synovitis, effusion, or erosions, loose bodies *(displaceable with dynamic evaluation)* Bicipitoradial bursitis Median nerve entrapment Distal biceps tendon tear Osteoarthritis: cartilage degeneration. Crystal deposition: gout *(deposition overlying cartilage)* vs. pseudogout *(deposition within cartilage)*
Lateral	Common extensor tendon Lateral collateral ligament complex Annular recess (radial head)	Tendinosis, tear, calcification, enthesitis[a] *(abnormal tendon features)* Ligament laxity or partial or complete tear Synovitis, effusion, or erosions
Medial	Common flexor tendon Medial olecranon joint Ulnar collateral ligament (UCL)	Tendinosis, tear, calcification, enthesitis[a] *(abnormal tendon features)* Synovitis, effusion, or erosions Ligament laxity or partial or complete tear of the anterior band of the UCL
Posterior	Triceps tendon Posterior joint recess Olecranon bursa Ulnar nerve	Tendinosis, tear, calcification, enthesitis[a] *(abnormal tendon features)* Synovitis, effusion, or erosions, loose bodies *(displaceable with dynamic evaluation)* Bursitis (hypoechoic thickening or anechoic compressible fluid) or nodules Thickening or hypoechogenicity of the ulnar nerve, entrapment, or subluxation *(dynamic maneuvers may confirm subluxation/snapping triceps syndrome)*

[a]Abnormal tendon features: *tendinosis*, echotexture, or tendon contour changes (e.g., loss of fibrillar pattern, hypoechogenicity, thickening). *Tear*: anechoic defect in two orthogonal planes; dynamic views of extensor tendon may confirm tear. Tear may have surrounding fluid or power Doppler signal. *Enthesitis:* color power Doppler signal may be noted within tendon or bony entheses. Cortical irregularities can be noted in chronic tendinitis or inflammatory spondyloarthropathy

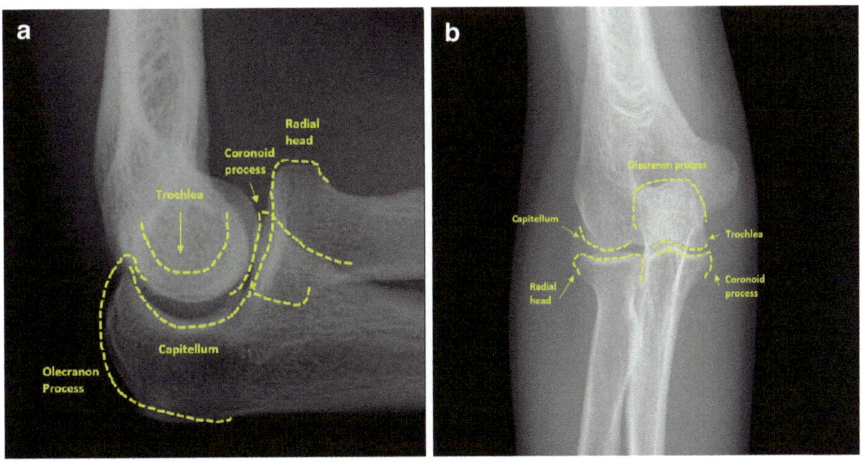

Fig. 4.1 Relevant bony landmarks of the elbow. (**a**) Lateral view. (**b**) Posterior view

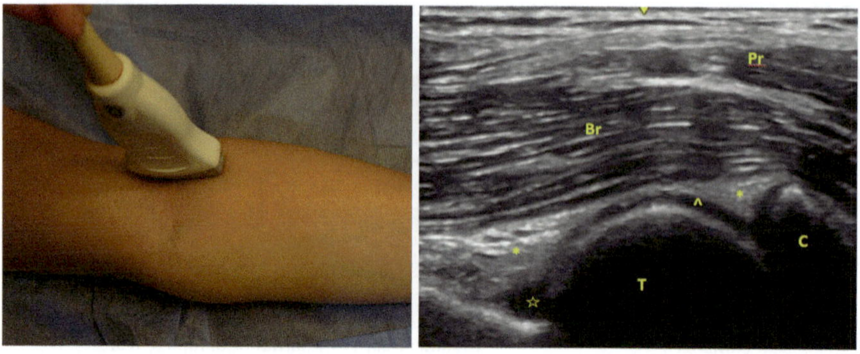

Fig. 4.2 Anterior longitudinal view of the humeroulnar or ulnotrochlear joint: probe positioning with ultrasound view. Trochlea (T), coronoid (C), brachialis muscle (Br), pronator teres muscle (Pr), fat pad (*), coronoid fossa (star), articular cartilage (^)

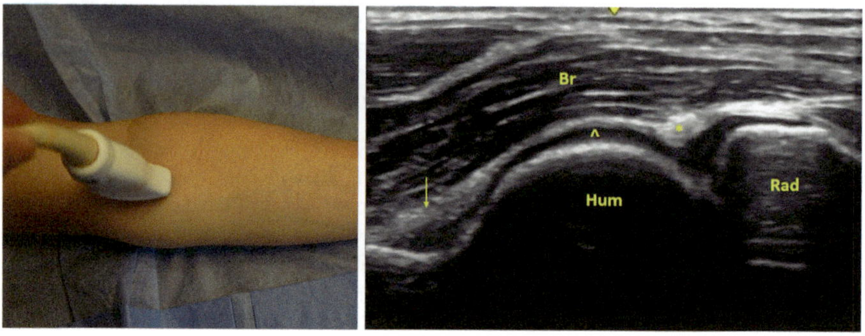

Fig. 4.3 Anterior longitudinal humeroradial or radiocapitellar joint: brachioradialis muscle (Br), humerus (Hum), radial head (Rad), coronoid fossa (arrow), cartilage (^), fat pad (*)

To evaluate the longitudinal view of the humeroulnar or ulnotrochlear joint, the probe is placed perpendicular to the elbow crease over the extended elbow medially. The bony landmarks to identify include the trochlea of the medial humerus articulating with the "peaked or triangular" coronoid process of the ulna (Fig. 4.2). Scanning the humeroulnar joint proximally will evaluate the coronoid fossa that is occupied by a triangular hyperechoic fat pad. Performing a heel-toe maneuver of the probe can assist in enhancing the distal bony contour of the coronoid process that angles sharply away from the joint space appearing as a "mountain peak." The brachialis muscle overlying the joint can be scanned distally to its insertion to the tuberosity of the radius.

Sweeping the probe laterally will display the lateral capitellum of the humerus articulating with the boxy-appearing radial head that conforms the humeroradial or radiocapitellar joint (Fig. 4.3). Physiologic hyperechoic fat will also overlie the cartilage at this site creating a "seagull" appearance over the joint cleft that is appreciated at the humeroulnar joint. In the presence of effusion or synovitis, this hyperechoic "seagull"-appearing fat pad may be distorted and shifted anteriorly [1].

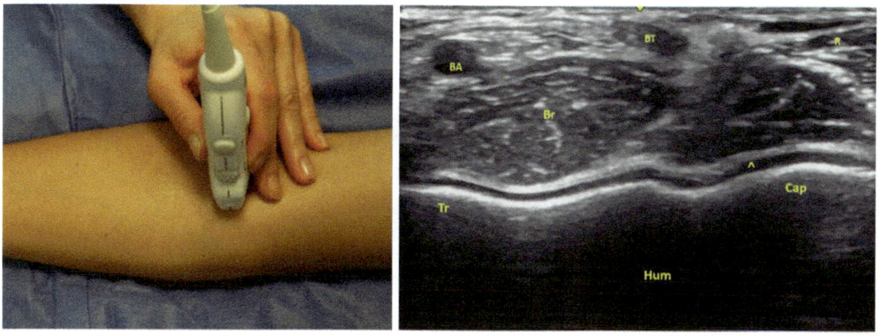

Fig. 4.4 Anterior transverse view. Humerus (Hum), trochlear portion of humerus (Tr), capitellar portion of humerus (Cap), brachialis muscle (Br), bicipital tendon (BT), brachial artery (BA), radial nerve (R), articular cartilage (^). Left is medial and right is lateral

Scanning the humeroradial joint proximally will identify the radial fossa and more distally the annular recess to evaluate for the presence of fluid. It is useful to dynamically assess the joint with supination and pronation to assist in the detection of loose bodies as well as identification of smaller fluid collections. The brachioradialis muscle is the muscle that runs over the humeroradial joint. Slightly distal, directly on top of the radial shaft, the supinator muscle can be visualized.

The probe can then be rotated 90 degrees almost parallel to the elbow crease with slight movements proximally and distally to evaluate the anterior transverse view of the elbow joint (Fig. 4.4). At this level, the distal humerus has a distinctive wavy appearance with a thick anechoic cartilage appearing similar to the surface of a "clam shell." One must be aware to avoid confusing this anechoic hyaline cartilage lying directly over the articulating bone for an effusion that is also anechoic at the same location. The echogenic joint capsule will lie directly on the hyaline cartilage of the distal humerus, whereas separation of the structures will be seen in the presence of an effusion or synovitis. Note the trochlear portion of the humerus on the left and the capitellum of the humerus laterally on the right. Sweeping the probe cranially will assess the radial and coronoid fossa that can identify fluid or abnormal synovium extending proximally. The brachialis muscle is located centrally over the humerus, the extensor carpi radialis and brachioradialis muscle lying superficially on the lateral aspect. The median nerve medially and radial nerve laterally can be seen between the muscles.

The anterior transverse windows also evaluate the biceps brachii tendon that lies lateral to the brachial artery and superficial to the brachialis muscle. The bicipitoradial and interosseous bursa which are virtual cavities that are only identified in cases of pathology can be evaluated through the anterior transverse elbow view. The integrity of the tendon can be assessed in short axis tracking its proximal and distal portions to the insertion to evaluate for tears of the tendon. The biceps brachii tendon can also be evaluated in long axis superficial to the brachialis muscle as a hyperechoic fibrillar structure located lateral to the brachial artery. As the biceps brachii tendon courses over the elbow joint, it takes a steep and slight oblique course

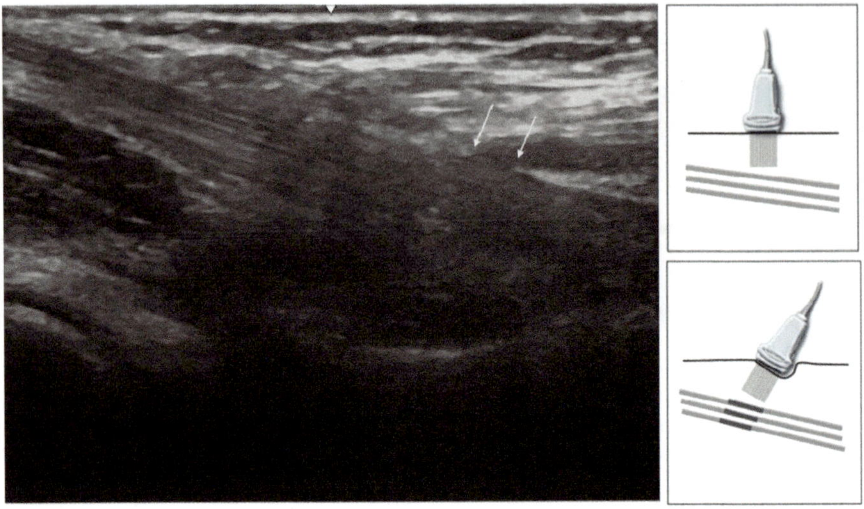

Fig. 4.5 Longitudinal view of the biceps tendon. Right side demonstrates "heel-toe" probe positioning maneuver applying increased pressure distally to overcome tendon anisotropy

making its appearance become more hypoechoic as it inserts onto the radial tuberosity. This hypoechoic effect of the tendon from anisotropy can be reduced by applying a heel-toe maneuver or adjusting the elbow position with mild flexion or extension to obtain a more conspicuous view of the distal tendon (Fig. 4.5). The use of beam steering function (allows a point on an image to be insonated from multiple angles from a single probe and a single position of the probe) available in some ultrasound machines may also improve the visibility of the tendon. Dynamic assessment with supination and pronation can enhance evaluation of the distal fibers that will disappear with supination [2].

Lateral Elbow

The lateral elbow is evaluated with the elbow flexed and the arm internally rotated. The common extensor tendon can be visualized placing the proximal probe over the bony prominence of the lateral epicondyle parallel to the tendon (Fig. 4.6). Assessment of the common extensor tendon integrity, width, echogenicity, presence of hyperemia, and bony irregularities at its bony attachment and distal evaluation of the myotendinous junction are among the features included in a comprehensive tendon evaluation. It is recommended to evaluate the most anterior portion of the tendon where abnormalities can be frequently encountered. The radial collateral ligament is viewed as a thin hyperechoic fibrillar structure lying deep to the extensor tendon connecting the humerus and radius. Distinction of the radial collateral ligament fibers from the common extensor tendon can be performed by following its course that extends distally to the radial head blending with the annular ligament fibers. In contrast, the common extensor tendon has a different course that is seen

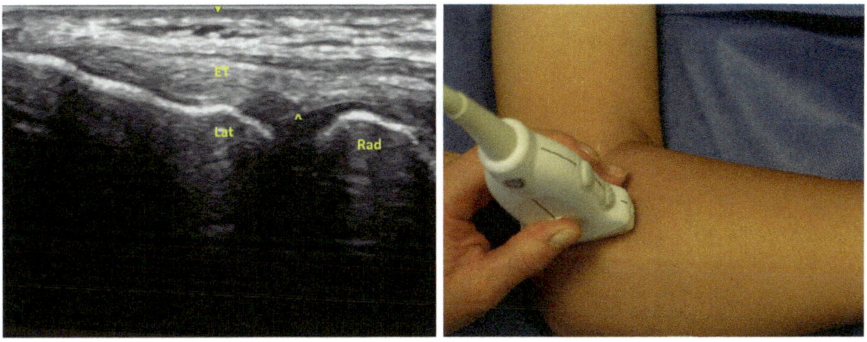

Fig. 4.6 Lateral longitudinal view. Lateral epicondyle (Lat), radial head (Rad), extensor tendon (ET), radial annular ligament (^)

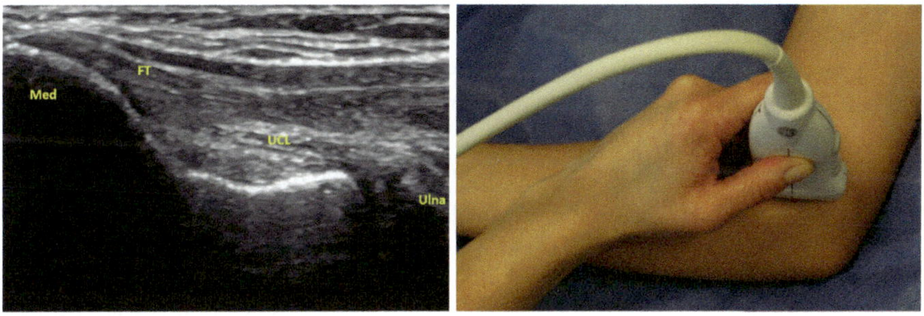

Fig. 4.7 Medial longitudinal view. Medial epicondyle (Med), ulna, flexor tendon (FT), ulnar collateral ligament (UCL)

superficially as a thicker fibrillar structure that extends distally to become muscle. The lateral radiocapitellar joint cleft is occupied by a triangular meniscus like synovial fold termed synovial fringe or posterolateral plica which may be symptomatic and misdiagnosed as lateral epicondylitis. At the radial neck, the annular recess is collapsed and poorly visualized in normal circumstances but will appear distended when occupied by synovium or fluid. The deep and superficial branches of the radial nerve can be identified transversely as a round hypoechoic structure between the fascial planes of the brachioradialis and brachialis anteriorly.

Medial Elbow

Scanning the medial elbow is best performed with the elbow extended or slightly flexed and the arm abducted in full supination. The probe is positioned in long axis with the proximal portion of the probe over the medial epicondyle (Fig. 4.7). The characteristic sloped appearance of the medial epicondyle can be easily identified as well as the superficial common flexor tendon overlying the anterior bundle of the ulnar collateral ligament. Evaluation of the same tendon features described above for the common extensor tendon should be assessed for the common flexor tendon.

The medial joint line between the humerus and the ulna is located distally deep to the ulnar collateral ligament. The ulnar collateral ligament is constituted by three components; the anterior band is functionally the most important and best visualized through ultrasound. The anterior band of the ulnar collateral ligament is seen as a compact hyperechoic fibrillar structure deep to the common flexor tendon that can be identified slightly shifting the probe off plane of the tendon to trace its attachment from the medial epicondyle of the humerus to the proximal ulna. Dynamic valgus stress with the elbow slightly flexed to disengage the olecranon from the olecranon fossa can aid in evaluating for injury of the ulnar collateral ligament [3].

Posterior Elbow

Positioning the arm with 90-degree flexion with the hand placed on the patients hip or a table will allow evaluation of the posterior elbow. The probe is placed proximal to the elbow in longitudinal plane with the tip of the probe supported over the olecranon process (Fig. 4.8). The superficial hyperechoic fibrillar triceps tendon overlying the olecranon fossa is evaluated for swelling, disruption, Doppler signal, calcifications, or bony irregularities at its insertion onto the olecranon. The bony contours of the olecranon, the joint cleft, and the pronounced concavity of the olecranon fossa can be clearly identified lying deep to the triceps muscle and tendon. The olecranon fossa is normally occupied by a hyperechoic posterior fat pad that is noted to be displaced superficially in the presence of an effusion. Dynamic flexion and extension can enhance evaluation of fluid or loose bodies at this site. Turning the probe 90 degrees to the triceps will image the transverse view of the olecranon recess (Fig. 4.9). Evaluation of the olecranon bursa that is only seen in abnormal conditions is best performed with the arm extended having caution to apply light pressure of the probe to avoid displacement of pathologic bursal fluid.

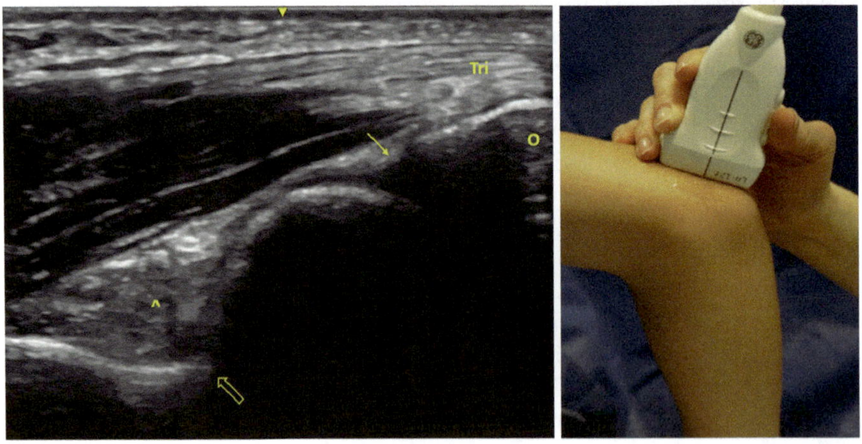

Fig. 4.8 Posterior longitudinal view. Olecranon process (O), triceps tendon (Tri), joint cleft (arrow), olecranon fossa (open arrow), fat pad (^)

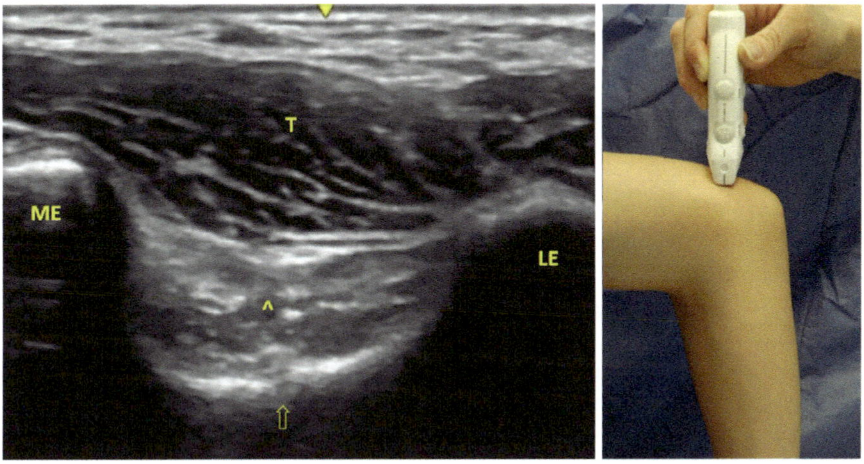

Fig. 4.9 Posterior transverse view. Triceps tendon (T), medial epicondyle of the humerus (ME), lateral epicondyle of the humerus (LE), olecranon fossa (open arrow), fat pad (^)

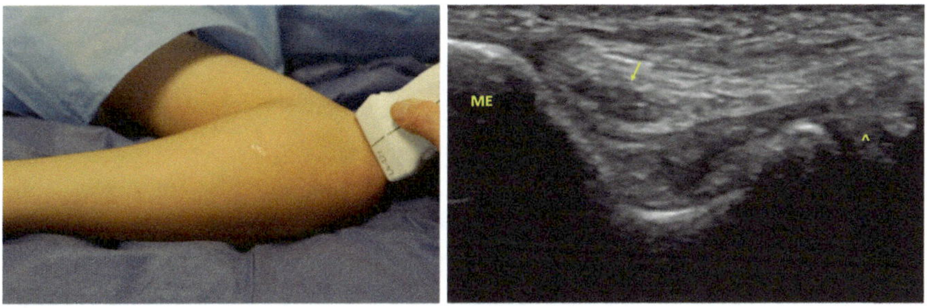

Fig. 4.10 Transverse view of the cubital tunnel. Medial epicondyle of the humerus (ME), ulnar nerve (arrow), medial joint cleft (^)

The probe can later be redirected bridging one end on the olecranon process and the other end at the medial epicondyle with the elbow turned outward to evaluate the cubital tunnel region. The ulnar nerve is visible as a speckled or honeycomb oval structure in close proximity to the medial epicondyle that can be evaluated for increased surface area indicative of swelling. Superficial to the ulnar nerve is the cubital tunnel retinaculum (or Osborne fascia) that is typically not seen in normal state. Dynamic assessment of the cubital tunnel in transverse view with elbow flexion and extension can reveal the presence of a subluxing ulnar nerve or a snapping triceps over the apex of the medial epicondyle (Fig. 4.10). Applying firm pressure with the transducer should be avoided as this may prevent displacement of the ulnar nerve from the ulnar tunnel. The examiner should also be cautious to evaluate for any space-occupying lesion within the cubital tunnel including bone spurs, ganglion cysts, effusion, or synovium that may compress or displace the ulnar nerve. Comparison with the asymptomatic side at the same level may also be utilized as an indicator of ulnar nerve swelling. Long axis of the ulnar nerve is performed by rotating the probe 90 degrees parallel to its tract which can reveal areas of nerve compression.

Rheumatologic Elbow Pathology

Synovial Pathology

Ultrasound is extremely useful for the detection of synovitis or effusion at the elbow where it has demonstrated to be more sensitive than physical exam and radiography in detecting effusions [4, 5]. Ultrasound evaluation of the elbow to identify synovial proliferation or effusion can be evaluated at various sites including the coronoid or radial fossa anteriorly, the annular joint recess laterally, and the medial joint cleft and the coronoid fossa posteriorly. Figures 4.11, 4.12, 4.13, 4.14, and 4.15 include examples of synovitis or effusion at each one of these sites. In these examples, it can

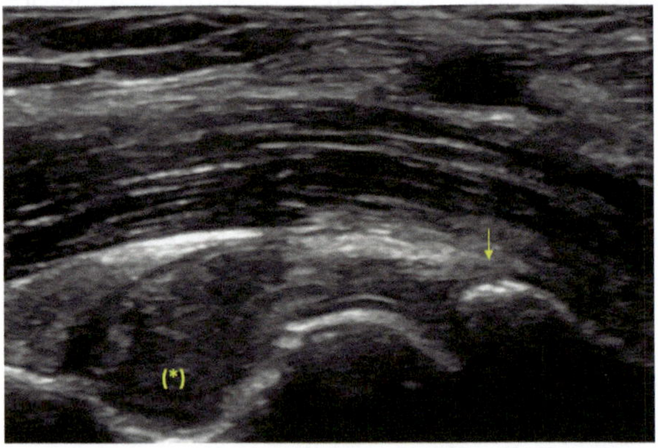

Fig. 4.11 Anterior longitudinal view demonstrating synovitis of the ulnotrochlear joint: coronoid fossa (*). Note the peak-like appearance of the ulna (arrow) to identify medial positioning of the probe

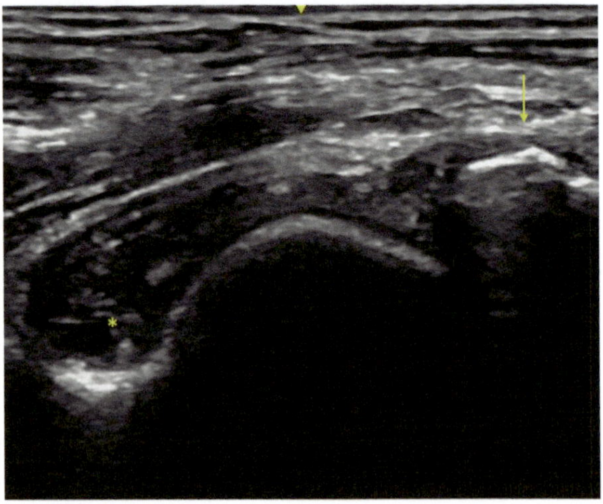

Fig. 4.12 Anterior longitudinal view of synovitis of the radiocapitellar joint: radial fossa (*). Note the "boxy appearance" of the radial head (arrow) to identify lateral positioning of the probe

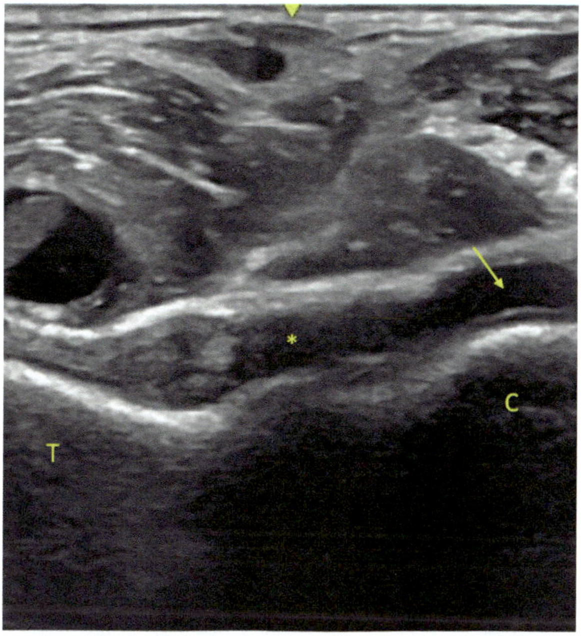

Fig. 4.13 Anterior transverse view of synovitis (*) of the elbow: trochlea (T) and capitellum (C). Notice the artifactual sharp hyperechoic thin interface sign (arrow) between the hyaline cartilage and overlying anechoic or hypoechoic material created by the difference in acoustic impedance between the two tissues

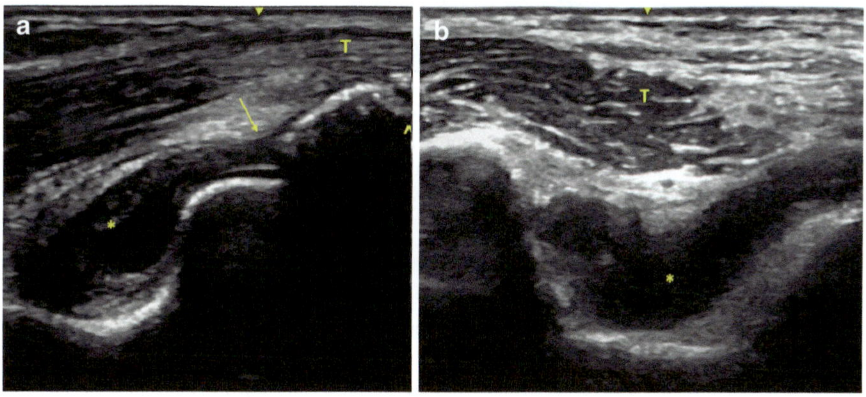

Fig. 4.14 Posterior longitudinal (**a**) and transverse (**b**) view of the elbow showing synovitis with effusion of the olecranon recess (*) in a patient with spondyloarthropathy. Triceps (T), olecranon (O), joint cleft (arrow)

be noted how the thickened synovium or fluid separates the joint capsule from the bone surface and displaces the fibrofatty tissue from the joint cleft.

Distinguishing synovial hypertrophy from an effusion may be challenging as both present as hypoechoic or anechoic tissue within the intra-articular space. However, synovial hypertrophy is not displaceable and poorly compressible and may or may not exhibit Doppler signal. In contrast, synovial effusion is more frequently anechoic and is displaceable and fully compressible and should not exhibit Doppler signal [6] (Fig. 4.16).

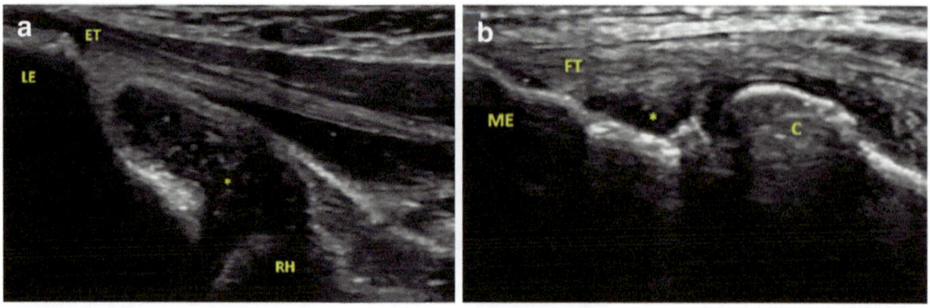

Fig. 4.15 Longitudinal views of synovitis (*) emerging from the lateral (**a**) and medial (**b**) joint cleft. Extensor tendon (ET), lateral epicondyle (LE), radial head (RH), flexor tendon (FT), medial epicondyle (ME), coronoid (C)

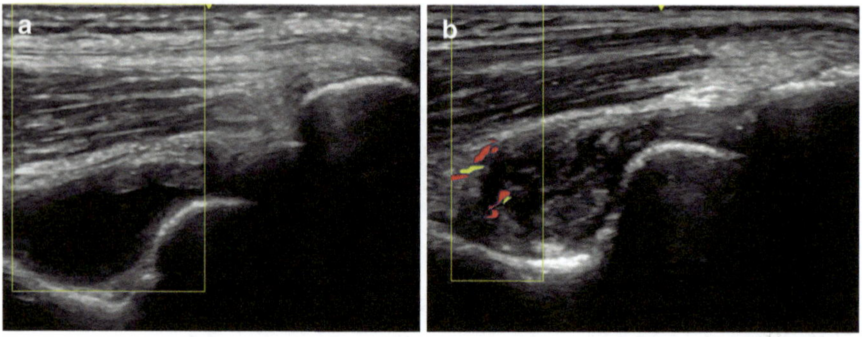

Fig. 4.16 Posterior longitudinal views of the olecranon fossa of two different cases. Picture (**a**) shows an anechoic effusion that is fully compressible and does not show Doppler signal. Contrast to picture (**b**) that shows hypoechoic synovium that is poorly compressible and may present Doppler signal. In both examples, the fat pad will be displaced anteriorly

Synovitis, on the other hand, is described as the presence of hypoechoic synovial hypertrophy regardless of the presence of effusion or any grade of Doppler signal. In many cases of inflammatory arthritis, the combination of both synovial hypertrophy and effusion is noted in conjunction (Fig. 4.17a, b). In contrast, an effusion (Fig. 4.16a) can be clearly distinguished from synovitis with power Doppler signal (Fig. 4.16b).

Small amounts of fluid initially collect in the olecranon fossa and are best visualized with the elbow in flexion. As the pathologic synovial process increases, there is elevation of the anterior and posterior fat pad creating a crescent-shaped appearance of the fat pad. On elbow extension, the fat pad will be compressed by the overlying brachialis muscle against the bone leading to less fluid collecting in the anterior coronoid and radial recess compared to elbow flexion. In markedly distended joints, anterior bulging of the joint cavity is noted and may extend down to the joint recess (Fig. 4.18b) [4, 7]. The recesses located inferiorly to the anterior fat pad, including the annular recess, tend to fill in cases of large amounts of joint effusion.

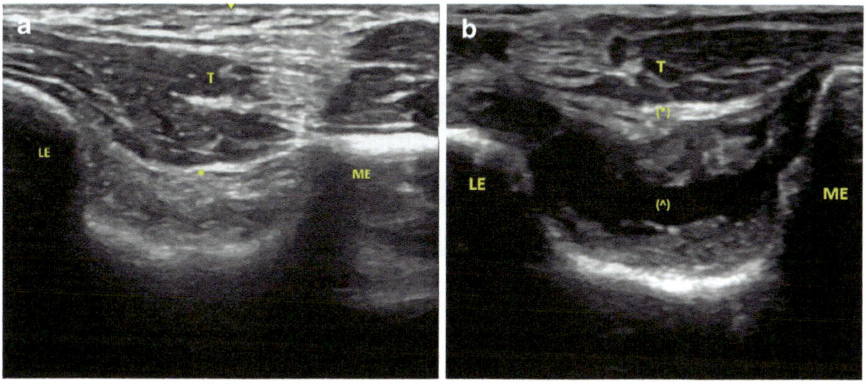

Fig. 4.17 (**a**) Transverse images over the posterior olecranon recess in a normal subject with normal hyperechoic fat occupying the fossa between the lateral (LE) and medial (ME) epicondyle. (**b**) Patient with an anechoic effusion (^) within hypoechoic synovium distending the olecranon recess (*). Fat pad should not be confused with synovitis or effusion. In doubtful cases, dynamic examination with elbow flexion and extension may help distinguish these conditions

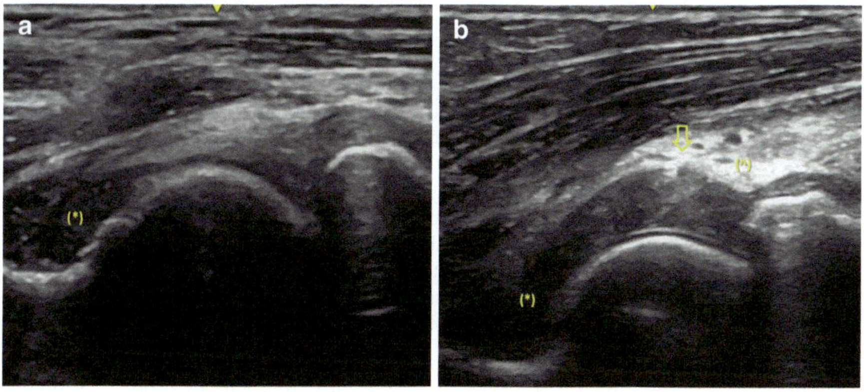

Fig. 4.18 Synovitis of the elbow: anterior longitudinal view. (**a**) Mild synovitis that is initially noted occupying the radial recess (*). (**b**) As joint fluid of synovium increases, the anterior fat pad is displaced anteriorly creating a characteristic crescent shape (^) with anterior bulging of the joint cavity more distally (open arrow)

Although ultrasound is optimal in identifying synovitis in evaluation of the elbow, there are no pathognomonic sonographic features that will distinguish among various forms of inflammatory arthritis. Nonetheless, there may be additional findings that may distinguish between different crystal-related arthropathies. The presence of tophus, double-contour sign, hyperechoic aggregates, and erosion are elementary lesions noted on ultrasound to have reliability in the diagnosis of gout [8–10] (Fig. 4.19).

In cases of calcium pyrophosphate deposition disease (CPPD), hyperechoic deposits of variable shape and size within the fibrocartilage or hyaline cartilage,

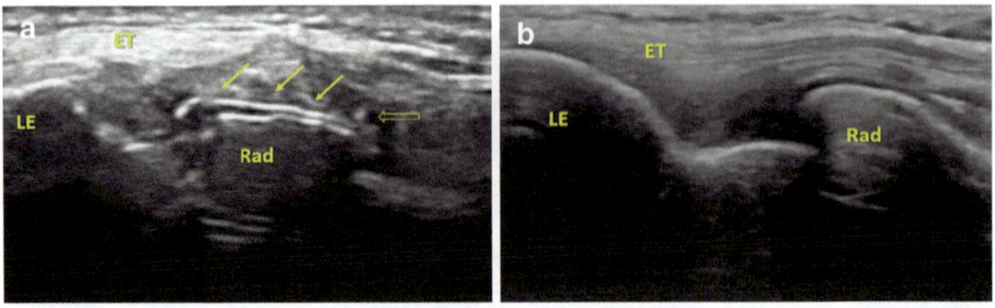

Fig. 4.19 Gouty-related findings of a lateral longitudinal elbow (**a**) distorted bony landmarks, hyperechoic aggregates (open arrow), and double-contour sign (arrows). Figure (**b**), normal lateral longitudinal elbow view. Lateral epicondyle (LE), extensor tendon (ET), radial head (Rad)

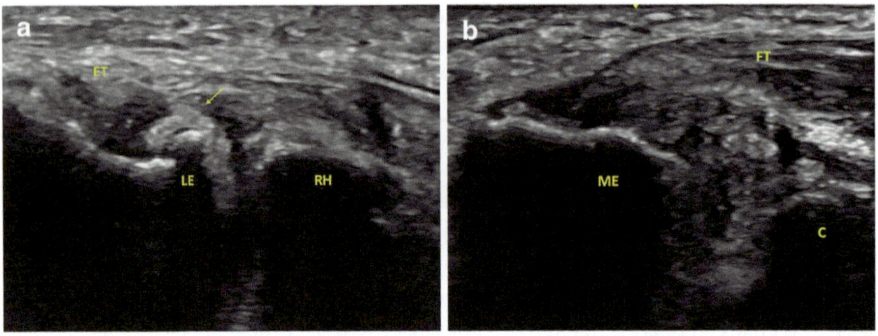

Fig. 4.20 Images of CPPD deposition. (**a**) Longitudinal view of the lateral elbow: there is a dense hyperechoic density in the intra-articular space over the lateral epicondyle (LE). (**b**) Longitudinal view of the medial elbow: bulkier hyperechoic densities at the joint cleft between the medial epicondyle (ME) and the coronoid (C). The flexor tendon exhibits hypoechoic swelling and thickening with anechoic gap from tear at the distal insertion. Note the smaller punctate hyperechoic CPPD densities scattered within the synovium in both images

linear deposits in tendons, or mobile punctate to large deposits in synovial fluid are among the various findings identified through sonography (Fig. 4.20). The medial meniscus and femoral condyle hyaline cartilage of the knee are considered the most frequently involved sites, but any joint, including the elbow, may be affected [11].

Bursal Pathology

The elbow has various bursae that are typically not visible through ultrasound in normal conditions. The most commonly visualizable olecranon bursa is evaluated with the elbow extended ideally floating the transducer with a thick layer of gel and minimal pressure to avoid displacing fluid from the field of view (Fig. 4.21). The olecranon bursa can be pathologically distended with fluid or synovium of variable echogenicity in cases of inflammatory or crystal-related arthritis, traumatic or septic bursitis, and possible concomitant soft tissue cellulitis (Fig. 4.22). Similar to what

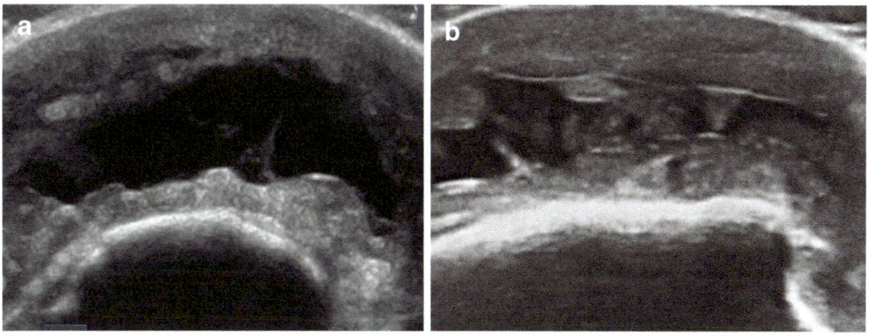

Fig. 4.21 (**a**) Olecranon bursitis with predominantly anechoic fluid and thickened synovial walls. (**b**) Chronic olecranon bursitis distended mostly by hypoechoic tissue hypertrophy and thickened bursal wall

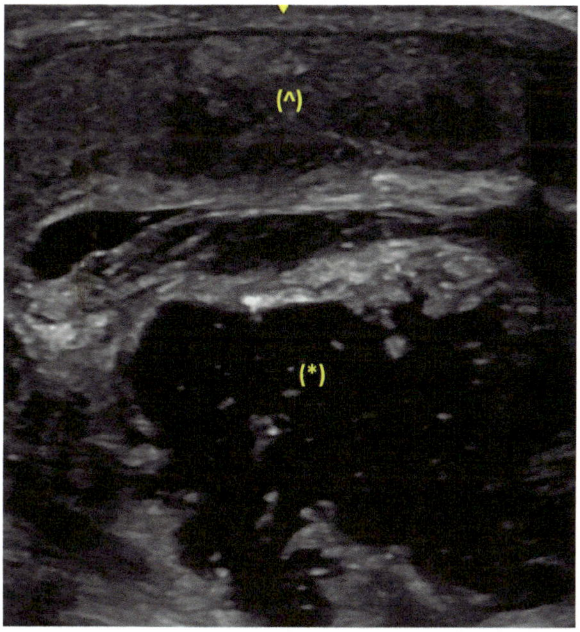

Fig. 4.22 Olecranon bursitis in a patient with severe rheumatoid arthritis. Transverse image reveals a painless heterogeneous soft-tissue mass (*) with mixed echotexture located in the subcutaneous tissue of the olecranon. Note the homogeneous rheumatoid nodule overlying the distended olecranon bursa

can be seen in the joint recess, hypoechoic complex fluid can be distinguished from tissue hypertrophy by the presence of compressibility, redistribution, or motion of bursal contents with transducer pressure and absence of Doppler flow. Identification of well-defined borders of a bursa and characteristic location may help differentiate a bursal collection from a joint effusion or abscess. Ultrasound features of olecranon bursitis are nonspecific, and there are no characteristic findings to definitively establish the etiology of bursal swelling. Sometimes a few crystals can be seen floating in effusion; however, aspiration is necessary to clarify whether fluid is infected and/or define crystalline contribution of bursitis. Ultrasound-guided aspirations can facilitate evacuation of fluid and loculated fluid collections or in cases where there is extensive tissue hypertrophy obstructing the needle.

A less frequently encountered bursa is the bicipitoradial bursa that does not communicate with the joint cavity and is found on the anterior aspect of the elbow adjacent to the distal biceps tendon attachment onto the radial tuberosity. Bicipitoradial bursitis presents as an anechoic formation surrounding the distal biceps tendon at the cubital fossa that can be accompanied by neurological symptoms caused by compression of the radial nerve. Ultrasound not only is useful in diagnosing the inflamed bursa but also can provide information about radial nerve injury and be used for guidance of therapeutic intrabursal aspiration and injection [12].

Tendon and Ligament Pathology

Lateral and medial epicondylitis is a misnomer that mostly describes degeneration, swelling, and at times microtearing of the common extensor/flexor tendon rather than true inflammation. It is a condition that can be diagnosed easily through physical exam, but ultrasound can aid by confirming the clinical diagnosis in doubtful or refractory cases, to qualitatively reveal the extent and severity of the disease and to monitor the response to therapy. The main ultrasound features noted are preinsertional hypoechoic swelling of the tendon with loss of the fibrillar pattern (tendinosis), fluid adjacent to the common tendon, ill-defined tendon margins, adjacent bone irregularity, and on occasions hyperechoic calcification. The extensor carpi radialis brevis component of the common extensor tendon located at the most anterior portion of the tendon is found to be the most commonly affected (Fig. 4.23). Sonographic findings of intratendinous calcification, tendon thickening, adjacent bone irregularity, focal hypoechoic regions, and diffuse heterogeneity have been proven to correlate with symptom severity [15] (see Figs. 4.23 and 4.24 for examples of these elementary lesions).

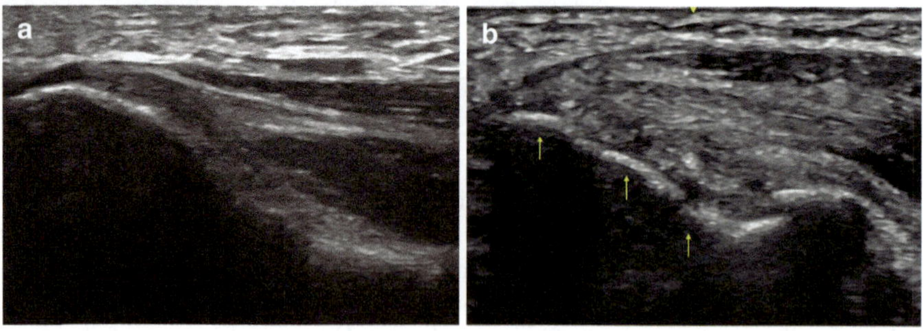

Fig. 4.23 Medial longitudinal view of the elbow. (**a**) Normal flexor tendon with linear fibrillar pattern of the tendon and attachment at bone is clearly delineated. (**b**) Hypoechoic thickening with loss of the fibrillar pattern of the tendon consistent with tendinosis. Note the increased convexity or bowing at the surface of the tendon caused by swollen fibers as well as small superimposed anechoic interstitial tears at portions of the tendon insertion (arrows)

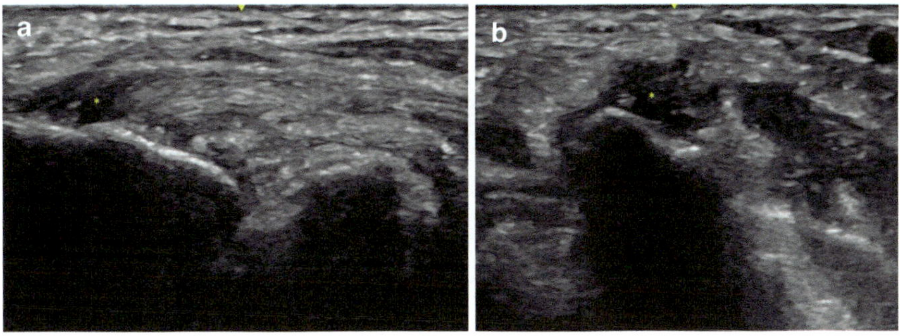

Fig. 4.24 Lateral extensor tendon insertional tear. (**a**) Longitudinal view of a common extensor tendon tear: anechoic interruption of the fibers at the superior attachment (extensor carpi radialis brevis component of the tendon) of the tendon that do not correct upon adjusting probe to exclude anisotropy. (**b**) Transverse view of a common extensor tendon tear for confirmation

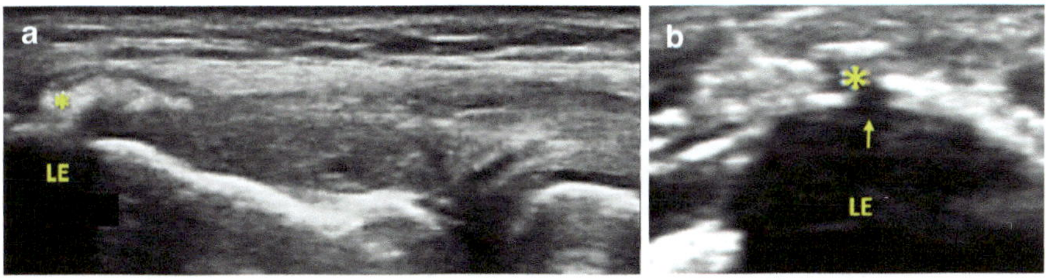

Fig. 4.25 Lateral extensor tendon calcification. Longitudinal (**a**) and transverse (**b**) view of a common extensor tendon showing linear calcification (*) that connects to the bone and can be seen in cases of chronic tendinosis. Note in image (**b**) acoustic shadowing (arrow) casted by the mature calcification

Intratendinous calcification or enthesopathy may be present in cases of chronic tendinosis (Fig. 4.25) [13, 14]. In cases of enthesophytes (Fig. 4.26), calcifications appear as hyperechoic spurs forming at a tendon insertion into the bone, growing in the direction of the natural pull of the tendon involved. Distinguishing mechanical vs. inflammatory calcifications may be challenging, and at times, it may be necessary to seek additional inflammatory features as well as correlate findings with clinical history and exam for a more conclusive assessment.

An additional feature of non-inflammatory "epicondylitis" is the presence of neovascularization noted as Doppler signal within the tendon substance that is a consequence of an angiofibroblastic hyperplasia with an immature reparative response (Fig. 4.27) In high-grade tendinosis, the angiofibroblastic infiltration secondary to migration of fibroblasts and vascular granulation tissue within the tendon substance causes a striking hypervascular pattern of the intratendinous hypoechoic areas [16] that should not be misinterpreted as enthesitis seen in inflammatory arthritis.

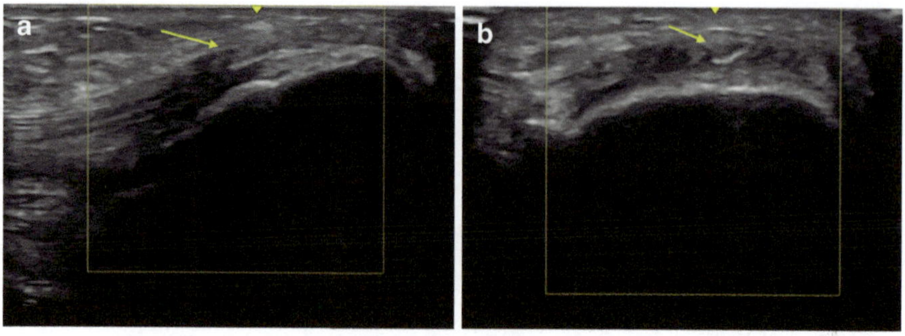

Fig. 4.26 Enthesophyte near triceps tendon of a patient with spondyloarthropathy. Posterior longitudinal (**a**) and transverse (**b**) view of a triceps tendon showing an enthesophyte appearing like a calcification (arrow); however, bony formation is seen connected to bony enthesis along the natural pull of the tendon

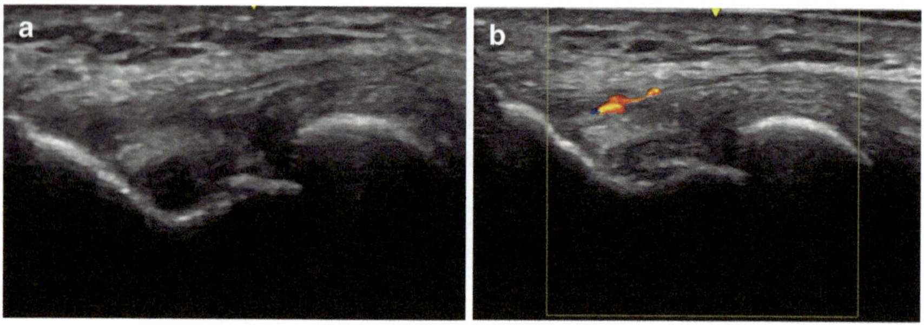

Fig. 4.27 (**a**) Lateral longitudinal view of a common extensor tendon at the lateral epicondyle showing hypoechoic tendinosis swelling of the tendon with anechoic interstitial tears. (**b**) View of the same tendon demonstrates power Doppler signal at the anechoic gaps from neovascularity signaling the tendons attempt to regenerate

Enthesitis is sonographically defined as hypoechoic and/or thickened insertion of the enthesis close to the bone (within 2 mm from the bony cortex) which exhibits Doppler signal if active and that may show erosions and enthesophytes/calcifications as sign of structural damage [8]. The detection of enthesitis with ultrasound is far more sensitive and specific than clinical examination in evaluating patients for spondyloarthropathies (SpA) [17]. Furthermore, ultrasound evaluation for enthesitis is reproducible and provides the means to quantify disease severity [18]. Various studies have included the triceps tendon or the common flexor or extensor tendon of the elbow as areas to evaluate for enthesitis in evaluating for SpA. The validity of ultrasound assessment evaluating elemental lesions of enthesis thickness, structure, calcifications, erosions, bursae, and power Doppler signal has been described for the diagnostic classification of SpA [19]. Distinction of non-inflammatory Doppler signal related to reparative neovascularization from that seen in inflammatory arthritis can be elusive at times. Detailed comparative studies of enthesis features in normal controls and patients with SpA have demonstrated absent power Doppler signal

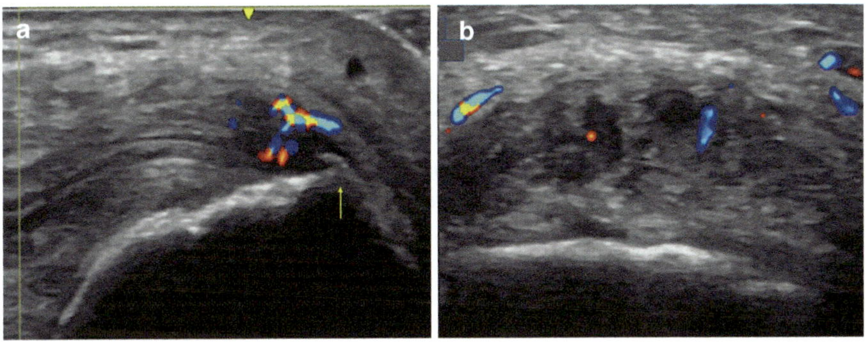

Fig. 4.28 Triceps tendon enthesitis in a patient with spondyloarthropathy. (**a**) Posterior longitudinal view of the triceps tendon showing heterogeneous thickening of the tendon with vascularization and cortical irregularities at its insertion to the olecranon. A small enthesophyte (arrow) noted as a hyperechoic spur forming at a tendon insertion into the bone growing in the direction of the natural pull of the tendon. (**b**) Same triceps tendon insertion changes on posterior transverse view

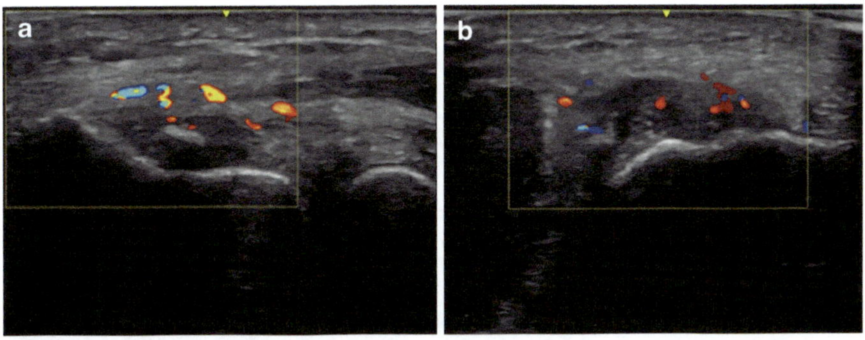

Fig. 4.29 Enthesitis of the common extensor tendon in a patient with psoriatic arthritis. (**a**) Longitudinal lateral view of the common extensor tendon at the lateral epicondyle showing tendon thickening with decreased echogenicity, positive power Doppler signal, and early cortical irregularities. (**b**) Transverse lateral view of the extensor tendon showing anechoic gaps, hypoechoic swelling, and positive power Doppler signal

of the abnormal entheses in control patients, whereas Doppler signal was seen in 81% of abnormal entheses of SpA patients. In patients with SpA, vascularization was usually detected at the cortical bone insertion and at times also in the bursa with no difference observed in the distribution of enthesis pattern between the distinct SpA subtypes [20] (see Figs. 4.28 and 4.29 for examples of enthesitis).

Ligaments of the elbow that can be evaluated by ultrasound include the anterior band of the ulnar collateral ligament (UCL) medially and laterally the lateral collateral ligament (LCL) and radial collateral ligament (RCL). A focal tear of the ligament may appear as focal hypoechoic heterogeneity and laxity with thickening of the ligament without complete ligament fiber disruption. In cases of complete tears, widening of the adjacent joint space can be noted with soft tissue falling into the distracted articular space with surrounding effusion slightly posterior and deep to the medial or lateral epicondyle. Comparative dynamic imaging with contralateral elbow demonstrating joint instability and ligament laxity can be exerted through valgus and varus stress for evaluation of UCL and varus LCL injury, respectively [15]. It is of interest to include evaluation of the overlying tendon as concomitant tears of the flexor or extensor tendon can occur as a result of the same forces or overuse mechanisms on adjacent structures.

Bony Pathology

Erosions seen in cases of inflammatory arthritis are usually seen as an intra-articular discontinuity of the bone surface that is visible in two perpendicular planes [8] (see Figs. 4.30 and 4.31).

Ultrasound of the elbow has been demonstrated to be useful for the detection of early changes in rheumatoid arthritis (Fig. 4.32). In early disease, soft tissue alterations and early erosions are better detected by sonography than by conventional

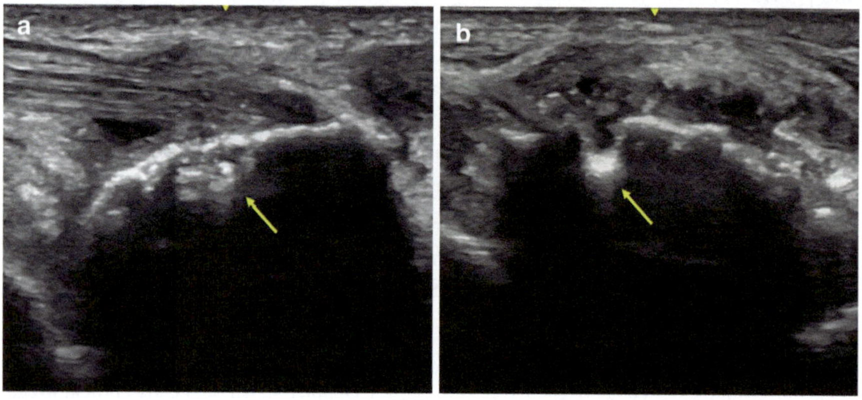

Fig. 4.30 Triceps tendon enthesitis and erosion in orthogonal planes. Longitudinal (**a**) and transverse (**b**) views of the triceps tendon enthesitis with a large punched out erosion (arrow) at the insertion of the tendon. Figure (**b**) shows a transverse view of the erosion and extensive cortical bone disruption observed at the level of the triceps insertion

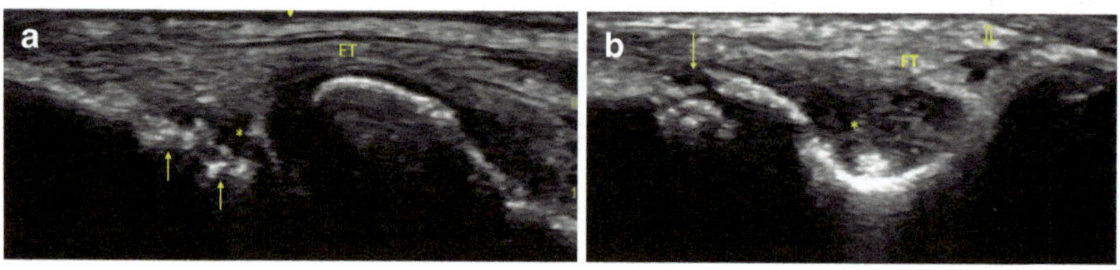

Fig. 4.31 Bony erosions (arrow) adjacent to site of emerging synovitis (*) from the lateral (**a**) and medial (**b**) joint cleft in a patient with rheumatoid arthritis. Flexor tendon *FT*, extensor tendon *ET*. Note in Figure b the presence of a tendon tear of the flexor tendon (open arrow)

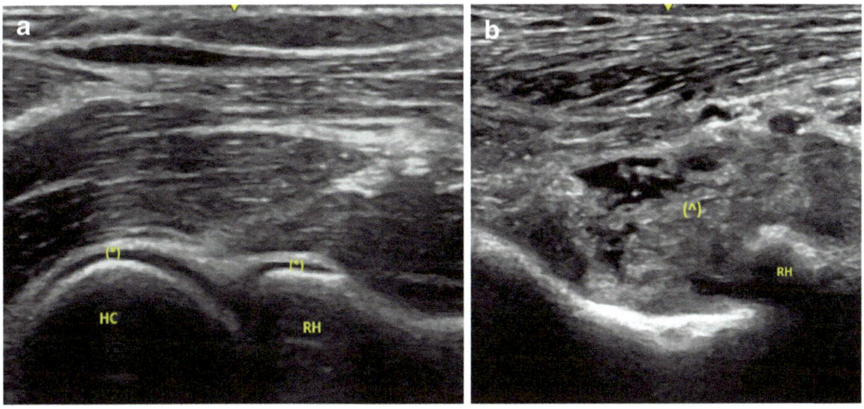

Fig. 4.32 Anterior longitudinal view of the radiocapitellar joint. (**a**) Normal. The articular cartilage (*) and the normal profile of the bone of the humeral capitellum (HC) and radial head (RH) can be clearly identified. (**b**) Destructive pannus in rheumatoid arthritis = grade 5 in a patient with severe rheumatoid arthritis. Note the complete loss of the cartilage and the eroded humeral capitellum (HC) and loss of the bony contours of the radial head (RH) distorting the classic bony landmarks. Proliferative synovial pannus (^) is noted on the surface of the joint distending the annular recess

radiography. A sonographic classification of rheumatoid joint destruction at the elbow to stage disease and identify early destructive process for both the prognosis and treatment strategy has been described: grade 0, normal condition; grade 1, joint effusion with capsular distension; grade 2, small erosion of the radial head with an irregular floor and joint cyst filled with pannus; grade 3, cortical defect of the humeral capitellum, joint effusion, and joint space narrowing; grade 4, cortical defect of the radial head and humeral capitellum; and grade 5, cortical destruction and loss of articular guide structures [21] (Fig. 4.32, 4.33).

Osteoarthritis in the elbow is seen as in other joints presenting with osteophytes as a cardinal feature. Osteophytes have a characteristic sonographic appearance as an irregularity or protuberance of the bony cortex localized in the borders of articular surfaces (Fig. 4.33). In addition, loss of echotexture, width, and definition of the borders of the adjacent cartilage can be identified [22] (Fig. 4.34).

Intra-articular loose bodies can at times be confused with osteophytes if found in close proximity to the bone. These can appear as a hyperechoic fragment that may be ossified and produce acoustic shadowing depending on its level of ossification. Dynamic flexion and extension of the elbow will result in mobilization of fluid and loose bodies that can help differentiate them from local heterotopic ossification or an osteophyte. The elbow is the second most common site of intra-articular bodies after the knee, where they typically present in dependent portions of the olecranon or coronoid fossa that can result in intermittent locking and loss of extension of the joint (Fig. 4.35) [16].

High-resolution ultrasound can be useful in detecting occult fractures missed on conventional radiography. Occult fractures will present as a "step-off" bone disruption or discontinuity of the bone surface (Fig. 4.35). Further diagnostic imaging with computed tomography or magnetic resonance may be considered for

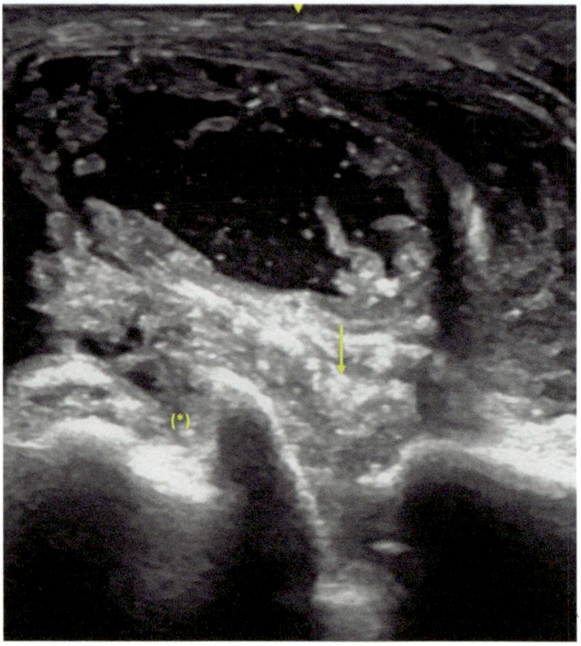

Fig. 4.33 Lateral longitudinal elbow view of a patient with rheumatoid arthritis showing synovitis with effusion. The lateral collateral ligament is not visualized and has been replaced by synovium protruding through the joint cleft between the lateral epicondyle and the radial head (arrow). Note the large erosion (*) of the lateral epicondyle giving the appearance of an osteophyte

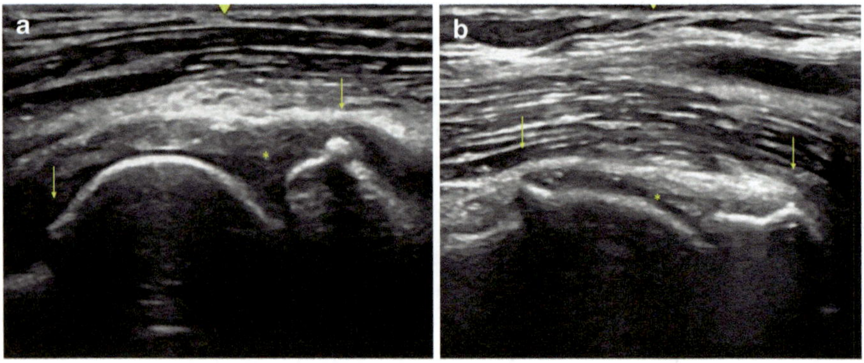

Fig. 4.34 Anterior longitudinal views of (**a**) humeroradial joint and (**b**) humeroulnar joint. Early osteophytic protuberance at the humeral head in both images with cartilage loss and osteophyte (arrows) at the radial head (**a**) and early deformity of the coronoid process in (**b**)

confirmation of fracture in suspected cases, particularly to clarify avulsion fracture. The hip, elbow, and ankle are the most common sites of avulsion fractures.

Soft Tissue Pathology

The posterior elbow is a common location to encounter various nodular lesions. The sonographic characteristics that distinguish gouty tophi from rheumatoid nodules

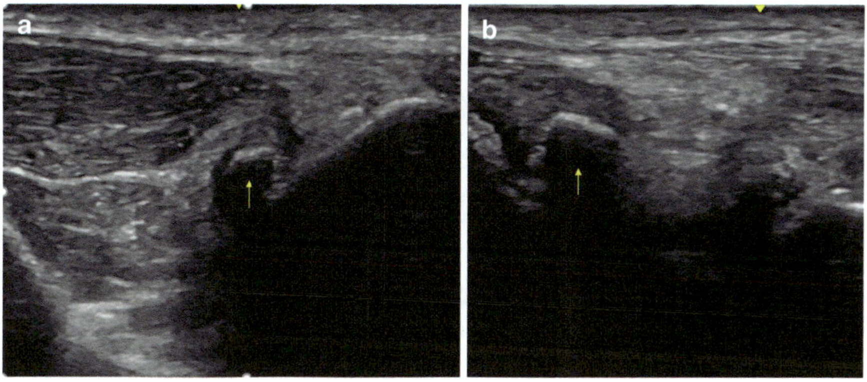

Fig. 4.35 Posterior longitudinal (**a**) and transverse (**b**) views of an intra-articular loose body (arrows) within the posterior fossa. Notice the posterior acoustic shadowing casted by the hyperechoic ossified loose body. There is no connection of the loose body to the olecranon. Dynamic maneuver with flexion and extension of the elbow can show a loose body may be displaceable, while an osteophyte will remain attached to the bone

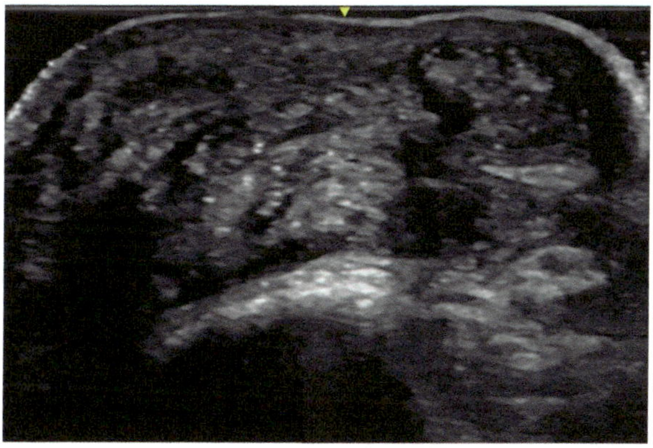

Fig. 4.36 Gouty tophus. Heterogeneous mass with ill-defined borders: hyperechoic punctate tophi admixed with hypoechoic areas thought to be due to chalky liquid material

have been well described. Gouty tophi will generally appear as irregularly shaped heterogeneous masses with the presence of hyperechoic densities from tophi that can occasionally show posterior acoustic shadowing in cases of calcified tophi from long established gout (Fig. 4.36). Cortical bone erosions adjacent to tophi can more frequently be noted in gout compared to rheumatoid nodules. In contrast, rheumatoid nodules appear as oval, generally homogeneous masses with hyperechogenic walls that are attached in close proximity to the bone and have less frequently associated erosive changes. Rheumatoid nodules can frequently present with a centrally sharp demarcated hypoechoic area that is thought to correspond to central necrosis (Fig. 4.37) [23].

Other soft tissue masses, including ganglion cysts and lymph nodes, and tumors, including and lipomas and sarcomas, can be found in various regions of the elbow. MRI and/or biopsy may be necessary for further investigation.

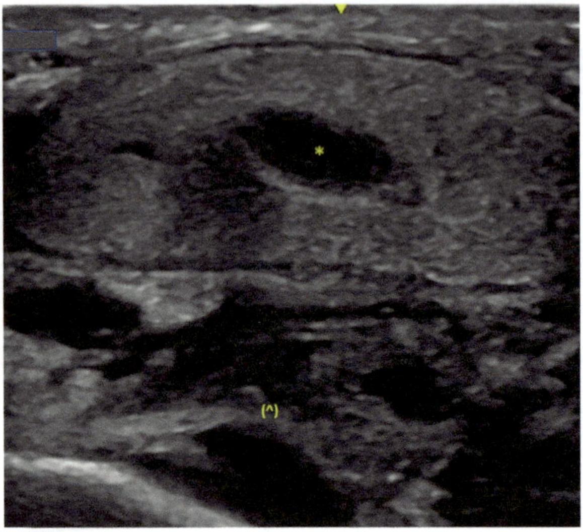

Fig. 4.37 Rheumatoid nodule. Homogeneous mass with well-defined borders and characteristic hypoechoic center (*) presumed to be due to central necrosis. In this case, the rheumatoid nodule is not in close proximity to the bone as typically described as it is overlying a distended olecranon bursa (^)

Nerve Pathology

Ultrasound is a feasible tool to evaluate the pathology of the ulnar nerve at the elbow. Entrapment of the ulnar nerve at the cubital tunnel is the second most common entrapment syndrome of the upper limb after carpal tunnel syndrome. The cubital tunnel encased superiorly by the retinaculum (Osborne's fascia) is identified transversely by placing one end of the probe on the medial epicondyle and the other end at the distal olecranon. Ulnar nerve entrapment can be seen as enlargement of the ulnar nerve just proximal to the cubital tunnel with hypoechoic swelling with loss of the normal speckled pattern of the nerve and, in some cases, hypervascularity with power Doppler imaging. A recent metanalysis "assessing" the ulnar nerve cross-sectional area (CSA) for the diagnosis of cubital tunnel syndrome concluded that a CSA of 10 mm^2 is a cutoff point for diagnosing ulnar nerve entrapment at the elbow region [24]. Ultrasound can also identify among several causes of ulnar nerve impingement, including bone abnormalities (fracture-related bony deformities, medial osteophytes, loose bodies, or heterotopic ossification), as well as the presence of space-occupying lesions, including invasive synovium, ganglia, lipoma, and cases of accessory anconeus epitrochlearis muscle that occurs in 23% of the population. (Figs. 4.38 and 4.39).

It is important to dynamically assess for subluxation of the ulnar nerve over the medial epicondyle with flexion and extension. This condition may predispose to nerve injury and irritation or in 20% be an asymptomatic condition, highlighting the importance of clinical correlation [18]. This maneuver at the same location can also help diagnose snapping triceps syndrome that may be accompanied by nerve subluxation (Fig. 4.40) [25].

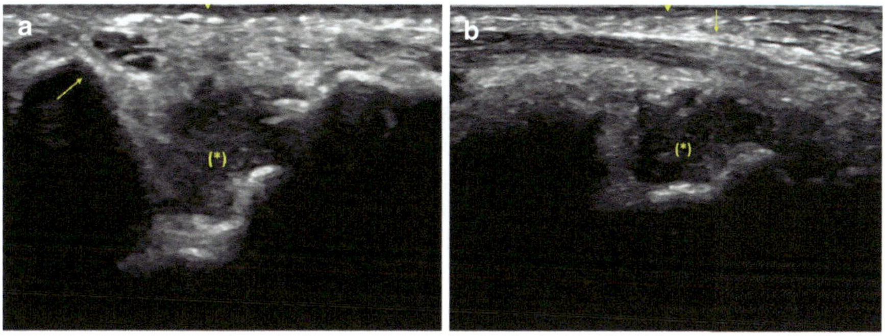

Fig. 4.38 Posteromedial view of the ulnar tunnel of the elbow: (**a**) transverse and (**b**) longitudinal views showing ulnar nerve (arrow) compression and displacement by synovial proliferation (*). Note in Figure (**b**) the area of pre-stenotic swelling and loss of fascicular pattern of the nerve as it enters the cubital/ulnar tunnel

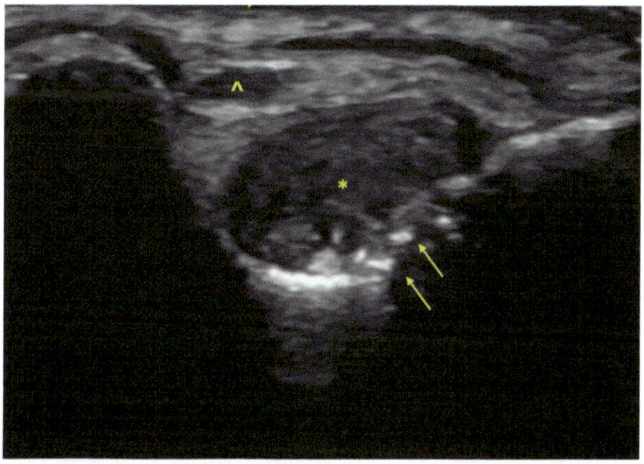

Fig. 4.39 Transverse view of the cubital tunnel of the elbow with compressed ulnar nerve (^) from synovial proliferation (*) from calcium-related arthropathy (arrows)

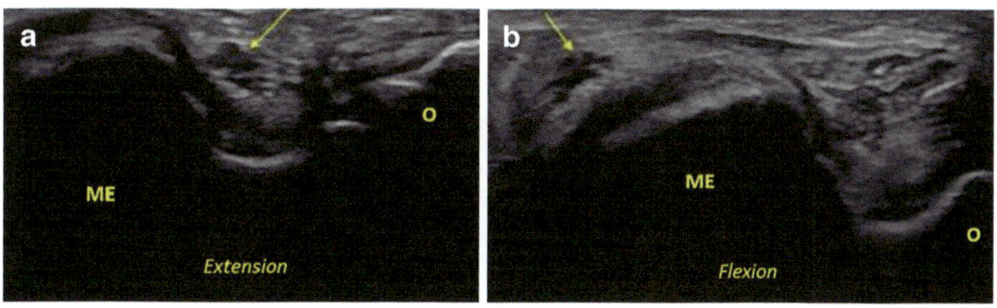

Fig. 4.40 Ulnar nerve subluxation. (**a**) Nerve within the ulnar tunnel with elbow in extension. (**b**) Translocation of the nerve over the medial epicondyle with elbow in full flexion

Ultrasound-Guided Procedures at the Elbow

Injection or aspiration of the elbow joint has been traditionally performed using clinical anatomic landmarks. Few studies have assessed the accuracy of palpation-guided injections (PGI) with that of ultrasound-guided injections (USGI) [26, 27]. A small study by Kim and colleagues reported an accuracy rate of 100% of USGI by posterior approach compared to 77.5% accuracy rate of PGI after confirmation by fluoroscopy in elbows of patients with osteoarthritis [29]. Available literature favors the posterior approach as the posterior olecranon recess is the most sensitive location to identify fluid [4], and there is less risk of vascular or nerve injury when approaching posteriorly. Posterior elbow joint injection is performed with the elbow flexed 90 degrees introducing the needle in plane longitudinally targeting the olecranon fossa or the needle can be introduced via transverse approach laterally to target the olecranon fossa (Fig. 4.41).

In refractory cases of lateral epicondylosis where conventional therapy is ineffective, ultrasound (US)-guided injection therapies have become of increasing interest. Positioning of the patient for USGI of the common extensor tendon is with the elbow flexed 90 degrees with the forearm prone with the transducer placed at the long axis of the tendon. The needle is advanced from distal to proximal direction. Depending on the injectate, the needle target may vary from peritendinous to intratendinous (Fig. 4.42).

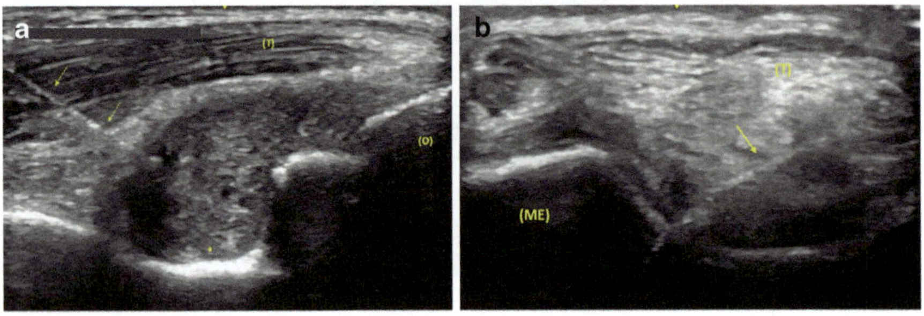

Fig. 4.41 Ultrasound-guided elbow injection through posterior longitudinal (**a**) and transverse (**b**) approaches

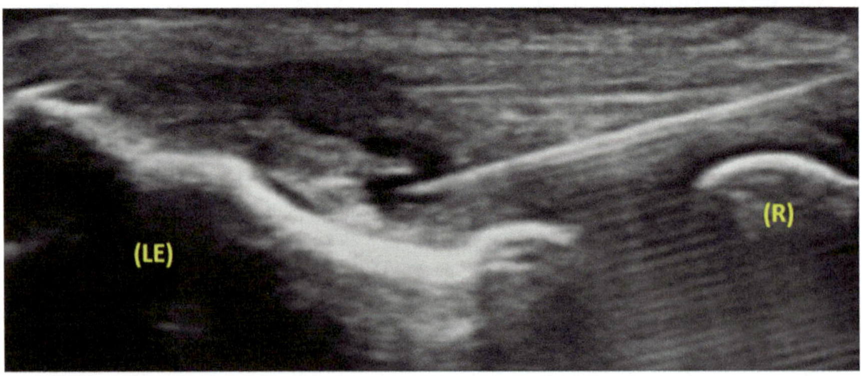

Fig. 4.42 Example of common extensor injection through in-plane lateral longitudinal approach

The literature regarding efficacy of individual approaches of US-guided treatment including needle tenotomy, prolotherapy, autologous whole blood injection (AWB), platelet-rich plasma (PRP) injection, and steroid injection is currently unclear. A systematic review of needle tenotomy demonstrated improvement in pain, but studies have not included placebo or control groups. McShane and colleagues have demonstrated superior results of US-guided tenotomy without administration of corticosteroid after tendon fenestration after a prior trial by the same group that was followed routinely by corticosteroid injection [28, 29]. PRP therapy has demonstrated a statistically significant improvement in pain and functionality for refractory lateral epicondylitis in a systematic review performed in 2013. AWB injection has been evaluated through well-designed studies to show statistically significant reductions in pain. Prolotherapy studies have also reportedly been of some benefit, although a recent study looking at prolotherapy in combination with physiotherapy vs. physiotherapy alone showed no significant differences in pain and function [30]. Nonetheless, no clear conclusions can be drawn at this time of a preferred approach among these methods for the management of degenerative tendon pathology [31]. Notably, corticosteroid injections for lateral epicondylitis, while once standard of care and helpful in short-term symptoms, have fallen out of favor and may lead to worse outcomes in long-term management with results showing inferior outcome and higher recurrence rate at 1 year [32].

Aspiration or injection of the olecranon bursa can often be easily performed without needle guidance. However, ultrasound can assist in successfully guiding needle placement in cases where there is significant synovial thickening and septations to ensure maximal drainage and accurate corticosteroid placement when indicated (Fig. 4.43).

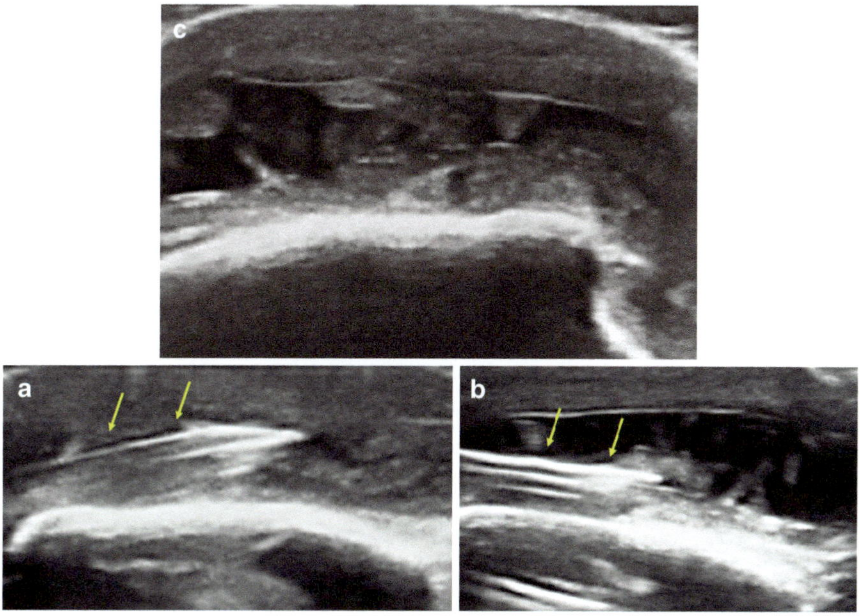

Fig. 4.43 (**a**) Olecranon bursitis, (**b**) needle placement during aspiration, (**c**) successful evacuation of fluid

Conclusion

Ultrasound is an invaluable tool that can be used to evaluate for various elbow pathologic conditions. The spectrum of additional information that can be obtained in various rheumatic conditions exceeds that obtained from radiography, and the costs and convenience are preferable over magnetic resonance. Complementing evaluation with elbow sonography can enhance diagnostic and procedural accuracy leading to improved management and outcomes of elbow disorders.

Review Questions

1. The following longitudinal view of the elbow demonstrates distention of which of the following joint recesses/fossa?

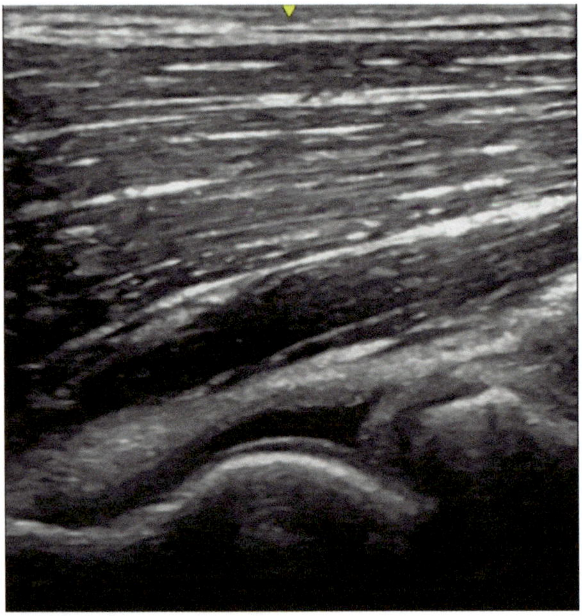

   (a) Olecranon fossa
   (b) Annular fossa
   (c) Radial fossa
   (d) Coronoid fossa

2. Identify the site of the effusion in this posterior longitudinal view of the elbow.

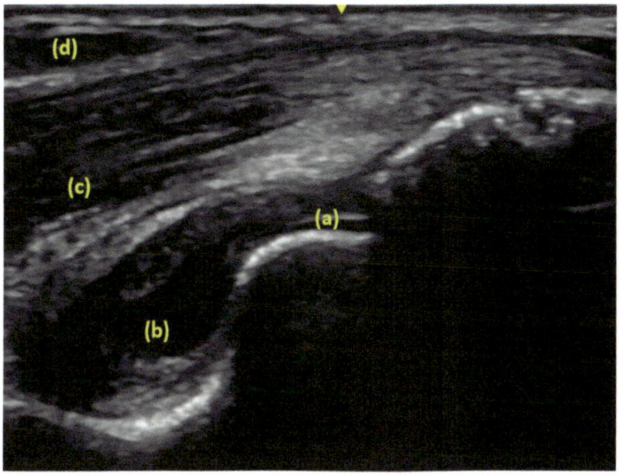

3. Identify the descriptive features of this soft tissue abnormality at the olecranon with its associated diagnosis.

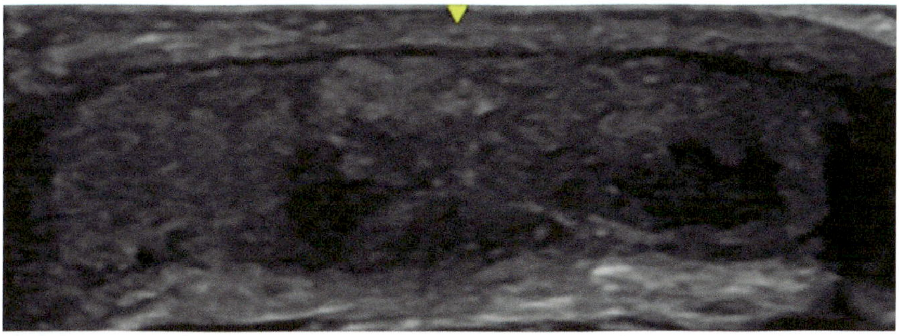

(a) Subcutaneous hypoechoic/anechoic compressible material: olecranon bursa effusion
(b) Heterogeneous irregular mass with hyperechoic densities: tophus
(c) Diffuse thickening of the dermis with edema and anechoic fat stranding: cellulitis
(d) Homogeneous well-defined mass with hypoechoic center: rheumatoid nodule

4. The following image is viewed by which of the following probe positions?

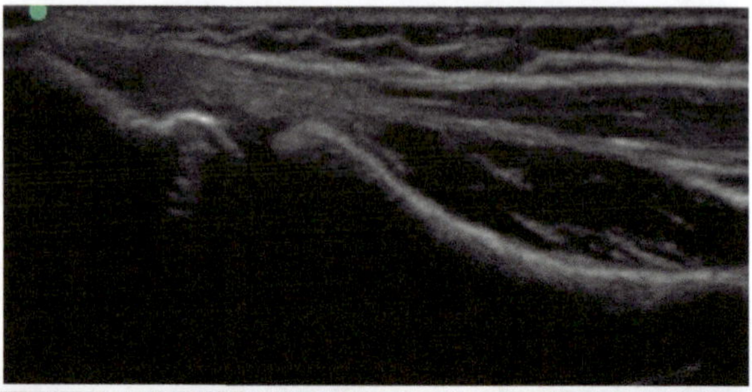

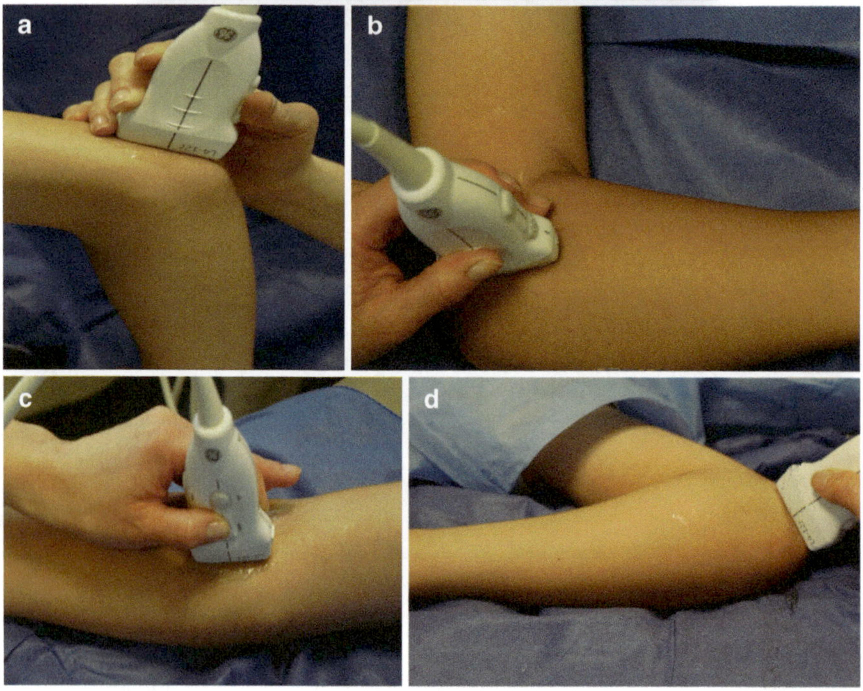

5. Which of the following markings is *not* associated properly with the corresponding anatomical structure on this anterior transverse view of the elbow?

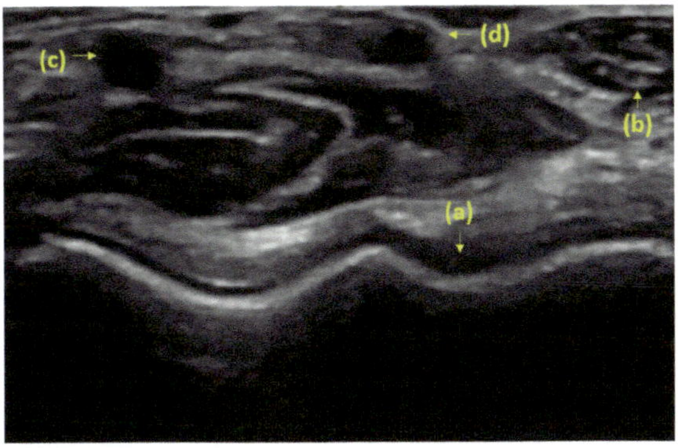

Med Lat

(a) Articular cartilage
(b) Brachialis muscle
(c) Brachial artery
(d) Biceps brachii tendon

6. Identify the dynamic maneuver that will enhance the detection of a tear of the radial collateral ligament.
(a) Flexion extension
(b) Valgus stress
(c) Supination pronation
(d) Varus stress

7. Which feature of this longitudinal view of the lateral extensor tendon is most suggestive of inflammatory enthesitis?

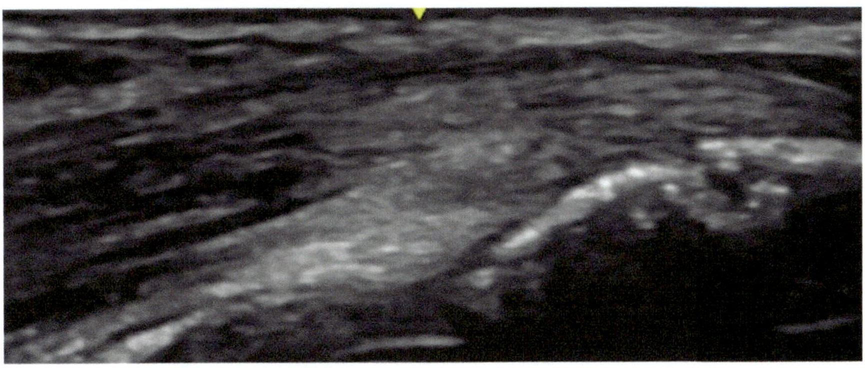

(a) Diffuse thickening of the tendon
(b) Loss of tendon fibrillar pattern
(c) Erosion at the tendon insertion
(d) Disruption of the tendon fibers

8. The presence of which of the mentioned characteristics of abnormal intra-articular material in this anterior transverse view of the elbow joint will *not* be seen in an effusion and may be seen in synovitis?

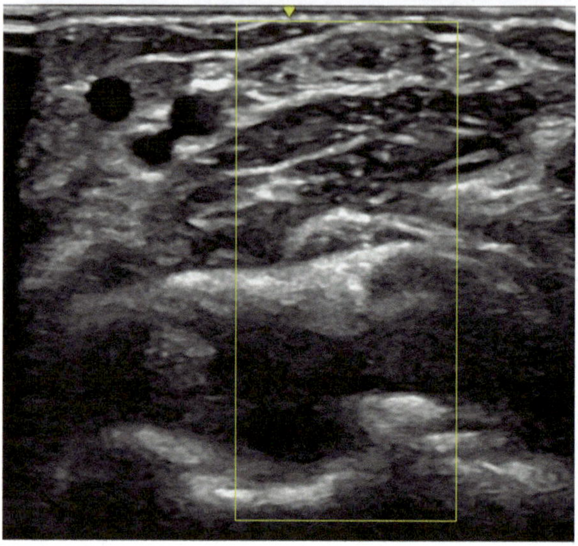

   (a) Compressibility
   (b) Varying echogenicity
   (c) Presence of Doppler signal
   (d) Displacement of fat pad
9. Select the option that can best optimize the visibility of the distal insertion of the biceps brachii tendon in this anterior longitudinal view of the elbow.

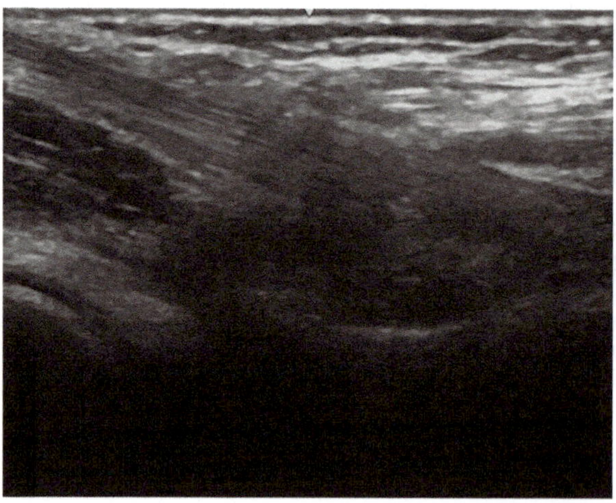

(a) Increasing the pressure at the distal end of the probe (heel-toe)
(b) Increasing the depth of the image
(c) Tilting the probe side to side (rock the probe)
(d) Decreasing the gain of the image

10. The following image of the posterior elbow longitudinal (left image) and transverse (right image) view is demonstrating?

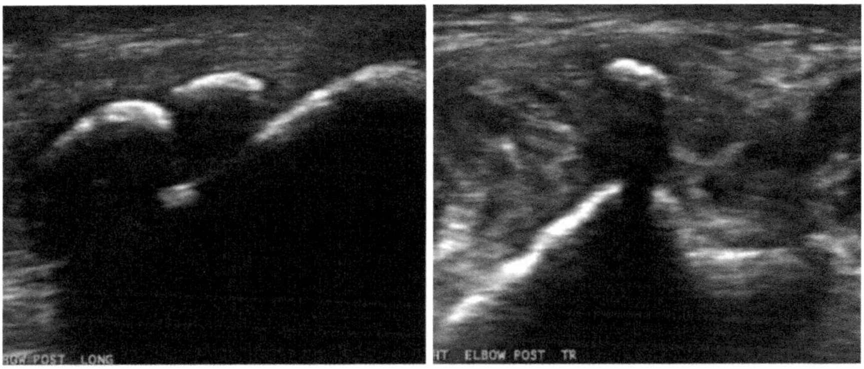

(a) Degenerative osteophyte
(b) Tendon enthesophyte
(c) Intra-articular loose body
(d) Double-contour sign: gout

Answers

1. (d) Coronoid fossa
2. (b)
3. (d) Homogeneous well-defined mass with hypoechoic center: rheumatoid nodule
4. (b)
5. (b) Brachialis muscle
6. (d) Varus stress
7. (b) Erosion at the tendon insertion
8. (c) Presence of Doppler signal
9. (a) Increasing the pressure at the distal end of the probe (heel-toe)
10. (c) Intra-articular loose body

References

1. Miles KA, Lamont AC. Ultrasonic demonstration of the elbow fat pads. Clin Radiol. 1989;40(6):602–4.
2. Jacobson J. Elbow ultrasound. In: Fundamentals in musculoskeletal ultrasound. 3rd ed. Philadelphia: Elsevier; 2017. p. 127–67.

3. De Smet AA, Winter TC, Best TM, Bernhardt DT. Dynamic sonography with valgus stress to assess elbow ulnar collateral ligament injury in baseball pitchers. Skeletal Radiol. 2002;31(11):671–6.
4. De Maeseneer M, Jacobson JA, Jaovisidha S, Lenchik L, Ryu KN, Trudell DR, Resnick D. Elbow effusions: distribution of joint fluid with flexion and extension and imaging implications. Invest Radiol. 1998;33(2):117–25.
5. Luukkainen R, Sanila MT, Saltyshev M, Huhtala H, Koski JM. Relationship between clinically detected joint swelling and effusion diagnosed by ultrasonography in elbow joints in patients with rheumatoid arthritis. Clin Rheumatol. 2005;24(3):228–31.
6. Wakefield RJ, Balint PV, Szkudlarek M, et al. Musculoskeletal ultrasound including definitions for ultrasonographic pathology. J Rheumatol. 2005;32(12):2485–7.
7. O'Neill J. The elbow. In: Musculoskeletal ultrasound: anatomy and technique. New York: Springer; 2008. p. 77–101.
8. Bruyn GA, Iagnocco A, Naredo E, et al. OMERACT definitions for ultrasonographic pathologies and elementary lesions of rheumatic disorders 15 years on. J Rheumatol. 2019;1. Epub ahead of print.
9. Thiele RG, Schlesinger N. Diagnosis of gout by ultrasound. Rheumatology. 2007;46(7):1116–21.
10. Cazenave T, Martire V, Reginato AM. Reliability of OMERACT ultrasound elementary lesions in gout: results from a multicenter exercise. Rheumatol Int. 2019;39(4):707–13.
11. Filipppou G, Scire C, Damjanov N, et al. Definition and reliability assessment of elementary ultrasonographic findings in calcium pyrophosphate deposition disease: a study by the OMERACT calcium pyrophosphate deposition disease ultrasound task force. J Rheumatol. 2017;44(2):1744–9.
12. Draghi F, Gregoli B, Sileo C. Sonography of the bicipitoradial bursa: a short pictorial essay. J Ultrasound. 2012;15(1):39–41.
13. Levin D, Nazarian LN, Miller TT, O'Kane PL, Feld RI, Parker L, McShane JM. Lateral epicondylitis of the elbow: US findings. Radiology. 2005;237(1):230–4.
14. Connell D, Burke F, Coombes P, et al. Sonographic examination of lateral epicondylitis. AJR Am JRoentgenol. 2001;176(3):777–82.
15. Konin GP, Nazarian LN, Walz DM. US of the elbow: indications, technique, normal anatomy, and pathologic conditions. Radiographics. 2013;33(4):E125.
16. Bianchi S, Martinoli C. Elbow. In: Bianchi S, Martinoli C, eds. Ultrasound of the musculoskeletal system, New York, : Springer, 2007; pp 349–408.
17. Balint PV, Kane D, Wilson H, McInnes IB, Sturrock RD. Ultrasonography of entheseal insertions in the lower limb in spondyloarthropathy. Ann Rheum Dis. 2002;61:905–10. 9.
18. Alcalde M, Acebes JC, Cruz M, Gonzalez-Hombrado L, Herrero-Beaumont G, Sanchez-Pernaute O. A Sonographic Enthesitic Index of lower limbs is a valuable tool in the assessment of ankylosing spondylitis. Ann Rheum Dis. 2007;66:1015–9.
19. de Miguel E, Cobo T, Muñoz-Fernández S, et al. Validity of enthesis ultrasound assessment in spondyloarthropathy. Ann Rheum Dis. 2009;68(2):169–74.
20. D'Agostino MA, Said-Nahal R, Hacquard-Bouder C, Brasseur JL, Dougados M, Breban M. Assessment of peripheral enthesitis in the spondyloarthropathies by ultrasonography combined with power Doppler. A cross-sectional study. Arthritis Rheum. 2003;48:523–33. 10.
21. Lerch K, Borisch N, Paetzel C, Grifka J, Hartung W. Sonographic evaluation of the elbow in rheumatoid arthritis: a classification of joint destruction. Ultrasound Med Biol. 2003;29(8):1131–5.
22. Guinsburg M, Ventura-Ríos L, Bernal A, Hernández-Díaz C, Pineda C. Usefulness, validity, and reliability of ultrasound in the diagnosis of osteoarthritis: a critical review of the literature. Gac Med Mex. 2013;149(5):509–20.
23. Nalbant S, Corominas H, Hsu B, Chen LX, Schumacher HR, Kitumnuaypong T. Ultrasonography for assessment of subcutaneous nodules. J Rheumatol. 2003;30(6):1191–5.

24. Chang KV, Wu WT, Han DS, Özçakar L. Ulnar nerve cross-sectional area for the diagnosis of cubital tunnel syndrome: a meta-analysis of ultrasonographic measurements. Arch Phys Med Rehabil. 2018;99(4):743–57.
25. Jacobson JA, Jebson PJ, Jeffers AW, Fessell DP, Hayes CW. Ulnar nerve dislocation and snapping triceps syndrome: diagnosis with dynamic sonography: report of three cases. Radiology. 2001;220(3):601–5.
26. Balint PV, Kane D, Hunter J, et al. Ultrasound guided versus conventional joint and soft tissue fluid aspiration in rheumatology practice; a pilot study. J Rheumatol. 2002;29(10):2209–13.
27. Kim TK, Lee JH, Park KD, et al. Ultrasound versus palpation guidance for intra-articular injections in patients with degenerative osteoarthritis of the elbow. J Clin Ultrasound. 2013;41(8):479–85.
28. McShane JM, Shah VN, Nazarian LN. Sonographically guided percutaneous needle tenotomy for treatment of common extensor tendinosis in the elbow: is a corticosteroid necessary? J Ultrasound Med. 2008;27(8):1137–44.
29. McShane JM, Nazarian LN, Harwood MI. Sonographically guided percutaneous needle tenotomy for treatment of common extensor tendinosis in the elbow. J Ultrasound Med. 2006;25(10):1281–9.
30. Yelland M, Rabago D, Ryan M, et al. Prolotherapy injections and physiotherapy used singly and in combination for lateral epicondylalgia: a single-blinded randomised clinical trial. BMC Musculoskelet Disord. 2019;20:509.
31. Shergill R, Choudur HN. Ultrasound-guided interventions in lateral epicondylitis. J Clin Rheumatol. 2019;25(3):e27–34.
32. Smidt N, van der Windt DA, Assendelft WJ, et al. Corticosteroid injections, physiotherapy, or a wait and see policy for lateral epicondylitis: a randomised controlled trial. Lancet. 2002;359(9307):657–62.

Ultrasound of the Shoulder

5

Midori Jane Nishio and Gurjit Singh Kaeley

Key Points

- Shoulder pain is common as an outpatient complaint.
- Ultrasound by an experienced operator or clinician can be as reliable as MRI or surgery in diagnosing common causes of shoulder pain.
- The shoulder ultrasound should be systematic and concentrate on structures that lend themselves to good ultrasound resolution.
- The cause of pain should not automatically be assigned to sonographic findings, but take into consideration the clinical history and other imaging information.
- Detailed scan of the shoulder requires an intimate knowledge of the sonoanatomy as well as the dynamic function of the shoulder.
- In order to depict many of the structures, the patient needs to be positioned in order to create sonographic windows to examine the relevant structure.

Introduction

Shoulder pain is a common complaint that prompts patients to seek care. In one estimate, it is the third most common musculoskeletal pain following low back and knee pain [1]. The rheumatologist will frequently need to decide if a shoulder complaint represents new activity of the rheumatic disorder versus other causes of pain.

M. J. Nishio (✉)
Rheumatology, Walnut Creek, CA, USA
e-mail: midori.nishio_md@johnmuirhealth.com

G. S. Kaeley
Division of Rheumatology, University of Florida College of Medicine, Jacksonville, FL, USA
e-mail: Gurjit.Kaeley@jax.ufl.edu

M. J. Kohler (ed.), *Musculoskeletal Ultrasound in Rheumatology Review*,
https://doi.org/10.1007/978-3-030-73555-5_5

Treatment recommendations also are more nuanced as mechanical and age-related shoulder conditions will co-exist with inflammatory pathology.

Ultrasound can be used to image many of the shoulder structures in high resolution without ionizing radiation. Ultrasound examination by the provider evaluating the complaint (point-of-care ultrasound) has the advantage of immediate correlation with historical and dynamic information. The goals of the rheumatologist using shoulder ultrasound are to provide insight into the likelihood that orthopedic intervention will improve the pain and functionality of the joint, to facilitate rheumatic diagnoses incorporating ultrasound definitions, and to reveal pathology that can be treated by the rheumatologist.

Many asymptomatic individuals have sonographic findings ranging from bursitis to rotator cuff alterations. It is therefore important not to assign the cause of pain to an abnormal structure without careful consideration of clinical findings [2]. Ultrasound of the shoulder does not image subcortical bone or give complete anatomic information about the joint; therefore, correlative plain X-rays will complement the examination especially in individuals with a history of trauma or who are more than 50 years old [3]. Subcortical pathology may require MRI or CT imaging as well. Orthopedic consultation may be required to complete treatment of a painful shoulder in some cases.

Shoulder pain evaluation benefits from a full systematic examination. The following chapter will describe the relevant sonoanatomy as well as techniques in acquiring these scans. Shoulder pathology relevant to rheumatic diagnoses will also be presented.

Sonoanatomy

The glenohumeral joint is a ball (head of the humerus) and socket (glenoid depression of the scapular and cartilaginous labral extension) joint. The joint volume appears to vary with height and sex but at baseline is estimated at 15–25 ml. In keeping with the relative lack of restrictive external ligaments, the joint volume can increase in pathologic states to over 100 ml [4].

Relevant bony landmarks are the lesser and greater tuberosities of the humerus separated by the bicipital groove (Fig. 5.1). The ultrasonographer uses these landmarks to locate the four rotator cuff tendon insertions and their muscles. As the joint is dynamically manipulated during scanning, the landmarks are always a reference point to standardize imaging (Fig. 5.2).

The subscapularis tendon inserts on the lesser tuberosity, while the supraspinatus, infraspinatus, and teres minor tendons insert on facets of the greater tuberosity.

The long head of the biceps tendon originates on the superior and posterior glenoid labrum and tubercle which is within the glenoid joint capsule and then exits the joint into the bicipital groove between the lesser and greater tuberosities (Figs. 5.1 and 5.3).

The humerus articulates with the glenoid concavity which is not well visualized by sonography. The edge of the joint and adjacent labrum, especially on the

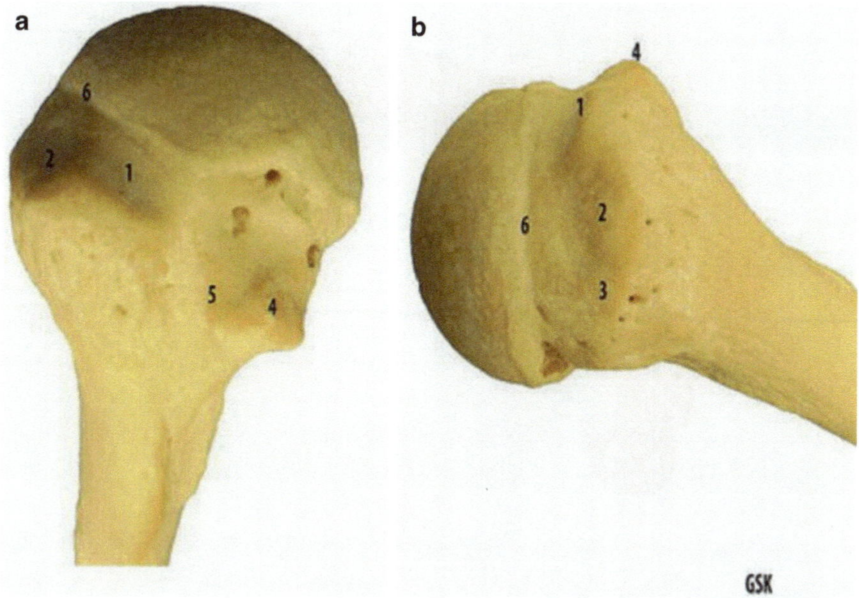

Fig. 5.1 Anatomy of the the shoulder. **(a)** Superolateral view of the humerus. **(b)** Posterior view of the humerus. Greater tuberosity facets: *1*—supraspinatus insertion, *2*—infraspinatus insertion, *3*—teres minor insertion. Lessor tuberosity facet: *4*—lesser tuberosity and insertion for subscapularis, 5—bicipital groove, *6*—anatomical neck

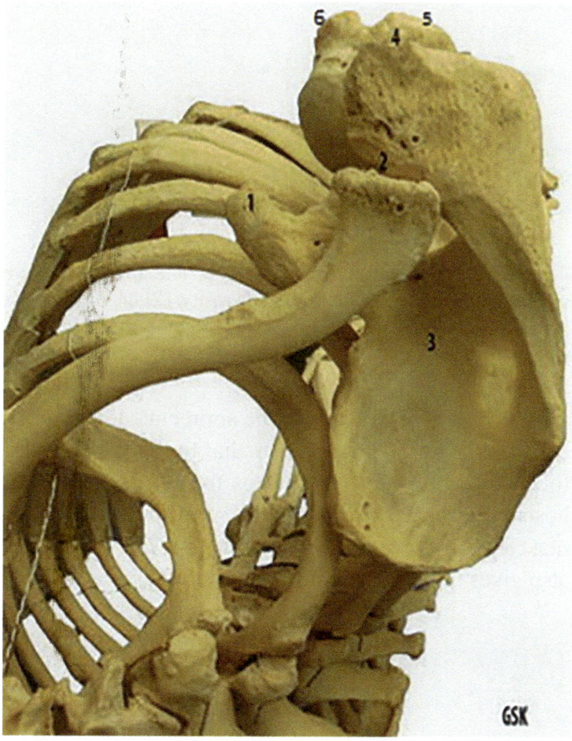

Fig. 5.2 Shoulder Bone Anatomy. Superior view of the shoulder complex. (1) Coracoid process, (2) acromio-clavicular joint, (3) suprascapular fossa and origin for supraspinatus, (4) acromion, (5) greater tuberosity (6) lessor tuberosity

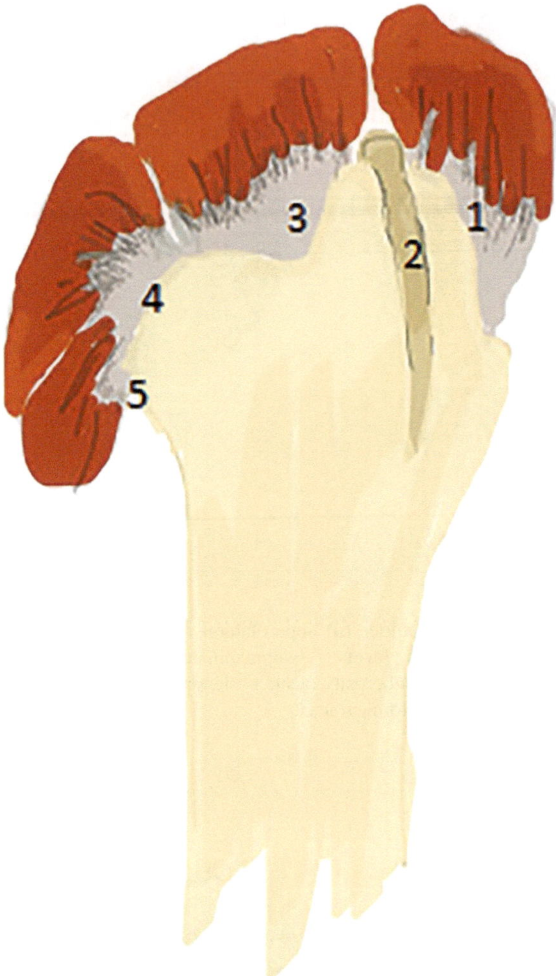

Fig. 5.3 Rotator Cuff Anatomy. Anterior lateral view of the rotator cuff tendon insertions. (1) subscapularis tendon at the lessor tuberosity, (2) bicipital groove and long head of the biceps tendon, (3) supraspinatus tendon at the anterior greater tuberosity facet, (4) infraspinatus tendon at the posterior greater tuberosity facet, (5) teres minor insertion

posterior joint, however, can be appreciated. An important anterior landmark is the coracoid process which lies medial to the lesser tuberosity and is the site of origin for the short head of the biceps muscle as well as coracobrachialis. The scapula hosts superiorly the origin of the supraspinatus muscle, anteriorly the subscapularis muscle, and posteriorly the infraspinatus and teres minor muscles. Posteriorly, it also gives the origin to the posterolateral portions of the deltoid muscle.

Standard Scanning Protocol

Standard scans of the shoulder have been described by several international groups, and shoulder scanning has been the subject of multiple publications. The protocols vary in their emphasis on mechanical and overuse or traumatic causes of symptoms. The following approach is described for the purposes of an outpatient, rheumatic-oriented scan that can reveal soft tissue pathology and also inform the rheumatologist about the presence of inflammatory pathology (Table 5.1) in a stepwise, time efficient approach.

This approach allows the ultrasonographer to efficiently position the patient working from the front of the patient, over the top of the shoulder, to the back of the shoulder and lastly to reposition into the appropriate positions to view the supraspinatus tendon enthesis. It is desirable that a sonographer adopt the sequence of the scans to an individual protocol to reinforce completion of a minimum number of standard scans. In this fashion, the rotator cuff tendons, the subdeltoid bursa, the long head of the biceps tendon, the glenohumeral joint space, and the acromioclavicular joint can be assessed for the majority of reasons for shoulder pain in a rheumatology clinic (Fig. 5.4).

Additional views which can be added are included in Table 5.2.

Anterior Transverse and Longitudinal Scans: Biceps Tendon and Subscapularis Tendon

It is essential that the patient be correctly in a neutral position at the start of the scan (Fig. 5.4). The patient is seated with the corresponding elbow bent to 90 degrees and

Table 5.1 Standard ultrasound scans for commonly encountered pathology causing shoulder pain

Ultrasound scan view	Positioning	Structure
Anterior transverse – Biceps	Neutral position	Biceps tendon at bicipital groove-transverse axis, transverse ligament
Anterior longitudinal – Biceps	Neutral position	Long head of biceps tendon Longitudinal axis
Anterior longitudinal – subscapularis	External rotation	Subscapularis tendon Longitudinal axis
Anterior transverse – subscapularis	External rotation	Subscapularis tendon Transverse axis
Acromioclavicular joint	Superior longitudinal	Acromioclavicular joint
Posterior longitudinal	Internal rotation	Infraspinatus tendon in longitudinal axis
	External rotation	Posterior glenohumeral joint Transverse to joint
Anterior longitudinal supraspinatus	Crass or modified crass	Supraspinatus tendon Longitudinal axis
Anterior transverse supraspinatus	Modified Crass or Crass	Supraspinatus tendon Transverse axis

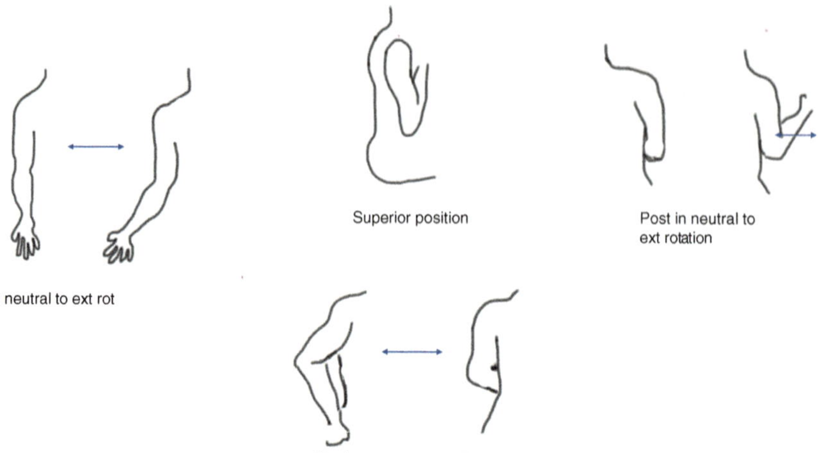

Fig. 5.4 Patient Positioning

Table 5.2 Supplemental ultrasound scans for specific diagnoses

Ultrasound scan view	Positioning	Structure
Dynamic impingement	Probe placed lateral to acromioclavicular joint with active abduction of the arm (dynamic maneuver)	Demonstration of possible impingement of subdeltoid bursa
Posterior transverse	Internal or external rotation	Teres minor transverse and infraspinatus transverse
Axillary-longitudinal	With patient lying down, arm above the head to give access to axilla	Glenohumeral joint
Suprascapular notch – transverse	Internal or neutral rotation	Suprascapular nerve
Anterior medial with probe longitudinal to subscapularis (transverse position on body)	External rotation	Anterior glenohumeral joint anterior and subcoracoid bursa/recess

placed on the ribs with the palm facing up. From this position, the sonographer is able to move the forearm into external rotation while keeping the elbow at the ribs, thus eliminating introduction of oblique views.

The neutral and external rotation positions are useful to create the most advantageous patient position to help the sonographer to locate the landmark of the bicipital groove and then to reveal the subscapularis tendon (Figs. 5.5 and 5.6). The following steps illustrate an efficient approach to the anterior shoulder ultrasound exam.

Evaluating the image while moving from neutral to external rotation will also help clarify areas of subscapularis tendon anisotropy vs. true tendon pathology. Cortical irregularities underlying the tendon are often observed at this site and are not currently correlated with clinically significant rotator cuff pathology. It can also

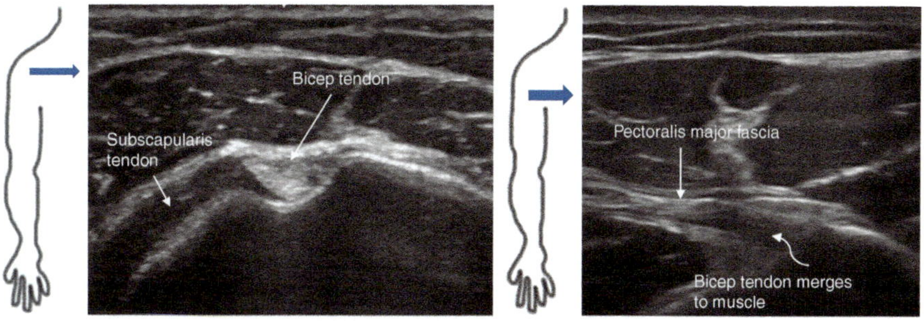

Fig. 5.5 Transverse Long Head of the Biceps Tendon (Step 1). Patient positioning for the anterior biceps tendon scan has the patient seated with elbow flexed, shoulder in neutral position, and palm up. It is important that the bicipital groove is orientated anteriorly, and placing the patient's hand on the thigh will result in some internal rotation, making the exam more difficult. The probe is first placed in short axis over the greater and lesser tuberosities proximally and then gradually swept down to the level of the pectoralis major insertion. It is important to rock the probe to overcome anisotropy. If fluid or tissue thickening is detected, then power Doppler should be employed. Finally, the probe should be placed at the level of the tuberosities in transverse view, and patient asked to internally and externally rotate the arm. Attention should be paid to see if there is subluxation of the biceps tendon. If it is subluxed, its position relative to the subscapularis tendon should be noted

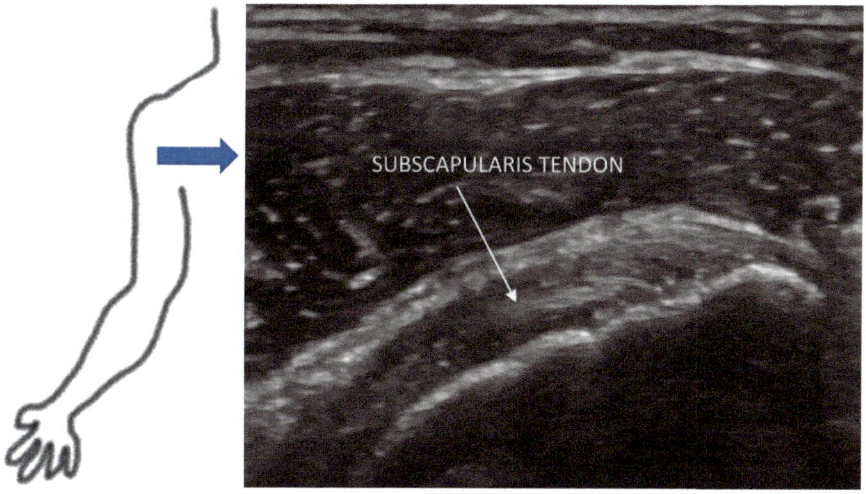

Fig. 5.6 Longitudianl Subscapularis Tendon (Step 2). The subscapularis tendon is a multipennate muscle which originates from the anterior aspect of the scapula. In neutral position, most of the tendon is oblique and not visible by sonography. The patient needs to be placed in external rotation in order to view the tendon. It is advisable that the patient is asked to internally and externally rotate the arm to inspect for sub-coracoid impingement as well as presence of fluid in the sub-coracoid bursa or the subacromial subdeltoid bursa. Since the axis of the tendon insertion is horizontal, the probe postion from Step 1 transverse to the bicep tendons will actually be in the longitudianl axis of the subscapularis tendon. The tendon inserts upon the lesser tuberosity in a beak-like fashion

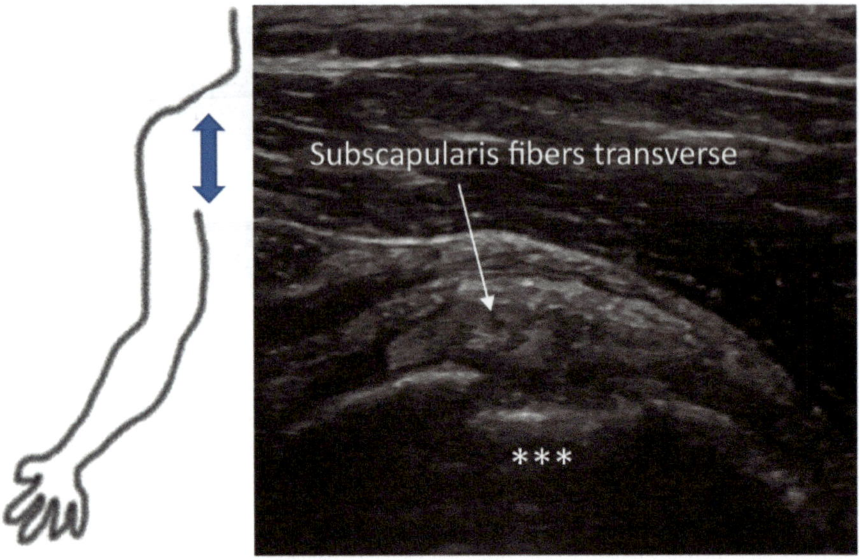

Fig. 5.7 Subscapularis Tendon Transverse (Step 3). The probe is rotated into a sagittal plane to view the tendon in transverse axis. The probe should be rocked to overcome anisotropy of the tendon fibers which are formed within the multipennate muscle. *** indicates a symptomatic cortical irregularity

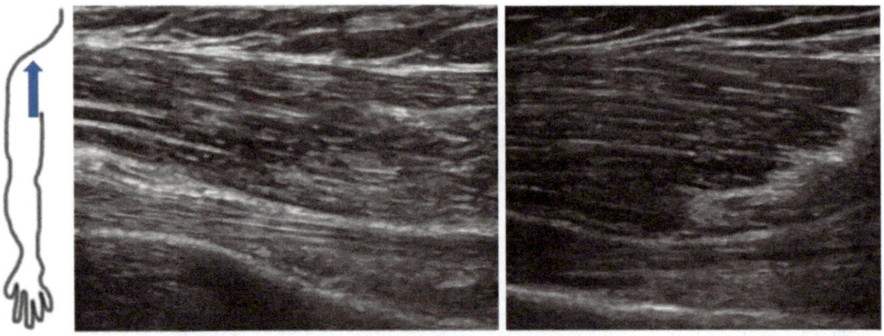

Fig. 5.8 Long Head of the Biceps Tendon (Step 4). Continuing the medial to lateral sweep of the probe will reveal the medial border of the bicipital groove, then the biceps tendon in its longitudinal axis lying in the groove itself. In long axis, in addition to placing the probe in the intertubercular groove, there is an additional requirement of heel-toeing the probe in order to make it parallel to the tendon. The tendon should be followed to the musculotendinous junction. As in the transverse view, power Doppler should be employed if fluid or tissue thickening is detected. The long head of the biceps tendon exits the glenohumeral joint capsule as it sits in the bicipital groove of the humerus. The tendon is anchored to the superior and posterior glenoid labrum and the supraglenoid tubercle. It runs through the glenohumeral joint: thus, as it exits the joint into the groove, it will carry a reflection of the joint capsule with it. Where there is a glenohumeral joint process, this anterior reflection can be enlarged and easily seen (Figs. 5.8 and 5.9). This joint capsular reflection will taper off giving a clear impression of its relationship to joint rather than a separate tendon sheath

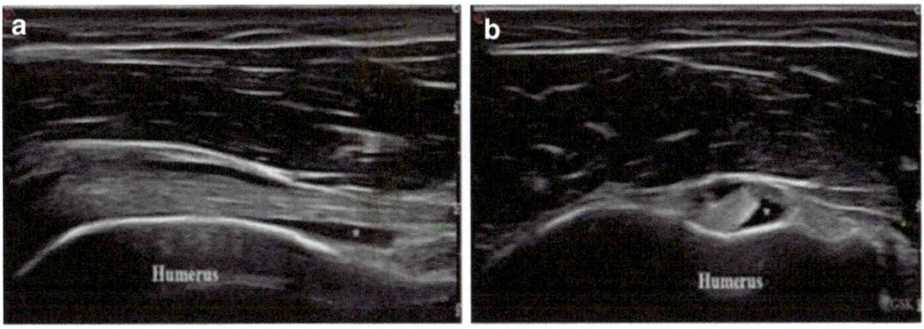

Fig. 5.9 Fluid around the proximal biceps tendon consistent with tenosynovitis. Glenohumeral joint effusion surrounding the biceps tendon as it exits from joint cavity

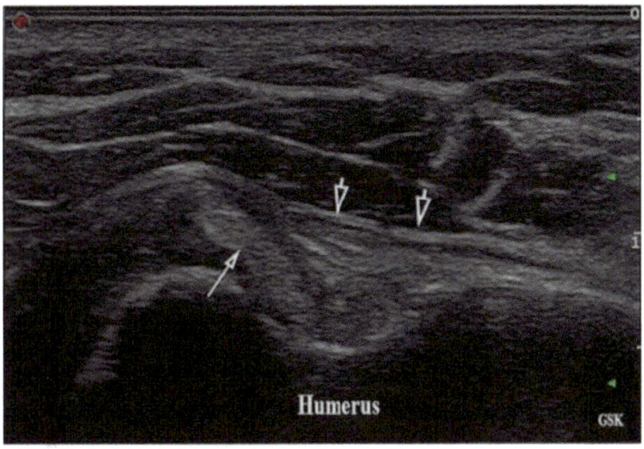

Fig. 5.10 Subluxation of the Biceps Tendon. Biceps tendon subluxation (long arrow). Note partial discontinuity of the transverse humeral ligament medially (arrow heads)

reveal subluxation of the biceps tendon due to damage to the stabilizing ligaments of the rotator cuff interval. In these views, the sonographer can also see the anterior portion of the subdeltoid bursa. The bursa may be variably thickened and should also be assessed at the border between the deltoid muscle and the underlying rotator cuff structures. The probe should be swept superiorly and inferiorly to inspect all of the tendon (Fig. 5.7).

The biceps tendon is anchored in the groove by the coracohumeral ligament and the superior glenohumeral ligament. These ligaments merge with the external joint capsule of the shoulder joint and are closely associated with stabilizing the biceps tendon as well as the joint. While trauma can disrupt the external shoulder capsular ligaments acutely, the more gradual processes of inflammatory arthritis and aging can also contribute to tearing of these ligaments [6]. The biceps tendon is subluxed when it overlies the tip of the lesser tuberosity (Fig. 5.9), and it is dislocated when it is out of the bicipital groove (Fig. 5.10). When the coracohumeral ligament is torn and the subscapularis tendon is intact, the tendon can dislocate superficial to the subscapularis. However, if the subscapularis tendon and the coracohumeral ligament are both torn, then the biceps tendon may be displaced deep to the remaining subscapularis fibers (Fig. 5.11). Abnormal movement of the biceps tendon implies dysfunction of the anatomic rotator cuff interval. The interval is relevant as a

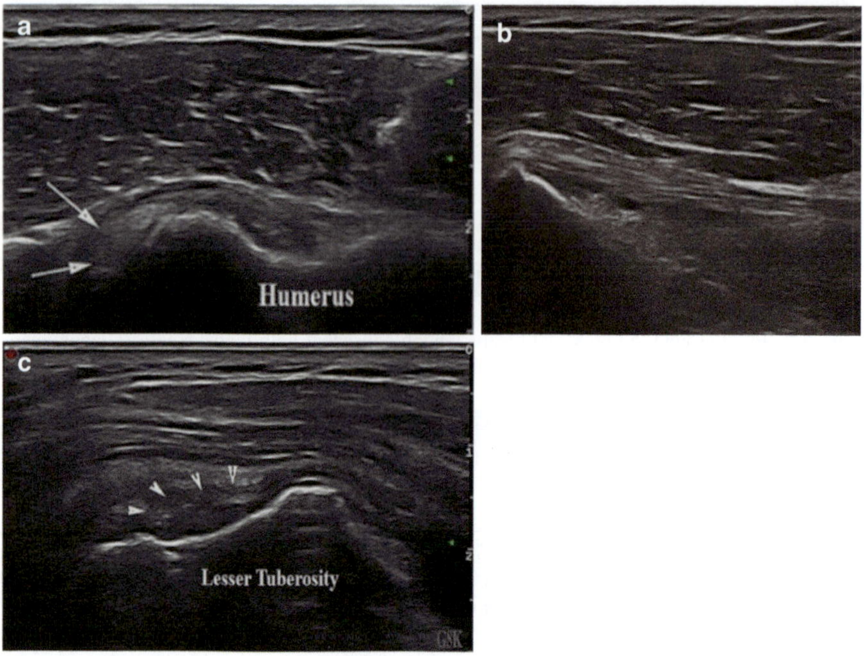

Fig. 5.11 Displacement of the Biceps Tendon. (**a**) Biceps tendon dislocation seen in short (long arrows) and (**b**) long axis, with accompanying subscapularis tear (**c**) depicted by arrowheads

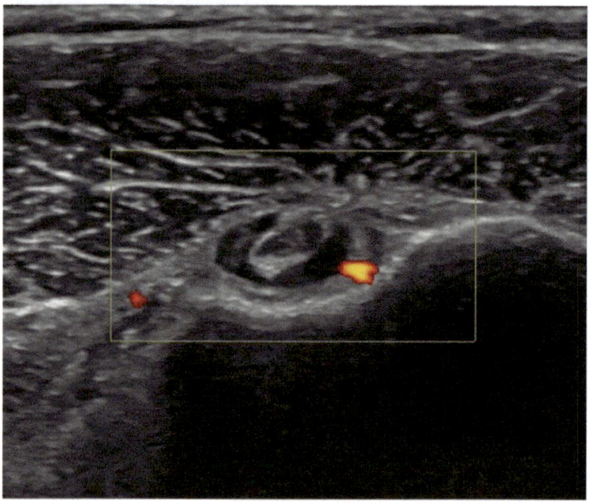

Fig. 5.12 Circumflex humeral artery Doppler signal in the bicipital groove. Although there is an anechoic collection around the bicep tendon, the visualized vessel is in the expected position for the anterior lateral branch of the anterior circumflex artery supplying the biceps tendon

repairable anatomic brake to glenohumeral motion, and awareness of its impact on normal shoulder range of motion comes from the orthopedic literature [7].

For the rheumatologist, color power Doppler assessment of pathology can always be added bearing in mind that vascularity of joint synovium in this location has not been specifically studied as a predictor of natural history in this location (Figs. 5.12 and 5.13).

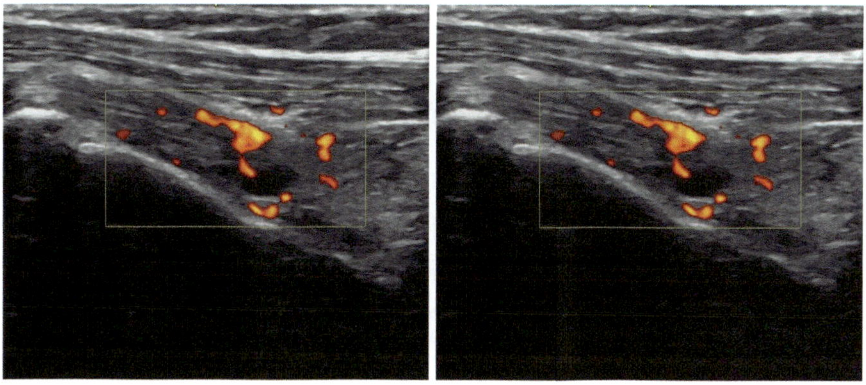

Fig. 5.13 Pathologic Doppler signal of the biceps tendon. Pathologic Doppler signal associated with the biceps tendon is seen in the bicipital groove. Transverse and longitudinal views of Doppler positive synovitis in the biceps tendon sheath related to glenohumeral synovitis of the shoulder in a rheumatoid arthritis patient

Superior Scan: Acromioclavicular Joint

The acromioclavicular (AC) joint can easily be scanned after the initial anterior scans with the patient in the same neutral position. The probe is placed in front of the clavicle in the anterior transverse position and drawn up over the top of the shoulder into a superior coronal location over the joint where a view of the acromioclavicular articulation is revealed. Taking advantage of sweeping motions while scanning eliminates having to stop to palpate for anatomic landmarks. Developing the skill of orienting the probe footprint over the structure of interest can be enhanced if the sonographer scans a continuous area rather than interrupting the scan by taking the probe off the patient (Fig. 5.14).

The AC joint has a firm meniscus in its normal state which can degenerate and extrude leaving a potential pathway into the overlying soft tissue for subacromial pathology to collect. If the underlying supraspinatus tendon is ruptured and there is a chronic, inflammatory process of the shoulder joint, a synovial collection can track through this joint. The external Geyser sign is an example of this [8]. Crystalline deposits can also be seen in the meniscus of the joint (Fig. 5.15). The most common changes to be seen at this joint are degenerative changes depicted by bordering osteophytes, although spondyloarthropathies and rheumatoid arthritis can develop inflammatory synovitis in this joint.

AC joint instability can be demonstrated by positioning the patient's arm from the neutral position to across their chest with the hand reaching for the opposite shoulder. Widening of the joint can be appreciated by contralateral comparison (Fig. 5.16). Further assessment of AC joint separation requires orthopedic consultation.

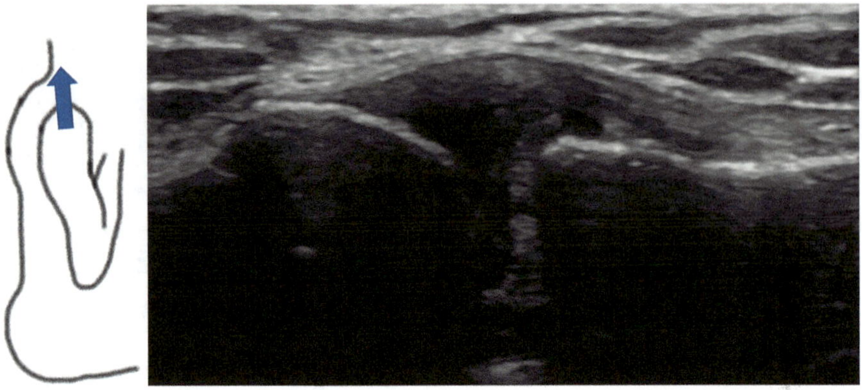

Fig. 5.14 Acromioclavicular Joint Transverse (Step 5). Superior scans: The acromioclavicular joint can be visualized by placing the probe superiorly on the acromioclavicular joint in a coronal plane. The joint is inspected for smooth cortical margins as well as a homogeneous interosseous portion

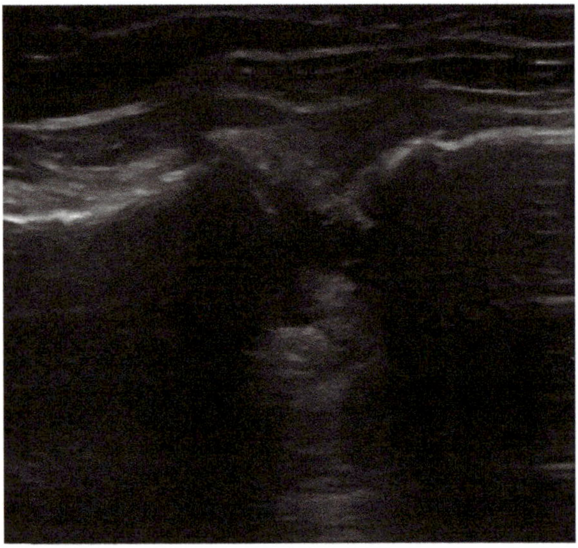

Fig. 5.15 Crystalline deposits in acromioclavicular joint. Hyperechoic deposit in the acromioclavicular meniscus in a patient with advanced shoulder osteoarthritis

Posterior Longitudinal Scans in Internal and External Rotation: Infraspinatus Tendon, Posterior Glenohumeral Joint, and Posterior Labrum

The examination is continued from the top of the shoulder and acromioclavicular joint to the posterior and lateral areas of the shoulder by continuing the sweep with the ultrasound probe.

The posterior scans are important for visualization of the infraspinatus, posterior recess, posterior glenoid labrum, as well as surface of the humerus. The neutral

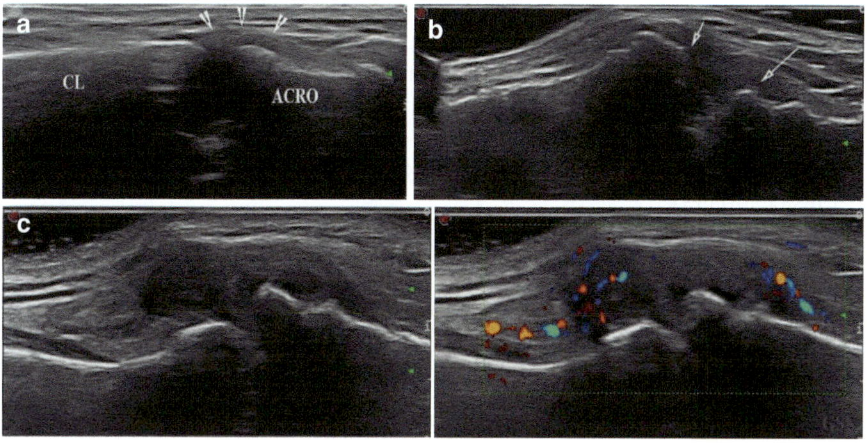

Fig. 5.16 Acromioclavicular Joint Pathology. (**a**) Normal acromioclavicular joint formed by the articulation of the clavicle (CL) and acromion (ACRO). Arrowheads delineate the capsule. (**b**) Osteoarthritic acromioclavicular joint with bony proliferation and osteophyte formation (arrows). (**c**) B-mode and power Doppler of synovial hypertrophy at the acromioclavicular joint

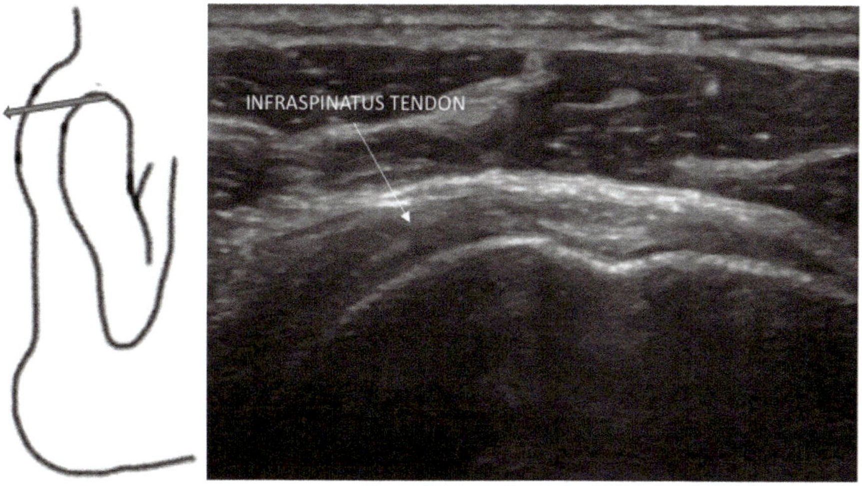

Fig. 5.17 Infraspinatus Tendon Longitudinal (Step 6). From the superior acromioclavicular location the probe is moved behind the shoulder joint where a transverse view of the glenohumeral joint is identified as well as a view of the infraspinatus tendon. The probe is then moved laterally along the long axis of the infraspinatus tendon to find its insertion. The infraspinatus tendon inserts on the middle facet of the greater tuberosity

position with the arm adducted is used. The probe is placed obliquely with the medial edge of the probe slightly caudal to visualize the bony landmarks of the posterior humeral head and glenoid. The probe is slid anterolaterally to examine the infraspinatus insertion (Fig. 5.17).

The infraspinatus is then observed dynamically by rotating the shoulder from neutral to external rotation and back. During this motion, attention to bursal distension, tendon calcifications, and infraspinatus tearing are the focus of the scan. The humeral surface should be inspected for depressions or erosions. The presence of a shallow wedge-shaped defect just proximal to the infraspinatus insertion suggests a Hill-Sachs lesion which occurs due to osteochondral compression in anterior shoulder dislocation [9].

The probe is recentered transversely over the glenohumeral joint to inspect its posterior recess and posterior labrum. The labrum appears as a homogeneous, hyperechoic triangular structure. A 2-mm hypoechoic zone at the base of the labrum may be seen in normal individuals. If the labrum cannot be viewed sufficiently, then the patient is asked to place the hand on the contralateral shoulder, thus stretching the structures and enabling better view of the labrum (Fig. 5.18). The adjacent spinoglenoid notch should also be examined for the presence of a paralabral cyst which occurs most commonly in this location [10].

The posterior recess is constituted by a loose capsule posteriorly. In the presence of fluid, the capsule is lifted superficially. While performing external rotation, the area directly anterior to the glenoid labrum should be observed (Fig. 5.18). In the presence of fluid, the infraspinatus tendon can be displaced by a hypoechoic collection (Fig. 5.19). The normal value of the maximal perpendicular distension in external rotation has historically been described as less than 3 mm [11]. The sensitivity of ultrasound in detecting a glenohumeral joint effusion compared to MRI arthrography at the posterior location has been estimated at 100% [12].

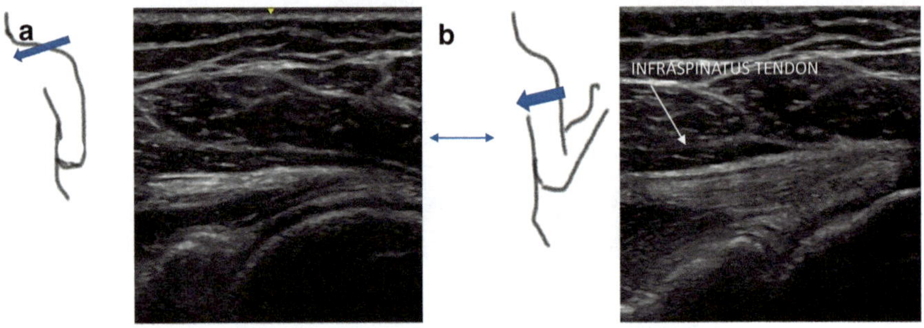

Fig. 5.18 Glenohumeral Joint Posterior Transverse (Step 7). The probe is moved medially after examing the infraspinatus tendon and recentered over the posterior glenohumeral joint. The view is transverse to the joint. The medial edge of the probe can be moved slightly caudal so the probe is in a shallow oblique angle to visualize the glenoid and labrum optimally. In (**a**), the shoulder is in a neutral position. In (**b**), the shoulder is in external rotation. Note the labral borders, position of the infraspinatus inferior border, and lack of a hypoechoic collection around the labrum or displacing the infraspinatus tendon by performing dynamic scanning of the joint. The infraspinatus tendon inferior border, superior joint capsule line, and subtle pattern changes in the infraspinatus muscle must be used to appreciate bulging of a joint collection

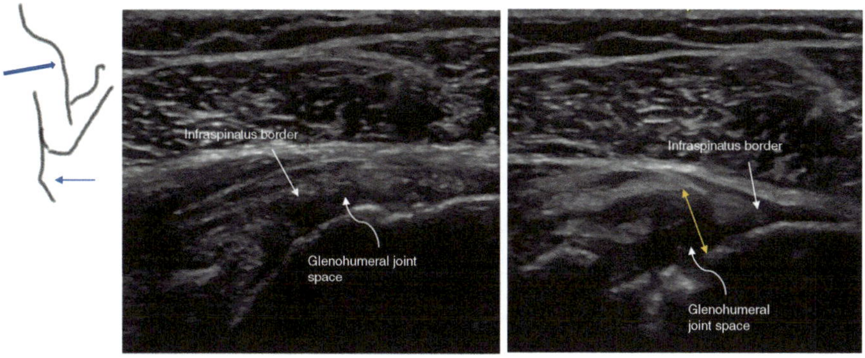

Fig. 5.19 Evaluation of Joint Effusion. Posterior joint effusion revealed by external rotation. A hypoechoic bisected space representing effusion forms around the labrum with external rotation of the glenohumeral joint

Anterior Longitudinal and Transverse Supraspinatus Tendon Scans: Supraspinatus Tendon and Subacromial Bursa

In neutral position, the supraspinatus tendon is largely hidden by the acromion. By extending and internally rotating the humerus, the greater tuberosity can be brought anterior to the acromion to allow examination of the supraspinatus tendons. Two standard positions are available which vary the degrees of tension upon the supraspinatus tendon. In the Crass position, the patient is asked to place the hand as far as they can reach in the lower back, although this may not be possible for some patients. The modified Crass position, where the palm of the hand is placed on the upper gluteal region and elbow tucked posteriorly, is achievable by most patients (Fig. 5.20). It is important to note that due to the variability of patient positioning, the starting positions of the probes are a guide, and probe adjustment may be necessary to obtain true orthogonal views of the supraspinatus tendon.

The supraspinatus tendon needs to be examined in orthogonal planes as well as sweeping over all the available tendon. The longitudinal scan is started medially. If the biceps tendon can be visualized, it is used to ensure that the probe is parallel to it and then to the supraspinatus tendon. The probe is then slid posteriorly to image the longitudinal fibrillar attachment to the superior facet of the greater tuberosity. Care must be taken to overcome anisotropy of the distal fibers by heel-toeing the probe (Fig. 5.21). As the probe is slid posteriorly over the surface of the supraspinatus tendon, it is important to continue to visualize the curved portion of the humeral head at the same time as seeing the greater tuberosity to ensure that the probe is parallel to the tendon (Fig. 5.22).

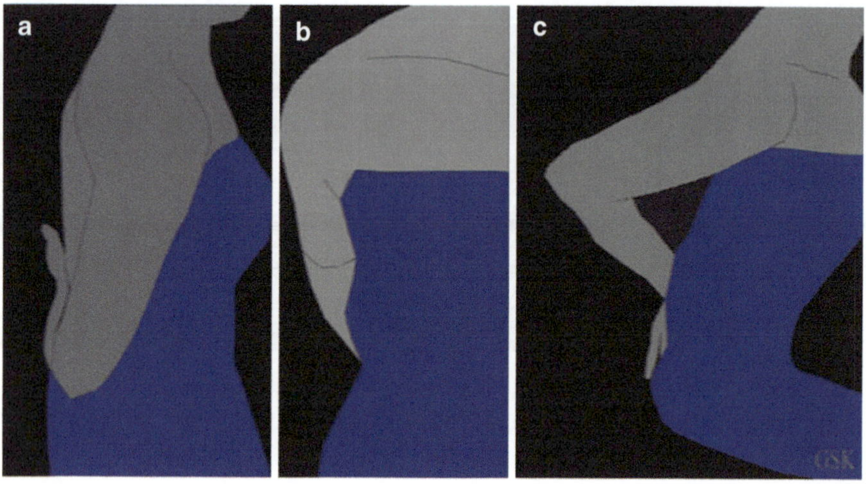

Fig. 5.20 Pictorial images of crass positioning for the supraspinatus tendon. (**a**) Full Crass position. (**b**) Anterior view of full Crass position. (**c**) Modified Crass position. Note the supraspinatus tendon insertion will be brought forward out from under the acromio-clavicular shadow

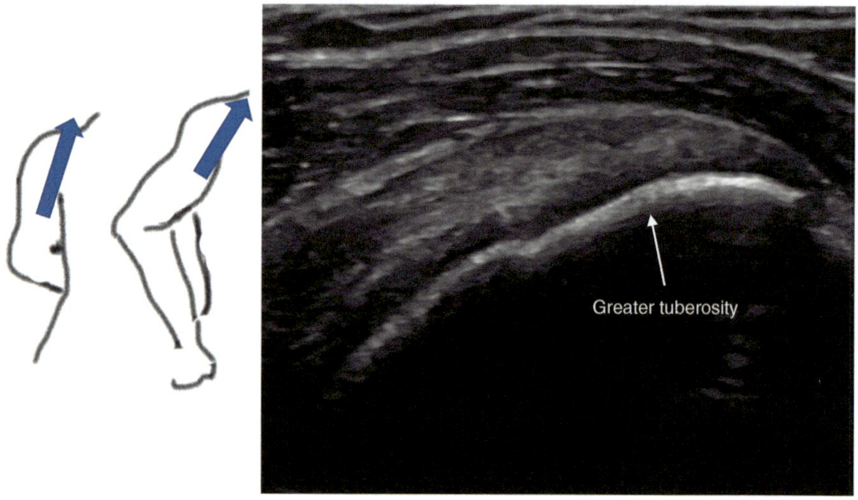

Fig. 5.21 Supraspinatus Tendon Longitudinal (Step 8). In the Crass or modified Crass position the probe is oriented longitudinally or in line with the direction of the tendon fibers with the medial pedge of the probe roughly pointing towards the ipsilateral ear. The Crass position increases tension on the supraspinatus tendon accentuating the appearance of tears

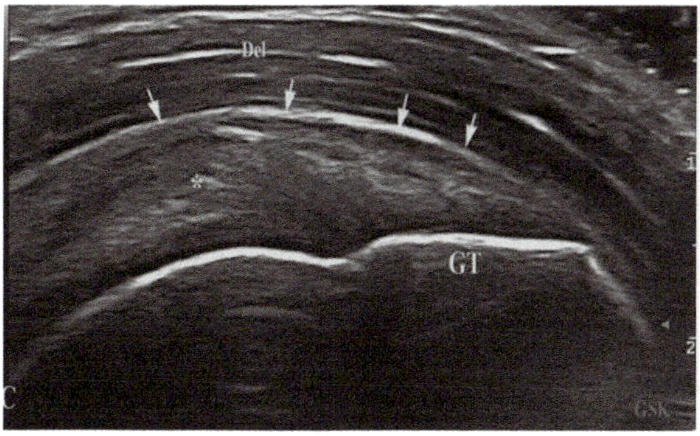

Fig. 5.22 Posterior Supraspinatus Tendon Longitudinal. Crass view of supraspinatus tendon in longitudinal axis. The probe is swept from the anterior (bicep tendon) border posteriorly. Posteriorly the angle of the greater tuberosity (GT) flattens and overlapping fibers of the infraspinatus appear (*). Note the deltoid muscle (Del) and peribursal fat stripe (arrows)

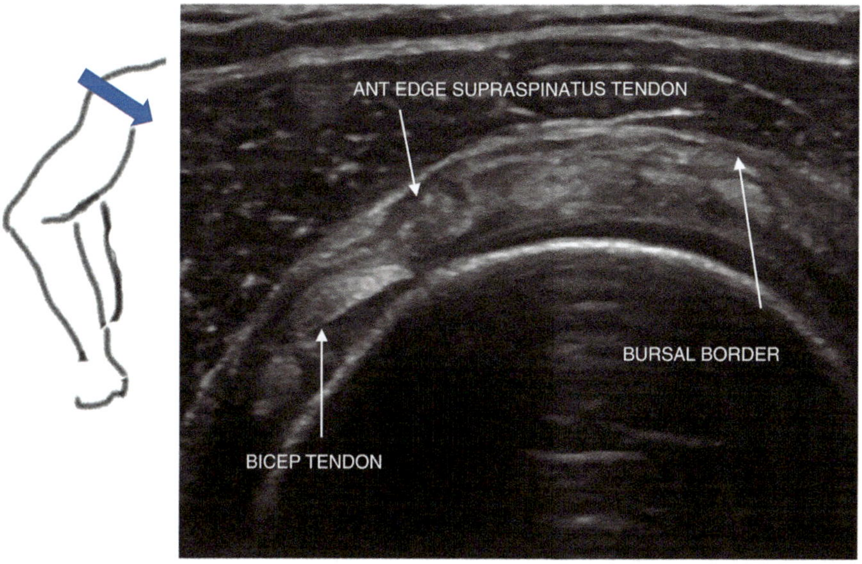

Fig. 5.23 Supraspinatus Tendon Transverse in Modified CRASS (step 9). The transverse view of the supraspinatus tendon requires the probe to be placed obliquely on the anterior superior humerus while the patient is in the modified CRASS position. This is best acheived by inspecting the top of the shoulder and visualizing the course of the tendon from its suprascapular origin to its insertion on the humerus. The probe is placed across the tendon with the medial edge of the probe pointed towards the nipple. With the hand fixed, the patient's elbow can be moved in an anterior-posterior arc to reveal the biceps tendon and true anterior edge of the supraspinatus tendon. The importance of identifying the supraspinatus tendon at the medial border for tearing cannot be overlooked [5] (Fig. 5.23)

The probe needs to be swept proximally and distally. As the probe is swept distally, it is important to also note the change in the shape of the bone (Fig. 5.24). The probe can be moved posteriorly until the junction of the infraspinatus tendon which can be recognized by anisotropy due to fiber interdigitation. The width of the

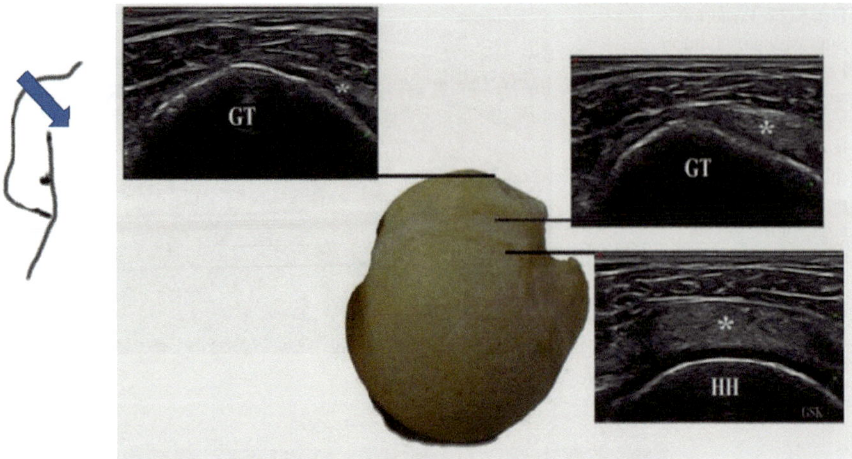

Fig. 5.24 Transverse supraspinatus tendon caudad to cranial

supraspinatus tendon is reported to be between 13 and 15 mm [9, 13]. If the supraspinatus tear exceeds this dimension, then the infraspinatus needs to also be examined carefully for extension of rotator cuff tear.

Examination of the supraspinatus tendon should be systematic with inspection of the bursal layer to inspect for signs of deltoid or bursal depression, evaluation of the tendon substance for tears, and calcification. The articular portion should also be evaluated for tears and finally the insertion and smoothness of the cortex at the greater tuberosity. The presence of overlying subacromial/subdeltoid bursitis should be noted. The supraspinatus is vital to shoulder abduction. In the initiation of abduction, it acts as a humeral depressor to allow the greater tuberosity to clear under the humerus. The shoulder can be examined for external impingement by placing the probe on the lateral aspect of the shoulder and asking the patient to abduct the arm. Smooth excursion of the greater tuberosity underneath the acromion should be observed. If the patient is unable to clear the greater tuberosity, or has pain then impingement may be occurring.

Sonopathology

Long Head Biceps Tendon

Bicipital Tendon Sheath Effusion

The long head of the biceps originates from the intra-articular supraglenoid tubercle and glenoid labrum and has a synovial sheath that extends from the articular joint capsule as a reflection into the bicipital groove leaving a bare tendon to join the musculotendinous junction at the pectoralis major. Fluid may be found in the sheath, which may be dependent and occur inferiorly, hence the importance of

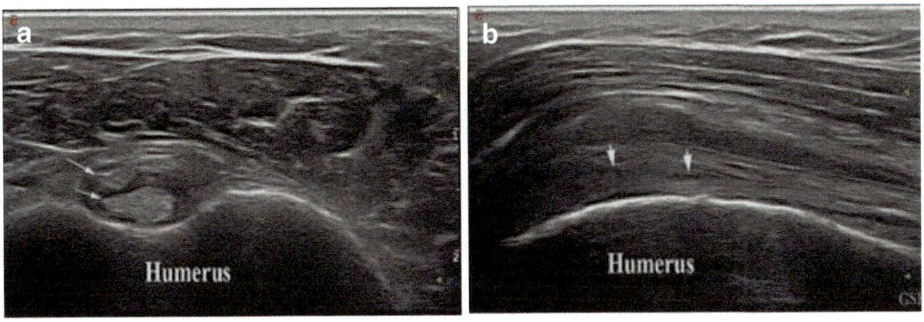

Fig. 5.25 Biceps tendon tear. Biceps tendon splitting seen in short (long arrows) and long axis (arrow heads), with surrounding tenosynovial fluid

systematically scanning distal to the bicipial groove to the pectoralis major insertion (Fig. 5.9). The biceps tendon sheath has been found to have 97% sensitivity as a site supporting the presence of a joint effusion compared to a gold standard of MR arthrography [12].

Although some authors suggest that biceps tendon sheath fluid may correlate with various shoulder pathologies [14, 15] as noted earlier, many subjects can have asymptomatic findings on shoulder US examination [2]. It is prudent to carefully examine the shoulder for other pathologies since bicipital tenosynovitis rarely occurs in isolation [15]. The presence of power Doppler in the tendon sheath suggests an inflammatory etiology to the effusion as power Doppler signal is not often seen in purely degenerative processes [16] (Fig. 5.12).

Biceps Tendon Tears

Biceps tendon tears may occur at the level of the intertubercular groove, at the musculotendinous junctions, or in subjects that use anabolic steroids at the tendon labrum junction [17]. If the tendon is ruptured at the level of intertubercular groove, it may not fully retract due to the presence of vinculae (band of connective tissue arising from mesotendon) [18]. Clues to a tendon tear include loss of fibrillar echotexture especially on long-axis viewing and presence of fluid at the distal musculotendinous junction. Only rarely is an empty bicipital groove depicted. Biceps tendon splitting can also be depicted (Fig. 5.25).

Rotator Cuff

Rotator Cuff Tears

Rotator cuff alterations are commonly encountered in painful shoulders. Ultrasound by experienced operators can depict full and partial thickness tears with high accuracy compared to MRI or operative findings [5]. Chronic rotator cuff tears lead to muscle atrophy. Compared to MRI, ultrasound is also relatively reliable in depicting muscle atrophy based on its hyperechoic appearance [19]. The supraspinatus is the most common tendon affected by tears. It has a relatively avascular distal tendon. Most of the degenerative tears occur 15–16 mm posterior to the biceps tendon, near the infraspinatus and supraspinatus junction [20]. Tears larger than 20 mm should prompt a careful examination of the other rotator cuff tendons for tears. The definitions of tendon tears are given in Table 5.3. Image examples of tears can be seen in Figs. 5.26, 5.27, and 5.28. If the patient is a surgical candidate, then the location, size in two planes of the tear, and distance from the biceps tendon should be recorded as well as the echogenicity of the relevant rotator cuff muscle.

Tendon fiber discontinuity is the most reliable sign of a tendon tear and is best seen in the presence of fluid in the joint. The presence of fluid may also give rise to an interface sign (Fig. 5.28). Tears of the supraspinatus are also associated with greater tuberosity irregularity. In an ultrasound study of 50 consecutive shoulders, the presence of joint fluid and greater tuberosity irregularity had the most reliability in diagnosing a full-thickness supraspinatus tendon tear. The presence of greater tuberosity cortical irregularity, interface sign, or tendon nonvisualization were the most important findings in diagnosing full- or partial-thickness tears [21].

Scanning through the anterior to posterior width of the supraspinatus tendon is necessary to show the extent of the tear (see Fig. 5.29).

Table 5.3 Shoulder tendon tear definitions

Type of tear	Definition
Complete tear	All the tendon substance is absent (Fig. 5.26)
Full-thickness tear	The tear extends from the bursal surface to the articular surface (Fig. 5.27)
Partial thickness Tear	Bursal – volume loss on the bursal side of the tendon often with deltoid and bursal invagination Articular – volume loss at the articular portion of the tendon (Fig. 5.28)
Rim rent tear	Tear at the footprint of the tendon insertion

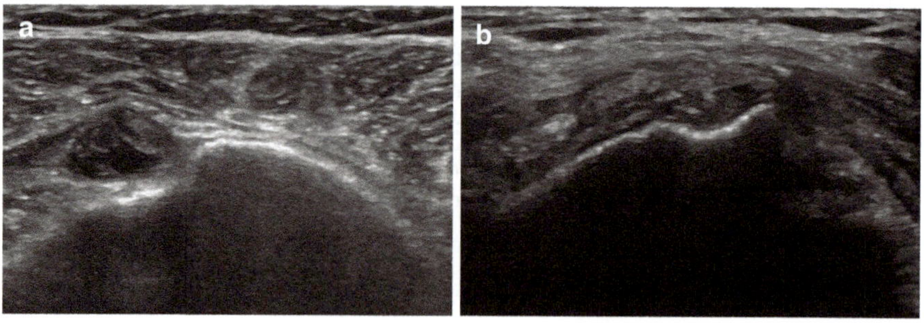

Fig. 5.26 Complete or massive supraspinatus tendon tear. (**a**) Transverse view of complete supraspinatus tendon tear. (**b**) Longitudinal view of complete supraspinatus tendon tear showing no recognizable fibers and remodeling of the greater tuberosity

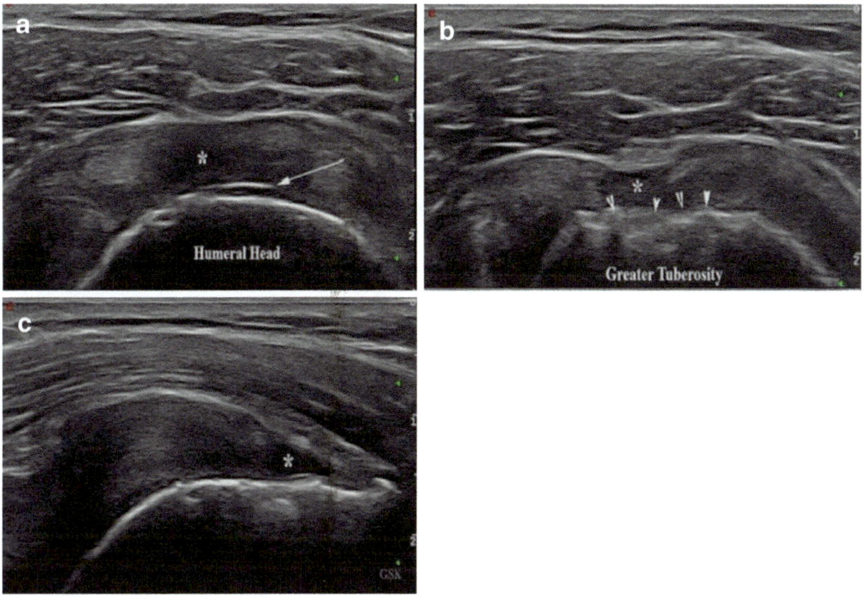

Fig. 5.27 Full thickness tear supraspinatus tendon. Full thickness supraspinatus tear (**a**) at level of humeral head, depicting interface sign (arrow) and focal discontinuity, (**b**) at level of greater tuberosity in short axis depicting osseous irregularity (arrow heads), and (**c**) in long axis

Rotator Cuff Calcifications

Ultrasound can depict calcifications in the rotator cuff tendons. These are more often likely basic calcium phosphate (BCP) deposits rather than calcium pyrophosphate deposits (CPPD). The morphology of these calcifications can vary from amorphous fluffy collections with poorly defined borders to discrete, homogeneous collections with well-described borders [22]. The poorly defined collections may be sonolucent. Discrete collections may appear eggshell-shaped or as hyperechoic punctate areas within the tendon (Fig. 5.30). Ultrasound can be as sensitive as plain X-rays for large, slurry, or bursal calcifications [23]. However, based on plain X-rays, rotator cuff calcifications may be found in 8–20% of patients, and of these, pain may be attributed to the calcification in up to 30% of these patients. In a study of 62 patients with calcific rotator cuff tendinopathy, positive power Doppler signal around the calcification and bursal distension was associated with pain [24]. Corticosteroid injection into the bursa adjacent to the calcification performed equally in the short term with ultrasound-guided percutaneous needle fragmentation (needle tenotomy or barbotage) followed by corticosteroid injection.

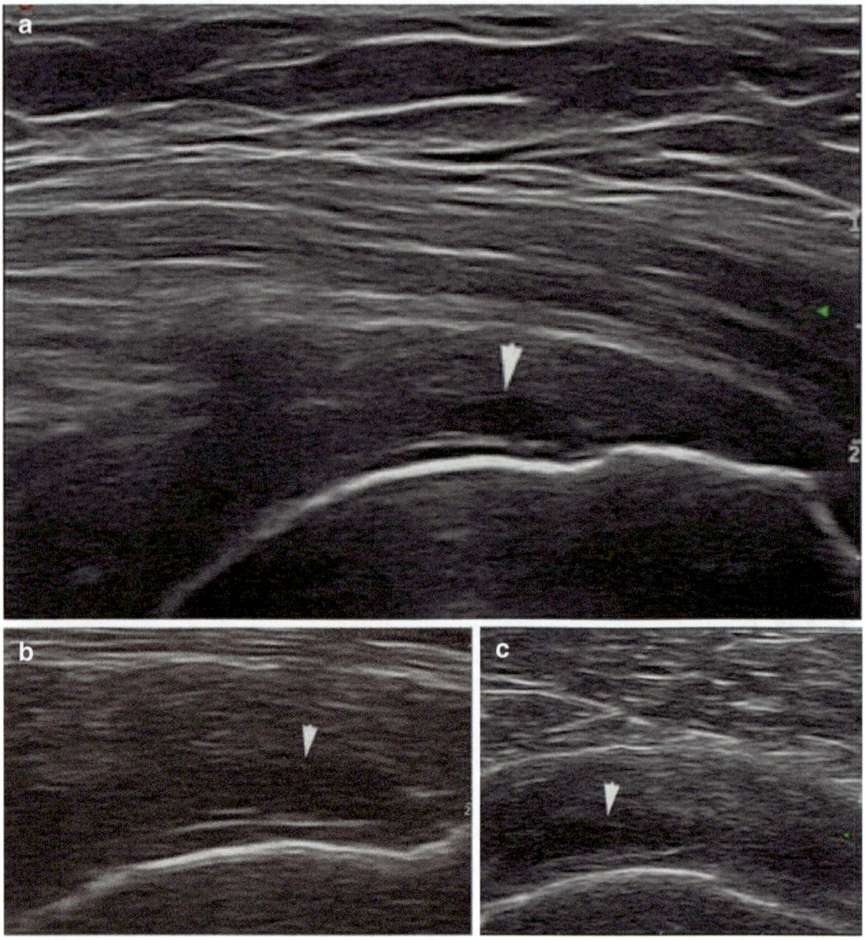

Fig. 5.28 Articular surface partial tear supraspinatus tendon. (**a**) Articular surface tear (arrow head) with accompanying interface sign, high magnification views in long axis (**b**), and in short axis (**c**)

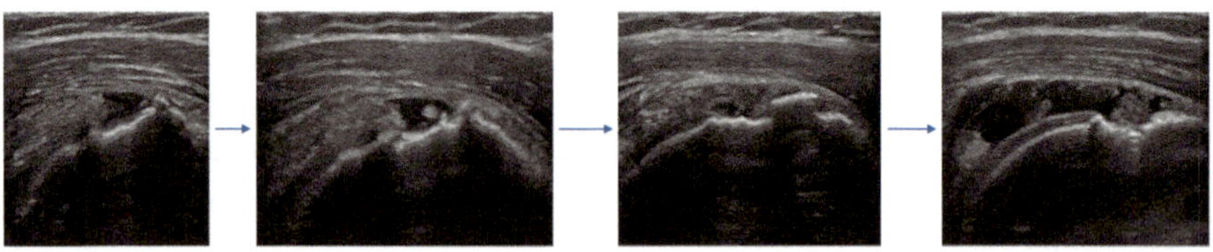

Fig. 5.29 Supraspinatus tear from anterior to posterior. Scanning in the longitudinal plane moving the anterior edge of the supraspinatus tendon to the more posterior portion of the tendon demonstrates the extent of the tear

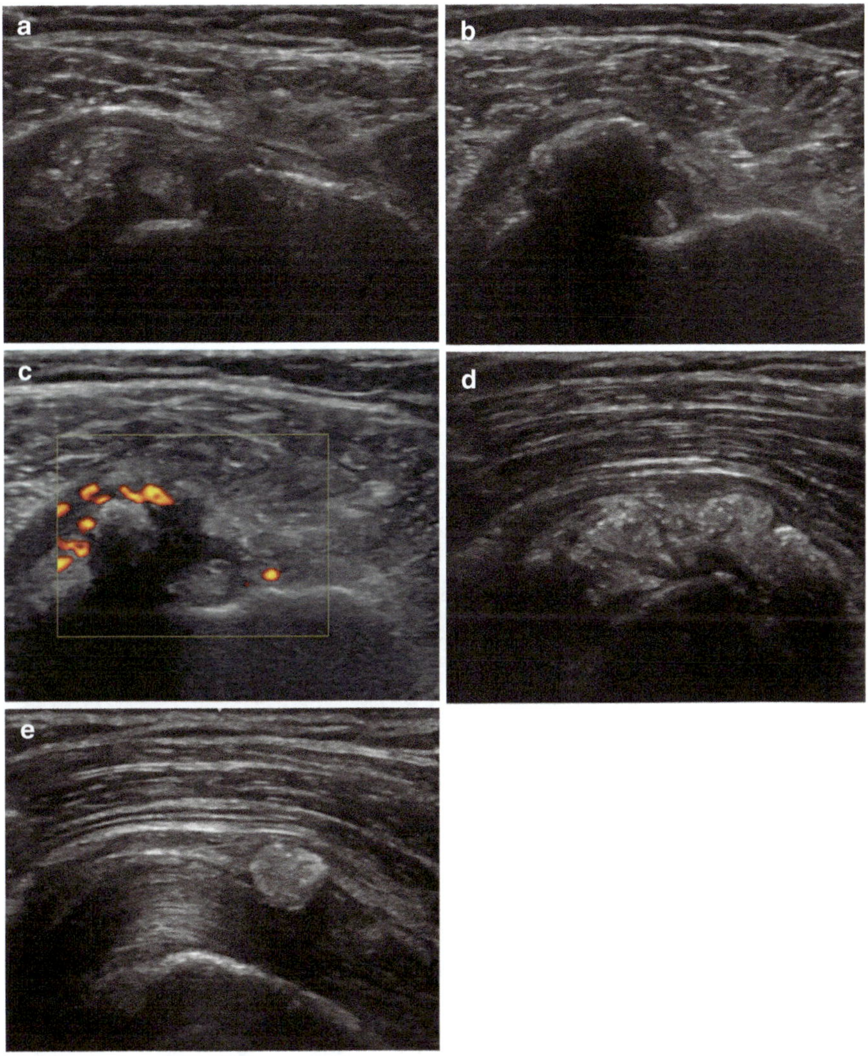

Fig. 5.30 Basic calcium phosphate deposition. (**a**) Transverse view of amorphous basic calcium phosphate (BCP) deposit in subscapularis next to bicep tendon. (**b**) Transverse view of same calcific deposit showing different linear pattern with acoustic shadow. (**c**) Doppler signal around the BCP deposit. (**d**) Longitudinal view of subscapular amorphous BCP deposit. (**e**) Migration of BCP nodule into subacromial bursa

Subacromial/Subdeltoid Bursitis

The subacromial and subdeltoid bursa is a large bursa that lies superficial to the rotator cuff tendons. It is lined by synovium and allows smooth gliding of the shoulder. It may enlarge in various forms of inflammatory and mechanical conditions (Fig. 5.31) and may show extensive findings to mere thickening. Although bursal thickening is associated with subacromial impingement, impingement does not necessarily milk fluid from the bursa to the lateral aspect [25]. It is important to recognize that one of the most important causes of external impingement is supraspinatus dysfunction or tear. The function of the supraspinatus as a humeral depressor in the first 30° of abduction allows the greater tuberosity to clear the acromion. With supraspinatus dysfunction, the bursa is caught between the greater tuberosity and the acromion, and irritation results in bursal effusion. The distension or thickening of the bursa is variable and ranges from anterior to anterolateral locations. The bursa may be accessed with ultrasound guidance for aspiration and injection (Fig. 5.32).

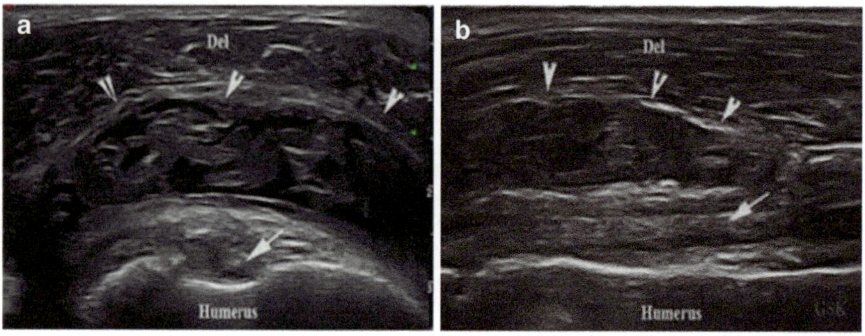

Fig. 5.31 Bursitis. Large subacromial bursal process (*arrowheads*) seen in short (**a**) and long (**b**) axis with hypoechoic and anechoic material

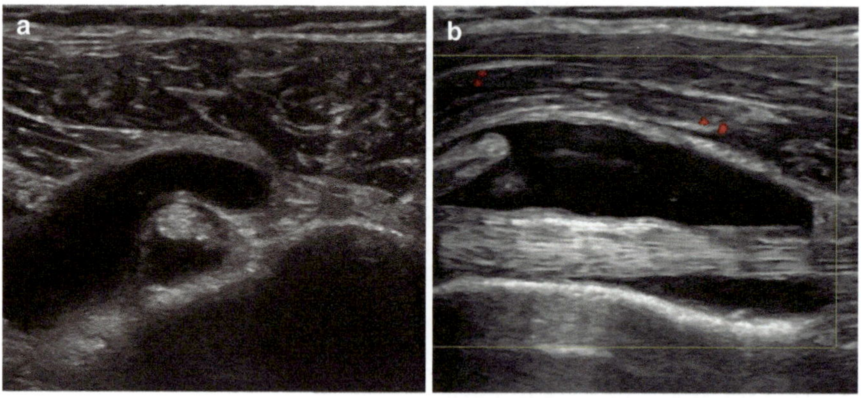

Fig. 5.32 Subdeltoid bursitis. (**a**) Subdeltoid bursitis shown in transverse orientation as distinct from an effusion around the biceps tendon. (**b**) Longitudinal view of the same

Glenohumeral Effusion

Glenohumeral effusions are encountered in a variety of inflammatory and non-inflammatory conditions. Clinical examination has poor agreement with imaging-based diagnosis of glenohumeral effusions [26]. Detection and aspiration of fluid are important if septic arthritis is being considered. The shoulder joint has three main recesses, as well as the long head of the biceps tendon sheath for fluid to collect in. The characteristics of these recesses are summarized in Table 5.4. Of note, the most reliable recess to examine is the posterior recess in external rotation [27] and the biceps tendon sheath [12]. A distension of more than 3 mm from the bone to the underneath surface of the infraspinatus is considered abnormal [11] (Figs. 5.33

Table 5.4 Ultrasound views of glenohumeral joint recesses

Recess	Patient Position	Characteristics
Anterior recess	Arm in neutral to internal rotation	Poorest reliability with US to detect fluid between humerus and coracoid process. Should not be confused with subcoracoid bursitis which is superficial to the subscapularis
Long head biceps tendon sheath	Arm in neutral position	Scan from level of bicipital groove to level of pectoralis major. Presence of power Doppler may suggest inflammatory etiology
Posterior recess	Arm in external rotation	Bulging of >3 mm of infraspinatus is suggestive of effusion
Axillary recess	Arm on patient's head	Positioning the patient leads to collapse of the recess, and fluid will be detected only when large effusions are present
Subacromial-subdeltoid bursa	Multiple	The bursa does not normally communicate with the glenohumeral joint. In the presence of a rotator cuff tear, fluid from the joint communicates with the bursa

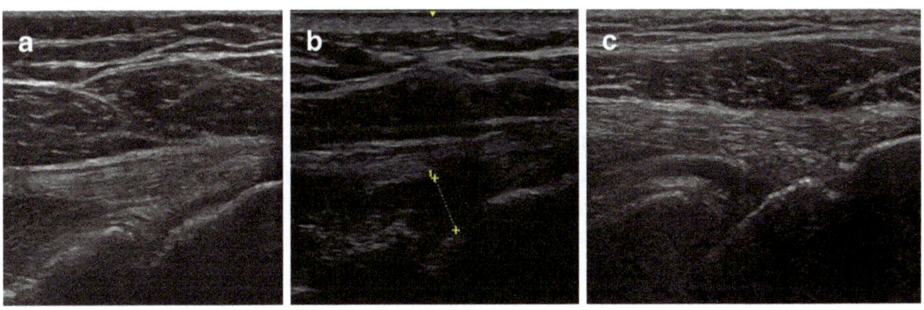

Fig. 5.33 Shoulder joint effusion: (**a**) Normal joint in external rotation (**b**) Bulging fluid collection around glenoid (>3 mm) in osteoarthritis patient (**c**) Bulging fluid collection in rheumatoid arthritis patient

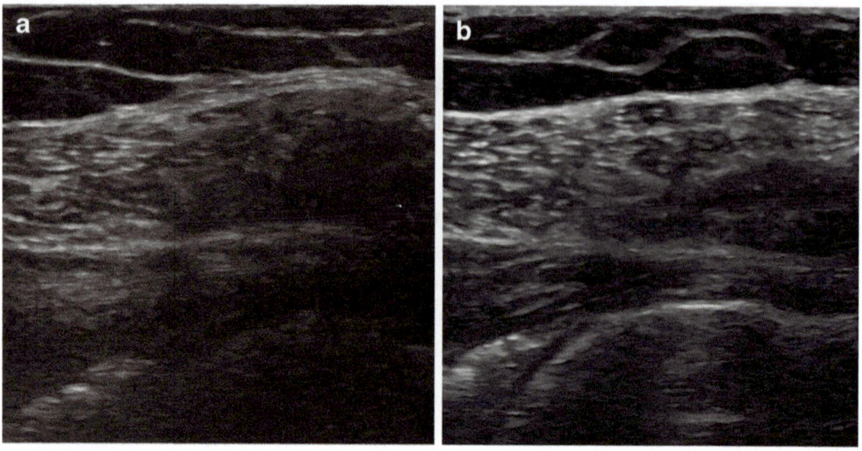

Fig. 5.34 Pitfalls for shoulder joint effusion. When technical limitations often related to body habitus occur, misinterpretation of a joint effusion may occur. (**a**) Inability to visualize the inferior surface and muscle body of the infraspinatus tendon. (**b**) Repositioning and clarifying the appearance of the joint capsule and infraspinatus tendon by slightly caudal shift of medial probe edge. Machine adjustments in probe frequency, dynamic range, or gray scale can should also be employed

and 5.34). The glenohumeral joint process may represent an effusion or may represent synovial hypertrophy. Dynamic imaging techniques or the presence of Doppler signal can help distinguish the two.

Inflammatory Arthritis

Rheumatoid Arthritis

Rheumatoid arthritis (RA) is a symmetric autoimmune arthropathy that is associated with destructive changes in joints. The shoulder is often affected in RA. Literature from the prebiologic era suggests that osseous abnormalities can occur bilaterally after 5 years of disease and only up to 10% of patients may have normal plain shoulder X-rays throughout the course of their disease [28]. Care must be exercised in defining erosions since cortical defects of >1 mm were found in 23% of healthy adults between ages 20 and 60 [11]. Rheumatoid erosions most frequently occur superiorly, adjacent to the greater tuberosity, followed by anterior and posterior humeral surfaces [28, 29] (Fig. 5.35). Due to the lack of a sonographic window, glenoid erosions cannot be detected by ultrasound. In other areas, ultrasound is more sensitive than plain X-rays and similarly sensitive to MRI for the detection of erosions [30].

Sonographic studies of RA patients commonly show synovitis, bursitis, and bicipital tenosynovitis (Fig. 5.36) in high frequencies in symptomatic and asymptomatic patients with RA [30–32]. Doppler signal can be detected in synovial hypertrophy in the shoulder area (Fig. 5.37). It is important to understand the

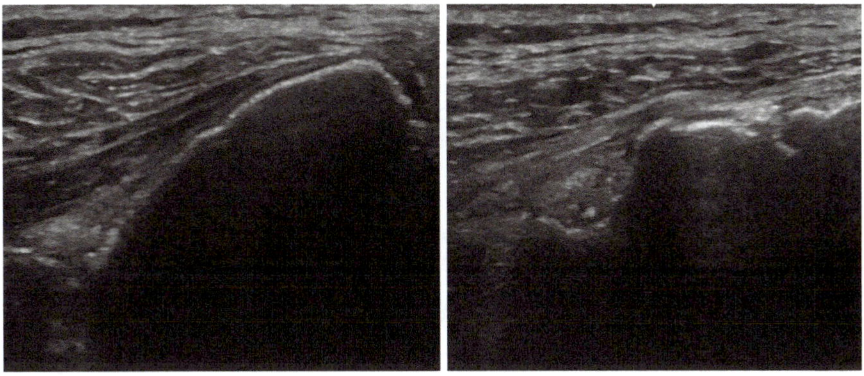

Fig. 5.35 Rheumatoid Arthritis. Advanced rheumatoid arthritis. Posterior views of a patient with longstanding rheumatoid arthritis showing a remodeled glenoid with poor labral cartilage definition and an isoechoic process likely synovial hyperplasia in the joint in external rotation

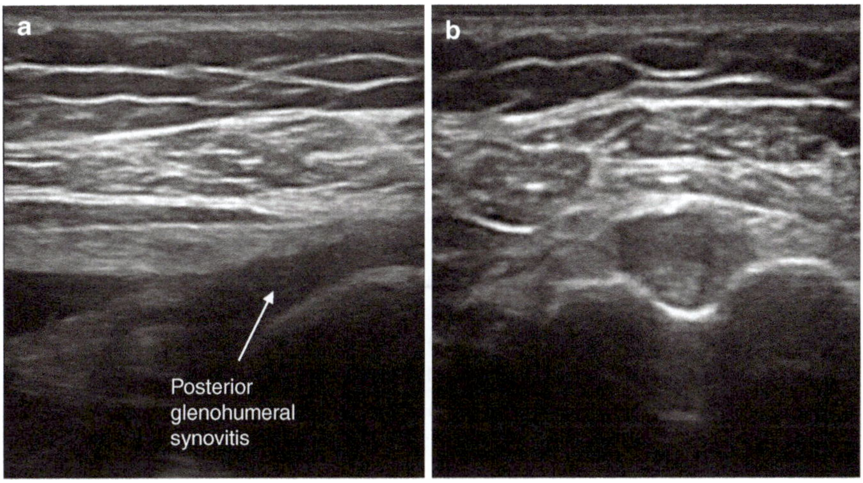

Fig. 5.36 Synovial hypertrophy in rheumatoid arthritis: (**a**) Posterior glenohumeral synovitis in a patient with RA also seen in the (**b**) anterior view of the biceps tendon sheath. The anechoic quality of collection can mimic an effusion

physics of Doppler settings as they influence negative results. In general, principles of lowering the frequency, lowering the wall filter, lowering the scale (PRF), and maximizing gain should be followed but need to be adjusted for depth [33]. Power Doppler signal appears to be most commonly seen in the biceps tendon joint capsule extension and may be a distinguishing finding in RA versus degenerative arthritis [15, 16]. Shoulder ultrasound is less comprehensive than MRI in detecting synovitis and tenosynovitis [34]. Ultrasound thus offers an efficient method of assessing involvement of the shoulder in RA, but negative studies or technically insufficient studies should consider further evaluation with MRI.

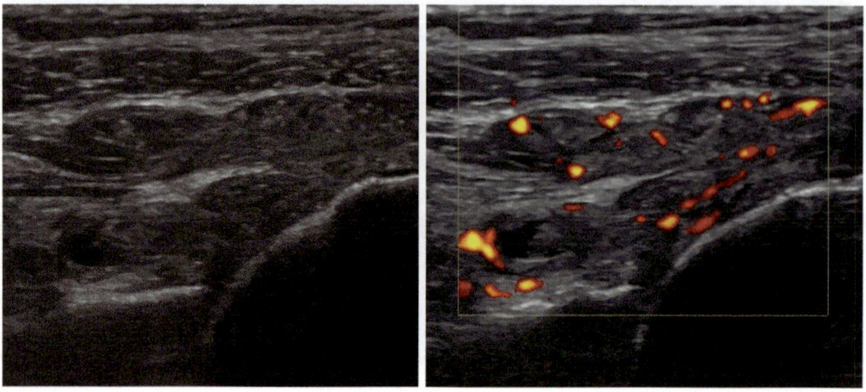

Fig. 5.37 Glenohumeral synovitis with power Doppler signal. Posterior glenohumeral synovitis with power Doppler signal in a patient with rheumatoid arthritis. Note the ruptured infraspinatus tendon and extension of the synovial collection cranially with loss of joint margins and labral architecture

Polymyalgia Rheumatica

Polymyalgia rheumatica (PMR) is an inflammatory disorder that affects older individuals. It has cardinal upper and lower limb girdle stiffness and can be associated with giant cell arteritis. The diagnosis is made clinically, with elevation of acute phase reactants adding circumstantial evidence for the condition. No other serological tests exist to confirm the diagnosis. The major differential diagnoses are RA and CPPD. In view of the difficulty in defining this condition with high specificity, classification criteria have been developed. The 2012 EULAR/ACR classification criteria included ultrasound findings of shoulder and hip periarthritis in the criteria [35]. Specifically, in addition to clinical criteria, imaging criteria included the presence of shoulder bursitis, glenohumeral effusion, and/or biceps tendon tenosynovitis as well as hip trochanteric bursitis or joint synovitis (see Table 5.5).

In the original classification cohort, the criteria performed better at distinguishing PMR from all comparison subjects than with RA subjects. Adding ultrasound increased sensitivity to 66% and specificity to 81% in patients of age > 50 presenting with shoulder pain and without corticosteroid treatment [35]. However, ultrasound-based classification highly correlated with steroid response at 4 weeks [36]. In subsequent cohorts, the ultrasound-based criteria were able to improve specificity from 81.5% to 91.3% compared to patients in an early RA clinic and to improve discrimination of PMR from RA, but the specificity went down if only patients with shoulder pain were compared [37]. Ultrasound findings are more commonly seen in the shoulders than the hips.

Table 5.5 2012 ACR/EULAR classification criteria for PMR [35]

Criteria	Points
Morning stiffness duration >45 minutes	2
Hip pain or limited range of motion	1
Absence of RF or ACPA	2
US 1: 1 shoulder[a] and 1 hip[b] involvement	1
US 2: bilateral shoulder[a] involvement	1

Mandatory criteria: age > 50 years, bilateral shoulder pain, elevated ESR/CRP
Clinical criteria: 4 of 6 points (US points not counted)
Clinical + US criteria: 5 of 8 points
RF rheumatoid factor, *ACPA* anti-citrullinated polypeptide antibody
[a]US shoulder findings: subdeltoid bursitis and/or biceps tenosynovitis and/or glenohumeral synovitis (either posterior or axillary)
[b]US hip findings: hip with synovitis and/or trochanteric bursitis

Conclusion

Ultrasound examination of the shoulder can be extremely useful as a point of care tool in the evaluation of rheumatology patients with shoulder pain; in experienced users it can be as reliable as MRI. Care must be taken to fully scan the shoulder in a systematic manner for identification of tendon tears and other pathology. All visualized pathology must be clinically correlated and should not automatically be attributed to the cause of the patient's symptoms.

Review Questions

1. The rotator cuff interval is defined by which of the following tendons:
   (a) Supraspinatus and infraspinatus
   (b) Supraspinatus and teres minor
   (c) Supraspinatus and subscapularis
   (d) Infraspinatus and subscapularis
2. The following structures retain the long head of the biceps tendon in its position *except*
   (a) Coracohumeral ligament
   (b) Coracoacromial ligament
   (c) Transverse humeral ligament
   (d) Pectoralis major insertion
3. Which of the following does *not* predispose to long head of biceps tendon subluxation?
   (a) Congenitally shallow intertubercular sulcus
   (b) Coracohumeral ligament tear
   (c) Medial supraspinatus tear
   (d) Subscapularis tear

4. The best position of the patient for examination of the rotator cuff and the coracohumeral ligament is
   (a) Neutral position with palm facing up
   (b) In internal rotation with palm facing up
   (c) In external rotation with palm facing up
   (d) In the modified Crass position
5. The use of ultrasound in classification criteria of polymyalgia rheumatica is associated with which of the following?
   (a) Better specificity in distinguishing PMR from RA than from other types of arthritis
   (b) A higher rate of hip involvement than shoulder involvement
   (c) Higher rates of synovitis in the shoulder bursitis of PMR patients than RA patients
   (d) Superior specificity than previous classification criteria
6. Ultrasound is most sensitive at detecting fluid at which of the following recesses?
   (a) Anterior recess
   (b) Posterior recess
   (c) Axillary recess
   (d) None of the above
7. Sonography best visualizes the
   (a) Posterior labrum
   (b) Anterior labrum
   (c) Superior labrum
   (d) Inferior labrum
8. Hill Sachs abnormality occurs when
   (a) The shoulder dislocates posteriorly.
   (b) The posterolateral humeral head strikes the antero-inferior glenoid rim during dislocation.
   (c) The antero-humeral head strikes the inferior glenoid rim during dislocation.
   (d) The rotator cuff tendons are avulsed during dislocation.
9. In rheumatoid arthritis shoulders, erosions most commonly occur
   (a) Anteriorly adjacent to the lesser tuberosity
   (b) Posteriorly
   (c) Superiorly adjacent to the greater tuberosity
   (d) Inferiorly

Answers

1. (c) Supraspinatus and subscapularis
2. (b) Coracoacromial ligament
3. (c) Medial supraspinatus tear
4. (d) In the modified Crass position
5. (d) Superior specificity than previous classification criteria

6. (b) Posterior recess
7. (a) Posterior labrum
8. (b) The posterolateral humeral head strikes the antero-inferior glenoid rim during dislocation.
9. (c) Superiorly adjacent to the greater tuberosity

References

1. Urwin M, Symmons D, Allison T, Brammah T, Busby H, Roxby M, et al. Estimating the burden of musculoskeletal disorders in the community: the comparative prevalence of symptoms at different anatomical sites, and the relation to social deprivation. Ann Rheum Dis. 1998;57(11):649–55.
2. Girish G, Lobo LG, Jacobson JA, Morag Y, Miller B, Jamadar DA. Ultrasound of the shoulder: asymptomatic findings in men. Am J Roentgenol. 2011;197(4):W713–9.
3. Nazarian LN, Jacobson JA, Benson CB, Bancroft LW, Bedi A, McShane JM, et al. Imaging algorithms for evaluating suspected rotator cuff disease: Society of Radiologists in ultrasound consensus conference statement. Radiology. 2013;267(2):589–95.
4. Dietz SO, Barti C, Magosch P, Lechenberg S, Habermeyer P. Intra-articular volume assessment in glenohumeral instability. Knee Surg Sports Traumatol Arthrosc. 2006;14(2):189–92.
5. Teefey SA. Shoulder sonography: why we do it. J Ultrasound Med. 2012;31(9):1325–31.
6. Frank R, Taylor D, Verman N, Romeo A, Mologne T, Provencher M. The rotator interval of the shoulder. Orthop J Sports Med. 2015;3(12):1–10.
7. Harryman DT, Sidles JA, Harris SL, Matsen FA. The role of the rotator interval capsule in passive motion and stability of the shoulder. J Bone Joint Surg Am. 1992;74:53–66.
8. Cooper HJ, Milillo R, Klein DA, DiFelice GS. The MRI geyser sign: acromioclavicular joint cysts in the setting of a chronic rotator cuff tear. Am J Orthop. 2011;40(6):E118–21.
9. Mochizuki T, Sugaya H, Uomizu M, Maeda K, Matsuki K, Sekiya I, et al. Humeral insertion of the supraspinatus and infraspinatus. New anatomical findings regarding the footprint of the rotator cuff. J Bone Joint Surg Am. 2008;90(5):962–9.
10. Martinoli C, Bianchi S, Prato N, Pugliese F, Zamorani MP, Valle M, et al. US of the shoulder: non-rotator cuff disorders. Radiographics. 2003;23(2):381–401. quiz 534
11. Schmidt WA, Schmidt H, Schicke B, Gromnica-Ihle E. Standard reference values for musculoskeletal ultrasonography. Ann Rheum Dis. 2004;63(8):988–94.
12. Zubler V, Mamisch-Saupe N, Pfirrmann CW, Jost B, Zanetti M. Detection and quantification of glenohumeral joint effusion: reliability of ultrasound. Eur Radiol. 2011;21(9):1858–64.
13. Karthikeyan S, Rai SB, Parsons H, Drew S, Smith CD, Griffin DR. Ultrasound dimensions of the rotator cuff in young healthy adults. J Shoulder Elb Surg. 2014;23(8):1107–12.
14. Chang KV, Chen WS, Wang TG, Hung CY, Chien KL. Associations of sonographic abnormalities of the shoulder with various grades of biceps peritendinous effusion (BPE). Ultrasound Med Biol. 2014;40(2):313–21.
15. Stegbauer J, Rump LC, Weiner SM. Sites of inflammation in painful rheumatoid shoulder assessed by musculoskeletal ultrasound and power Doppler sonography. Rheumatol Int. 2008;28(5):459–65.
16. Strunk J, Lange U, Kurten B, Schmidt KL, Neeck G. Doppler sonographic findings in the long bicipital tendon sheath in patients with rheumatoid arthritis as compared with patients with degenerative diseases of the shoulder. Arthritis Rheum. 2003;48(7):1828–32.
17. Ejnisman B, Monteiro GC, Andreoli CV, de Castro Pochini A. Disorder of the long head of the biceps tendon. Br J Sports Med. 2010;44(5):347–54.

18. Gothelf TK, Bell D, Goldberg JA, Harper W, Pelletier M, Yu Y, et al. Anatomic and biomechanical study of the biceps vinculum, a structure within the biceps sheath. Arthroscopy. 2009;25(5):515–21.
19. Wall LB, Teefey SA, Middleton WD, Dahiya N, Steger-May K, Kim HM, et al. Diagnostic performance and reliability of ultrasonography for fatty degeneration of the rotator cuff muscles. J Bone Joint Surg Am. 2012;94(12):e83.
20. Kim HM, Dahiya N, Teefey SA, Middleton WD, Stobbs G, Steger-May K, et al. Location and initiation of degenerative rotator cuff tears: an analysis of three hundred and sixty shoulders. J Bone Joint Surg Am. 2010;92(5):1088–96.
21. Jacobson JA, Lancaster S, Prasad A, van Holsbeeck MT, Craig JG, Kolowich P. Full-thickness and partial-thickness supraspinatus tendon tears: value of US signs in diagnosis. Radiology. 2004;230(1):234–42.
22. Gazzola S, Bleakney RR. Current imaging of the rotator cuff. Sports Med Arthrosc. 2011;19(3):300–9.
23. Farin PU, Jaroma H. Sonographic findings of rotator cuff calcifications. J Ultrasound Med. 1995;14(1):7–14.
24. Le Goff B, Berthelot JM, Guillot P, Glemarec J, Maugars Y. Assessment of calcific tendonitis of rotator cuff by ultrasonography: comparison between symptomatic and asymptomatic shoulders. Joint Bone Spine. 2010;77(3):258–63.
25. Daghir AA, Sookur PA, Shah S, Watson M. Dynamic ultrasound of the subacromial-subdeltoid bursa in patients with shoulder impingement: a comparison with normal volunteers. Skelet Radiol. 2012;41(9):1047–53.
26. Luukkainen R, Sanila MT, Luukkainen P. Poor relationship between joint swelling detected on physical examination and effusion diagnosed by ultrasonography in glenohumeral joints in patients with rheumatoid arthritis. Clin Rheumatol. 2007;26(6):865–7.
27. Bruyn GA, Naredo E, Moller I, Moragues C, Garrido J, de Bock GH, et al. Reliability of ultrasonography in detecting shoulder disease in patients with rheumatoid arthritis. Ann Rheum Dis. 2009;68:357–61.
28. Lehtinen JT, Belt EA, Lyback CO, Kauppi MJ, Kaarela K, Kautiainen HJ, et al. Subacromial space in the rheumatoid shoulder: a radiographic 15-year follow-up study of 148 shoulders. J Shoulder Elb Surg. 2000;9(3):183–7.
29. Alasaarela E, Suramo I, Tervonen O, Lahde S, Takalo R, Hakala M. Evaluation of humeral head erosions in rheumatoid arthritis: a comparison of ultrasonography, magnetic resonance imaging, computed tomography and plain radiography. Br J Rheumatol. 1998;37(11):1152–6.
30. Amin MF, Ismail FM, El Shereef RR. The role of ultrasonography in early detection and monitoring of shoulder erosions, and disease activity in rheumatoid arthritis patients; comparison with MRI examination. Acad Radiol. 2012;19(6):693–700.
31. Sanja MR, Mirjana ZS. Ultrasonographic study of the painful shoulder in patients with rheumatoid arthritis and patients with degenerative shoulder disease. Acta Reumatol Port. 2010;35(1):50–8.
32. Coari G, Paoletti F, Iagnocco A. Shoulder involvement in rheumatic diseases. Sonographic findings. J Rheumatol. 1999;26(3):668–73.
33. Torp-Pedersen ST, Terslev L. Settings and artefacts relevant in colour/power Doppler ultrasound in rheumatology. Ann Rheum Dis. 2008;67:143–9.
34. Hermann KGA, Backhaus M, Schneider U, Labs K, Loreck D, Zuhlsdorf S, Schink T, Fischer T, Hamm B, Bollow M. Rheumatoid arthritis of the shoulder joint comparison of conventional radiography, ultrasound, and dynamic contrast-enhanced magnetic resonance imaging. Arthritis Rheum. 2003;48(12):3338–49.
35. Dasgupta B, Cimmino MA, Kremers HM, Schmidt WA, Schirmer M, Salvarani C, et al. Provisional classification criteria for polymyalgia rheumatica: a European League Against

Rheumatism/ American College of Rheumatology collaborative initiative. Arthritis Rheum. 2012;64(4):943–54.

36. Matteson EL, Maradit-Kremers H, Cimmino MA, Schmidt WA, Schirmer M, Salvarani C, et al. Patient-reported outcomes in polymyalgia rheumatica. J Rheumatol. 2012;39(4):795–803.
37. Macchioni P, Boiardi L, Catanoso M, Pazzola G, Salvarani C. Performance of the new 2012 EULAR/ ACR classification criteria for polymyalgia rheumatica: comparison with the previous criteria in a single-centre study. Ann Rheum Dis. 2014;73(6):1190–3.

Ultrasound of the Hip

6

Mark A. Matza and Naina Rastalsky

Key Points

- Ultrasound of the hip is easy to perform in the office setting and adds important diagnostic information to the physical exam of the hip.
- Ultrasound facilitates diagnosis of mechanical, degenerative, and inflammatory pathologies in the hip and can be used to guide hip joint aspiration/injection as well as trochanteric bursa injection.
- Correct positioning of the patient and correct probe placement are key for optimal imaging of the hip joint as well as the abductor mechanism in the lateral hip.
- The use of low-frequency transducers may be necessary for optimal image acquisition in obese or muscular patients. The highest frequency possible for the depth of the structures should be used.

Introduction

Musculoskeletal ultrasound of the hip is a very useful clinical tool that aids the clinician in diagnosis and treatment of a wide array of hip conditions. Hip pain is a nonspecific complaint that can be caused by inflammatory, degenerative, overuse, or traumatic causes. Clinical evaluation of the hip is often limited due to the

M. A. Matza (✉)
Division of Rheumatology, Allergy, and Immunology, Department of Medicine, Massachusetts General Hospital, Harvard Medical School, Boston, MA, USA
e-mail: mmatza@mgh.harvard.edu

N. Rastalsky
SQZ Biotechnologies, Watertown, MA, USA
e-mail: naina.rastalsky@sqzbiotech.com

M. J. Kohler (ed.), *Musculoskeletal Ultrasound in Rheumatology Review*,
https://doi.org/10.1007/978-3-030-73555-5_6

depth of the hip joint and limited number of maneuvers for examination. Ultrasound allows for visualization of the anterior, lateral, and posterior aspects of the hip. In particular, bony irregularities such as osteophytes, synovial hypertrophy, synovial effusions, bursitis, tendon pathology, and periarticular soft tissue lesions can all be diagnosed. The 2012 American College of Rheumatology report on reasonable use of musculoskeletal ultrasonography in rheumatology reports that ultrasound evaluation is reasonable for evaluation of a patient with pain or mechanical symptoms at the hip in search of joint effusion and intraarticular and periarticular soft tissue pathology. Guidance for diagnostic and therapeutic articular or periarticular aspiration and injections is also considered to be of reasonable use [1].

Technical Requirements

The best resolution for evaluation of the hip is obtained with linear transducers with frequencies of 9–15 MHz; however, due to the depth of the structures, convex 3.5–5 MHz transducers are often required in obese or very muscular patients. Using a combination of probes may be necessary for optimal imaging.

Standard Views and Normal Ultrasound Findings

Table 6.1 shows standard views of the hip [2–4].

Table 6.1 Standard views of the normal hip [2–4]

Location	Orientation	Positioning	Structures
Anterior	*Longitudinal*	Supine, hips and knees extended, hip in 10–15° external rotation	Acetabulum, labrum, femoral head, femoral neck, synovial capsule, iliopsoas muscle, and tendon
	Transverse	Supine, hips and knees extended, hip in 10–15° external rotation	Acetabulum, femoral head articular cartilage, neurovascular structures
Lateral	*Longitudinal*	1. Supine 2. Lateral decubitus with the hip flexed 20°	Long-axis views of greater trochanter, gluteus medius tendon, gluteus minimus tendon, iliotibial band, subgluteus maximus (trochanteric) bursa (only visible if thickened or filled with fluid)
	Transverse	Lateral decubitus	Short-axis views of greater trochanter, gluteus medius tendon, gluteus minimus tendon, iliotibial band, subgluteus maximus (trochanteric) bursa (only visible if thickened or filled with fluid)

Anterior Hip

The patient lies in a supine position with the hips and knees extended and the hip in 10–15° of relaxed external rotation. An overview of the structures of the hip joint is obtained with the anterior longitudinal view. For this view, the probe is placed parallel to the long axis of the femoral neck in a cranial-medial to caudal-lateral orientation (Fig. 6.1a). From cranial to caudal, this brings into view the anterior acetabular rim, the anterosuperior portion of the acetabular labrum, the femoral head with femoral cartilage, the femoral neck, and the overlying anterior joint recess (Fig. 6.1b, c). The anterior joint recess which lies between the femoral neck and the iliopsoas fascia measures approximately 5 mm in the normal joint, *generally less than 7 mm*, and is formed by an anterior and posterior fibrous layer which together form a hyperechoic band and are only visualized as separate layers in the presence of a hip joint effusion [5]. Cranial to the anterior joint recess, the anterosuperior portion of the fibrocartilaginous labrum is seen as a hyperechoic triangular extension to the acetabular rim. Sometimes the iliofemoral ligament can be detected as a thin fibrillar structure superficial to the acetabular labrum, blending into the anterior layer of the synovial capsule. Deep muscle layers on the anterior view from medial to lateral include the iliopsoas, with its tendinous portion medially, the rectus femoris, and the vastus lateralis muscles. If the probe is moved laterally over the anterior superior iliac spine (Fig. 6.1d), the origin of the tensor fasciae latae can be seen (Fig. 6.1e).

For the anterior transverse view, the probe is placed at a 90° angle to the long axis of the femoral neck (Fig. 6.2a). When placing the probe at the level of the joint space, this brings into view from medial to lateral the neurovascular bundle with the femoral vein, the femoral artery, and the femoral nerve and the articular cartilage of the femoral head. Muscular structures from medial to lateral are the iliopsoas muscle with its tendon posteriorly and the rectus femoris muscle (Fig. 6.2b). The iliopsoas tendon lies superficial to the anterior joint recess. *Deep to* it, between the tendon and the joint capsule, is the iliopsoas bursa *which cannot be visualized* in the normal non-distended state.

Lateral Hip

Standard lateral (*greater* trochanter) views are obtained with the patient lying on the contralateral side with the greater trochanter facing upward and the hip flexed about 20°. This allows for evaluation of the greater trochanter, the gluteus medius and minimus tendons, as well as the superficial trochanteric bursa (also called the subgluteus maximus bursa), the deep subgluteus medius bursa, and the proximal iliotibial band. To assess for fluid in the trochanteric bursa, it may be prudent to obtain an initial overview of the lateral hip with the patient in supine position, as small fluid collections may dissipate and can sometimes be missed once the patient is

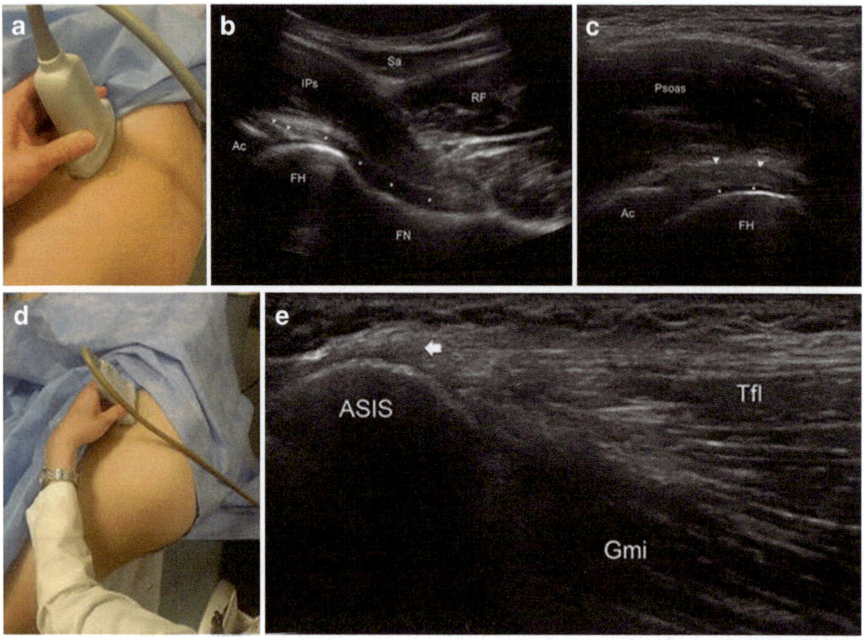

Fig. 6.1 (**a**) Probe placement for anterior longitudinal view. (**b**) Normal anterior longitudinal view of the hip. Anterior recess of the hip joint (*asterisks*) anterior to the femoral neck (*FN*) and deep to the iliopsoas muscle (*IPs*). The recess appears hypoechoic in this image, due to anisotropy. *Arrowheads* indicate the anterior limits of the hyperechoic triangular acetabular labrum extending from the acetabular rim and covering the articular cartilage of the femoral head (FH). *Sa* sartorius muscle. *RF* rectus femoris. Image obtained with 5–2 MHz curvilinear probe. (**c**) Normal anterior longitudinal view (15–6 MHz probe). Anterosuperior fibrocartilaginous labrum (*arrowheads*) overlying the articular cartilage (rhombi) of the femoral head (FH). *Ac* acetabulum. (**d**) Probe placement for tensor fasciae latae at ASIS. (**e**) Normal ultrasound of tensor fasciae latae. Tensor fasciae latae tendon (*arrow*) and muscle (*Tfl*) at the anterior superior iliac spine (ASIS). Observe the normal fibrillar pattern of the healthy tendon. *Gmi* gluteus minimus

placed in the lateral decubitus position. However, for visualization of the gluteal tendons and iliotibial band, the lateral decubitus position is the optimal position. Probe positioning is oriented along the anterior, lateral, and superoposterior facets of the greater trochanter [4]. A lateral longitudinal view over the lateral facet of the greater trochanter brings into view the insertion of the lateral and anterior portion of the gluteus medius tendon (Fig. 6.3a, b). This is where gluteus medius tendinopathy, oftentimes in the most anterior fibers of the tendon, is commonly seen. Probe alignment over the superoposterior facet of the greater trochanter is achieved by moving the probe proximally from the lateral facet and rotating it posteriorly at about a 30° angle to the lateral longitudinal view. This brings into view the superoposterior portion of the gluteus medius tendon which is oftentimes also involved by tendinopathy (Fig. 6.3c, d). For optimal visualization of the gluteus minimus tendon, the probe is

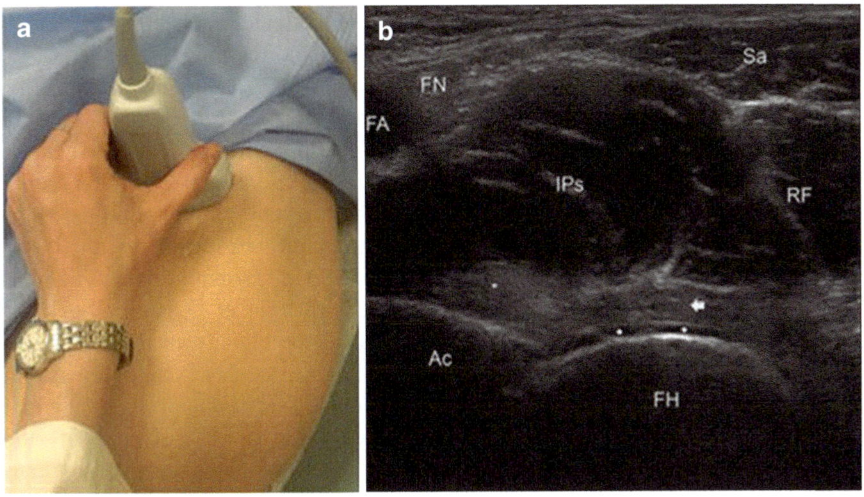

Fig. 6.2 (**a**) Probe placement for anterior transverse view. (**b**) Anterior transverse hip normal ultrasound image (15–6 MHz probe). Note the synovial capsule (*arrow*) anterior to the femoral head cartilage (rhombi) and deep to the iliopsoas muscle (*IPs*) with its tendon (*asterisk*). *FH* femoral head. *Ac* acetabulum. *RF* rectus femoris. *Sa* sartorius. *FA* femoral artery. *FN* femoral nerve

rotated anteriorly at about a 30° angle to the lateral longitudinal view onto the anterior surface of the greater trochanter. Additional heel-toe maneuver helps to avoid anisotropy by orienting the probe in a parallel plane to the oblique course of the gluteus minimus tendon. When the probe is positioned correctly, the axis of the gluteus minimus tendon will appear at approximately a 20° angle to the overlying fascia lata (Fig. 6.3e, f). Care must be taken not to mistake anisotropy of this particular tendon for tendinopathy.

A transverse view over the greater trochanter will show short-axis views of the gluteus minimus and lateral and posterior portions of the gluteus medius tendon with the overlying iliotibial band and confirm any cortical irregularities, tendinopathy, and bursal fluid collections in an orthogonal plane (Fig. 6.4a, b).

Posterior Hip

In addition to the standard anterior and lateral views of the hip, the posterior views allow for visualization of the proximal hamstring tendons (Figs. 6.5 and 6.6) and posterior gluteal muscles, including the piriformis muscle and sciatic nerve. The patient is placed in the prone position with the hip and knees extended to visualize the posterior hip area under ultrasound. A low-frequency linear or curvilinear transducer is placed over the ischial tuberosity, which is a palpable bony prominence near the midline of the horizontal gluteal crease. The transducer can be placed transversely between the greater trochanter and ischial tuberosity (Fig. 6.5a). Here, the proximal hamstring muscles and tendons (long head of the biceps femoris, semimembranosus, and semitendinosus) can be visualized as they insert onto the ischial tuberosity (Fig. 6.5b and c). The semitendinosus and the long head of biceps insert as a conjoint tendon on the medial aspect of the ischial tuberosity. The semimembranosus attaches on the lateral aspect of the ischial tuberosity. The tendons can be evaluated in both transverse and longitudinal views to assess for tendinosis, tear, and ischial-gluteal bursitis. Additionally, the posterior gluteal muscles can be visualized under ultrasound by having the patient lay prone on the stomach and placing a curvilinear transducer horizontally (transverse) over the posterior superior iliac spine. Here, the gluteus maximus, medius, and minimus muscles can be seen from superficial to deep, respectively. As the probe is positioned more caudally, the greater sciatic foramen appears from which the piriformis muscle arises (Fig. 6.6a). The tendinous portion of the piriformis can be visualized by directing the lateral end of the transducer toward the greater trochanter or caudally. The ischial spine will appear by positioning the transducer even further caudally at which point the sciatic nerve can be seen medially as it enters the greater sciatic foramen under the piriformis muscle (Fig. 6.6b). Finally, the sacroiliac joint can be imaged using ultrasound, which will allow for ultrasound-guided sacroiliac joint injection. For this view, the curvilinear or low frequency linear transducer is placed in the transverse orientation over the sacral region to to view the midline sacral hiatus and sacral cornu and then moved laterally over the sacral foramina to view the lateral edge of the sacrum. Next, the transducer should be moved cephalad to identify the ileum (Fig. 6.7a). The posterior aspect of the sacroiliac joint is identified as the cleft between the sacrum and ileum (Fig. 6.7b) [27, 28].

Fig. 6.3 (**a**) Probe placement longitudinal view lateral facet of greater trochanter (lateral gluteus medius tendon). (**b**) Longitudinal view of lateral facet normal ultrasound image. *Arrows* show the lateral portion of the gluteus medius tendon inserting on the lateral facet of the greater trochanter (GT). *Gme* gluteus medius muscle at tendon junction. *Gmax* gluteus maximus muscle at iliotibial band junction. *ITB* iliotibial band. (**c**) Probe placement longitudinal view of superoposterior facet (Fig. 6.3) (continued) of greater trochanter (superoposterior gluteus medius tendon). (**d**) Longitudinal view of superoposterior facet normal ultrasound image. *Arrows* indicate the superoposterior portion of the gluteus medius tendon inserting on the superoposterior facet of the greater trochanter (GT). *Gme* gluteus medius muscle at tendon junction. *Gmax* gluteus maximus at iliotibial band junction. *ITB* iliotibial band. (**e**) Probe placement longitudinal view of anterior facet (gluteus minimus tendon). (**f**) Longitudinal view of anterior facet normal ultrasound image. *Arrows* show gluteus minimus tendon insertion on the anterior facet of the greater trochanter (GT). Note the approximate 20° angle between the gluteus minimus tendon and the iliotibial band (ITB). *Tfl* tensor fasciae latae

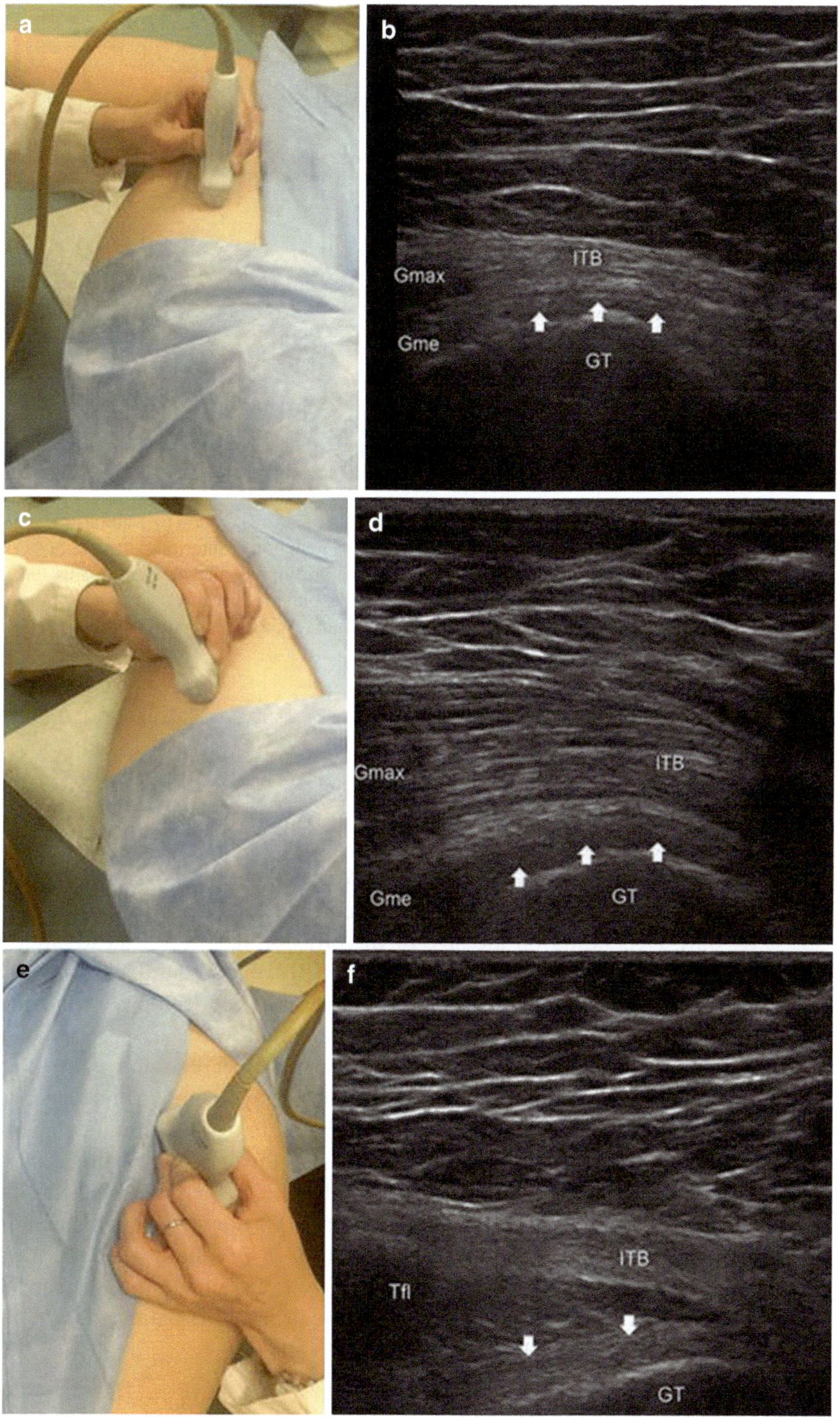
a
b
ITB
Gmax
Gme
GT
c
d
Gmax
ITB
Gme
GT
e
f
ITB
Tfl
GT

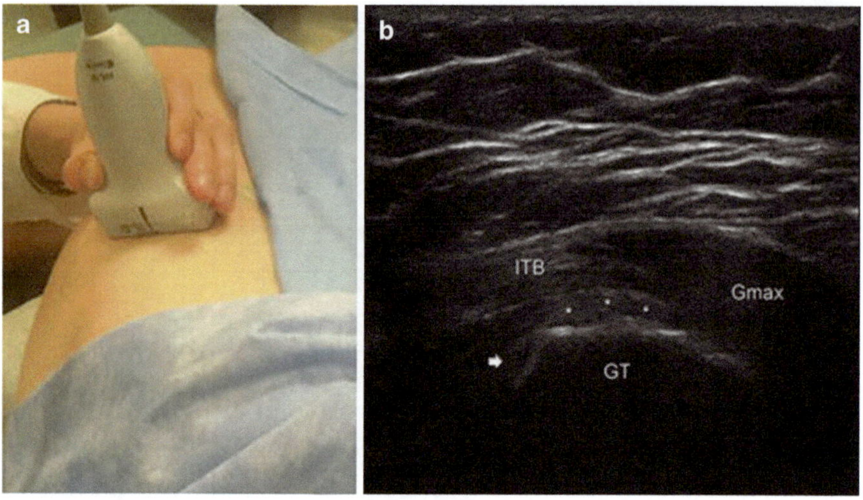

Fig. 6.4 (**a**) Probe placement lateral transverse view greater trochanter. (**b**) Lateral transverse view greater trochanter normal ultrasound image. Image orientation is anterior to the *left*, posterior to the *right*. *Asterisks* indicate the lateral and posterior portions of the gluteus medius tendon inserting onto the greater trochanter (GT). *Arrow* shows the gluteus minimus tendon at its insertion on the anterior facet of the greater trochanter (GT). *Gmax* gluteus maximus muscle. *ITB* iliotibial band

Pathology Relevant to the Hip

Hip Joint Effusion and Synovitis

A hip joint effusion appears as an anechoic or hypoechoic compressible collection that results in separation of the posterior and anterior layers of the hip joint capsule (Fig. 6.8). Depending on the size of the effusion this may lead to anterior bulging of the capsule, creating a convex shape [5]. Ultrasound does not distinguish between septic and aseptic effusions although the echogenicity of the effusion may vary depending on the nature of the fluid. In the case of synovial hypertrophy, the synovium appears thickened and hypoechoic and is noncompressible (Fig. 6.9). When an effusion is present or the synovium is thickened, the femoral neck to capsule distance increases to ≥7 mm, or to >1–1.5 mm compared with the contralateral side [6]. To measure capsule thickness, it is important to avoid internal rotation of the hip joint as it may lead to thickening of the capsule. Care should be taken not to mistake the anterior and posterior layers of the joint capsule for an effusion as these may appear falsely hypoechoic when the ultrasound beam is not perpendicular to the joint capsule. Differentiating the capsule from a hip joint effusion can become more difficult in obese patients due to the

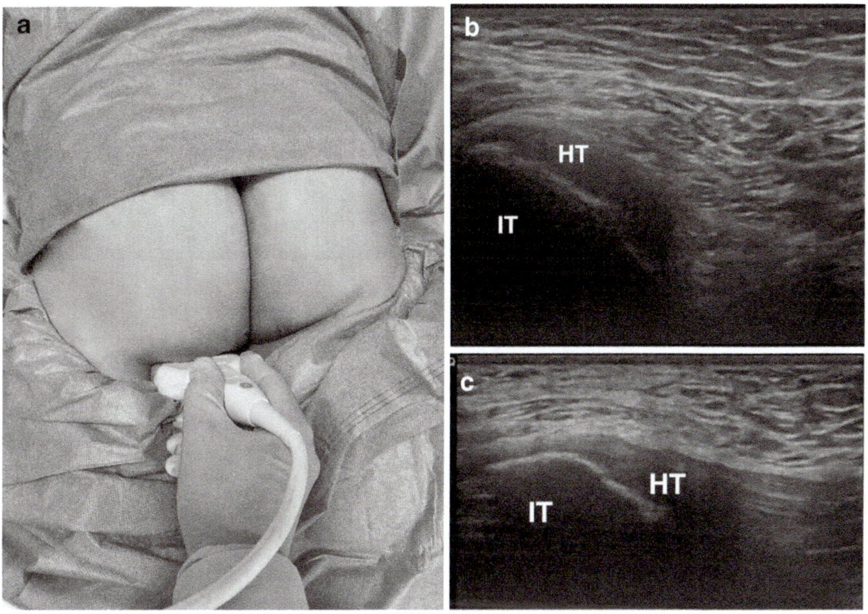

Fig. 6.5 Transverse (**a**) and longitudinal (**b**) views of the posterior hip demonstrating the proximal hamstring tendons (HT) originating from the ischial tuberosity (IT). (Courtesy of Joanne Borg-Stein, MD)

depth of the joint and loss of resolution when using lower-frequency probes [7]. Evaluation for synovial perfusion and hyperemia with color power Doppler (CPD) ultrasound has been shown to be feasible in the hip joint and correlated well with histopathologic findings [8]. However, this technique depends on the particular Doppler capabilities of the ultrasound equipment and may have its limitations in obese patients.

Arthritis/Osteonecrosis of the Hip

While ultrasound performs well in the assessment of synovial thickening and effusion, it is not the optimal imaging modality to assess the extent of structural bony or cartilaginous damage in osteoarthritis or inflammatory arthritis because it does not provide a window beyond the acetabular rim and because it does not allow for evaluation of the entire circumference of the hip joint. Nonetheless, cortical irregularities/osteophytes as seen in degenerative disease of the hip are often found at the anterolateral femoral head-neck junction and acetabular rim (Fig. 6.10). Erosions, as seen in rheumatoid arthritis, are more typically found along the femoral head. In advanced osteoarthritis or avascular necrosis, the femoral head may appear collapsed and flattened.

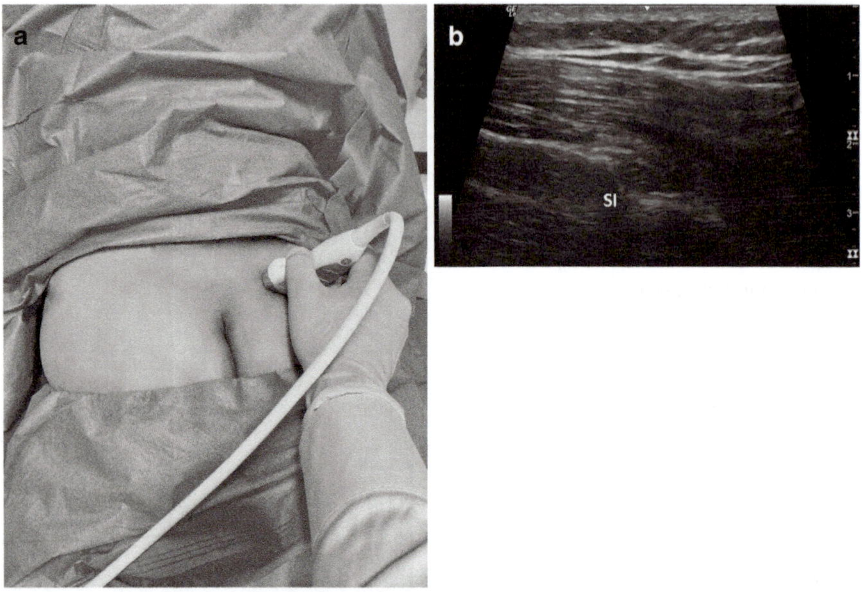

Fig. 6.6 Transverse view of the right sacroiliac joint (SI)

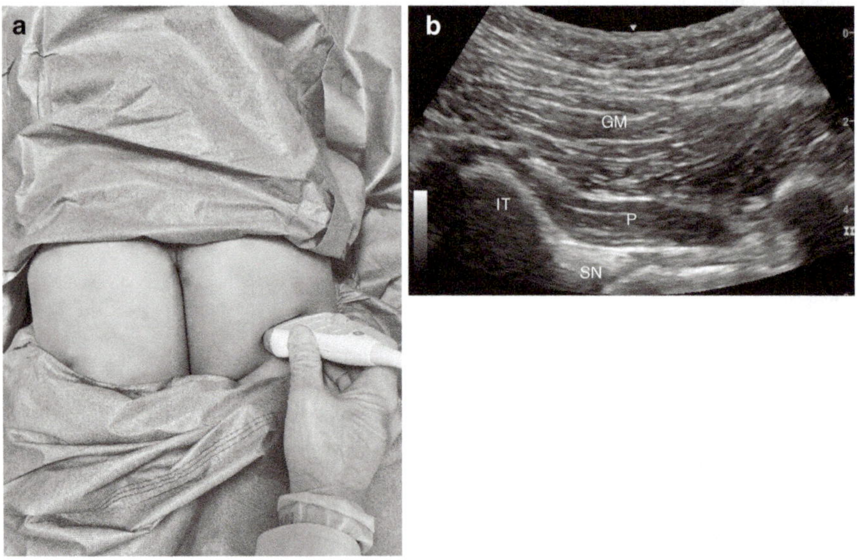

Fig. 6.7 Longitudinal view of the right piriformis muscle (P) abutting the ischial tuberosity (IT), with the gluteus maximum (GM) above and the sciatic nerve (SN) below

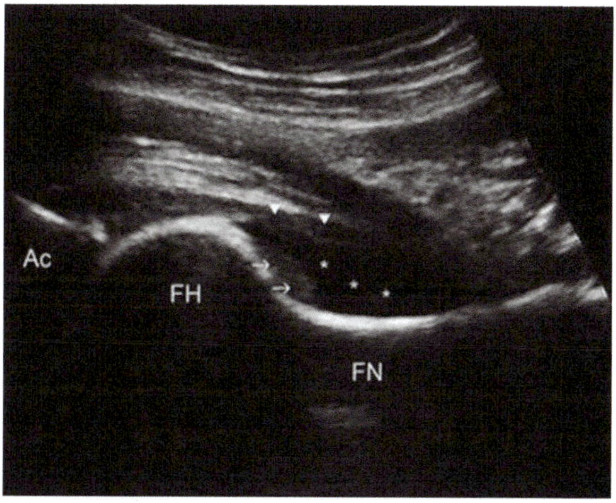

Fig. 6.8 Hip joint effusion. Anechoic hip joint effusion (*asterisks*) separating the anterior (*arrows*) and posterior (*arrowheads*) joint capsule. *Ac* acetabulum. *FH* femoral head. *FN* femoral neck

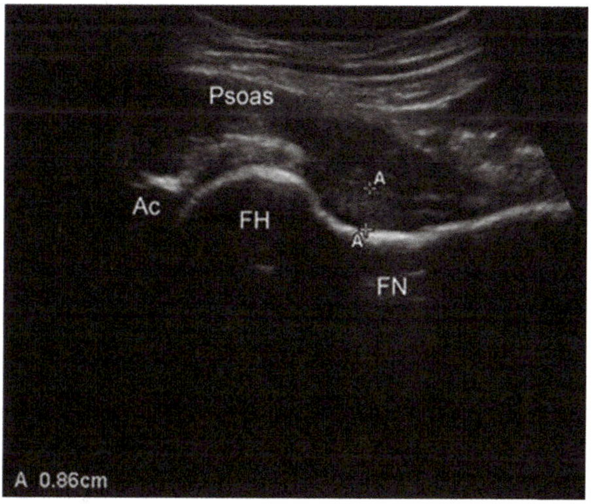

Fig. 6.9 Hip synovial thickening. Distention of the hip joint capsule measuring 0.86 cm at the femoral neck (FN). *Ac* acetabulum. *FH* femoral head

Labral Tears and Paralabral Cysts

Labral tears commonly occur in the anterosuperior portion of the acetabular labrum. In slender patients, ultrasound may delineate a tear as a hypoechoic cleft or fissure within the triangular structure of the labrum (Fig. 6.11). Anterior to the labrum, paralabral ganglion cysts can form as hypoechoic, noncompressible, lobulated structures filled with mucoid material that communicate with the labral tear; these cysts sometimes can evolve into palpable groin masses. Ultrasound has limited utility in the diagnosis of labrum tears, and MRI and particularly MR arthrogram remain the diagnostic modalities of choice for this indication.

Prosthetic Joint

Ultrasound offers a distinct advantage over computed tomography and magnetic resonance imaging in the evaluation of the periprosthetic soft tissues after hip arthroplasty because it is not limited by metal artifacts. It is therefore an excellent imaging tool to evaluate for complications of hip arthroplasty, such as joint effusions and extra-articular fluid collections, iliopsoas tendonitis and bursitis, and gluteal tendon pathology at the site of tenotomy [9]. However, prosthetic components or periprosthetic bones are not well visualized by ultrasound beyond their superficial borders.

Iliopsoas Bursitis

Iliopsoas bursitis can be due to overuse, trauma, total hip arthroplasty, or secondary to hip osteoarthritis or inflammatory arthritis. Increased intra-articular pressure from a hip joint effusion or small defects in the synovial lining can result in communication of the joint cavity with the iliopsoas bursa.

In the normal state, the iliopsoas bursa cannot be visualized by ultrasound. When distended, it becomes visible as a hypoechoic or anechoic fluid-filled compressible space between the anterior capsule of the hip and the iliopsoas muscle, sometimes extending medially toward the neurovascular bundle (Fig. 6.12) [10]. In chronic iliopsoas bursitis, the bursa can take on an echogenic appearance. Rarely, a large iliopsoas bursa can extend proximally into the pelvis and be mistaken for an intra-abdominal cyst or mass [11].

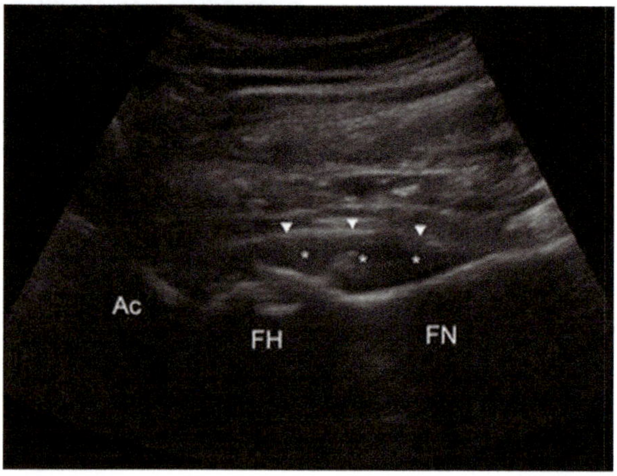

Fig. 6.10 Osteoarthritis of the hip. Note the marked cortical irregularity on the femoral head (FH) and distended joint capsule (*asterisks*) with mixed hyperechoic and hypoechoic signal. *Arrowheads* outline the anterior margin of the anterior joint recess. *Ac* acetabulum. *FN* femoral neck

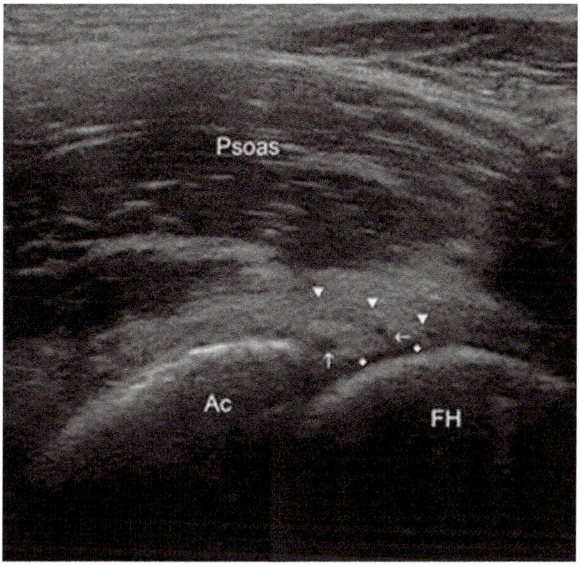

Fig. 6.11 Labral tear. *Arrowheads* indicate the anterior margin of the hyperechoic triangular labrum overlying the articular cartilage (rhombi) of the femoral head (FH). *Arrows* point to hypoechoic clefts on the acetabular and articular sides of the labrum in this patient with anterosuperior labrum tear. *Ac* acetabulum

Snapping Iliopsoas Tendon

Snapping iliopsoas tendon, also referred to as internal snapping hip syndrome, is due to snapping of the iliopsoas tendon over the iliopectineal eminence typically when moving the hip from a flexed, abducted, and externally rotated position into an extended, adducted, and internally rotated position or vice versa. The abrupt movement of the tendon from lateral to medial, or medial to lateral, can be visualized with dynamic ultrasound, placing the probe medially to the femoral head, parallel to the iliopectineal eminence. The patient is then asked to perform the maneuver that produces the snapping sensation while visualizing the abrupt movement of the tendon in short-axis view over the iliopectineal eminence [12].

Greater Trochanteric Pain Syndrome

The main findings in patients presenting with lateral hip pain are tendinopathy of the abductor tendons, tendinopathy in the proximal iliotibial band, and trochanteric bursitis. Ultrasound enables the examiner to differentiate these conditions, which cannot be distinguished by clinical exam alone. The typical patient is a middle-aged or elderly woman who presents with pain in the lateral hip that is exacerbated by lying on the affected side and by weight bearing. Greater trochanteric pain syndrome is somewhat less common in men and in people of younger age. It is increasingly recognized that the majority of patients with greater trochanteric pain syndrome have tendinopathy predominantly in the gluteus medius tendon [13]. The sonographic findings are thickening and hypoechogenicity with loss of fibrillar

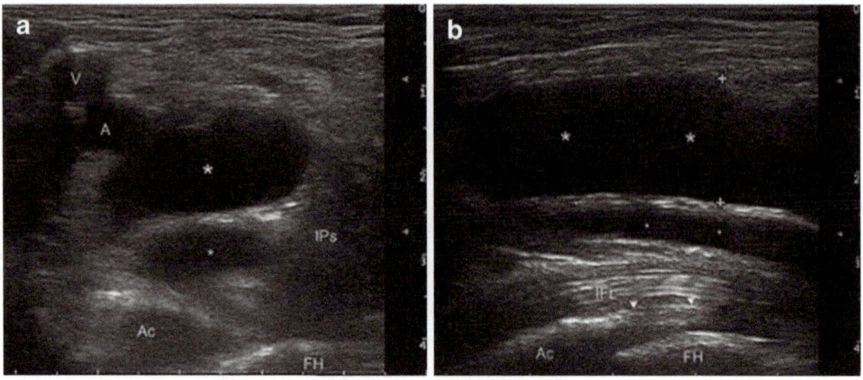

Fig. 6.12 Iliopsoas bursitis in transverse (**a**) and longitudinal (**b**) views. *Large* and *small asterisks* indicate two communicating compartments of the distended iliopsoas bursa. *V* femoral vein. *A* femoral artery. *Ac* acetabulum. *FH* femoral head. *IPs* iliopsoas muscle and hyperechoic tendon. *IFL* iliofemoral ligament. *White arrowheads* indicate the margins of the acetabular labrum. (Original pictures are courtesy of Wolfgang Schmidt)

pattern in the anterior portion of the tendon more commonly than the posterior and superoposterior portions of the tendon (Fig. 6.13). In the case of calcific tendinopathy, ultrasound demonstrates hyperechoic densities of variable size within the tendon substance (Fig. 6.14). Partial-thickness tears appear as anechoic defects within or at the undersurface of the tendon (Fig. 6.15). In the case of full-thickness tears, the tendon may be retracted proximally and the full-thickness defect replaced with debris or compressible fluid (Fig. 6.16). Tendinopathy and partial- or full-thickness tears can also be seen in the gluteus minimus tendon (Fig. 6.17) although pathology in the gluteus minimus tendon is less common than in the gluteus medius tendon and care must be taken to avoid anisotropy when imaging the gluteus minimus tendon, due to its oblique course on the anterior facet of the greater trochanter [31].

Abnormalities of the proximal iliotibial band include thickening, tendinopathy, and rarely ~~also~~ partial-thickness tears. Trochanteric or subgluteus maximus bursitis is far less common than previously thought to be the case in greater trochanteric pain syndrome [14]. It can be an associated finding when tendinopathy of the abductor mechanism is present, or less commonly it is found in isolation as an anechoic or hypoechoic compressible fluid collection laterally and posteriorly to the gluteus medius tendon, deep to the gluteus maximus muscle and iliotibial band (Fig. 6.18). Of note, fluid in the subgluteus maximus bursa may best be visualized in a supine position as small fluid collections can dissipate away from the field of view when the patient is placed in the lateral decubitus position with the affected hip facing upward. In chronic trochanteric bursitis, the bursal space may appear hyperechoic and thickened, without compressible fluid, and occasionally may take on a calcified appearance as can be seen in calcific bursitis.

An important advantage of ultrasound over other imaging modalities that applies particularly to the evaluation of greater trochanteric pain syndrome is that imaging findings can be correlated to the patient's clinical symptoms and area of tenderness.

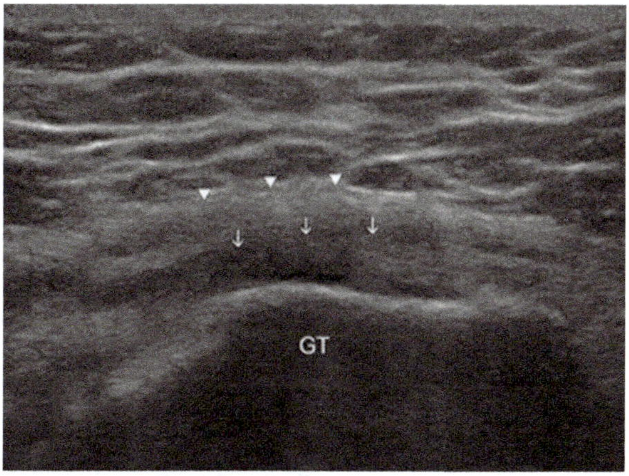

Fig. 6.13 Gluteus medius tendinopathy. Note the diffuse hypoechogenicity and loss of fibrillar pattern in the lateral portion of the gluteus medius tendon (*arrows*). *Arrowheads* point to the overlying iliotibial band which also appears diffusely hypoechoic, indicating edema

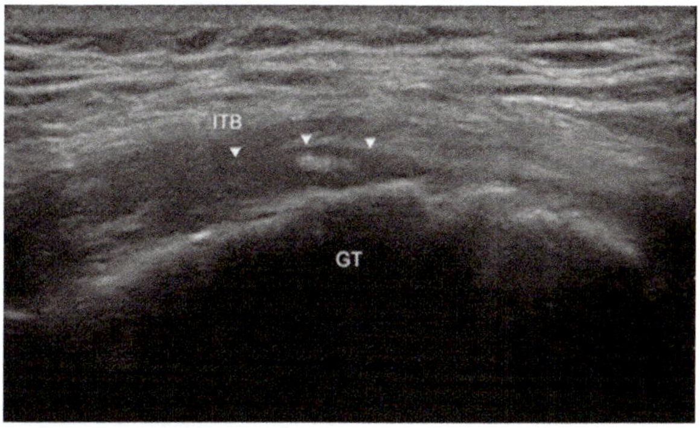

Fig. 6.14 Gluteus medius calcific tendinopathy. Amorphous hyperechoic deposit representing calcification within the diffusely hypoechoic gluteus medius tendon. *GT* greater trochanter. *ITB* iliotibial band

Tensor Fasciae Latae Tendinopathy

Tensor fasciae latae tendinopathy is an overuse tendinopathy common in runners, but can also occur as a result of degenerative enthesopathy. It should be suspected when a patient presents with point tenderness just below and slightly laterally to the anterior superior iliac spine (ASIS). Ultrasound shows thickening and hypoechogenicity with loss of fibrillar pattern at the origin of the tendon at the ASIS [15] (Fig. 6.19). Ultrasound has a higher sensitivity compared to physical exam in detecting enthesopathy; however, further studies are needed to determine the prognostic value of ultrasound findings predicting clinical enthesitis [16].

Piriformis Muscle Syndrome

The sciatic nerve can be seen medially as it enters the greater sciatic foramen under the piriformis muscle. It is here that swelling of the piriformis muscle can impinge

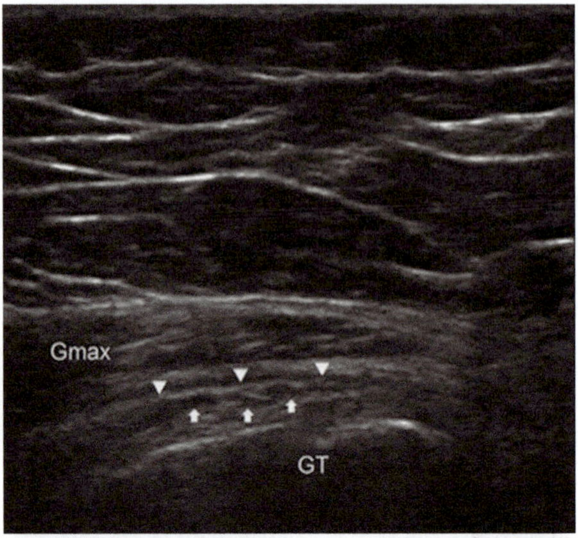

Fig. 6.15 Gluteus medius partial-thickness tear. Irregular shaped traumatic partial-thickness tear (*arrows*) extending through the lateral gluteus medius tendon. *Arrows* outline the anterior margin of the gluteus medius tendon. *GT* greater trochanter. *Gmax* gluteus maximus muscle at iliotibial band junction

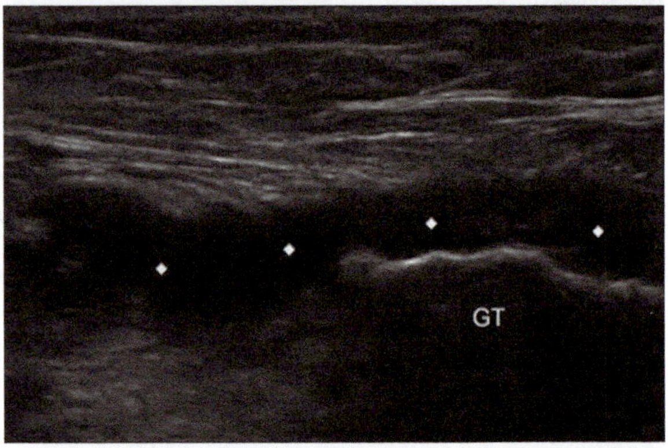

Fig. 6.16 Gluteus medius full-thickness tear. Complete full-thickness tear of the gluteus medius tendon replaced with compressible anechoic fluid. Note the absence of tendon fibers on the greater trochanter (GT)

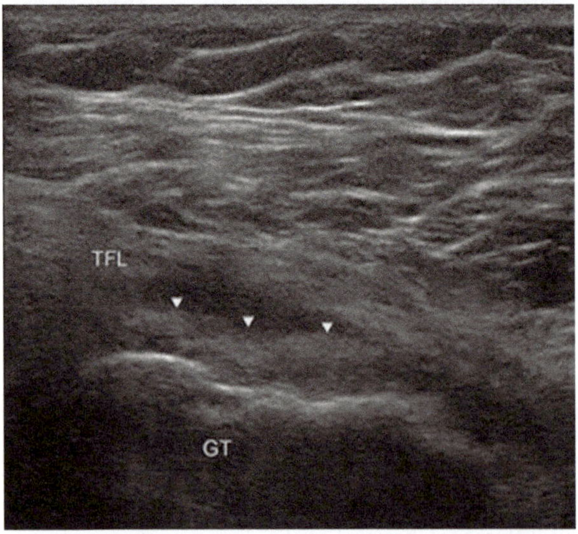

Fig. 6.17 Gluteus minimus tendinopathy. *Arrowheads* indicate the anterior margin of the hypoechoic gluteus minimus tendon on the anterior facet of the greater trochanter (GT), deep to the tensor fasciae latae (TFL)

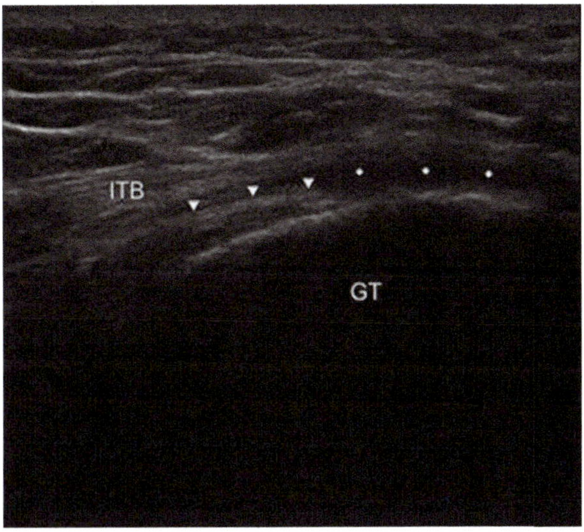

Fig. 6.18 Trochanteric bursitis. Rim of anechoic fluid (rhombi) between the gluteus medius tendon (*arrowheads* indicate anterior margin) and iliotibial band (ITB). *GT* greater trochanter

on the sciatic nerve causing sciatica of the ipsilateral leg, termed piriformis syndrome. This area is amenable to injection by placing the transducer along the long axis of the piriformis. The sciatic nerve and ascending branches of the inferior gluteal artery located deep to the gluteus maximus muscle (identified with doppler) should be avoided. The needle can be inserted in plane from medial to lateral at the most painful point which is generally at the tendinous portion of the piriformis between the gluteus maximus and ilium (Fig. 6.20).

Ultrasound of the Hip Joint in Rheumatologic Diseases

While correlation has been demonstrated between symptoms in the hip joint and the extent of cortical irregularity and synovial thickening or effusion on ultrasound, such findings have not yet shown to be disease-specific for osteoarthritis versus rheumatoid arthritis or the spondyloarthropathies. Hyperemia, as evidenced by positive CPD signal, is rarely reported in ultrasound of hip joints in patients with inflammatory arthropathies. In one case series of 100 hip joints in patients with rheumatoid arthritis examined by ultrasound, only one case was found to have positive CPD signal [17]. Changes of joint inflammation and damage furthermore did not correlate with disease activity scores although the extent of erosions found by ultrasound did correlate with disease duration. In a series of 130 hip joints in patients with psoriatic arthritis, synovial effusion with or without synovial hypertrophy and osteophytes was demonstrated in 20% of the cases, with only one case that showed positive CPD signal and none with evidence of erosions [18]. Similar prevalence of joint effusions and synovial hypertrophy were found in 56 patients with ankylosing spondylitis, and these correlated with levels of pain and markers of systemic inflammation, though not with other measures of disease activity. None of the patients had evidence of hyperemia in the hip joint by CPD [19].

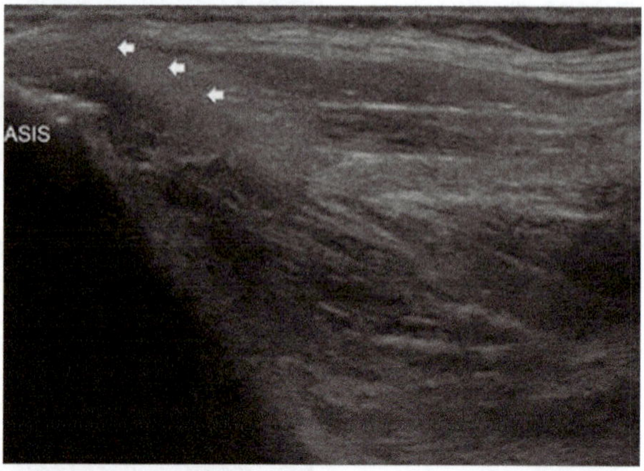

Fig. 6.19 Tensor fasciae latae tendinopathy. Hypoechogenicity and loss of fibrillar pattern of the tensor fasciae latae tendon (arrows) at its origin on the anterior superior iliac spine (ASIS). Note cortical irregularity on the ASIS

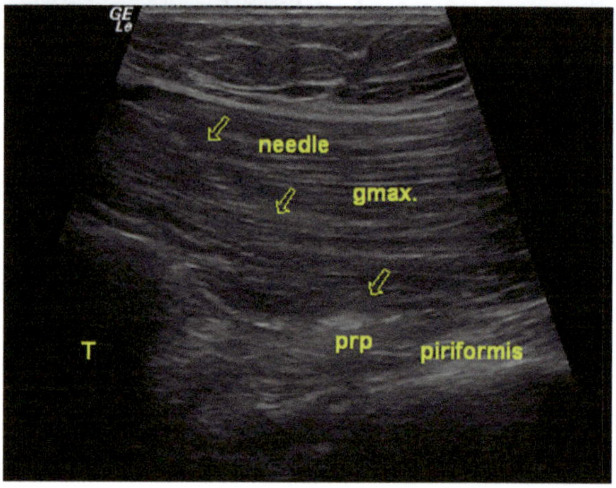

Fig. 6.20 Injection of the piriformis muscle (piriformis) with platelet-rich plasma (PRP) showing the needle track (needle, arrows). T (Ischial tuberosty). gmax (gluteus maximus). (Courtesy of Joanne Borg-Stein, MD)

A standardized ultrasound score to determine the degree of inflammation in large joints including the hips called the SOLAR (sonography of large joints in rheumatology) score has been introduced and evaluated in clinical practice as a tool to monitor disease activity with treatment. During an observation period of 12 months, gray-scale ultrasound (GSUS) scores were significantly improved with treatment in a cohort of 199 patients with rheumatoid arthritis. Power Doppler ultrasound (PDUS) scores were low at baseline compared with other joints, and although these improved with treatment as well, this was not statistically significant [20]. The SOLAR score has also been evaluated in patients with psoriatic arthritis and ankylosing spondylitis with similar performance in a cohort of 83 patients during longitudinal follow-up over 6 months. GSUS scores improved significantly with treatment, but improvements in baseline low PDUS scores were not statistically significant [21].

Polymyalgia Rheumatica

Ultrasound evaluation of the hips and shoulders has been included in the 2012 European League Against Rheumatism (EULAR)/American College of Rheumatology (ACR) classification criteria for polymyalgia rheumatica (PMR). Specifically, the finding of either a hip effusion or trochanteric bursitis, in addition to shoulder abnormalities (glenohumeral joint effusion, subacromial bursitis, or bicipital tenosynovitis), and/or the finding of abnormalities in both shoulders can each add a point to the scoring algorithm used for classification. Including ultrasound did not improve the sensitivity but modestly increased the specificity of the criteria for the classification of PMR (81% compared with 78% for clinical criteria without ultrasound). It performed well in differentiating PMR from non-inflammatory conditions but not as well in differentiating PMR from rheumatoid arthritis [22].

Gout and Pseudogout

While the hip is not a frequent site of gouty arthritis, ultrasound evaluation of the hips can be used to help confirm the diagnosis of gout. In a series of 40 patients who met the 2015 ACR/EULAR classification criteria for gout, ultrasound revealed imaging evidence of gout in at least one hip in 42.5% of patients, including crystalline aggregates, tophus, and double-contour sign [30]. In addition, ultrasound has been shown to be effective in the diagnosis of calcium pyrophosphate deposition disease or pseudogout, and its use has been encouraged in the EULAR recommendations for the diagnosis of pseudogout. In one such study, US confirmed the presence of CPPD crystals in 90% of definite pseudogout cases, yielding a sensitivity and specificity of 90% and 85%, respectively [29].

Ultrasound-Guided Aspiration and Injection of the Hip Joint

Ultrasound allows for hip joint aspiration and injections to be performed at the point of care in the office setting. Ultrasound-guided intra-articular injections of the hip joint have been shown to be accurate using fluoroscopy as a reference standard [23]. Using ultrasound for procedural guidance offers several advantages over fluoroscopy, such as visualization of periarticular and neurovascular structures, lack of ionizing radiation, accessibility, and possibly less procedure-related pain [24]. Aspiration or injection of the hip joint is usually performed using an axial approach along the femoral neck [25]. The patient is placed in a supine position and an anterior longitudinal view of the hip joint obtained with the transducer placed in the longitudinal oblique plane. The needle is then advanced from distal to proximal toward the femoral head-neck junction under direct ultrasound guidance in an in-plane approach until the needle tip is visualized in the anterior synovial joint recess (Fig. 6.21).

Ultrasound-Guided Injection of the Trochanteric Bursa/Gluteus Medius Peritendinous Space

Ultrasound guidance can be used to direct injection treatment for greater trochanteric pain syndrome. Whether ultrasound guidance increases the accuracy of local injection therapy compared with palpation-guided injection has not been shown. Both lateral longitudinal and transverse approaches are used in clinical practice for ultrasound-guided injection of the trochanteric bursa. For the more commonly used lateral longitudinal approach, the patient is placed in the lateral decubitus position with the symptomatic side facing up and the hip slightly flexed. A lateral longitudinal view of the greater trochanter and gluteus medius insertion is obtained and the needle advanced from distal to proximal toward the greater trochanter until its tip is visualized in the trochanteric bursa/gluteus medius peritendinous space under the iliotibial band [26] (see Fig. 6.22).

Common Pitfalls in Hip Ultrasonography

- With internal rotation of the hip, the anterior joint recess may falsely measure >7 mm, falsely indicating a joint effusion or synovitis when none actually is present. The hip should rather be placed in 10–15 degrees of external rotation.
- The transducer must be placed along the correct long axis of the femoral neck in order to accurately visualize the synovium and anterior joint recess; otherwise, it may appear hypoechoic in nature and simulate a joint effusion. Additionally, in order to best visualize the anterior joint recess, increased pressure should be placed at the more caudal end of the probe by using a heel-toe maneuver.
- When present, a paralabral cyst can easily be misdiagnosed as a joint effusion.

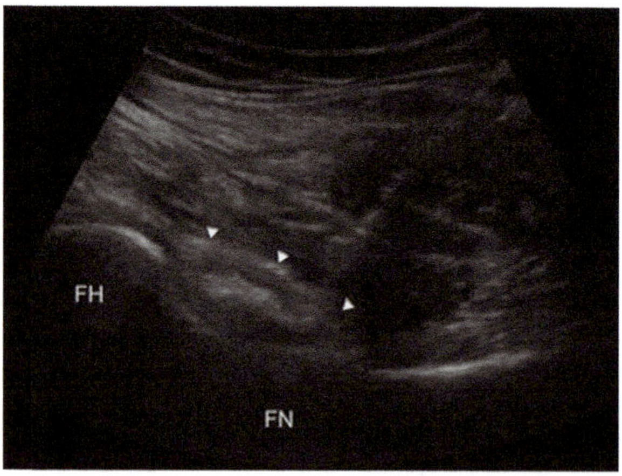

Fig. 6.21 Hip joint injection. *FH* femoral head. *FN* femoral neck. *Arrowheads* indicate the superficial margin of the anterior joint capsule

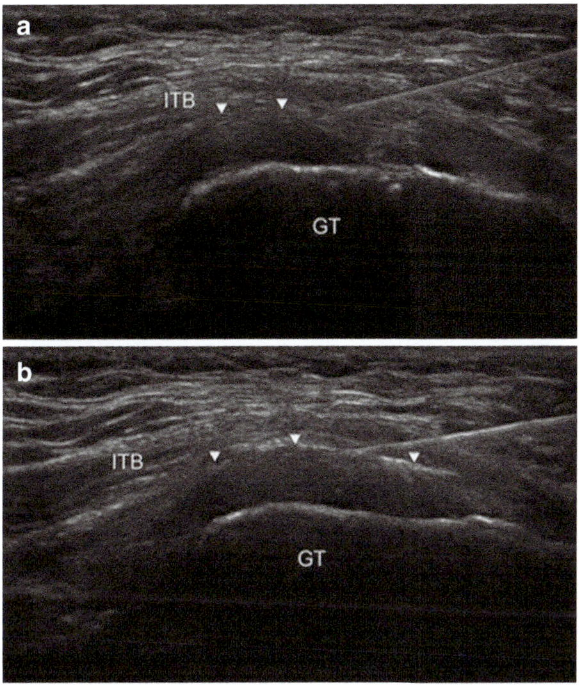

Fig. 6.22 Ultrasound-guided trochanteric bursa injection. (**a**) pre-injection, (**b**) post-injection. Note the needle tip in the bursal space between the gluteus medius tendon (*arrows* indicate superficial margin of the tendon) and the iliotibial band (ITB). *GT* greater trochanter

Conclusion

The hip is a deep-structured joint with bony as well as many soft tissue and periarticular structures that can be affected by mechanical, degenerative, and inflammatory pathology. The hip is amenable to ultrasonographic diagnosis and injection guidance and has the potential for early identification of inflammatory disease and treatment monitoring. A clear understanding of the normal anatomy, pathologic presentations, and their implications is essential to the successful use and interpretation of ultrasound images of the hip.

Review Questions

1. Synovitis or effusion in the hip joint is probable when:
   (a) The anterior joint capsule measures ≥5 mm in thickness and takes on a concave shape.
   (b) The anterior joint capsule measures ≥5 mm in thickness, or there is asymmetric distention of the joint capsule of ≥1 mm compared to the opposite hip.
   (c) The anterior joint capsule measures ≥7 mm in thickness, or there is asymmetric distention of the joint capsule of ≥1 mm compared to the opposite hip.
   (d) The anterior joint capsule measures ≥9 mm in thickness and takes on a convex shape.

2. Which of the following structures is not seen on the anterior longitudinal view of the hip?
   (a) Acetabulum
   (b) Labrum
   (c) Iliopsoas tendon
   (d) Tensor fasciae latae
3. Positive color power Doppler ultrasound is a common finding in inflammatory arthritis of the hip joint.
   (a) True
   (b) False
4. In patients with rheumatoid arthritis, synovial thickening in the hip joint has been shown to improve with disease-modifying treatment.
   (a) True
   (b) False
5. Which of the following findings could be missed on lateral longitudinal views of the hip with the patient placed in the lateral decubitus position?
   (a) Subgluteus maximus bursitis
   (b) Gluteus medius tendinopathy
   (c) Gluteus minimus tendinopathy
   (d) Iliotibial band tendinopathy
6. The gluteus medius tendon inserts on the
   (a) Anterior facet of the greater trochanter
   (b) Lateral facet of the greater trochanter
   (c) Superoposterior facet of the greater trochanter
   (d) (b) and (c)
7. Which of the following tendons is most prone to anisotropy, due to its oblique course relative to the surface of the skin?
   (a) Gluteus medius tendon
   (b) Iliopsoas tendon
   (c) Gluteus minimus tendon
   (d) Iliotibial band
8. The needle path during ultrasound-guided hip joint injection using a long-axis approach to the femoral neck from distal to proximal includes all of the following except:
   (a) Rectus femoris
   (b) Tensor fasciae latae
   (c) Iliopsoas
   (d) Anterior hip joint capsule
9. The following structures exhibit anisotropy except
   (a) Anterior hip joint capsule
   (b) Gluteus medius tendon
   (c) Iliopsoas tendon
   (d) Femoral head cartilage

10. Which of the following ultrasound findings constitutes part of the scoring system in the 2012 European League Against Rheumatism (EULAR)/American College of Rheumatology (ACR) provisional classification criteria for polymyalgia rheumatica (PMR)?
    (a) Unilateral hip effusion or trochanteric bursitis, in addition to unilateral glenohumeral joint effusion, subacromial bursitis, and biceps tenosynovitis
    (b) Hip effusion alone
    (c) Trochanteric bursitis alone
    (d) Bilateral hip effusion or trochanteric bursitis

Additional Questions

11. The appropriate positioning of the patient for ultrasound evaluation of the anterior hip is with
    (a) The patient in supine position with hip and knee extended and the leg in 10–15 degrees of internal rotation
    (b) The patient in supine position with hip and knee extended and the leg in 10–15 degrees of external rotation
    (c) The patient in supine position with hip and knee extended and the leg in neutral position
    (d) The patient in the lateral decubitus position with the hip in 30 degrees of flexion and the knees in slight flexion as well
12. If the ultrasonographer is unable to clearly visualize the anterior hip joint recess, he or she should first try
    (a) Heel-toe maneuver with increased pressure/depth of the caudal or distal aspect of the probe
    (b) Switching from a curvilinear to linear probe for increased frequency
    (c) Rotating the probe 20–30 degrees in the cranial-lateral and caudal-medial direction
    (d) Externally rotating the leg an additional 10 degrees
13. In patients with gout and pseudogout, monosodium urate crystal deposition and calcium pyrophosphate crystal deposition, respectively, have been identified frequently in the hip joint.
    (a) True
    (b) False
14. In patients with lateral hip pain and physical exam findings of trochanteric bursitis or greater trochanteric pain syndrome, fluid within the trochanteric bursa or subgluteus maximus bursa
    (a) Is frequently visualized
    (b) Is rarely visualized
15. In patients with lateral hip pain, the more commonly seen pathology with ultrasound is
    (a) Gluteus maximus tendinopathy
    (b) Gluteus medius tendinopathy
    (c) Gluteus minimus tendinopathy
    (d) Subgluteus maximus bursitis

16. In the anterior view of the hip, the structures identified from medial to lateral are
    (a) Femoral artery, femoral head, femoral nerve, femoral vein
    (b) Femoral nerve, femoral vein, femoral artery, femoral head
    (c) Femoral head, femoral nerve, femoral artery, femoral vein
    (d) Femoral vein, femoral artery, femoral nerve, femoral head
17. In patients with sciatica deemed to be due to piriformis syndrome, an injection closest to the _____ can be most beneficial.
    (a) Sciatic nerve
    (b) Gluteus maximus muscle
    (c) Piriformis muscle
    (d) Gluteus medius muscle

Answers

1. (c) The anterior joint capsule measures ≥7 mm in thickness or there is asymmetric distention of the joint capsule of ≥1 mm compared to the opposite hip.
2. (d) Tensor fasciae latae
3. (b) False
4. (a) True
5. (a) Subgluteus maximus bursitis
6. (d) (b) and (c)
7. (c) Gluteus minimus tendon
8. (b) Tensor fasciae latae
9. (d) Femoral head cartilage
10. (a) Unilateral hip effusion or trochanteric bursitis, in addition to unilateral glenohumeral joint effusion, subacromial bursitis, and biceps tenosynovitis
11. (b) The patient in supine position with hip and knee extended and the leg in 10–15 degrees of external rotation
12. (a) Heel-toe maneuver with increased pressure/depth of the caudal or distal aspect of the probe
13. (a) True
14. (b) Is rarely visualized
15. (b) Gluteus medius tendinopathy
16. (d) Femoral vein, femoral artery, femoral nerve, femoral head
17. (c) Piriformis muscle

References

1. McAlindon T, Kissin E, Nazarian L, Ranganath V, Prakash S, Taylor M, et al. American College of Rheumatology report on reasonable use of musculoskeletal ultrasonography in rheumatology clinical practice. Arthritis Care Res (Hoboken). 2012;64(11):1625–40.
2. Backhaus M, Burmester GR, Gerber T, Grassi W, Machold KP, Swen WA, et al. Guidelines for musculoskeletal ultrasound in rheumatology. Ann Rheum Dis. 2001;60(7):641–9.
3. Schmidt WA, Hauer RW, Banzer D, Bohl-Bühler M, Braun J, Mellerowicz H, et al. Technik und Stellenwert der Arthrosonographie in der rheumatologischen Diagnostik. Teil 2: Sonographie der Hueftregion. Z Rheumatol. 2002;61:180–8.

4. Pfirrmann CW, Chung CB, Theumann NH, Trudell DJ, Resnick D. Greater trochanter of the hip: attachment of the abductor mechanism and a complex of three bursae – MR imaging and MR bursography in cadavers and MR imaging in asymptomatic volunteers. Radiology. 2001;221:469–77.
5. Robben SG, Lequin MH, Diepstraten AF, den Hollander JC, Entius CA, Meradji M. Anterior joint capsule of the normal hip and in children with transient synovitis: US study with anatomic and histologic correlation. Radiology. 1999;210:499–507.
6. Koski JM, Anttila PJ, Isomaki HA. Ultrasonography of the adult hip joint. Scand J Rheumatol. 1989;18(2):113–7.
7. Weybright PN, Jacobson JA, Murry KH, Lin J, Fessell DP, Jamadar DA, et al. Limited effectiveness of sonography in revealing hip joint effusion: preliminary results in 21 adult patients with native and postoperative hips. Am J Roentgenol. 2003;181(1):215–8.
8. Walther M, Harms H, Krenn V, Radke S, Kirschner S, Gohlke F. Synovial tissue of the hip at power Doppler US: correlation between vascularity and power Doppler US signal. Radiology. 2002;225:225–31.
9. Long S, Surrey D, Nazarian L. Common sonographic findings in the painful hip after hip arthroplasty. J Ultrasound Med. 2012;31:301–12.
10. Wunderbaldinger P, Bremer C, Schellenberger E, Cejna M, Turetschek K, Kainberger F. Imaging features of iliopsoas bursitis. Eur Radiol. 2002;12(2):409–15.
11. Bianchi S, Martinoli C, Keller A, Bianchi-Zamorani MP. Giant iliopsoas bursitis: sonographic findings with magnetic resonance correlations. J Clin Ultrasound. 2002;30(7):437–41.
12. Pelsser V, Cardinal E, Hobden R, Aubin B, Lafortune M. Extraarticular snapping hip: sonographic findings. Am J Roentgenol. 2001;176(1):67–73.
13. Klauser AS, Martinoli C, Tagliafico A, Bellmann-Weiler R, Feuchtner GM, Wick M, et al. Greater trochanteric pain syndrome. Semin Musculoskelet Radiol. 2013;17(1):43–8.
14. Long SS, Surrey DE, Nazarian LN. Sonography of greater trochanteric pain syndrome and the rarity of primary bursitis. Am J Roentgenol. 2013;201(5):1083–6.
15. Bass CJ, Connel DA. Sonographic findings of tensor fascia lata tendinopathy: another cause of anterior groin pain. Skelet Radiol. 2002;31:143–8.
16. Ruta S, Gutierrez M, Pena C, García M, Arturi A, Filippucci E, et al. Prevalence of subclinical enthesopathy in patients with spondyloarthropathy: an ultrasound study. J Clin Rheumatol. 2011;17(1):18–22.
17. Di Geso L, Filippucci E, Riente L, Sakellariou G, Delle Sedie A, Meenagh G, et al. Ultrasound for the rheumatologist XL. Sonographic assessment of the hip in rheumatoid arthritis. Clin Exp Rheumatol. 2012;30(4):464–8.
18. Riente L, Delle Sedie A, Sakellariou G, Filippucci E, Meenagh G, Iagnocco A, et al. Ultrasound imaging for the rheumatologist XXXVIII. Sonographic assessment of the hip in psoriatic arthritis patients. Clin Exp Rheumatol. 2012;30(2):152–5.
19. Sakellariou G, Iagnocco A, Meenagh G, Riente L, Filippucci E, Delle Sedie A, et al. Ultrasound imaging for the rheumatologist XXXVII. Sonographic assessment of the hip in ankylosing spondylitis patients. Clin Exp Rheumatol. 2012;30(1):1–5.
20. Hartung W, Kellner H, Strunk J, Sattler H, Schmidt WA, Ehrenstein B, et al. Development and evaluation of a novel ultrasound score for large joints in rheumatoid arthritis: one year of experience in daily clinical practice. Arthritis Care Res. 2012;64(5):675–82.
21. Schäfer VS, Fleck M, Kellner H, Strunk J, Sattler H, Schmidt WA, et al. Evaluation of the novel ultrasound score for large joints in psoriatic arthritis and ankylosing spondylitis: six month experience in daily clinical practice. BMC Musculoskelet Disord. 2013;14:358.
22. Dasgupta B, Cimmino MA, Kremers HM, Schmidt WA, Schirmer M, Salvarani C, et al. 2012 provisional classification criteria for polymyalgia rheumatica: a European League Against Rheumatism/American College of Rheumatology collaborative initiative. Arthritis Rheum. 2012;64(4):943–54.
23. Smith J, Hurdle MF, Weingarten TN. Accuracy of sonographically guided intra-articular injections in the native adult hip. J Ultrasound Med. 2009;28:329–35.
24. Byrd JW, Potts EA, Allison RK, Jones KS. Ultrasound-guided hip injections: a comparative study with fluoroscopy-guided injections. Arthroscopy. 2014;30(1):42–6.

25. Fessell DP, Jacobson JA, Craig J, Habra G, Prasad A, Radliff A, et al. Using sonography to reveal and aspirate join effusions. AJR Ann J Roentgenol. 2000;174:1353–62.
26. Labrosse JM, Cardinal E, Leduc BE, Duranceau J, Rémillard J, Bureau NJ, et al. Effectiveness of ultrasound-guided corticosteroid injection for the treatment of gluteus medius tendinopathy. AJR Am J Roentgenol. 2010;194(1):202–6.
27. Becciolini M, Bonacchi G, Bianchi S. Ultrasound features of the proximal Hamstring muscle-tendon-bone unit. J Ultrasound Med. 2019;38(5):1367–82.
28. Chang KV, Wu WT, Lew HL, Özçakar L. Ultrasound imaging and guided injection for the lateral and posterior hip. Am J Phys Med Rehabil. 2018;97(4):285–91.
29. Di Matteo A, Filippucci E, Cipolletta E, Musca A, Carotti M, Mashadi Mirza R, Jesus D, Martire V, Pierucci D, Di Carlo M, Salaffi F, Grassi W. Hip involvement in patients with calcium pyrophosphate deposition disease: potential and limits of musculoskeletal ultrasound. Arthritis Care Res (Hoboken). 2018; https://doi.org/10.1002/acr.23814.
30. Di Matteo A, Filippucci E, Cipolletta E, Musca A, Di Donato E, Martire V, Jesus D, Salaffi F, Grassi W. Ultrasound and clinical features of hip involvement in patients with gout. Joint Bone Spine. 2019; pii: S1297-319X(19)30030-2.
31. Docking SI, Cook J, Chen S, Scarvell J, Cormick W, Smith P, Fearon A. Identification and differentiation of gluteus medius tendon pathology using ultrasound and magnetic resonance imaging. Musculoskelet Sci Pract. 2019;41:1–5.

Ultrasound of the Knee

7

Catherine J. Bakewell, Gary A. Kunkel, and Amanda E. Nelson

Key Points

- The knee joint is amenable to ultrasonographic imaging for diagnostic, therapeutic, and monitoring purposes.
- Correct positioning and probe placement are keys for image interpretation.
- Abnormalities at the knee can be seen in many rheumatologic conditions, including osteoarthritis, rheumatoid arthritis, spondyloarthropathies, and crystalline arthropathies.

Introduction

The knee is a highly accessible and relatively straightforward joint for the use of musculoskeletal ultrasound, which allows assessment of the bone, cartilage, synovium, joint effusion, tendons, ligaments, and peripheral menisci, as well as associated pathologies. Table 7.1 illustrates important anatomic landmarks that can be visualized using ultrasound. Structures are identified according to their anterior,

C. J. Bakewell (✉)
Rheumatology, Intermountain Medical Group, Salt Lake Clinic, Salt Lake City, UT, USA
e-mail: bakewell@uw.edu

G. A. Kunkel
Division of Rheumatology, University of Utah, Salt Lake City, UT, USA
e-mail: Gary.Kunkel@hsc.utah.edu

A. E. Nelson
Thurston Arthritis Research Center and Division of Rheumatology, Allergy, and Immunology, University of North Carolina at Chapel Hill, Chapel Hill, NC, USA
e-mail: aenelson@med.unc.edu

M. J. Kohler (ed.), *Musculoskeletal Ultrasound in Rheumatology Review*,
https://doi.org/10.1007/978-3-030-73555-5_7

Table 7.1 Standard views in the normal knee based on Backhaus et al. [5]

Location	Orientation	Positioning	Structures
Anterior			
Suprapatellar	*Longitudinal*	~30° flexion	Patella, femur, suprapatellar pouch, quadriceps tendon
	Transverse	~30° flexion	Quadriceps tendon, femur
	Transverse	Maximal flexion	Femur, articular cartilage
Infrapatellar	*Longitudinal, proximal*	Neutral	Patella, patellar ligament, femur
	Longitudinal, distal	Neutral	Tibial tuberosity, patellar ligament
	Transverse	Neutral	Patellar ligament, infrapatellar bursa
Medial			
Medial	*Longitudinal*	Neutral	Femur, tibia, joint line, medial collateral ligament, meniscus
Lateral			
Lateral	*Longitudinal*	Neutral	Femur, tibia, joint line, lateral collateral ligament, iliotibial band
Posterior			
Posterior	*Transverse*	Extension	Femur, gastrocnemius, semimembranosus, popliteal vessels

medial, lateral, or posterior location (Table. 7.1). The American College of Rheumatology recently published a report on the reasonable use of musculoskeletal ultrasonography (MSUS) in rheumatology clinical practice based on expert opinion using RAND/UCLA methodology [1]. Specific to the knee, reasonable use of MSUS included evaluation of articular pain, swelling, or mechanical symptoms without definitive diagnosis on clinical examination; evaluation of monoarthralgia or oligoarthralgia without definitive diagnosis on clinical examination; evaluation of disease activity, structural damage, and alternate causes in a patient with known inflammatory arthritis and new or ongoing symptoms; assessment of tendon and soft tissue pathologies in patients with periarticular pain; evaluation of inflammation, tendon, or soft tissue pathologies in patients with regional mechanical symptoms; facilitation of clinical assessment at symptomatic sites whose "evaluation is obfuscated by adipose or other local derangements of soft tissue"; and guidance of articular and periarticular aspiration or injection at synovial, tenosynovial, bursal, peritendinous, and perienthesal areas [1]. In addition, ultrasound examination of the knee is often a useful "second scan" joint area in suspected spondyloarthritis or crystalline arthritis, due to the high frequency of knee involvement in these diseases and characteristic ultrasound findings, which may add sensitivity to an equivocal or indeterminate primary foot and ankle scan [2–4].

Standard Views in the Normal Knee

Table 7.1 shows standard views of the knee [5].

Anterior

Suprapatellar

Suprapatellar Longitudinal View

The probe should be placed parallel to the quadriceps tendon, with the distal end over the patellar insertion (Fig. 7.1a). Observable landmarks include the femur, the patella, and the quadriceps tendon itself (Fig. 7.1b). As with the views to follow, it is essential to sweep with the probe medially and laterally to evaluate for effusions that may not be in the midline. Quadriceps contraction can help push fluid into the

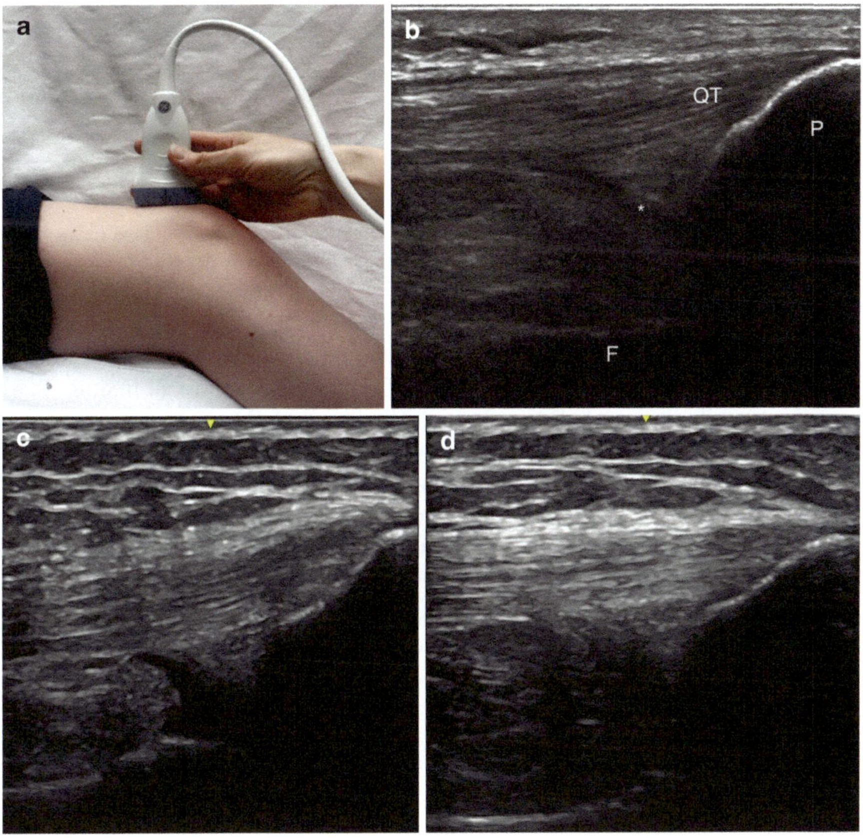

Fig. 7.1 Suprapatellar longitudinal image. (**a**) Probe placement for suprapatellar longitudinal image. (**b**) Normal suprapatellar longitudinal ultrasound view. Key visualized structures include the Quadriceps Tendon (QT), Patella (P), Synovial recess (*) and Femur (F). (**c**) Additional flexion on the knee can bring distal femur (DF) into view and sharpen boundaries of synovial recess (*). Additional structures shown include the Quadriceps fat pad (**) and the Prefemoral Fat Pad (***). (**d**) Quadriceps contraction can draw effusion out from under the patella (not visualized) or highlight gray scale abnormalities of the quadraceps enthesis or tendon body (such as tears or tendinosis)

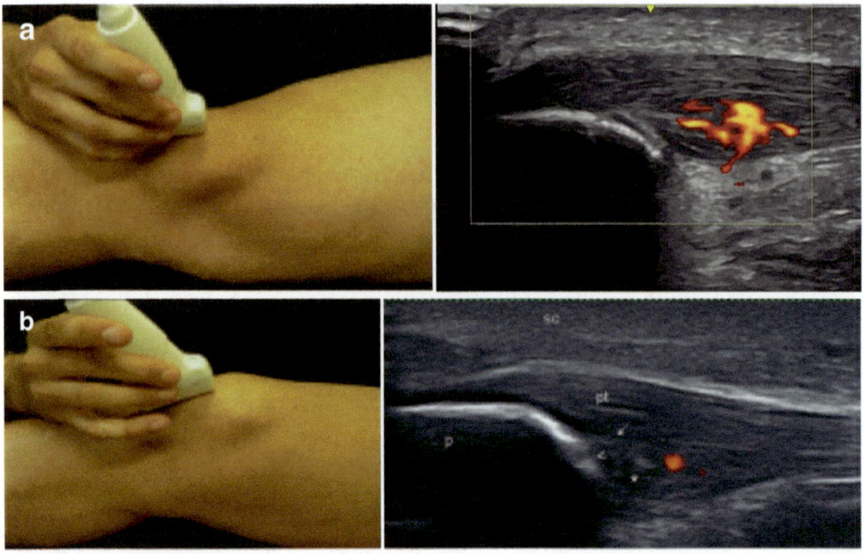

Fig. 7.2 Patellar tendon enthesitis (**a**) extended position, patellar tendon with significant power Doppler signal, (**b**) 30 degrees flexed position, patellar tendon with less power Doppler signal

suprapatellar recess, increasing the sensitivity to detect effusion [6]. It is important to note that too much pressure on the transducer may shift otherwise visible effusion away from view. The presence of 2–4 mm of fluid may be a normal finding [7, 8], and suprapatellar synovial plica, appearing as a hyperechoic separation of the synovial membrane, are typically asymptomatic.

The suprapatellar longitudinal view should be performed with the knee in 30° of flexion. In a study of 45 knees with active inflammatory arthritis which had ultrasound imaging in full extension, full extension with quadriceps contraction, 30° of flexion, and 90° of flexion, the views in 30° of flexion had the greatest sensitivity for detection of effusion [9]. However, Doppler imaging for enthesitis of the quadriceps tendon may be more sensitive in the extended position where less tension is placed on the intratendinous vessels [10] (Fig. 7.2).

Suprapatellar Transverse View

The probe should be placed over the quadriceps tendon proximal to the patellar insertion, scanning proximal to distal up to the insertion (Fig. 7.3a). Observable landmarks include the femur, the synovial fold, and the quadriceps tendon (Fig. 7.3b). Scanning proximal to distal and also medial to lateral can increase sensitivity for detecting effusion.

Parapatellar Views (Nonstandard)

The probe position is transverse to the long axis of the femur, over the superior portion to midway down the length of the patella, with the anterior end of the transducer at the medial or lateral border of the patella, and the posterior end at the femur

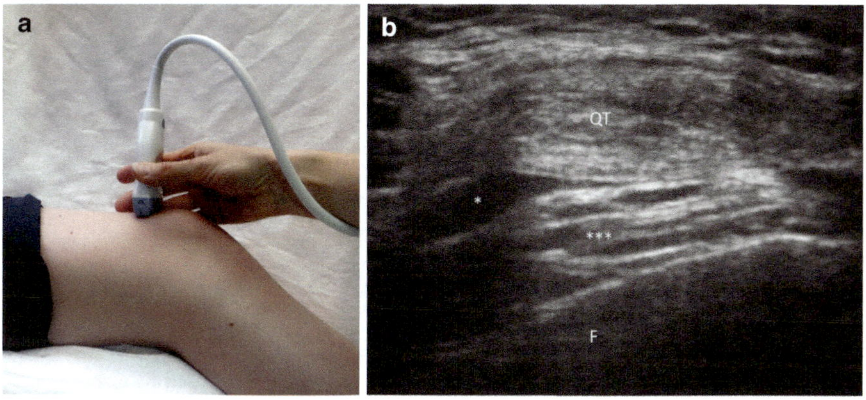

Fig. 7.3 Suprapatellar transverse image. (**a**) Probe placement for suprapatellar transverse image. (**b**) Normal suprapatellar transverse ultrasound view

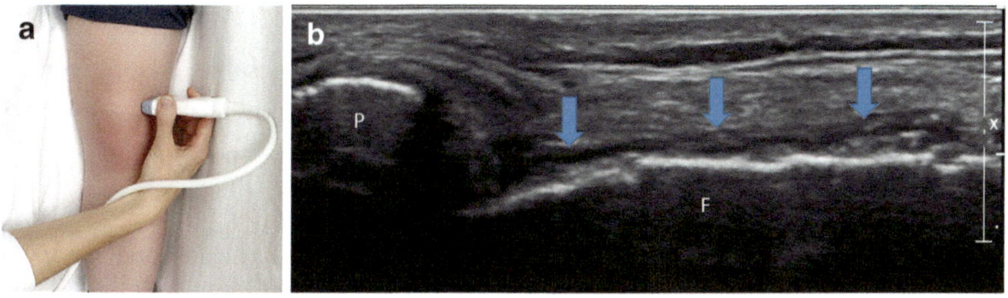

Fig. 7.4 Lateral Parapatellar Recess. (**a**) Probe placement on patient. (**b**) Lateral parapatellar recess (arrows) is seen emerging underneath the Patella (P) and layering along the femur (F)

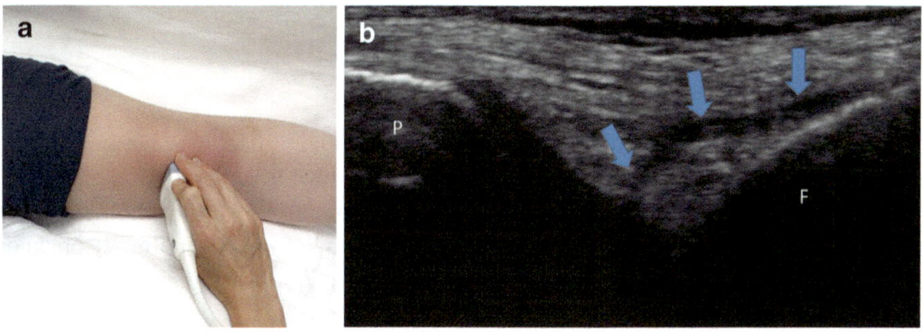

Fig. 7.5 Medial Parapatellar Recess. (**a**) Probe placement on patient. (**b**) Medial parapatellar recess (arrows) is seen emerging underneath the Patella (P) and layering along the femur (F)

(Figs. 7.4 and 7.5). The landmarks medially will include the patella and femur. Sweeping from the midpatellar position proximally and distally will increase sensitivity for finding the maximal amount of effusion or synovial proliferation. In the lateral parapatellar view, small, dependent effusions may be seen quite posteriorly

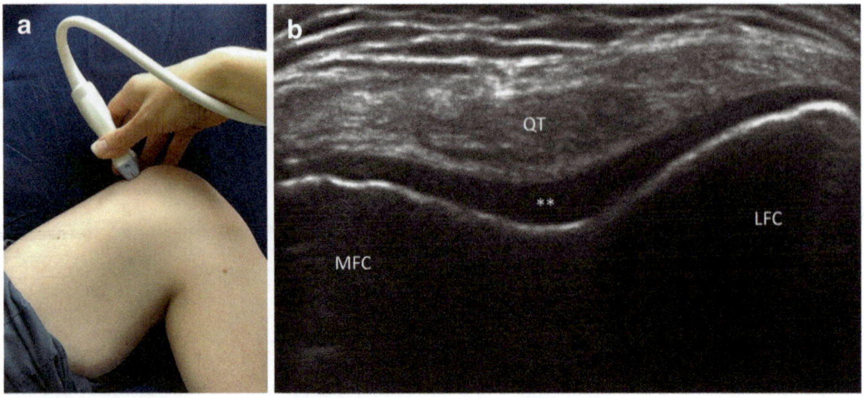

Fig. 7.6 Suprapatellar Maximum Flexion. (**a**) Demonstration of probe placement on patient. (**b**) Normal suprapatellar Maximum Flexion transverse view. Key visualized structures include the Quadriceps Tendon (QT), Hyaline cartilage (**) and Medial and lateral femoral condyles (MFC, LFC)

over the femur, so sliding the transducer posteriorly is advisable. Also, given the relatively superficial position of the parapatellar recesses, avoidance of excess transducer pressure is critical for detecting effusion.

Suprapatellar Transverse in Maximum Flexion View

The probe position is the same as in the standard suprapatellar transverse view, but now with the knee in maximum flexion (Fig. 7.6a). The landmarks will include the femoral condyles and overlying anechoic articular cartilage, as well as the quadriceps tendon (Fig. 7.6b). This view is best suited for evaluation of the cartilage itself, and less so for evaluation of effusion or synovitis.

Infrapatellar

There are two images of the patellar ligament, as many machines are not able to visualize the full extent of the ligament in a single view. In general, 30-degree flexion of the knee is preferable for assessment of tendon integrity and pathology, as the ligament tends to become lax and with variable anisotropy ("rippling") on knee extension (Fig. 7.7). But as in the suprapatellar views, Doppler imaging of the patellar ligament is best performed with the knee extended.

Infrapatellar Longitudinal-Proximal

The probe should be placed with the proximal end on the patella and the distal end extending along the tibia (Fig. 7.8a). Landmarks include the patella and the patellar ligament superficially and, deeper, the surfaces of the femur proximally and the tibia distally (Fig. 7.8b). Given the significant width of patellar ligament, medial to

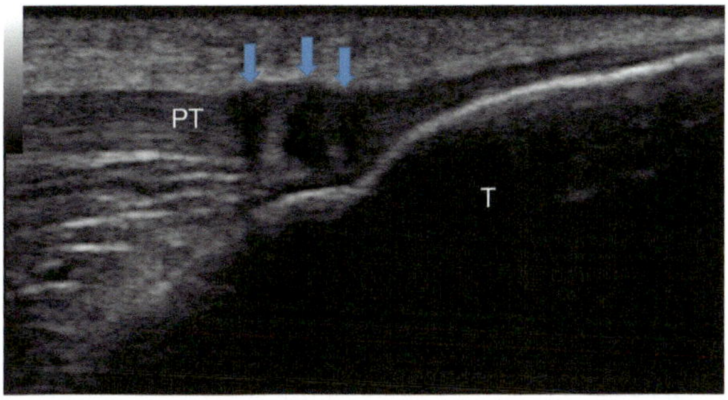

Fig. 7.7 Infrapatellar tendon laxity. A patellar tendon (PT) with considerable laxity on its insertion to the tibia (T) demonstrating hypoechoic regions mimicking tendinosis or even tears (arrows)

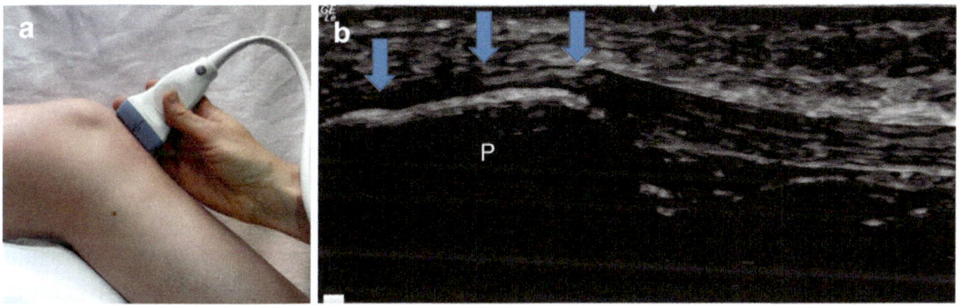

Fig. 7.8 Infrapatellar Long, Proximal. (**a**) Demonstration of probe placement on patient. (**b**) Normal Proximal Infrapatellar longitudinal view. Key visualized structures include the Patella (P) and origin of the Patellar ligament (arrows)

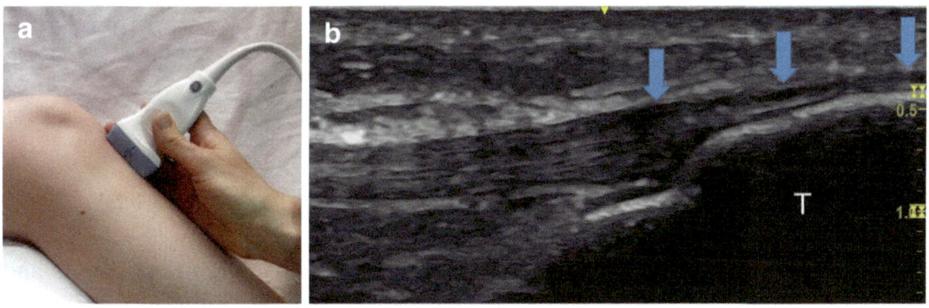

Fig. 7.9 Infrapatellar long, Distal. (**a**) Demonstration of probe placement on patient. (**b**) Normal Distal Infrapatellar longitudinal view. Key visualized structures include the Tibia (T) and insertion of the Patellar ligament (arrows)

lateral sweeping of the transducer will increase sensitivity for detecting ligament injury, enthesitis, or crystalline deposits. Avoidance of excess transducer pressure is critical for detecting prepatellar bursal swelling over the patella.

Infrapatellar Longitudinal-Distal

This image is obtained by moving the probe distally along the patellar ligament to the insertion of the ligament on the tibial tuberosity (Fig. 7.9a). Landmarks

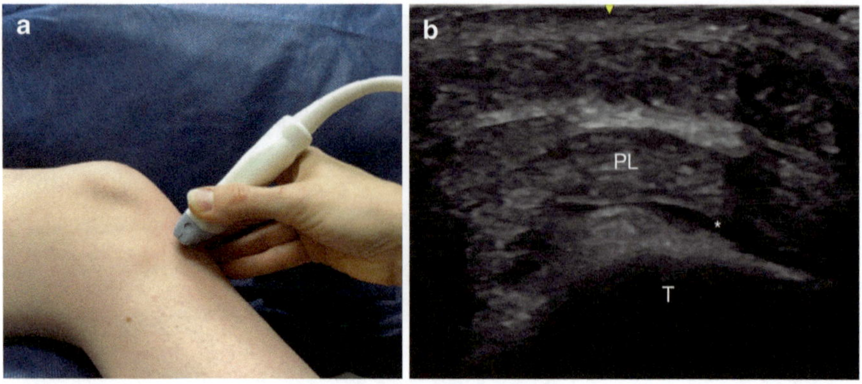

Fig. 7.10 Infrapatellar Transverse. (**a**) Demonstration of probe placement on patient. (**b**) Normal Distal Infrapatellar transverse view. Key visualized structures include the Tibia (T) and Patellar Ligament (PL). A small amount of fluid is appreciated in the deep infrapatellar bursa (*)

include the patellar ligament, tibial tuberosity, and infrapatellar fat pad superficially, as well as the surface of the tibia deeper in the image (Fig. 7.9b). As emphasized above, light transducer pressure and medial to lateral sweeping are important for increasing the sensitivity for infrapatellar bursal swelling or patellar ligament pathology.

Infrapatellar Transverse

By rotating the probe 90° between the proximal and distal longitudinal positions, a cross section of the patellar ligament can be identified over the surface of the tibia (Fig. 7.10a). This is the location of the deep infrapatellar bursa (Fig. 7.10b).

Medial

Medial Longitudinal

The probe should be placed along the medial joint line, medial to the patella and patellar ligament (Fig. 7.11a). Observable landmarks include the distal femur, proximal tibia, medial edge of the medial meniscus, and medial collateral ligament (Figs. 7.11b and 7.12). These are generally superficial structures requiring some machine adjustments to improve resolution. The origin of the medial collateral ligament can be found from a transverse-to the-femur transducer position (similar to the medial parapatellar view), with movement of the transducer posteriorly until the triangular bony prominence of the medial femoral epicondyle is seen. The ligament can be seen arising from the posterior aspect of the epicondyle (Fig. 7.13). As noted previously, it is essential to scan with the probe anterior to posterior to identify any

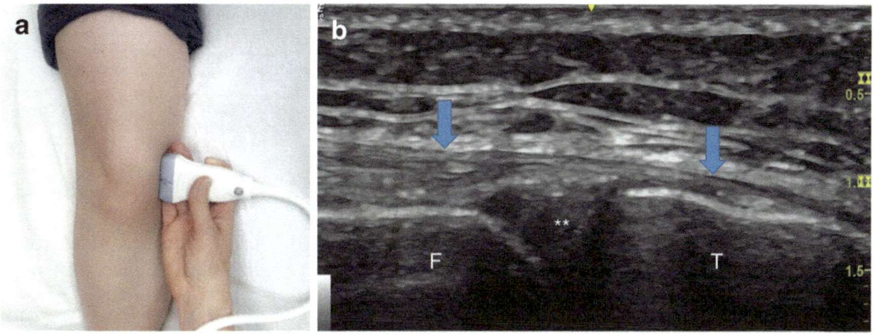

Fig. 7.11 Medial longitudinal. (**a**) Demonstration of probe placement on patient. (**b**) Normal Medial longitudinal view. Key visualized structures include the Medial collateral ligament (arrows), meniscus (**), Femur (F) and Tibia (T)

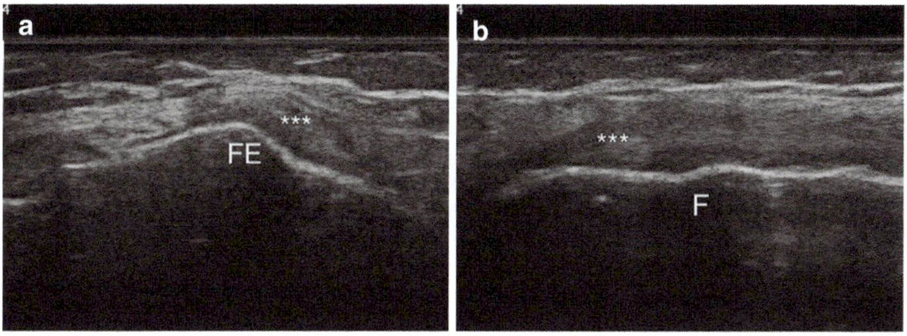

Fig. 7.12 Medial scan MCL takeoff. (**a**) Medial femoral epicondyle (FE) in transverse. The MCL (***) can be seen arising from posterior aspect of this bony landmark. (**b**) Longitudinal view of the origin of the MCL (***) on the femur (F)

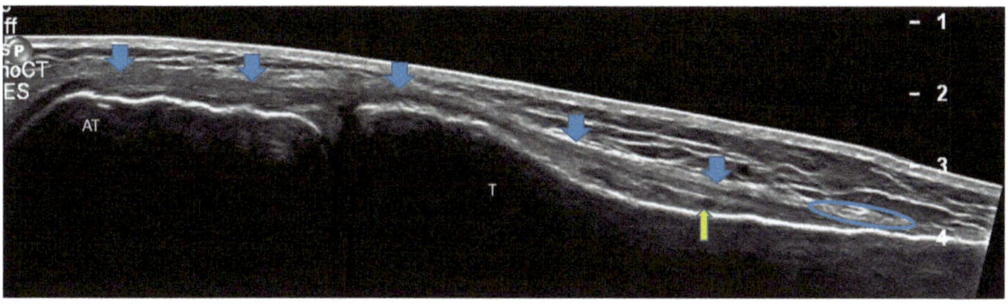

Fig. 7.13 Medial Long. Extended view Medial Knee: Medial Collateral Ligament (MCL, thick blue arrows) from Adductor tubercle (AT) to insertion distally onto Tibia (T). The medial inferior genicular artery can be visualized just deep to the MCL insertion (thin yellow arrow). Distal and superior to MCL insertion is the region of Pes Anserine tendon insertion (oval)

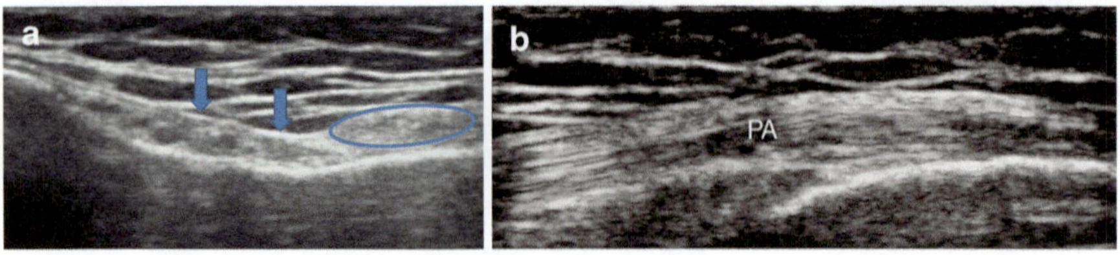

Fig. 7.14 Pes Anserine Insertion. (**a**) Longitudinal view of MCL insertion onto tibia (Arrows). The tendons of the pes anserine are seen in transverse (oval). (**b**) Angling the transducer posteriorly will bring in a longitudinal view of Pes Anserine (PA) tendons

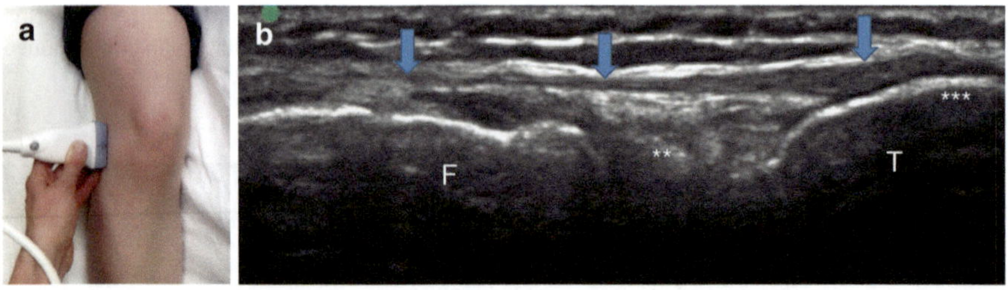

Fig. 7.15 Lateral Longitudinal View. (**a**) Demonstration of probe placement on patient. (**b**) Normal Lateral longitudinal view. Key visualized structures include the Iliotibial (IT) band (arrows), meniscus (**), Femur (F) and Tibia (T). The IT band inserts onto Gerdy's tubercle (***)

effusion or bony abnormalities in this region. The menisci are anisotropic structures, and care must be taken to ensure that they are bright on a normal knee image, allowing assessment of any pathology such as superficial tears or extrusion. Following the medial collateral ligament distally to the meniscus, the inferior medial geniculate artery can be seen, and just distal to this, the variably anisotropic oblique insertions of the pes anserine tendons are visible (Figs. 7.13 and 7.14).

Lateral

Lateral Longitudinal

The probe will be placed in a comparable position as for the medial view, but on the lateral side of the knee (Fig. 7.15a). In this case, if the probe is placed more anteriorly, the iliotibial band insertion on Gerdy's tubercle of the tibia will be seen (Fig. 7.15b), but if the probe is more posterior, the lateral collateral ligament insertion on the fibula will be visualized (Fig. 7.16). From the fibula, the lateral collateral

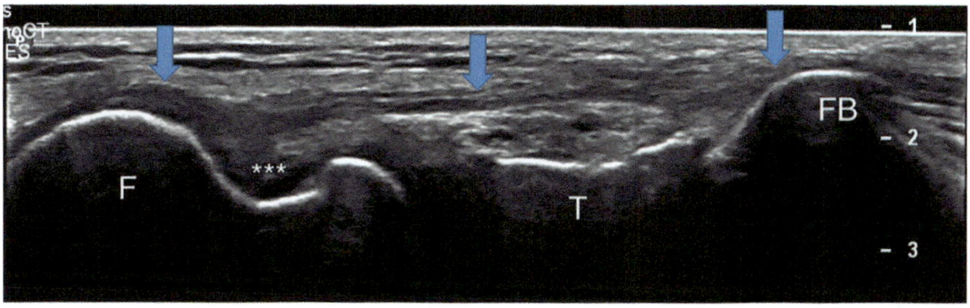

Fig. 7.16 Extended Posterior Lateral Long. Extended view of posterior lateral knee. Key visualized structures include the Lateral Collateral Ligament (blue arrows), Femur (F), Tibia (T) and Fibula (FB). The LCL inserts onto the fibular head, rather than the tibia. Note the groove for popliteus tendon (***)

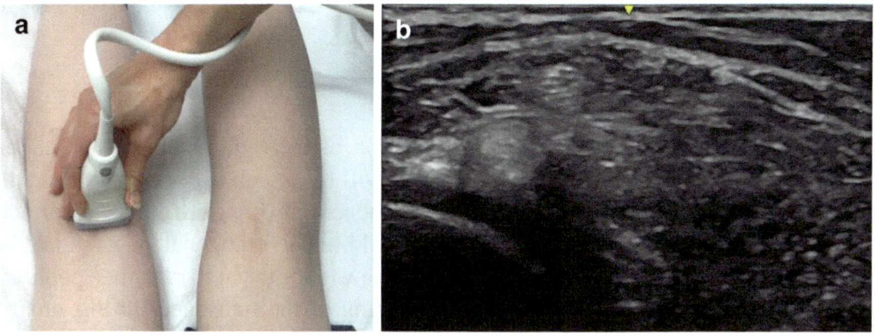

Fig. 7.17 Posterior Transverse. (**a**) Demonstration of probe placement on patient. (**b**) Normal Posterior Transverse View. Key visualized structures include the medial femoral condyle (MFC) with overlying cartilage (**), Semimembranosus tendon (SM), Semitendinosus tendon (ST), Medial head of the Gastrocnemius (G)

ligament can be followed proximally over the tibial groove for the popliteus tendon to its origin at the lateral epicondyle of the femur. The popliteus tendon displays significant anisotropy in the groove and can be mistaken for a parameniscal cyst or fluid. Other landmarks include the distal femur and proximal tibia at the joint line, and the lateral edge of the lateral meniscus.

Posterior

Posterior Transverse

The probe will be placed in the transverse orientation at the posterior knee crease, with the lateral edge essentially midline and the medial edge on the most medial aspect of the knee (Fig. 7.17a). Essential landmarks include the femur, the medial

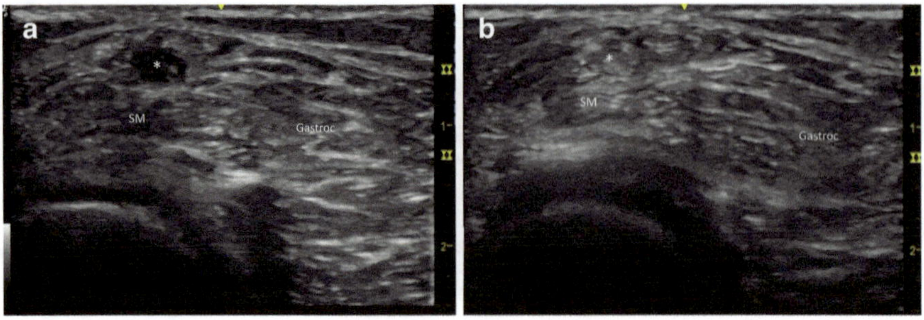

Fig. 7.18 Tendon anisotropy mimicking popliteal cyst: "pseudocyst". Panels (**a**, **b**) posterior transverse view, same patient. Panel (**a**) transducer rocked to produce anisotropy over semitendinosus tendon (*) producing pseudocyst appearance. SM semimembranosus, Gastroc gastrocnemius. Panel (**b**) transducer rocked to eliminate anisotropy demonstrating no cyst is present. Sonopalpation (to assess compressibility) is also a helpful technique for avoiding this pitfall [11]

head of the gastrocnemius, and a cross section of the semimembranosus tendon (Fig. 7.17b). If a popliteal cyst is present, it will be visualized between the semimembranosus and the medial head of the gastrocnemius (Fig. 7.18). If an abnormality is suspected, as with any other body areas, additional orthogonal views should be performed. A correctly positioned transverse view is sufficient to rule out a popliteal cyst for screening purposes. Rocking or fanning of the transducer in this area is critical to properly assess the tendons, as anisotropy of the tendons can often mimic a popliteal cyst (Fig. 7.18).

General Pathology Definitions and Structures Specific to the Knee

Effusion is defined as an abnormal hypoechoic or anechoic intra-articular material that is compressible and displaceable, without Doppler signal [12] (Fig. 7.19). At the knee, fluid greater than 3–4 mL can be visualized by ultrasound and is most frequently found in the suprapatellar pouch or the lateral or medial parapatellar regions. As noted previously, healthy persons may often have small detectable effusions. In extended knees with quadriceps contraction, one study of healthy patients detected a mean of 2.4 mm width of fluid in the suprapatellar recesses, with two standard deviations from the mean being up to 4.8 mm of fluid [35]. More fluid is typically seen in the lateral than medial parapatellar recesses, and more fluid is seen in the suprapatellar recess when the knee is flexed to 30 degrees or when the quadriceps is contracted. Cutoff values for abnormal fluid have been proposed at 1.8 mm

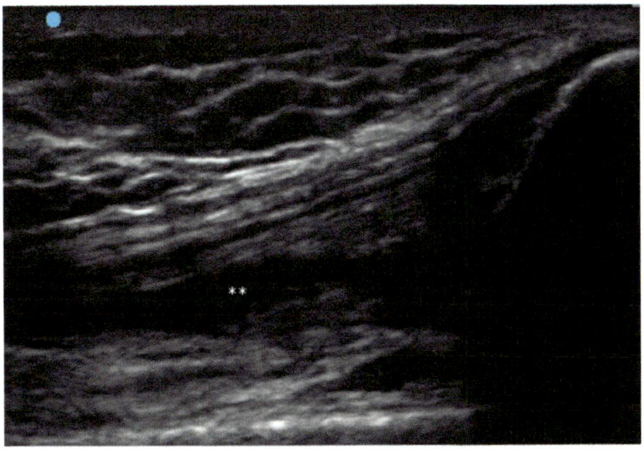

Fig. 7.19 Knee effusion in the suprapatellar longitudinal view. Effusion in an OA patient, seen as an anechoic area extending from the articular space (**)

and 2.7 mm in the lateral parapatellar recess to maximize sensitivity or specificity, respectively. Cutoff values for abnormal knee fluid in the suprapatellar recess have been proposed at 3.6 mm and 6 mm to maximize sensitivity or specificity, respectively [69]. It should be emphasized that as any mechanical or inflammatory knee pathology may promote effusion and because multiple knee pathologies may be present in the same patient, knee aspiration should be performed on effusions greater than normal when an inflammatory etiology is suspected.

Synovial hypertrophy is defined as abnormal hypoechoic intra-articular tissue that is non-displaceable and poorly compressible and may exhibit Doppler signal [12]. The knee can be a deep joint and does not always demonstrate Doppler signal. In a study of 200 knees with rheumatoid arthritis, of which 70% had effusion, 82% had visible synovial hypertrophy, but only 19% had power Doppler signal [13]. Theoretically the lateral parapatellar recess, which is more superficial, may be more amenable to Doppler examination. One small study of 26 patients with inflammatory knee pain found a stronger correlation of lateral parapatellar Doppler signal with synovial vascularity on pathological examination, when compared to suprapatellar or medial recesses [14].

Erosion is defined as intra-articular discontinuity of the bone surface visible in two perpendicular planes [12]. Ultrasound infrequently identifies erosions in the knee, partly due to the limited visualization of the femoral and tibial surfaces possible with this technology. In the same study of 200 knees with RA noted above, only 8% of knees had bone erosions [13].

Osteophytes were not included in the OMERACT definitions, but can be seen as an outgrowth of the bone in two perpendicular planes. Osteophytes in a knee with osteoarthritis can be readily seen on the medial or lateral longitudinal views for tibiofemoral osteoarthritis (Fig. 7.20a) or in the parapatellar views for patellofemoral osteoarthritis.

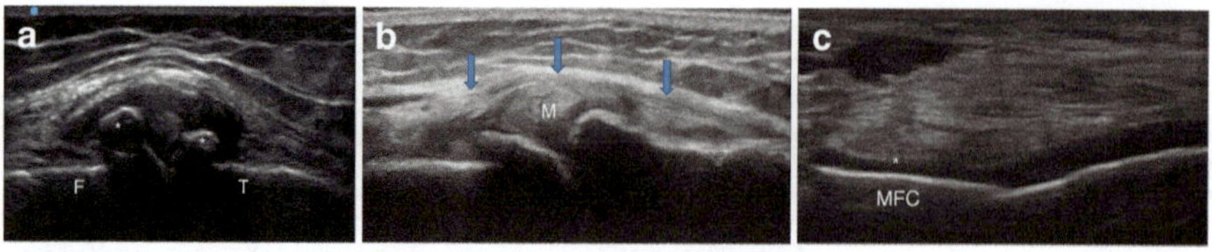

Fig. 7.20 Osteoarthritis. (**a**) Medial longitudinal view demonstrating Osteophytes (*) and joint space narrowing between the femur (F) and the Tibia (T). (**b**) Medial long view demonstrating meniscal extrusion (M) which in turn can be seen elevating the medial collateral ligament (arrows). (**c**) Suprapatellar max flex view demonstrating cartilage thinning (*) over the medial femoral condyle (MFC) only

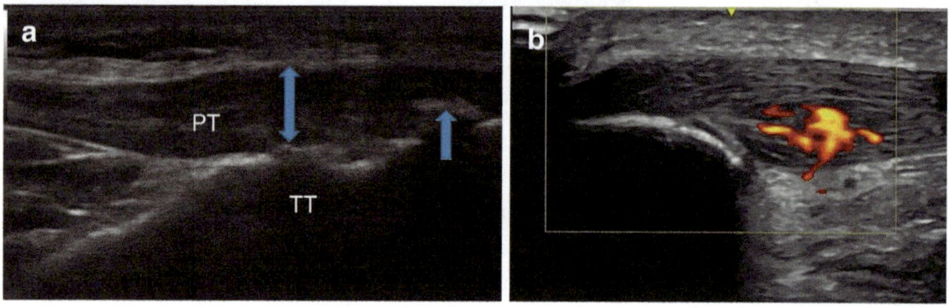

Fig. 7.21 Enthesopathy/ enthesitis in psoriatic arthritis patients. (**a**) Distal infrapatellar longitudinal view. Patellar Tendon (PT), Tibial Tuberosity (TT), Patella (P). Hypoechogenicity (loss of fibrillar echotexture), enthesophyte (arrow). (**b**) Proximal infrapatellar longitudinal view with thickening, positive power Doppler signal showing active inflammatory enthesitis. (Image b courtesy of Janeth Yinh MD, RhMSUS)

Enthesopathy is defined as abnormally hypoechoic and/or thickened tendon or ligament at a bony attachment, seen in two perpendicular planes. Doppler signal may be seen, as may bone changes such as enthesophytes, erosions, or bony irregularity (Fig. 7.21). Enthesopathy is a common finding in spondyloarthropathies, even in the absence of clinical findings, and may be seen in other inflammatory arthritides as well [15–17]. Calcific enthesopathy can be seen as thickening of the tendon with hyperechoic areas and may mimic a tear [18].

Popliteal cyst (Baker's cyst) is a common finding on ultrasound (Fig. 7.22a, b), seen in up to 20–60% of symptomatic knees [19–21]. Ultrasound can be utilized to identify and distinguish a cyst from thrombophlebitis or deep venous thrombosis and is as sensitive as magnetic resonance imaging for this purpose [22]. Patients with inflammatory arthritis such as rheumatoid arthritis (RA) are more prone to develop popliteal cysts, and often when these rupture, they can clinically mimic DVT. Figure 7.23 demonstrates a case of a patient with RA whose popliteal cyst became so enlarged that it was able to mimic DVT even in the unruptured state [23].

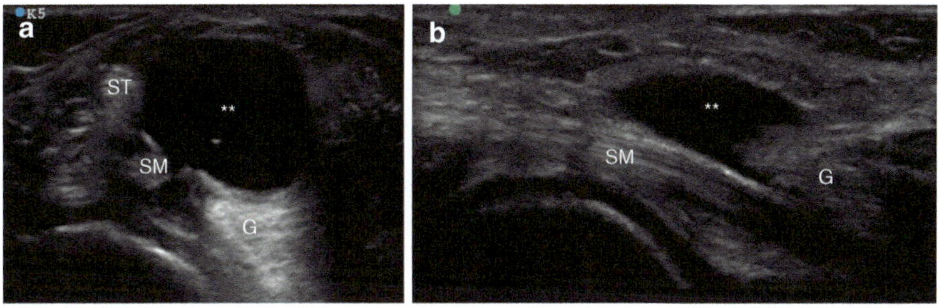

Fig. 7.22 Baker's/Popliteal Cyst. (**a**) Posterior transverse view demonstrating Baker's Cyst (**) arising between the Semimembranosis (SM) and medial head of the gastrocnemius (G). The Semitendinosis (ST) is visible as well. Due to posterior acoustic enhancement, the gastrocnemius appears significantly hyperechoic. (**b**) Posterior longitudinal view of Baker's Cyst (**). The criss-crossing pattern of the semimebranosis tendon (SM) and gastrocnemius (G) is apparent

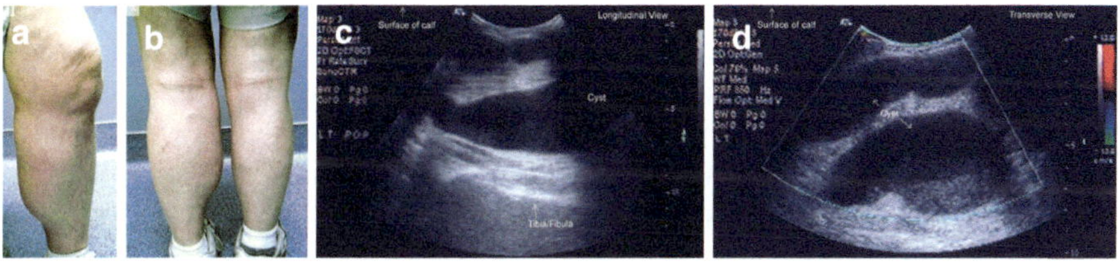

Fig. 7.23 Case of a Baker's cyst mimicking DVT. 45 year old male with rheumatoid arthritis who presented with 3 months of increasing pain and swelling in his left calf. Doppler studies were obtained to rule out DVT. No thrombosis was demonstrated, but rather a 16.8 × 10.5 cm tortuous fluid collection which communicated with the joint space, consistent with a popliteal cyst, also known as Baker's Cyst. (**a**) Lateral View. (**b**) Posterior View. (**c**) Longitudinal view. (**d**) Transverse View [23]

Popliteal cysts may contain fluid (which can be quite viscous), hypertrophic synovium, calcifications, or osteochondral fragments [17]. The cysts are generally rounded and smooth when intact but may demonstrate a more tapered appearance following rupture, when fluid may be seen extending into the calf along the gastrocnemius [24].

Disease-Specific Findings at the Knee

Rheumatoid Arthritis

Two studies found ultrasound to be superior to clinical exam for joint swelling in RA, finding that at the suprapatellar recess (Fig. 7.24), lateral and medial parapatellar recesses, and Baker's cyst locations, clinical exam significantly underestimated

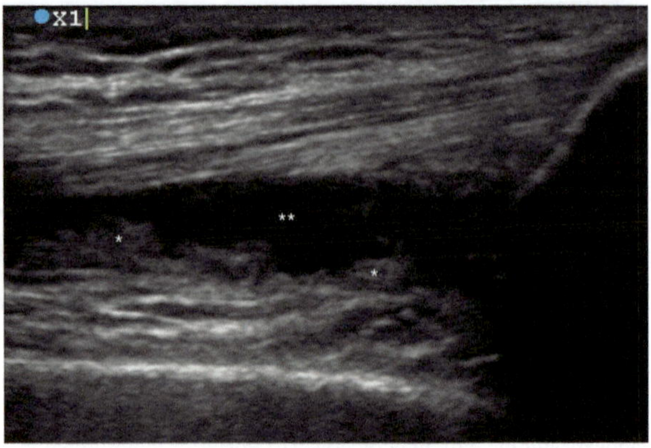

Fig. 7.24 Rheumatoid arthritis. Effusion in a patient with rheumatoid arthritis, seen as an anechoic area extending from the articular space (**). Note the synovial hypertrophy or pannus present as a thickened hypoechoic tissue surrounding the recess (*)

the amount of knee inflammation present compared with ultrasound [17]. In another study of 100 patients (200 knees) with RA, knee effusion was found in 70%, synovial hypertrophy in 82%, enthesopathy in 26%, bone erosions in 8%, and changes in cartilage in 73% [13]. Similarly in juvenile idiopathic arthritis, knees from patients demonstrated frequent effusion and significantly greater synovial thickness at the knee by ultrasound compared with age- and gender-matched control healthy children [25]. Ultrasound was comparable to MRI in assessing joint effusion, synovial proliferation, popliteal cysts, cartilage thickness, and tendinitis, with p values for concordance (by kappa coefficient) all less than 0.001 in 30 symptomatic adult RA knees [26].

Vreju et al. [27] used power Doppler to assess hypervascularity in knees from early RA patients and compared this to synovial biopsy specimens (on a subset of 35 patients) stained for VEGF (a promoter of angiogenesis such as that seen in RA synovitis) and its receptor, VEGF-R1. In this study, 59 of 65 patients were found to have abnormal hyperperfusion within at least one knee, which correlated strongly with VEGF and VEGF-R1 scores found on synovial biopsy and moderately with serum VEGF levels [27]. Similarly, Kondo et al. [28] found significant correlations in RA patient's knee joints between synovial fluid inflammatory cytokines such as IL-6 and sonographic synovial hypertrophy and between power Doppler vascularity and synovial fluid VEGF.

The usefulness of monitoring disease activity during RA treatment has been demonstrated in several studies looking at different therapeutic options. Over a 12-month period, etanercept demonstrated significant reductions in a US global score considering joint effusion, synovial proliferation, synovial hyperemia, tenosynovitis, bursitis, bone erosion, and cartilaginous abnormality at the second and fifth MCPs, third PIPs, wrists, and knees, with a p value of less than 0.0001 [29]. Adalimumab was studied in a similar fashion, over a 2-year period, with similar results [30]. Newer biologics such as tocilizumab have also been effective in showing an improvement in ultrasound findings in RA at multiple joints, including the knee, in small case series [31].

Osteoarthritis

Ultrasound is predictive of pain and joint replacement in knee osteoarthritis (OA). Baseline radiographic grade (hazard ratio [HR] 4.1 [95% CI 2.3–7.1]), ultrasonographic knee effusion (HR 2.6 [95% CI 1.7–4.1]), knee pain intensity (HR 1.8 [95% CI 1.2–2.8]), and disease duration (HR 1.6 [95% CI 1.1–2.5]) were independent predictors of knee joint replacement over 3 years in 531 adult patients with symptomatic knee OA [32]. In a study of 56 osteoarthritis patients with equal radiographic grades of OA in both knees, three ultrasound features were found to be more frequent in symptomatic knees compared with those that were asymptomatic: suprapatellar synovitis, suprapatellar effusion, and medial compartment synovitis. Frequencies of marginal osteophytosis, medial meniscal protrusion (Fig. 7.20b), and lateral compartment synovitis did not differ. Medial compartment synovitis was associated with pain by visual analog scale with movement and at rest and with pain by the WOMAC, more so with increasing severity of synovitis [33].

Ultrasound may predict response to therapeutic injection in OA. A small study of intra-articular corticosteroid injection for symptomatic knee OA found that the depth of synovial hypertrophy was significantly reduced after treatment (mean reduction 0.9 mm (SD 2.2), $p = 0.04$) and nonsignificantly reduced by saline placebo (mean reduction 1.0 mm (SD 3.7), $p = 0.91$) [34].

Articular cartilage at the knee has a normal thickness of approximately 3 mm [35]. In OA, the cartilage is asymmetrically thinned and can become less sharply defined (Fig. 7.20c). In a series of cadaveric knees, measurement of the articular cartilage in maximum flexion was reproducible within and between readers (ICC > 0.70) and was accurate when compared to direct anatomic measurements in knees with minimal to moderate damage. Ultrasound measurements were less accurate in more severely damaged knees [36]. Ultrasound measurement was also comparable in accuracy to arthroscopic measurements, particularly at the medial condyle [37].

Spondyloarthritis

The use of MSUS in evaluating inflammatory changes in spondyloarthropathies is well documented, as manifestations such as synovitis, erosions, and tenosynovitis do not differ from other inflammatory arthritides. However, enthesitis is observed with more frequency when evaluating patients with spondyloarthropathy, and this finding is well visualized on ultrasonography. Early studies done by Lehtinen et al. in 1994 [38] and Balint et al. in 2002 [39] revealed a high frequency of asymptomatic enthesitis in the lower limb. Balint et al. studied 35 spondyloarthritis patients (27 with ankylosing spondylitis, 7 with psoriatic arthritis, 1 with reactive arthritis) with ultrasound and clinical examination of the quadriceps tendon insertion, patellar ligament origin and insertion, Achilles tendon insertion, and plantar aponeurosis [39]. Abnormalities were detected by ultrasound in 56% of sites and by clinical examination in 22%; the most common findings were enthesophytes and tendon thickening [39]. OMERACT published in 2018 their final definition of enthesitis, which divides the features of enthesitis into inflammatory components (hypoechogenicity, thickening, and Doppler signal) and structural components (erosions, calcifications/enthesophytes), specifying that these elements should be present within the first 2 mm of the bony cortex to ensure specificity of enthesitis rather than tendinitis [40]. GRAPPA (Group for Research and Assessment of Psoriasis and Psoriatic Arthritis) ultrasound committee has proposed scoring separately in proximal and distal entheses (up to 5 mm from the bony cortex) as well as bursa. This was proposed to enable a data-driven approach to establishing the most sensitive and specific combination of findings associated with a diagnosis of spondyloarthropathy (SpA) at the patient level [41].

The use of Doppler specifically for enthesitis in spondyloarthropathies was reviewed by D'Agostino in 2010, who noted that the use of Doppler at entheses is not as reliable as used in the synovium due to less vascularization and the higher likelihood of visualizing artifact, stemming from reflection of nearby cortical bone [42]. Further complicating ultrasonographic findings of enthesitis are increased BMI, age >50, male gender, and increased biomechanical stress—each of which has been shown to increase scores on ultrasonographic enthesitis scoring systems [43–45]. However, extensive work in the field of enthesitis has been done, and several studies have demonstrated its utility in the detection of spondyloarthritis, as well as utility in monitoring of treatment response. D'Agostino has found that the detection of any vascularized enthesis has good sensitivity and specificity for the presence of underlying spondyloarthritis, and this technique is sensitive to change: there is a disappearance of vascularization with anti-TNF therapy and a reappearance with relapse [46]. There has also been work done to examine the relative specificity of each of the elementary lesions of enthesitis in patients with psoriatic arthritis (PsA)/SpA versus healthy controls. For example, in 2018, Tom et al. published that in up to a quarter of healthy controls, ultrasound could detect the presence of enthesophytes, thickening, and hypoechogenicity [41]. In contrast, other elementary lesions, including Doppler signal, bone proliferation, and erosions, were rarely found in healthy controls [41]. As with RA, treatment can be monitored for effectiveness with ultrasonography in patients with SpA. In a small study of 27 knees with either RA or PsA, a sustained regression in synovial thickening was achieved with the use of etanercept over a 12-month period [47]. Furthermore, superficial pannus and synovial villus hypervascularization was reduced after treatment with etanercept well before changes in synovial thickness were observed in both conditions [47].

Crystalline Arthropathies

Though there are many nonspecific signs of inflammation found on MSUS, including joint effusion, synovial proliferation, and hypervascularity, there are certain findings that are useful in distinguishing crystalline-related arthropathies from other conditions. In particular, findings of hyperechoic material overlying the superficial margin of the articular cartilage (double-contour sign in gout) or within the borders of the cartilage (as in CPPD) can be useful diagnostically (Fig. 7.25) [48]. It should be noted, however, that assessing whether

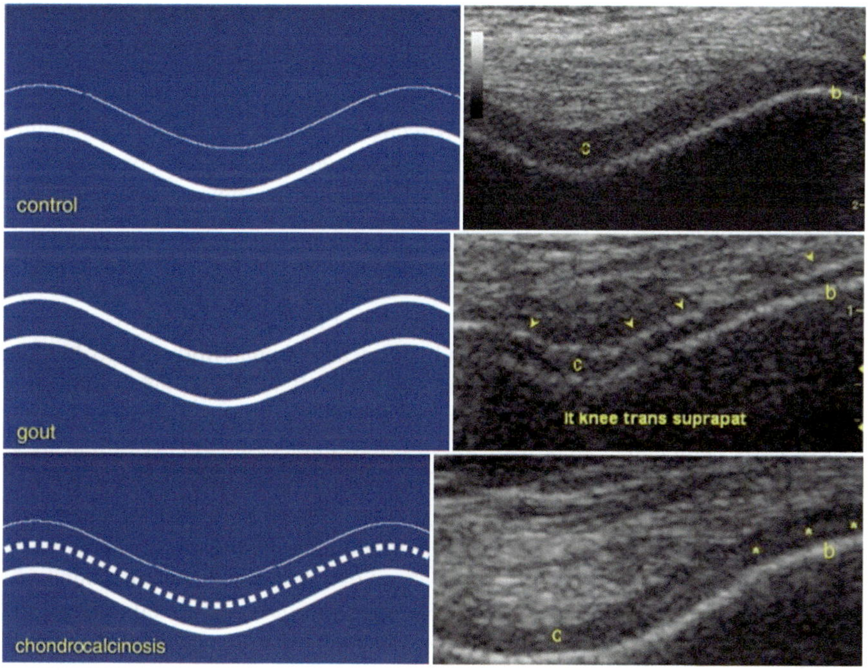

Fig. 7.25 Crystalline arthropathies. Comparison of sonographic appearance of normal control, gout, and chondrocalcinosis in knee joints. Suprapatellar, transverse view in flexion. Schematic illustrations on the left. Top: anechoic (*black*) layer of hyaline cartilage *c* overlying bony contour of distal femur *b*. *Middle*: double-contour sign. Hyperechoic (*bright*), slightly irregular layer of crystal deposits (*open arrowheads*) overlying anechoic hyaline cartilage *c* and bony contour of distal femur *b*. This patient had crystal-proven, untreated gouty arthritis. The hyaline cartilage is thin in this 88-year-old individual. Bottom: hyperechoic, crystalline material (*asterisks*) is layered in the center of the anechoic hyaline cartilage *c*. This layer parallels the outline of the bony cortex *b*. Calcium pyrophosphate crystals were found on aspiration [48]. (Reproduced with permission from Oxford University Press from Thiele and Schlesinger [48] by permission of Oxford University Press)

hyperechoic deposits are intracartilaginous or superficial to the cartilage is not always easy and that effusion may make the determination more difficult due to the anechoic appearance of both fluid and cartilage [49, 50]. Therefore, careful assessment of other findings such as tophi or meniscal calcification (see below) is important.

Thiele et al. studied 37 joints, including the knee, in patients with crystal-proven gout and found that 92% of patients, and no controls, displayed the double-contour sign [48]. Hyperechoic spots may be present within the synovial fluid as well, indicating the presence of monosodium urate (MSU) crystals. Other notable findings characterizing gout on ultrasound are the presence of tophi, represented by homogenously echoic echotexture, as seen in a soft tophus or, in the case of a hard tophus, a hyperechoic band resulting in a posterior acoustic shadow [51]. Recent reports using ultrasound and dual-energy computed tomography (DECT) have emphasized the tendon and peritendinous areas around the knee as key areas for identifying gout deposition in the form of hyperechoic aggregates or tophi [52, 53]. Most recently, Matteo et al. found the appearance of hyperechoic aggregates or tophi in and around the popliteus tendon at the popliteal groove was more sensitive than femoral cartilage double-contour sign and more specific than hyperechoic aggregates in the patellar ligament [54].

CPPD disease is distinct in that it may reveal a punctate pattern of hyperechoic rounded or amorphous shapes within fibrocartilage or tendons. Coari et al. were able to demonstrate hyperechoic inclusions in cartilage by ultrasound in 43 of 56 knees with known chondrocalcinosis, in both linear and punctiform patterns, while no such inclusions were seen in normal knees [55]. CPPD also tends to deposit crystals in a homogenous, hyperechoic nodular or oval pattern in bursae or articular recesses [56]. Filippou et al. provide a series of examples of CPPD at various locations in the knee as shown in Fig. 7.26 [57].

In a small study by Frediani et al. [58], 11 patients with chondrocalcinosis and joint effusion by US and 13 controls with OA and joint effusion were examined by X-ray and had synovial fluid examination by an observer blinded to ultrasound and X-ray results. Nine of the 11 patients had X-ray confirmation of chondrocalcinosis. Of the 11 patients identified by ultrasound as having chondrocalcinosis, all 11 had CPPD crystals on arthrocentesis, compared with 0 of 13 control patients [58]. Not only does ultrasound appear to be an accurate way to identify patients with chondrocalcinosis; its potential increased sensitivity relative to X-ray is highlighted in Fig. 7.27.

Unfortunately, there are not adequate studies regarding specific patterns of hydroxyapatite crystal deposition disease, but the condition is associated with hyperechoic deposits displaying posterior shadowing, more often at smaller sizes than would be seen with CPPD crystals [56].

As in other inflammatory arthropathies, treatment response in gout can be monitored by ultrasound. Specifically, response to urate-lowering therapy was studied in five patients (seven joints) by Thiele et al. [59]. The knee was the most frequent

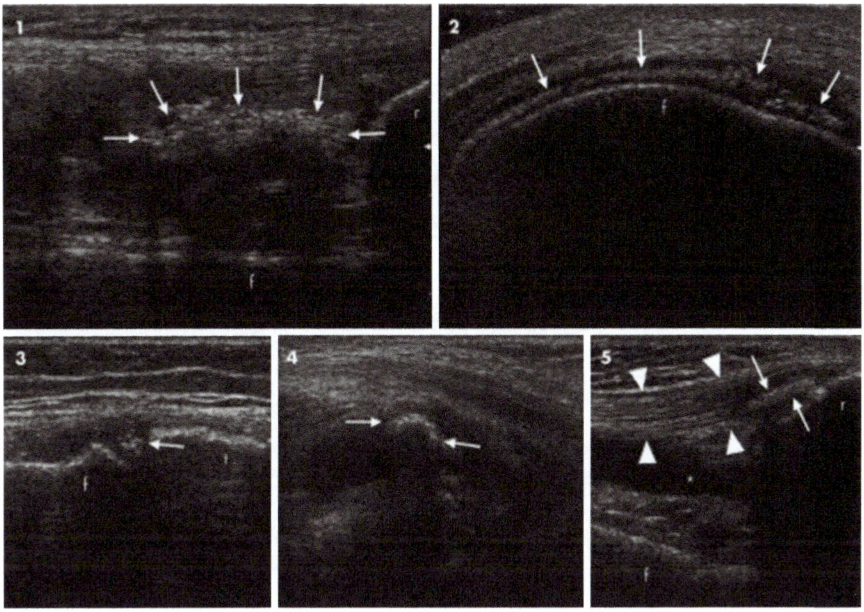

Fig. 7.26 Pseudogout. Hyperechoic deposits of CPPD in the knee. Hyperechoic deposits (*arrows*) are shown that are compatible with calcium pyrophosphate dihydrate (CPPD) calcifications in the context of the synovial membrane (*1*), hyaline cartilage of the femur (*2*), and meniscus (*3*), in the synovial fluid of a Baker's cyst (*4*), and in the insertional tract of quadriceps tendon (*5*); *arrowheads*, quadriceps tendon (purposely appearing hypoechoic at insertion—anisotropic artifact—to better highlight the CPPD deposits). Patterns *1*, *4*, and *5* are rare and generally occur when a large number of CPPD crystals are present in synovial fluid. In all cases, the deposits do not create an evident posterior shadow unless they reach moderate thickness. In such cases, a partial posterior shadow may be observed (photos *1* and *4*). *f* femur, *r* rotula (aka patella), *t* tibia, * (*asterisk*) joint effusion [57]. (Reproduced with Permission from BMJ publishing group from Filippou et al. [57], ©, with permission from BMJ Publishing Group Ltd.)

joint involved in this study, and conclusions drawn indicated that reducing serum urate levels to <6 mg/dl caused resolution of the double-contour sign seen upon initial enrollment, as well as a reduction in symptoms. Maintaining a serum urate concentration of ≥7 mg/dl was associated with a persistent double-contour sign and incomplete resolution of symptoms [59].

Tendon and Ligament Injuries

In addition to evaluating inflammatory findings, mechanical or degenerative tendon and ligament injuries at the knee can also be identified using ultrasound. Patellar tendinopathy, commonly associated with overuse in jumping or running activities,

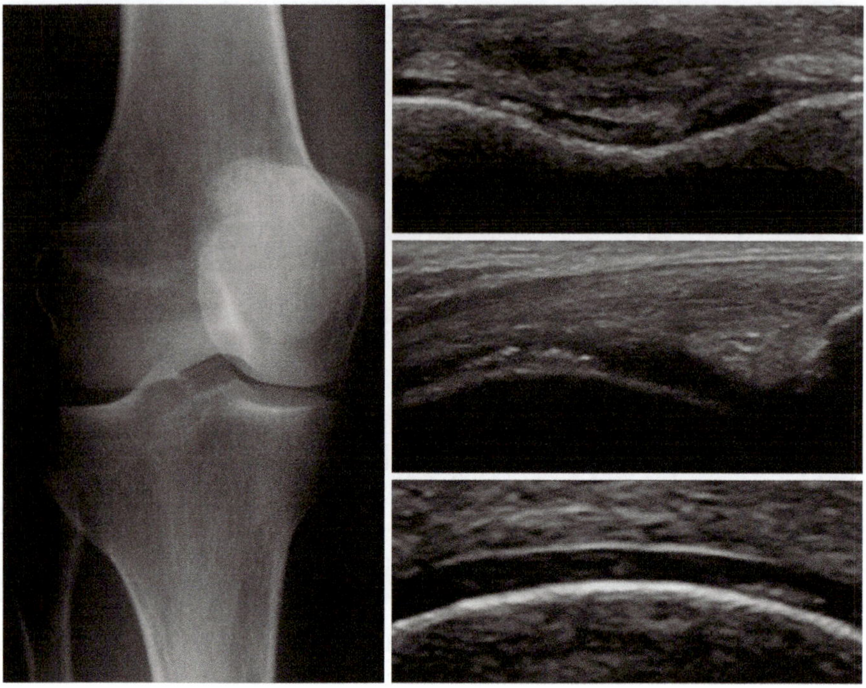

Fig. 7.27 Increased sensitivity of Ultrasound for CPPD detection relative to Conventional Radiography. Left: X-ray of a patient with knee pain demonstrating no cartilaginous abnormalities. Right: Ultrasound of same patient demonstrating intracartilagenous hyperechogenicities consistent w CPPD crystal deposition or pseudogout. (Images courtesy of Dr. Marwin Gutierrez, Professor of Rheumatology)

is seen as a thickened tendon with decreased echogenicity and altered fibrillar pattern with or without Doppler signal and is also associated with local tenderness. Ligament and tendon tears are seen as hypoechoic defects of either part (partial thickness) or full (full thickness) structure; associated debris, focal thickening, and retraction may be seen. In cases of suspected injury, comparison with the contralateral unaffected side is helpful [24].

Bursitis

Multiple bursae exist at the level of the knee, each of which can become distended from either mechanical, inflammatory, or infectious causes to produce fluid

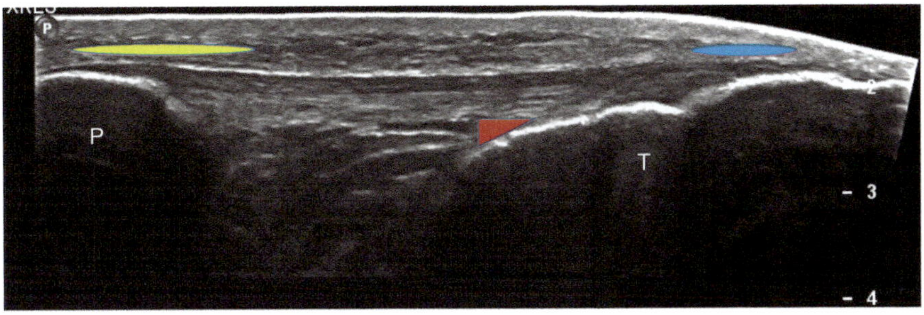

Fig. 7.28 Bursitis/Location of the patellar bursae. Entire Patellar Tendon (PT) from its origin on the patella (P) to insertion on the Tibia (T). The locations of the Patellar bursae are show as follows: Yellow oval = prepatellar bursa, Blue oval = superficial infrapatellar; Red triangle = Deep infrapatellar bursa

collections appreciable by ultrasound. The locations of the most commonly clinically involved bursae are depicted in Fig. 7.28. Bursitis at the knee can be seen at the prepatellar or infrapatellar bursae or the pes anserine bursa and can be differentiated on ultrasound from tendinopathy. A small amount of fluid may be appreciated in the deep infrapatellar bursa in the normal state, but only in the diseased state can fluid be seen in the prepatellar or superficial infrapatellar bursae or at the pes anserine bursa. Prepatellar bursitis, or "housemaid's knee," appears as a fusiform enlargement of the bursa with thickened synovium in the area superficial to the distal patella and the proximal third of the patellar ligament [24]. Pes anserine bursitis may be seen as a cystic mass adjacent and deep to the pes anserine tendon insertion (conjoined tendons of the sartorius, gracilis, and semitendinosus) [24]. In one study, pes anserine bursitis was present by MSUS in 20% of knees with symptomatic OA [60].

Reliability and Scoring Systems

Reliability of ultrasound has been assessed in a variety of conditions and clinical settings, although only a few studies focus specifically on the knee. In 60 outpatients fulfilling ACR criteria for knee OA, the agreement between two rheumatologists on a variety of features (meniscal extrusion, infrapatellar bursitis, effusion, popliteal cyst, and cartilage thickness) was moderate to good, with kappa values from 0.5 to 0.8. However, agreement on synovial hypertrophy was poor [61].

The sonography of large joints in rheumatology (SOLAR) study included 199 RA patients with large joint involvement and assessed longitudinal suprapatellar, dorsal, medial, and lateral knee views for gray-scale and power Doppler involvement (0–3 at each site, total score 0–12 for GS and PDUS at the knee). The baseline GS score was 5.2, with a significant decrease to 2.2 ($p < 0.001$) after 12 months of therapy; the PDUS score at baseline was 4.0, also decreasing significantly to 1.3 over 12 months. Reductions in DAS28 and ESR were also observed in the follow-up period. The intra-reader reliability for the SOLAR score at the knee was 0.7 [62].

Injections and Ultrasound Guidance at the Knee

A study comparing medial, midlateral, and superolateral approaches to US-guided knee injection in OA knees found that accuracy was highest for the superolateral approach (100%) followed by the midlateral (95%) and medial (75%) approaches [63]. Curtiss et al. compared palpation-guided and ultrasound-guided superolateral knee injections by both a fellow and an attending in cadaveric knees. Overall, US-guided injections were 100% accurate versus 78% accuracy for palpation-guided injections. However, the more experienced user was 100% accurate with either method, while the less experienced user was 100% accurate with US but 55% accurate using the palpation-guided method [64]. A review of five studies estimated the overall accuracy of knee injections at 96% with US and 78% without ($p < 0.001$) and was suggestive of greater clinical improvement and quality of life associated with US guidance [65]. Injections performed using US guidance are associated with reduced procedural pain, improved therapeutic response, and improved duration of response and may even be more cost-effective compared to palpation-guided injections [66, 67]. A systematic review of intra-articular knee injection including data on site of injection, image guidance (the vast majority being ultrasound guided), and provider experience from 23 publications found that injections at the superomedial patellar, medial midpatellar, superolateral patellar, and lateral suprapatellar sites were more accurate with image guidance than without. Although provider experience was associated with improved accuracy for blinded injections, this was not the case for image-guided injections [68]. Figure 7.29 demonstrates needle, transducer, and machine position for injection of the lateral aspect of the suprapatellar recess.

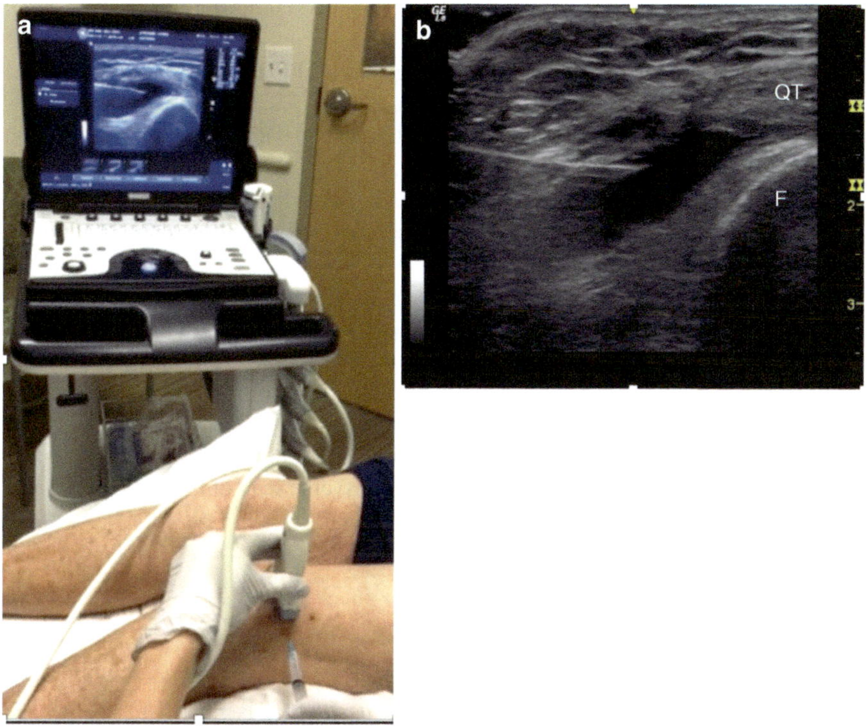

Fig. 7.29 Injection Guidance. (**a**) Correct alignment of patient, probe, needle and machine for knee aspiration (from suprapatellar transverse view). (**b**) Needle in the (lateral) suprapatellar recess (*), Femur (F), Quadriceps tendon (QT)

Conclusion

The knee is an accessible joint that is amenable to ultrasonographic diagnosis, injection guidance, and treatment monitoring. A clear understanding of the normal anatomy, pathologic presentations, and their implications is essential to the successful use and interpretation of ultrasound images of the knee.

Review Questions

1. To increase the sensitivity for the detection of effusions at the knee, suprapatellar imaging should be performed with the joint in
   (a) Full extension
   (b) 30° of flexion
   (c) 90° of flexion
   (d) Maximal flexion possible for the patient

2. MSU crystals can be distinguished from CPP crystal deposition on ultrasound imaging because
   (a) MSU crystals layer within cartilage and CPP crystals layer on top of cartilage.
   (b) MSU crystals layer on top of cartilage and CPP crystals layer within cartilage.
   (c) They cannot; both crystals may have the same appearance on ultrasound.
   (d) Only MSU crystals can be reliably seen on ultrasound imaging; CPP crystals cannot.
3. Ultrasound guidance for a knee aspiration may *not* be indicated if
   (a) Prior palpation-guided aspiration attempts have failed.
   (b) The patient is morbidly obese.
   (c) There is uncomplicated anatomy and prior palpation-guided attempts have been successful.
   (d) Aspiration is to be performed posteriorly for a popliteal cyst.
4. The essential landmarks on the posterior transverse scan of the knee to evaluate for popliteal cyst include
   (a) Semitendinosus
   (b) Popliteal vessels
   (c) Posterior collateral ligament
   (d) Medial head of the gastrocnemius
5. The OMERACT definition of synovial hypertrophy is
   (a) Abnormal hypoechoic intra-articular tissue that is non-displaceable and poorly compressible and may exhibit Doppler signal.
   (b) Abnormal hyperechoic intra-articular tissue that is non-displaceable and poorly compressible and may exhibit Doppler signal.
   (c) Abnormal hypoechoic intra-articular tissue that is non-displaceable and highly compressible and may exhibit Doppler signal.
   (d) Abnormal hyperechoic intra-articular tissue that is non-displaceable and highly compressible and may exhibit Doppler signal.
6. The articular cartilage of the knee is best characterized on which view?
   (a) Suprapatellar longitudinal
   (b) Posterior transverse
   (c) Suprapatellar transverse in maximal flexion
   (d) Medial longitudinal
7. The absence of Doppler signal indicates a lack of synovial inflammation.
   (a) True
   (b) False
8. Effusion at the knee is most readily detected in the
   (a) Suprapatellar pouch
   (b) Lateral or medial parapatellar regions
   (c) Either (a) or (b)
   (d) None of the above

9. Ultrasound assessment is a reliable method to monitor treatment response in several inflammatory diseases.
   (a) True
   (b) False
10. During examination of the entheses, what problem can arise when there is tension on tissues (as in flexed knee views)?
   (a) Obscured gray-scale findings of enthesitis
   (b) Obscured Doppler findings of enthesitis
   (c) Entheseal tears more difficult to evaluate
   (d) Obscured bursitis
11. When looking for pes anserine bursitis, what structure should be followed to its insertion?
   (a) Patellar ligament
   (b) Lateral collateral ligament
   (c) Medial collateral ligament
   (d) Popliteus tendon
12. Which of the following normal structures in the knee are anisotropic?
   (a) Patellar ligament
   (b) Medial meniscus
   (c) Articular cartilage
   (d) Tibia
   (e) (a) and (b)
   (f) None of the above

Answers

1. (b) 30° of flexion
2. (b) MSU crystals layer on top of cartilage and CPP crystals layer within cartilage.
3. (c) There is uncomplicated anatomy and prior palpation-guided attempts have been successful.
4. (d) Medial head of the gastrocnemius.
5. (a) Abnormal hypoechoic intra-articular tissue that is non-displaceable and poorly compressible and may exhibit Doppler signal.
6. (c) Suprapatellar transverse in maximal flexion
7. (b) False
8. (c) Either (a) or (b)
9. (a) True
10. (b) Tension may obscure Doppler findings, but gray-scale findings are unchanged or improved due to lessened anisotropy.
11. (c) Following the medial collateral ligament to its insertion, the pes anserine tendons will be visualized just superficial to this location.
12. (e), (a) and (b)

References

1. McAlindon T, Kissin E, Nazarian L, et al. American College of Rheumatology report on reasonable use of musculoskeletal ultrasonography in rheumatology clinical practice. Arthritis Care Res (Hoboken). 2012;64(11):1625–40.
2. D'Agostino M, Said-Nahal R, Hacquard-Bouder C, et al. Assessment of peripheral enthesitis in the spondyloarthropathies by ultrasonography combined with power Doppler: a cross-sectional study. Arthritis Rheum. 2003;48(2):523–33.
3. Mallinson P, Reagan A, Coupal T, et al. The distribution of urate deposition within the extremities in gout: a review of dual – energy CT cases. Skelet Radiol. 2014;43(3):277–81.
4. Peiteado D, De Miguel E, Villalba A, et al. Value of a short four-joint ultrasound test for gout diagnosis: a pilot study. Clin Exp Rheumatol. 2012;30(6):830–7.
5. Backhaus M, Burmester GR, Gerber T, et al. Guidelines for musculoskeletal ultrasound in rheumatology. Ann Rheum Dis. 2001;60(7):641–9.
6. Terslev L, D'Agostino MA, Brossard M, et al. Which knee and probe position determines the final diagnosis of knee inflammation by ultrasound? Results from a European Multicenter Study. Ultraschall Med. 2012;33(7):E173–8.
7. Naredo E, Cabero F, Palop MJ, et al. Ultrasonographic findings in knee osteoarthritis: a comparative study with clinical and radiographic assessment. Osteoarthr Cartil. 2005;13(7):568–74.
8. Hong BY, Lim SH, Cho YR, et al. Detection of knee effusion by ultrasonography. Am J Phys Med Rehabil. 2010;89(9):715–21.
9. Zayat AS, Freeston JE, Conaghan PG. Does joint position affect US findings in inflammatory arthritis? Rheumatology (Oxford). 2012;51(5):921–5.
10. Gutierrez M, Filippucci E, Grassi W, Rosemffet M. Intratendinous power Doppler changes related to patient position in seronegative spondyloarthritis. J Rheumatol. 2010;37(5):1057–9.
11. Kissin E, Demarco P, Malone D, Bakewell C et al. The rheumatologist. Sound feedback for ultrasound training. 2018.; https://www.the-rheumatologist.org/article/ultrasound-training-tips-pitfalls/
12. Wakefield RJ, Balint PV, Szkudlarek M, et al. Musculoskeletal ultrasound including definitions for ultrasonographic pathology. J Rheumatol. 2005;32(12):2485–7.
13. Riente L, Delle Sedie A, Filippucci E, et al. Ultrasound Imaging for the rheumatologist XXVII. Sonographic assessment of the knee in patients with rheumatoid arthritis. Clin Exp Rheumatol. 2010;28(3):300–3.
14. Najm A, Orr C, Gallagher L, et al. Knee joint synovitis: study of correlations and diagnostic performances of ultrasonography compared with histopathology. RMD Open. 2018;4(1):e000616.
15. Naredo E, Batlle-Gualda E, Garcia-Vivar ML, et al. Power Doppler ultrasonography assessment of entheses in spondyloarthropathies: response to therapy of entheseal abnormalities. J Rheumatol. 2010;37(10):2110–7.
16. Frediani B, Falsetti P, Storri L, et al. Ultrasound and clinical evaluation of quadricipital tendon enthesitis in patients with psoriatic arthritis and rheumatoid arthritis. Clin Rheumatol. 2002;21(4):294–8.
17. Vlad V, Iagnocco A. Ultrasound of the knee in rheumatology. Med Ultrason. 2012;14(4):318–25.
18. Dey A, Godsiff SP, Pandey R. Acute calcific tendinitis mimicking patella tendon rupture. Injury Extra. 2004;35(12):104–7.
19. Ward EE, Jacobson JA, Fessell DP, et al. Sonographic detection of Baker's cysts: comparison with MR imaging. AJR Am J Roentgenol. 2001;176(2):373–80.
20. Andonopoulos AP, Yarmenitis S, Sfountouris H, et al. Baker's cyst in rheumatoid arthritis: an ultrasonographic study with a high resolution technique. Clin Exp Rheumatol. 1995;13(5):633–6.
21. Rupp S, Seil R, Jochum P, Kohn D. Popliteal cysts in adults. Prevalence, associated intraarticular lesions, and results after arthroscopic treatment. Am J Sports Med. 2002;30(1):112–5.

22. Ostergaard M, Court-Payen M, Gideon P, et al. Ultrasonography in arthritis of the knee. A comparison with MR imaging. Acta Radiol. 1995;36(1):19–26.
23. Bakewell C, Dugowson C. Baker's cyst in a patient with rheumatoid arthritis. NEJM. 2009;361(11):1098.
24. Razek AA, Fouda NS, Elmetwaley N, Elbogdady E. Sonography of the knee joint. J Ultrasound. 2009;12(2):53–60.
25. Algergawy S, Haliem T, Al-Shaer O. Clinical, laboratory, and ultrasound assessment of the knee in juvenile rheumatoid arthritis. Clin Med Insights Arthritis Musculoskelet Disord. 2011;4:21–7.
26. Yucesoy C, Genc G, Bal A, et al. Ultrasonographic assessment of knee in patients with rheumatoid arthritis: is it an effective imaging method for initial evaluation? Arch Rheumatol. 2011;26(2):120–6.
27. Vreju F, Ciurea M, Rosu A, et al. Power Doppler sonography, a non-invasive method of assessment of the synovial inflammation in patients with early rheumatoid arthritis. Romanian J Morphol Embryol. 2011;52(2):637–43.
28. Kondo Y, Suzuki K, Inoue Y, et al. Significant association between joint ultrasonographic parameters and synovial inflammatory factors in rheumatoid arthritis. Arthritis Res Ther. 2019;21(1):14.
29. Iagnocco A, Perella C, Naredo E, et al. Etanercept in the treatment of rheumatoid arthritis: clinical follow-up over one year by ultrasonography. Clin Rheumatol. 2008;27(4):491–6.
30. Iagnocco A, Filippucci E, Perella C, et al. Clinical and ultrasonographic monitoring of response to adalimumab treatment in rheumatoid arthritis. J Rheumatol. 2008;35(1):35–40.
31. Epis O, Filippucci E, Delle Sedie A, et al. Clinical and ultrasound evaluation of the response to tocilizumab treatment in patients with rheumatoid arthritis: a case series. Rheumatol Int. 2014;34(5):737–42.
32. Conaghan PG, D'Agostino MA, Le Bars M, et al. Clinical and ultrasonographic predictors of joint replacement for knee osteoarthritis: results from a large, 3-year, prospective EULAR study. Ann Rheum Dis. 2010;69(4):644–7.
33. Wu PT, Shao CJ, Wu KC, et al. Pain in patients with equal radiographic grades of osteoarthritis in both knees: the value of gray scale ultrasound. Osteoarthr Cartil. 2012;20(12):1507–13.
34. Hall M, Doherty S, Courtney P, et al. Ultrasound detected synovial change and pain response following intra-articular injection of corticosteroid and a placebo in symptomatic osteoarthritic knees: a pilot study. Ann Rheum Dis. 2014;73(8):1590–1.
35. Schmidt WA, Schmidt H, Schicke B, Gromnica-Ihle E. Standard reference values for musculoskeletal ultrasonography. Ann Rheum Dis. 2004;63(8):988–94.
36. Naredo E, Acebes C, Moller I, et al. Ultrasound validity in the measurement of knee cartilage thickness. Ann Rheum Dis. 2009;68(8):1322–7.
37. Saarakkala S, Waris P, Waris V, et al. Diagnostic performance of knee ultrasonography for detecting degenerative changes of articular cartilage. Osteoarthr Cartil. 2012;20(5):376–81.
38. Lehtinen A, Taavitsainen M, Leirisalo-Repo M. Sonographic analysis of enthesopathy in the lower extremities of patients with spondyloarthropathy. Clin Exp Rheumatol. 1994;12(2):143–8.
39. Balint PV, Kane D, Wilson H, et al. Ultrasonography of entheseal insertions in the lower limb in spondyloarthropathy. Ann Rheum Dis. 2002;61(10):905–10.
40. Balint P, Terslev L, Aegerter P, et al. Reliability of a consensus-based ultrasound definition and scoring for enthesitis in spondyloarthritis and psoriatic arthritis: an OMERACT US initiative. Ann Rheum Dis. 2018;77(12):1730–5.
41. Tom S, Zhong Y, Cook R, et al. Development of a preliminary ultrasonographic enthesitis score in psoriatic arthritis – GRAPPA Ultrasound working group. J Rheumatol. 2019;46(4):384–90.
42. D'Agostino MA. Ultrasound imaging in spondyloarthropathies. Best Pract Res Clin Rheumatol. 2010;24(5):693–700.
43. Aydin S. 2018 GRAPPA (Group for Research and Assessment of Psoriasis and Psoriatic Arthritis Annual Meeting 2018, Toronto, Canada.

44. Solmaz D, Bakirci S, Kimyon G, et al. The impact of having family history of psoriasis or psoriatic arthritis on psoriatic disease. Arthritis Care Res. 2019; https://doi.org/10.1002/acr.23836.
45. Eder L, Jayakar J, Thavaneswaran A, et al. Is the Madrid Sonographic Enthesitis Index useful for differentiating psoriatic arthritis from psoriasis alone and healthy controls? J Rheumatol. 2014;41(3):466–72.
46. D'Agostino M, Olivieri I. Enthesitis. Best Prac Res Clin Rheumatol. 2006;20(3):473–86.
47. Fiocco U, Ferro F, Vezzu M, et al. Rheumatoid and psoriatic knee synovitis: clinical, grey scale, and power Doppler ultrasound assessment of the response to etanercept. Ann Rheum Dis. 2005;64(6):899–905.
48. Thiele RG, Schlesinger N. Diagnosis of gout by ultrasound. Rheumatology (Oxford). 2007;46(7):1116–21.
49. Löffler C, Sattier H, Peters L, et al. Distinguishing gouty arthritis from calcium pyrophosphate deposition disease and other arthritides. J Rheumatol. 2015;42(3):513–20.
50. Russell E, Checa A. Potential pitfalls in the diagnosis of crystal-induced arthritis and in the sonographic measurement of hyaline cartilage due to the presence of joint effusion. J Clin Rheumatol. 2013;19(2):98–100.
51. Thiele RG. Role of ultrasound and other advanced imaging in the diagnosis and management of gout. Curr Rheumatol Rep. 2011;13(2):146–53.
52. Fritz J, Henes J, Fuld M, et al. Dual-energy computed tomography of the knee, ankle, and foot: noninvasive diagnosis of gout and quantification of monosodium urate in tendons and ligaments. Semin Musculoskel Radiol. 2016;20(1):130–6.
53. Yuan Y, Liu C, Xiang X, Yuan TL, et al. Ultrasound scans and dual energy CT identify tendons as preferred anatomical location of MSU crystal depositions in gouty joints. Rheumatol Int. 2018;38(5):801–11.
54. Matteo A, Filippucci E, Cipolletta E, et al. The popliteal groove region: a new target for the detection of monosodium urate crystal deposits in patients with gout. An ultrasound study. Joint Bone Spine. 2019;86(1):89–94.
55. Coari G, Iagnocco A, Zoppini A. Chondrocalcinosis: sonographic study of the knee. Clin Rheumatol. 1995;14(5):511–4.
56. Delle Sedie A, Riente L, Iagnocco A, et al. Ultrasound imaging for the rheumatologist X. Ultrasound imaging in crystal-related arthropathies. Clin Exp Rheumatol. 2007;25(4):513–7.
57. Filippou G, Frediani B, Gallo A, et al. A "new" technique for the diagnosis of chondrocalcinosis of the knee: sensitivity and specificity of high-frequency ultrasonography. Ann Rheum Dis. 2007;66(8):1126–8.
58. Frediani B, Filippou G, Falsetti P, et al. Diagnosis of calcium pyrophosphate dihydrate crystal deposition disease: ultrasonographic criteria proposed. Ann Rheum Dis. 2005;64(4):638–40.
59. Thiele RG, Schlesinger N. Ultrasonography shows disappearance of monosodium urate crystal deposition on hyaline cartilage after sustained normouricemia is achieved. Rheumatol Int. 2010;30(4):495–503.
60. Uysal F, Akbal A, Gokmen F, et al. Prevalence of pes anserine bursitis in symptomatic osteoarthritis patients: an ultrasonographic prospective study. Clin Rheumatol. 2015;34(3):529–33.
61. Bevers K, Zweers MC, van den Ende CH, et al. Ultrasonographic analysis in knee osteoarthritis: evaluation of inter-observer reliability. Clin Exp Rheumatol. 2012;30(5):673–8.
62. Hartung W, Kellner H, Strunk J, et al. Development and evaluation of a novel ultrasound score for large joints in rheumatoid arthritis: one year of experience in daily clinical practice. Arthritis Care Res (Hoboken). 2012;64(5):675–82.
63. Park Y, Lee SC, Nam HS, et al. Comparison of sonographically guided intra-articular injections at 3 different sites of the knee. J Ultrasound Med. 2011;30(12):1669–76.
64. Curtiss HM, Finnoff JT, Peck E, et al. Accuracy of ultrasound-guided and palpation-guided knee injections by an experienced and less-experienced injector using a superolateral approach: a cadaveric study. PM R. 2011;3(6):507–15.
65. Berkoff DJ, Miller LE, Block JE. Clinical utility of ultrasound guidance for intra-articular knee injections: a review. Clin Interv Aging. 2012;7:89–95.

66. Sibbitt WL Jr, Peisajovich A, Michael AA, et al. Does sonographic needle guidance affect the clinical outcome of intraarticular injections? J Rheumatol. 2009;36(9):1892–902.
67. Sibbitt WL Jr, Band PA, Kettwich LG, et al. A randomized controlled trial evaluating the cost-effectiveness of sonographic guidance for intra-articular injection of the osteoarthritic knee. J Clin Rheumatol. 2011;17(8):409–15.
68. Maricar N, Parkes MJ, Callaghan MJ, et al. Where and how to inject the knee – a systematic review. Semin Arthritis Rheum. 2013;43(2):195–203.
69. Mandl P, Brossard M, Aegerter P, et al. Ultrasound evaluation of fluid in knee recesses at varying degrees of flexion. Arthritis Care Res (Hoboken). 2012 May;64(5):773–9.

Ultrasound of the Ankle and Foot

8

Jay B. Higgs

Key Points

- The sonographic anatomy of the ankle and foot is complex but very useful to the rheumatologist.
- Ultrasound of the ankle mortise is most useful for determining synovitis and effusion.
- Ultrasound is becoming the imaging modality of choice for tendon pathology due to its high resolution and dynamic imaging.
- Gout in the first metatarsophalangeal (MTP) joint has a characteristic but not pathognomonic appearance.
- Ultrasound is very sensitive for rheumatoid erosions; the specificity varies by erosion size and location.

Introduction

The ankle and foot are arguably the most intricate of musculoskeletal structures in the human body. The challenge of tremendous force generation and shock absorption is reflected in a complex, dynamic interplay of bones, joints, tendons, and ligaments. Similarly, this demand results in a wide spectrum of foot problems that present to the rheumatologist, either in isolation or within the context of systemic rheumatic disease. Careful study of ankle and foot ultrasound (US) can greatly enhance knowledge of anatomy and mechanics and provides the rheumatologist with additional armamentarium to diagnose and treat ankle and foot ailments [1, 2].

J. B. Higgs (✉)
Brooke Army Medical Center, Rheumatology SVC, MCHE-MDR, Houston, TX, USA
e-mail: jay.b.higgs.civ@mail.mil

M. J. Kohler (ed.), *Musculoskeletal Ultrasound in Rheumatology Review*,
https://doi.org/10.1007/978-3-030-73555-5_8

This chapter emphasizes the musculoskeletal ultrasound anatomy and pathology of greatest concern for the rheumatologist [3]. It does not include conditions of trauma, overuse, ligament pathology, nerve entrapment, foreign bodies, or neoplasia.

Standard Views in the Normal Ankle

The scanning technique for the ankle and foot largely mirrors that of other regions of the body. The standard views obtained for rheumatologic examinations are listed in Tables 8.1 and 8.2, modified after Backhaus et al. [4]. Most of the structures are superficial, allowing the use of high-frequency transducers and a shallow depth setting on the machine. Rather than taking a simple set of images, musculoskeletal ultrasound (MSKUS) of the ankle and foot often involves a dynamic study of the entire structure.

Good scanning technique involves variable pressure on the transducer to discern the deformability of the structures below. Accordingly, the transducer gel interface may vary from very thin to a thick band of gel used to "stand off" the skin surface (e.g., not touching the skin with the probe). The standoff technique allows visualization of the skin contour overlying structures of interest, shows deep structures without distortion, and avoids false-negative Doppler signal. Observing dynamic range of motion may enhance depiction of certain anatomy and pathology. For all of the ultrasound images in this chapter, the left side of the monitor is oriented to proximal, medial, or anterior. For clarity, the probe position figures omit gel in most cases. When setting up the examination, the patient and examiner should both be

Table 8.1 Standard views of the ankle [4]

Location	orientation	Most important structures
Dorsal		
	Longitudinal	Tibia, talus, anterior fat pad, tibialis anterior artery, extensor tendons
	Transverse	Tibia, talus, anterior fat pad, tibialis anterior artery, extensor tendons
Lateral	*Transverse*	Lateral malleolus, peroneus brevis, peroneus longus
	Longitudinal	Fibula, peroneus brevis, peroneus longus
	Inframalleolar longitudinal	Peroneus brevis insertion on fifth metatarsal
Medial	*Transverse*	Medial malleolus, tibialis posterior tendon, flexor digitorum, vascular bundle, tibialis posterior nerve, flexor hallucis longus
	Longitudinal	Tibialis posterior tendon
	Inframalleolar longitudinal	Tibialis posterior tendon insertion at navicular
Posterior	*Longitudinal*	Achilles tendon, paratenon, calcaneus fibrocartilage and Achilles insertion, retrocalcaneal bursa, retro-Achilles bursa (if present), Kager's fat pad

Reproduced and adapted by permission from Guidelines for musculoskeletal ultrasound in rheumatology in Annals of the Rheumatic Disease; Backhaus et al. [4], © 2001 with permission from BMJ Publishing Group Ltd

Table 8.2 Standard views of the foot [4]

Location	Orientation	Most important structures
Plantar fascia		
	Longitudinal	Calcaneus, plantar fascia
	Transverse	Used to confirm any pathology seen on longitudinal view
Subtalar joint	*Inferomedial*	Medial malleolus, talus with sustentaculum tali, subtalar joint, calcaneus
	Inferolateral	Fibula, talus, subtalar joint, calcaneus
	Anterolateral	Fibula, talus, sinus tarsi
Dorsal midfoot	*Longitudinal*	Talonavicular joint
	Transverse	To confirm pathology seen on longitudinal
MTP joint	*Dorsal longitudinal*	Metatarsal head, proximal phalanx, MTP joint, synovial recess, cartilage, extensor tendon
	Medial (lateral) longitudinal (MTP 1 and 5 only)	Metatarsal head, proximal phalanx, MTP joint, synovial recess
	Transverse	Metatarsal head, synovial recess
	Plantar longitudinal	Metatarsal head, proximal phalanx, MTP joint, synovial recess, flexor tendon
	Plantar transverse	Sesamoids, flexor tendon, limited image of MTP joint, intermetatarsal soft tissue

comfortably positioned. Most of the exam of the ankle and foot can be performed with the patient seated on the examination table. The foot can be placed plantar down on the exam table with the knee in 90° of flexion or the foot overhanging the edge of the table with the knee in full extension. The latter view can suffice for the entire exam including the posterior view. Rotating the leg will facilitate access to the lateral and medial views. The prone position, if possible, affords the best access to posterior and plantar anatomy.

Dorsal Ankle

Dorsal Longitudinal

The first view for the ankle is the dorsal longitudinal view of the ankle mortise (Fig. 8.1a, b). This view is most readily obtained by scanning over the distal tibia and then moving the transducer distally over the ankle mortise. The ankle should be comfortably plantar flexed. Moving the transducer medially and laterally will allow examination of the entire talar dome. Structures to note include the dorsal fat pad that extends to a point deep in the joint, the thin hypoechoic or anechoic cartilage, and the fat stripe just superficial to the cartilage. More superficially is the tibialis anterior artery which transitions to the dorsalis pedis artery as it passes under the extensor retinaculum. The extensor tendons also come into view, the most prominent of which is the tibialis anterior tendon.

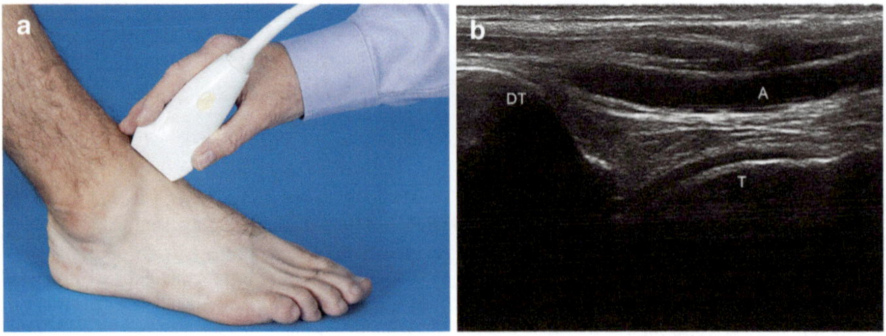

Fig. 8.1 Tibiotalar joint, dorsal longitudinal. (**a**) Probe placement. (**b**) Normal image. *T* talus, *DT* distal tibia, *A* tibialis anterior artery

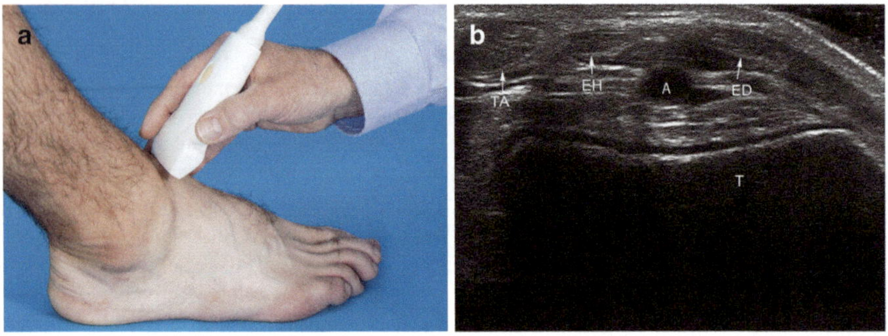

Fig. 8.2 Tibiotalar joint, transverse. (**a**) Probe placement. (**b**) Normal image. *T* talus, *A* tibialis anterior artery, *TA* tibialis anterior tendon, *EH* extensor hallucis longus tendon, *ED* extensor digitorum longus tendon

Dorsal Transverse

Turning the transducer 90° (moving the distal end of the transducer to the anatomic lateral according to the convention established earlier), the ankle mortise can be viewed in the anterior transverse plane (Fig. 8.2a, b). Similar to the longitudinal view, the most reliable way to bring this structure into view is to scan horizontally over the distal tibia and then move the transducer distally until the talar dome comes into view. In this transverse view, sliding the transducer between proximal and distal and changing the angle of insonation will allow the examination of both superficial and deep portions of the talar dome. In addition to the talar dome, the anterior transverse plane allows identification of the extensor tendons as they course deep to the proximal and distal retinacula: from medial to lateral, the *t*ibialis anterior, extensor *h*allucis longus (EHL), and extensor *d*igitorum longus (EDL) tendons (remembered by the mnemonic, *T*om hates *D*ick). The anterior tendons of the ankle do not normally have any detectable tenosynovial fluid. EHL and EDL may have a muscular component at this level, mimicking synovitis [5].

Lateral Ankle

Lateral Transverse

The lateral ankle anatomic structures of interest include the lateral malleolus (fibula), peroneus longus (PL), and peroneus brevis (PB) tendons. The most readily obtained view of the PL and PB is the lateral transverse view (Fig. 8.3a, b). The transducer is placed horizontally at the distal fibula, so that the left side of the monitor is anterior. PB is the tendon adjacent to the fibula (remembered by *b*revis next to the *b*one). PL is more posterior. There is otherwise some individual variation in how PB and PL relate to one another. It is normal to have a small hypoechoic rim around PB and PL [6], and the common peroneal sheath may contain a small amount of fluid [7]. There should be minimal or no color power Doppler (CPD) signal in this view. Peroneus quadratus (PQ) is an accessory muscle present in 22% of ankles [5]. Its origin is in the supramalleolar PB, and it inserts distally in PB or PL. PQ is important to recognize because the muscle can mimic tendinitis and the PQ tendon next to PB may be misinterpreted as a split tear in the PB. True tendinitis at this location is marked by tenosynovial swelling, local tenderness, tendon thickening, and sometimes increased CPD signal.

Lateral Longitudinal

Turning the transducer to the lateral longitudinal plane, the tendons may be more difficult to image (Fig. 8.4a, b). Aiming the transducer at the tendons from posterior to anterior, using extra gel as needed, will result in a better image. Attention to how PB and PL relate to each other in the transverse view can also assist in choosing the best angle of insonation in the long view.

Lateral Inframalleolar Longitudinal

Distally, PB continues on to the base of the fifth metatarsal. The easiest way to image the lateral inframalleolar longitudinal view of the distal PB is to palpate the

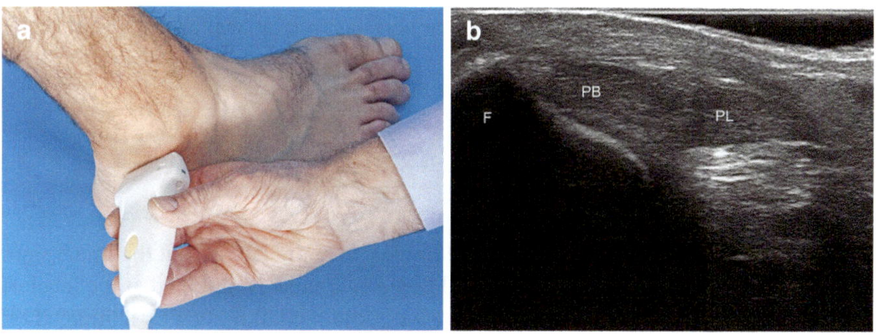

Fig. 8.3 Ankle, lateral transverse. (**a**) Lateral transverse probe placement. (**b**) Normal image. *F* fibula, *PB* peroneus brevis, *PL* peroneus longus

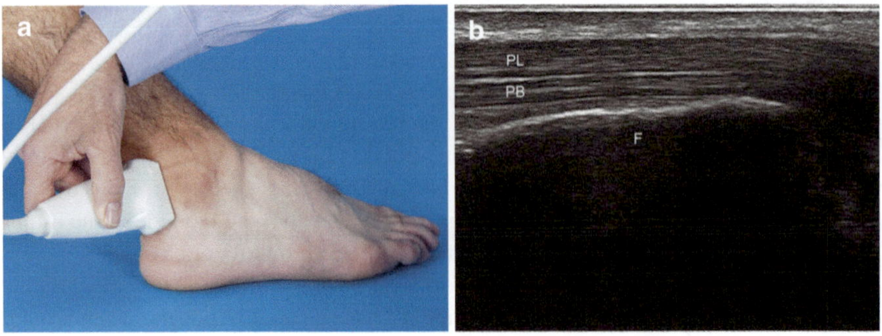

Fig. 8.4 Ankle, lateral longitudinal. (**a**) Probe placement. (**b**) Normal image. *F* fibula, *PB* peroneus brevis, *PL* peroneus longus

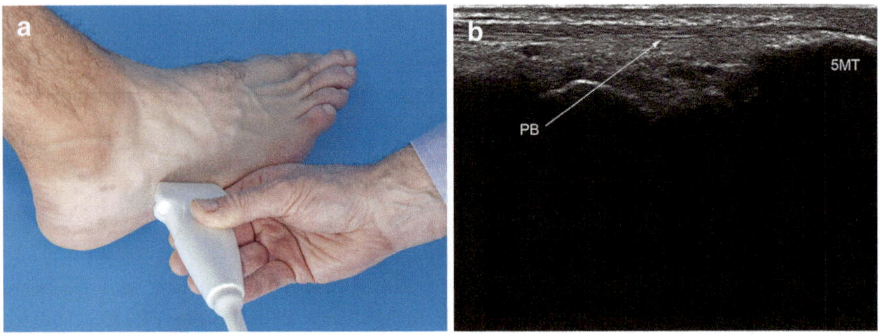

Fig. 8.5 Ankle, lateral inframalleolar longitudinal. (**a**) Probe placement. (**b**) Normal image. *5MT* base of fifth metatarsal, *PB* peroneus brevis

fifth metatarsal, image it on the right side of the monitor, and then adjust the proximal pole of the transducer toward the expected course of PB from the inferior malleolus (Fig. 8.5a, b). PB will appear less distinct as it traverses distally, because the tendon loses fibers to several branches proximal to the fifth metatarsal. When following both PB and PL from the medial malleolus distally, PL is the first to disappear as it takes a sharp dive into the plantar surface on its journey to its insertion on the navicular at the medial plantar arch.

Medial Ankle

Medial Transverse

The medial ankle is anatomically more complex than the lateral, but the images are obtained in a similar fashion. The medial transverse view is obtained at the level of the distal medial malleolus (Fig. 8.6a, b). First, the medial malleolus is imaged on the left side of the monitor, and then the posterior pole of the transducer is rotated until recognizable anatomic structures come into view. It is important to use

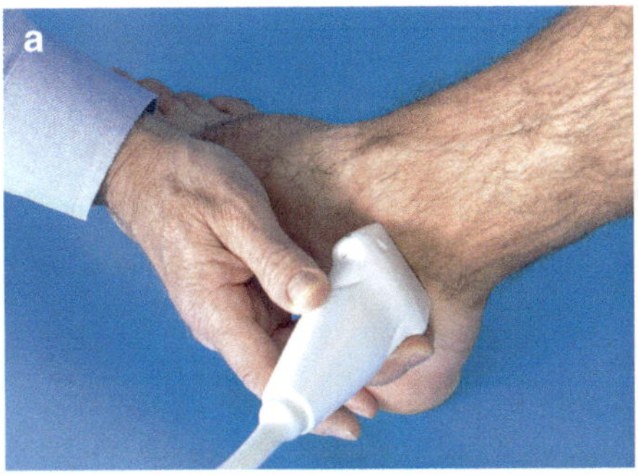

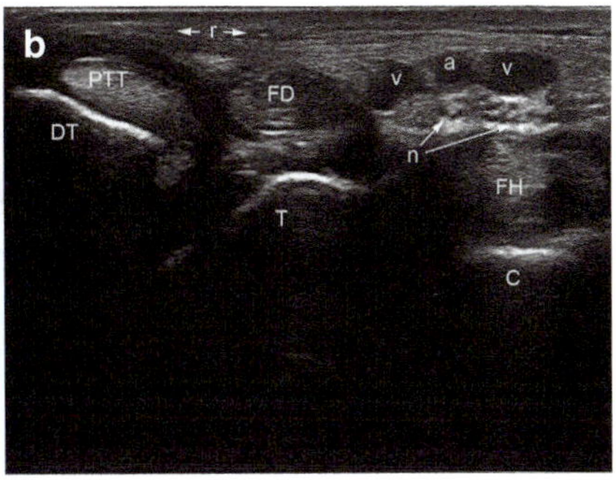

Fig. 8.6 Ankle, medial transverse. (**a**) Probe placement. (**b**) Normal image. *DT* distal tibia, *T* talus, *C* calcaneus, *PTT* posterior tibial tendon, *FD* flexor digitorum longus tendon, *v* veins, *a* artery, *n* posterior tibial nerve (two branches), *FH* flexor hallucis longus muscle, *r* flexor retinaculum

minimal pressure at this location so as to not distort the underlying soft tissue structures. The identifiable structures, from anterior (left side of monitor) to posterior, include the medial malleolus, the posterior *t*ibialis tendon, the flexor *d*igitorum longus tendon, the tibialis posterior *a*rtery with two *v*eins, the tibialis posterior *n*erve, and finally the flexor *h*allucis longus muscle or tendon. These structures can be remembered with the mnemonic, "*T*om, *D*ick *a*nd *v*ery *n*ervous *H*arry." The posterior tibialis tendon (PTT) is twice as large as the flexor digitorum longus (FDL) and travels along a fibrocartilaginous groove in the posterior tibia [8]. At the malleolus, PTT may normally have a small amount of tenosynovial fluid [7]. The tibialis posterior nerve has a typical honeycomb appearance but is small and may appear as more than one branch at this level. In this view, the flexor hallucis longus (FHL) may appear either tendinous or muscular, as the musculotendinous junction is near this location. If the FHL tendon or muscle cannot be readily identified, dynamic viewing during active flexion and extension of the great toe can reveal its location. In high-quality images, the flexor retinaculum can be seen superficial to these structures. Deep to the tendons, from anterior to posterior, the periostia of the tibia, talus, and calcaneus can be seen.

Medial Longitudinal

Of all the above structures, the PTT is one of the most relevant to rheumatologists. The PTT is viewed in the medial longitudinal view by first imaging the tibia and sliding the transducer posteriorly (Fig. 8.7a, b). The first tendon to come into view is the PTT. If this maneuver is not done, it is possible to end up over the FDL and mistake it for the PTT.

Medial Inframalleolar Longitudinal

The PTT can be followed distally to its insertion on the navicular bone. Along this course, the PTT branches off fibers to insert more medially in bones of the midfoot. Similar to PB, the PTT fans out to a broad insertion on the navicular [8], making its

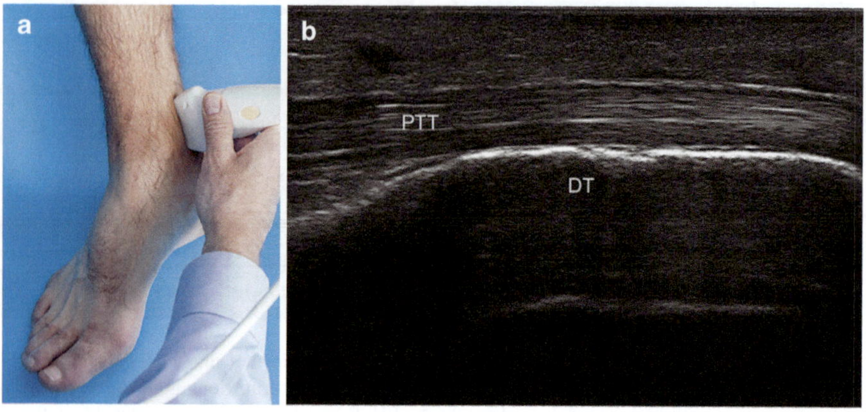

Fig. 8.7 Ankle, medial longitudinal. (**a**) Probe placement. (**b**) Normal image. *DT* distal tibia, *PTT* posterior tibial tendon

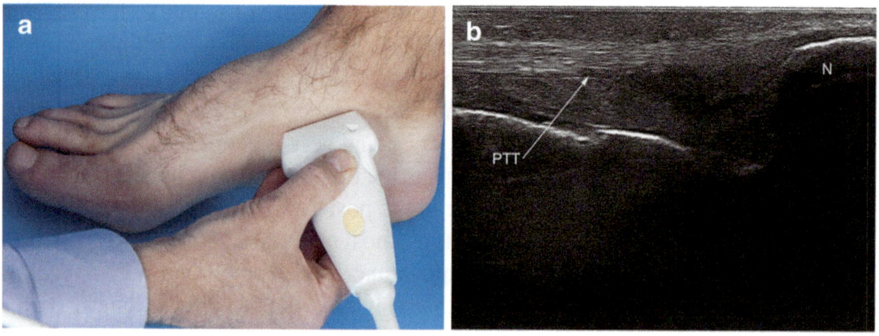

Fig. 8.8 Ankle, medial inframalleolar longitudinal. (**a**) Probe placement. (**b**) Normal image. *PTT* posterior tibial tendon, *N* navicular

image at this insertion in the medial inframalleolar longitudinal view difficult to obtain (Fig. 8.8a, b). Because PTT inserts into and traverses over the plantar-medial aspect of the navicular, this view can be optimized by aiming the transducer from plantar to cephalad in a direction approximately 45° from the perpendicular [32]. When the PTT cannot be easily followed to its insertion, the following technique may be used to image the insertion: (1) palpate the navicular bone, (2) place the probe over the plantar-medial aspect of the navicular aiming about 45° cephalad to image it on the right side of the screen, and (3) keeping the distal pole fixed on the navicular, swing the proximal pole in the expected course of the PTT as it emerges from the medial malleolus, keeping the transducer aimed cephalad as described earlier. One anatomic variant that may create additional confusion is an accessory navicular bone, which may lie between the medial malleolus and the navicular bone [8]. The PTT may course over the accessory navicular or partially insert into it. The accessory navicular bone may be misinterpreted as a tendon calcification or a

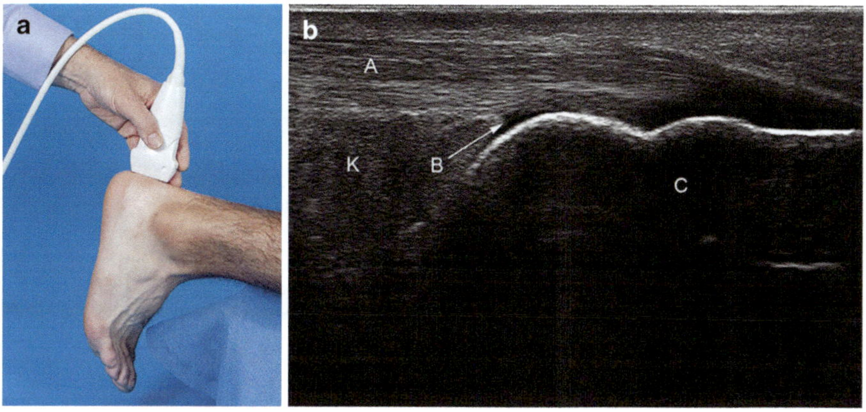

Fig. 8.9 Ankle, posterior longitudinal. (**a**) Probe placement. (**b**) Normal image. *A* Achilles tendon, *B* retrocalcaneal bursa, *C* calcaneus, *K* Kager's fat pad

navicular avulsion fragment. Finally, some fibers at the distal insertion may course over the navicular bone plantar-medially to insert on the base of the first cuneiform. The normal PTT should have minimal fluid or CPD signal surrounding it at the medial malleolus, and the distal portion does not have a tendon sheath.

Posterior Ankle

The posterior ankle is most easily imaged with the subject in the prone position, but with experience, it is possible to obtain high-quality images with the patient supine and the ankle overhanging the end of the examination table.

Posterior Longitudinal

The posterior longitudinal view of the ankle affords an excellent image of the Achilles tendon as it inserts into the calcaneus (Fig. 8.9a, b). The normal Achilles tendon is uniform and fibrillar. There is no tendon sheath around the Achilles, but there is a paratenon that can longitudinally stretch over 3 cm to facilitate smooth motion of the Achilles [9]. The distal aspect of the tendon appears hypoechoic due to anisotropy of the tendon fibers as they turn sharply and insert into the distal calcaneus. The tendon can be viewed with the ankle in dorsiflexion, in which case the fibers are most uniform but the CPD signal could be false-negative. For CPD assessment, having the ankle in slight plantar flexion with minimal or no transducer pressure will avoid false-negative signal.

The proximal portion of the calcaneus has a fibrocartilaginous surface. At the most proximal end of the calcaneus lies the retrocalcaneal bursa, which facilitates motion of the Achilles over the proximal calcaneus during flexion and extension. The horseshoe-shaped retrocalcaneal bursa [9] is thin and measures about 5 mm in both the longitudinal and transverse planes [6]. It should not, however, be distended more than 3 mm [7]. Deep to the Achilles proximally is Kager's fat pad.

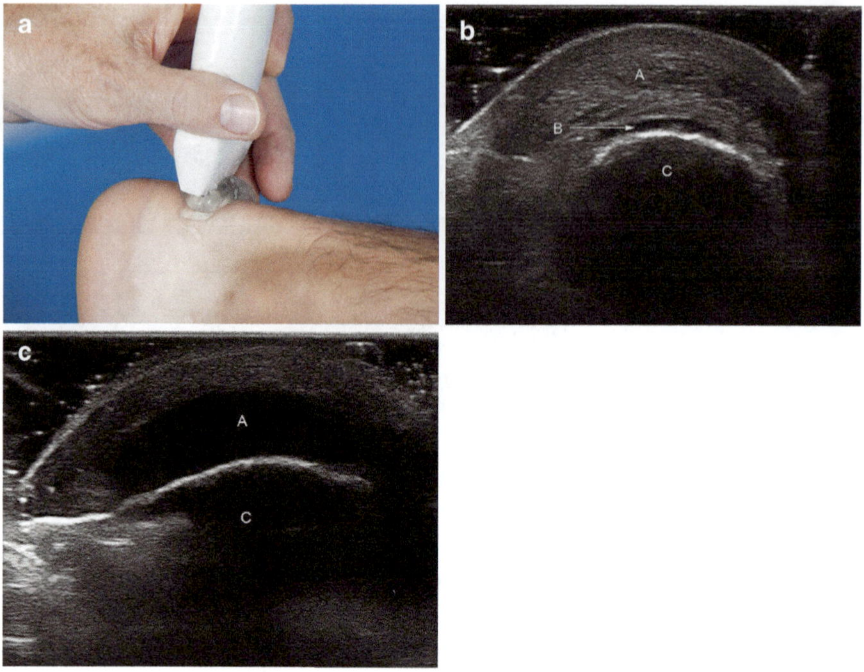

Fig. 8.10 Ankle, posterior transverse. (**a**) Probe placement. (**b**) Normal image at the level of the retrocalcaneal bursa; extra gel and a standoff technique are used to accommodate the convex skin. (**c**) Angling transducer yields Achilles tendon anisotropy, which better delineates the tendon margins. *A* Achilles tendon, *B* retrocalcaneal bursa, *C* calcaneus

Posterior Transverse

Turning the transducer horizontally yields the posterior transverse view (Fig. 8.10a–c). Because of the convex surface overlying the Achilles, the highest-quality image is obtained by placing a generous amount of gel on the center of the transducer and carefully indenting the gel into the posterior ankle until a standoff view is obtained (Fig. 8.10a). It is important in both planes to move the transducer as far as possible in each direction to examine the entire structure. The two standard recorded views will only represent a small fraction of the structure.

Standard Views of the Normal Foot

Plantar Fascia

Plantar Longitudinal

The plantar longitudinal view of the foot is mainly used to image the plantar fascia (Fig. 8.11a, b). This view may require machine adjustment, depending on the thickness of the callus at the heel. For a thick callus, lower frequency is required, at the cost of resolution. Placing US gel on the heel in advance of attempting the image

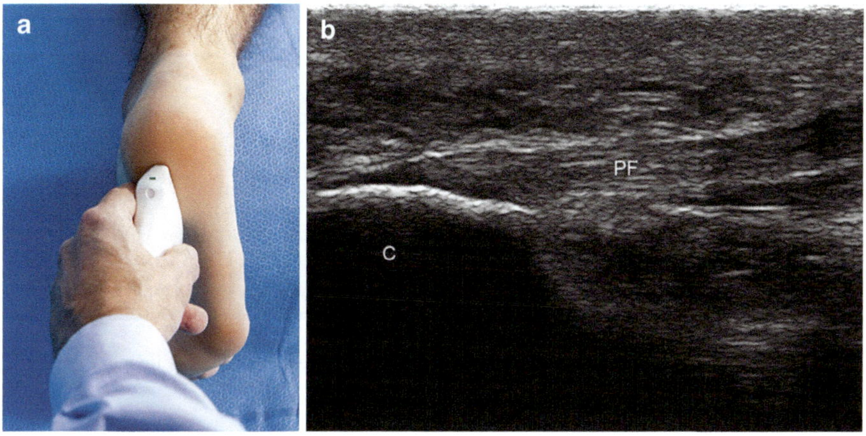

Fig. 8.11 Plantar fascia, plantar longitudinal view. (**a**) Probe placement. (**b**) Normal image. *C* calcaneus, *PF* plantar fascia

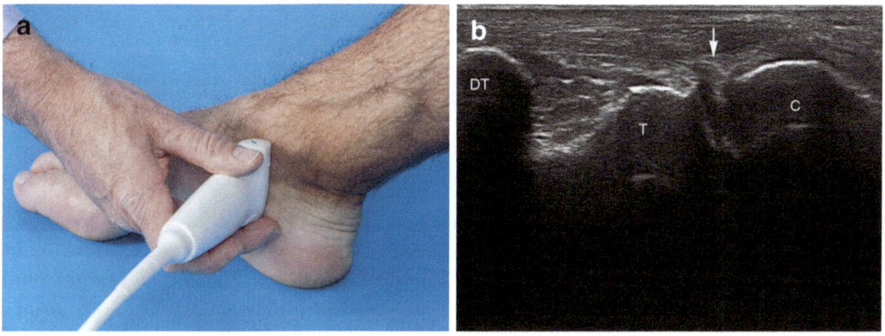

Fig. 8.12 Subtalar joint, inferomedial view. (**a**) Probe placement. (**b**) Normal image. *DT* distal tibia, *T* talus, *C* calcaneus, *Arrow* subtalar joint

may soften the skin and decrease surface reflection of the sound. The proximal pole of the transducer (left side of monitor) is placed over the medial calcaneal tubercle and the distal pole aimed in the direction of the fourth digit. From there, minor adjustments are needed to bring the plantar fascia origin at the calcaneus into optimal view. The maximum plantar fascia thickness is measured at the calcaneal origin and is normally 3–4.5 mm or less as described later.

Subtalar Joint

The subtalar joint may be imaged inferomedially, inferolaterally, or as the deep structure in the sinus tarsi anterolaterally. It should be noted that only the external margins of this complex joint can be seen by ultrasound. Inferomedially, the joint is best found with the transducer in the coronal plane distal to the malleolus (Fig. 8.12a, b). The distal aspect of the talus forms a joint with the prominent convex sustentaculum tali of

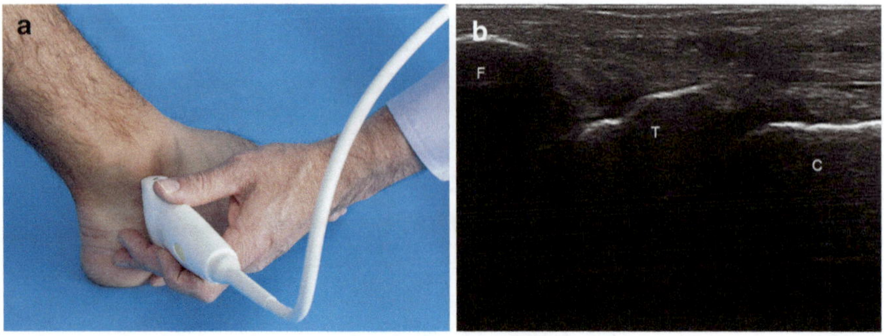

Fig. 8.13 Subtalar joint, inferolateral view. (**a**) Probe placement. (**b**) Normal image. *F* fibula, *T* talus, *C* calcaneus

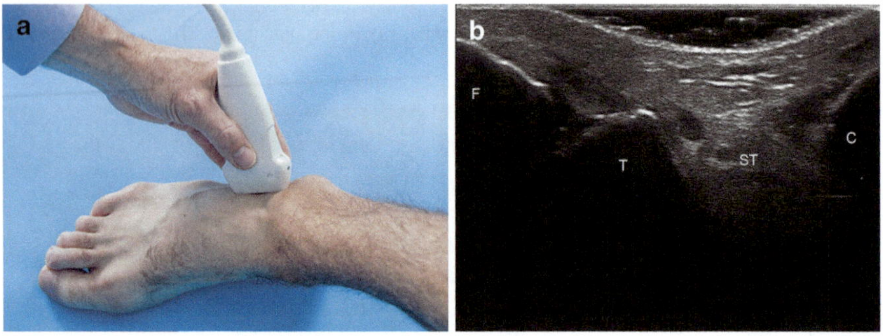

Fig. 8.14 Sinus tarsi, anterolateral view. (**a**) Probe placement. (**b**) Normal image. *F* fibula, *T* talus, *C* calcaneus, *ST* sinus tarsi

the calcaneus. Dynamic examination may be employed by placing valgus stress on the calcaneus to make this joint more apparent. The inferolateral view is similarly obtained in the lateral coronal plane (Fig. 8.13a, b). Anterolaterally, the sinus tarsi is easily identified by placing the proximal pole of the transducer on the anterior fibula and the distal pole in the anteroinferior direction of the fifth MTP (Fig. 8.14a, b). In this view, the subtalar joint lies deep in the sinus tarsi and cannot be directly seen. In the posterior longitudinal view of the ankle, the subtalar joint is just proximal to the calcaneus but is deep to Kager's fat pad and may be difficult to image. Pediatric subtalar joints are imaged more readily than those of adults due to the width of the developing joint and increased mobility in this population.

Dorsal Midfoot

MSKUS of the midfoot has traditionally been less commonly performed by the rheumatologist. While extensor tendon pathology is much less common than that of

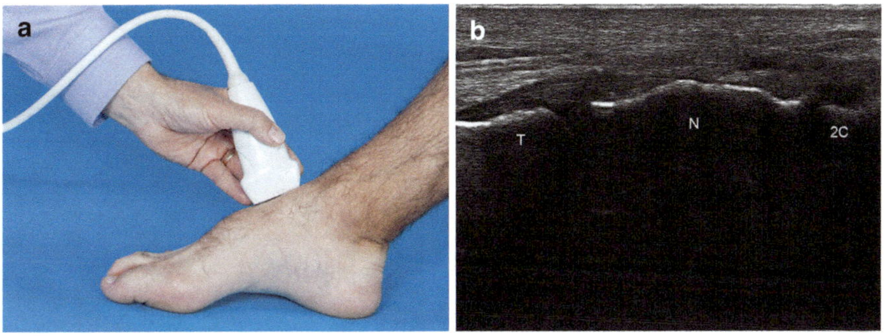

Fig. 8.15 Dorsal midfoot, longitudinal. (**a**) Probe placement. (**b**) Normal image. *T* talus, *N* navicular, *2C* second cuneiform

the flexors in inflammatory disease [7], important findings of tendinitis, synovitis, crystalline-induced pathology, and erosions may all be seen in the midfoot. In the dorsal longitudinal view, distal to the ankle mortise on the medial side is the talonavicular joint (Fig. 8.15a, b) and on the lateral side is the talocuboid joint. When normal, the midfoot joints will appear as small gaps between the tarsal bones, with no CPD signal.

Metatarsophalangeal Joints

In the forefoot, the metatarsophalangeal joints (MTP) are very important to the rheumatologist. The first and fifth MTP can be most thoroughly examined, owing to the ability to image the joints laterally in addition to the dorsal and plantar views.

Dorsal Longitudinal View

The dorsal longitudinal view may be obtained with the digit both in neutral position (Fig. 8.16a, b) and in plantar flexion, the former supplying a better view of the synovium and CPD imaging and the latter affording more complete imaging of the cartilaginous surface (Fig. 8.16c). As demonstrated in Fig. 8.16a, the neutral position image may be improved by a standoff view to show the overlying skin contour and avoid a false-negative CPD signal. Normal cartilage will often yield an "interface sign," a fine hyperechoic uniform line tapered at each end at the surface of the cartilage, which is a result of normal sound reflection. Differentiating this from the double-contour sign is discussed in the following pathology section. The first MTP commonly has a physiologic amount of fluid visible in the dorsal longitudinal view, creating a bone-capsule distance averaging 1.7 mm, with a range 0.2–4.8 [6]. The proximal reflection of the synovium covers much more bone than does the distal aspect.

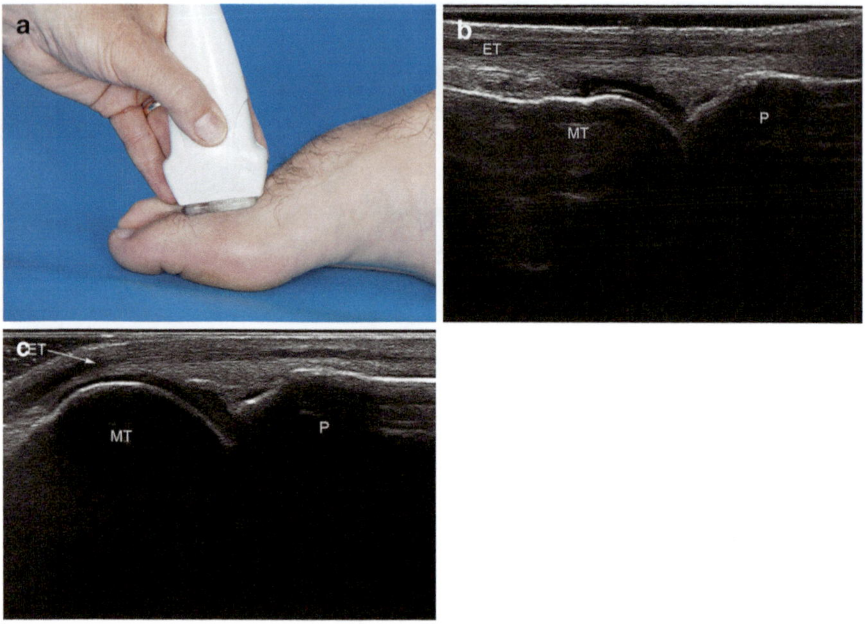

Fig. 8.16 First MTP, dorsal longitudinal, extra gel for standoff view. (**a**) Probe placement. (**b**) Normal image, standoff view demonstrating normal intra-articular fluid and interface reflex. (**c**) Same joint with toe in maximum flexion, no standoff technique, giving more complete view of cartilage and no interface reflex, but the intra-articular fluid is no longer apparent. *MT* first metatarsal, *P* proximal phalanx, *ET* extensor tendon

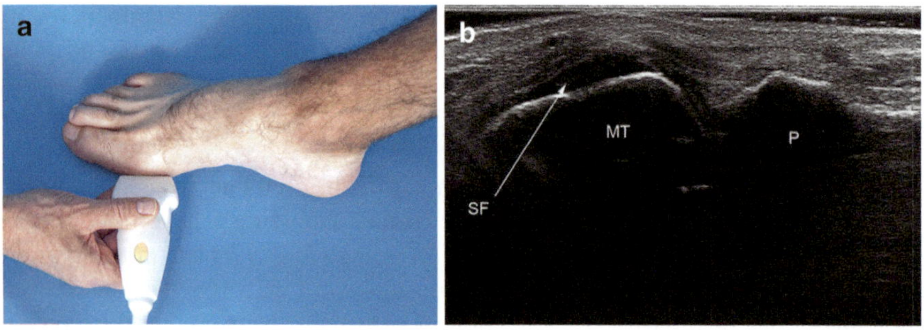

Fig. 8.17 First MTP, medial longitudinal. (**a**) Probe placement. (**b**) Normal image standoff view reveals normal synovial fluid. *MT* first metatarsal, *P* proximal phalanx

Medial and Lateral Longitudinal

The first MTP can be viewed medially (Fig. 8.17a, b) and the fifth MTP laterally. The other MTP medial and lateral views are very limited. Both views may be improved by a standoff view to show the overlying skin contour and avoid a false-negative CPD signal.

Transverse

The transverse view over the metatarsal head is performed dorsally and laterally (Fig. 8.18a, b). In both the longitudinal and transverse planes, it is important to move the transducer over all aspects of the joint for a complete examination. The transverse view can also be used to examine between the metatarsal heads, especially for Morton's neuroma as later described.

Plantar Longitudinal and Transverse

The plantar longitudinal view (Fig. 8.19a, b) may require extra gel and lower frequency, depending on the degree of deformity and plantar callus formation. The sesamoid bones limit the plantar view of the first MTP, but the flexor tendon can be imaged in plantar longitudinal and transverse planes (Fig. 8.20a, b).

Pathology

The most common ankle and foot pathologic findings encountered by the rheumatologist are listed in Table 8.3.

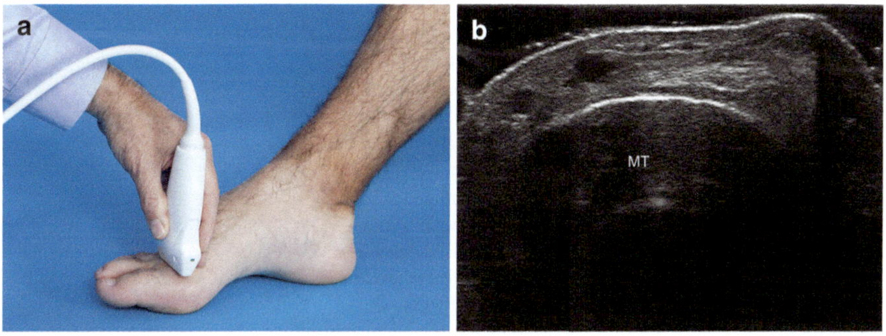

Fig. 8.18 First MTP, transverse. (**a**) Probe placement. (**b**) Normal image. Scanning the entire MT in transverse is useful to look for erosions. *MT* first metatarsal

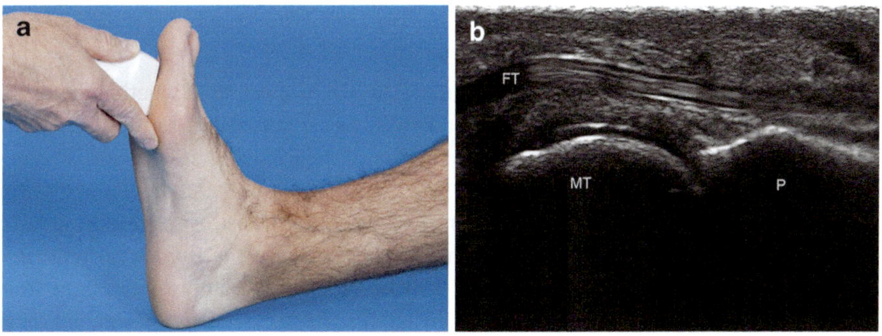

Fig. 8.19 First MTP, plantar longitudinal. (**a**) Probe placement. (**b**) Normal image. A lower frequency is required to obtain this image, resulting in less detail. An interface reflex at the cartilage surface is apparent

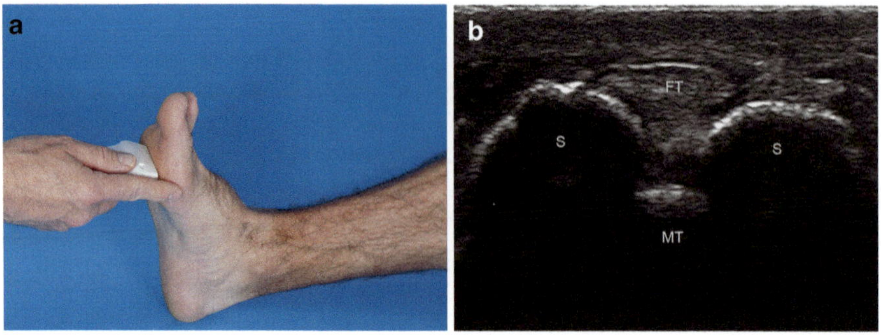

Fig. 8.20 First MTP, plantar transverse. (**a**) Probe placement. (**b**) Normal image. The sesamoids block most of the view of the joint. *S* sesamoids, *MT* first metatarsal head, *FT* flexor tendon

Table 8.3 Most common rheumatologic pathology of the ankle and foot

Site	Pathologic findings
Tibiotalar joint	Synovitis Effusion
Lateral ankle	Peroneus longus, peroneus brevis tendinitis Subtalar arthritis Peroneus brevis enthesitis
Medial ankle	Posterior tibial tendonitis Posterior tibial enthesitis
Posterior ankle	Achilles tendinopathy Achilles enthesitis Retrocalcaneal bursitis Retro-Achilles bursitis
Midfoot	Tibialis anterior tendinitis Midfoot arthritis
Forefoot	Metatarsophalangeal synovitis Microcrystalline deposition Metatarsophalangeal erosions Morton's neuroma

Tibiotalar Joint

At the ankle mortise, MSKUS is particularly useful to determine whether synovitis or synovial effusion is present. The fat pad of the ankle normally forms a sharp point between the tibia and talus at the deepest aspect of the joint. When effusion or synovitis is present, this fat pad will rise up out of the joint and become blunted (Fig. 8.21a, b). To determine the presence of fluid, the transducer pressure can be varied (ballottement) to alternately compress and release the fluid with real-time dynamic imaging. Synovial thickening will be much less compressible than free-flowing fluid [10]. CPD signal will be increased in the inflamed synovium, but there should be no CPD signal within synovial fluid. As always, CPD imaging requires minimal or no transducer pressure, and no motion between the transducer and subject. In B-mode, it is important to move the transducer around to image the entire joint in both the longitudinal and transverse views. Small pockets of fluid may be located laterally or medially and escape detection if only part of the joint is studied. The cartilage of the talar dome is normally thin and hypoechoic. A double-contour sign may be present in chronic gout, but the fat stripe superficial to the cartilage should not be mistaken for a double-contour sign. The fat stripe is uniform and smooth, and the irregular grainy double contour of urate will move with the cartilage in dynamic motion of the joint. Similarly, the interface reflex of normal cartilage is a smooth thin line on the surface of the cartilage; it tapers at each end and does not move with motion of the joint.

Lateral and Medial Ankle

Peroneal tendinitis is readily detected by ultrasonography. Tendon enlargement and loss of fibrillar pattern indicate tendinosis. Peritendinous fluid, as seen in Fig. 8.22a, b, and increased CPD signal, best seen on the transverse views, indicate tendinitis. Increased CPD signal at the distal PB insertion on the base of the fifth metatarsal

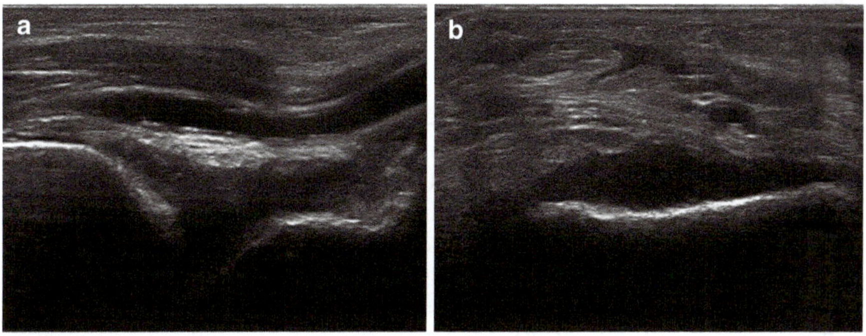

Fig. 8.21 Dorsal longitudinal and transverse. (**a**) Dorsal longitudinal view of the ankle shows blunting of the fat pad consistent with synovial thickening or effusion. (**b**) Dorsal transverse. Ballottement confirmed this was fluid

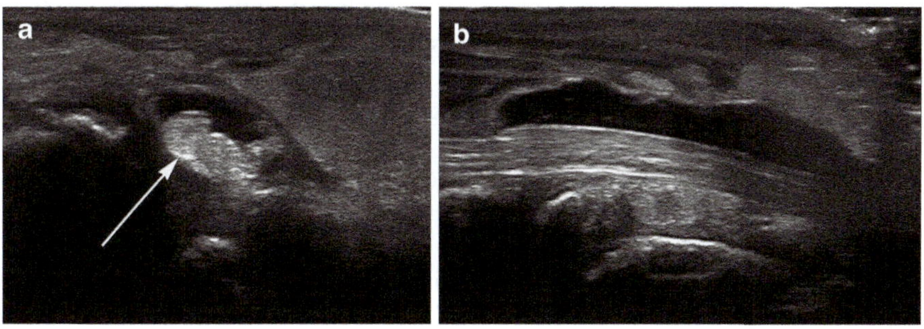

Fig. 8.22 Tenosynovitis of PB and PL tendons. (**a**) Transverse; PB and PL tendons (*arrow*) surrounded by excess fluid. (**b**) Longitudinal showing excess tenosynovial fluid

may represent enthesitis, but clinical correlations of this structure have not been well studied and the OMERACT definition of enthesitis is still under debate. Similarly, the medial views may show posterior tibial tendinosis or tendinitis, and the inflamed distal PTT insertion on the navicular bone may have increased CPD signal in enthesitis. In one study of the PTT, using criteria of (a) intratendinous blood flow by CPD, (b) increased proximal tendon diameter causing rounding of the tendon, and (c) inhomogeneity of the tendon, US yielded 80% sensitivity and 90% specificity for PTT tendinosis, using MRI as the standard [11]. Another US study of the distal PTT enthesis found patients with rheumatoid arthritis and spondyloarthropathy had a 5.1- and 3.6-fold increase vs. controls, respectively, in PTT abnormalities, including fiber disruption, tenosynovial effusion, and Doppler signal [32].

The PB/PL and PTT were included in the OMERACT consensus-based US score for tenosynovitis in rheumatoid arthritis [12]. Consensus-based grading was on a scale of 0–3, for normal, minimal, moderate, and severe abnormalities. Abnormalities in B-mode considered important were tendon sheath widening, effusion, and tenosynovial hypertrophy. Peritendinous CPD signal in two planes, excluding feeder vessels, was considered abnormal only if there were concomitant B-mode abnormalities.

Posterior Ankle

The posterior views of the ankle may be abnormal for a variety of reasons. The Achilles tendon is the most commonly injured tendon in the ankle, with the relatively avascular portion 2–6 cm proximal to the calcaneus being the most vulnerable [7, 9]. Mechanical disruption of the Achilles tendon causing tendinosis and partial- or full-thickness tendon rupture is reflected with partial or full loss of the fibrillar pattern of the tendon. The tendon, which normally has minimal vascularity, may develop increased CPD signal when disrupted. However, pathologic correlation with intratendinous Achilles CPD signal does not necessarily reflect true inflammation [9]. Hence, tendinosis is a better term than tendinitis for intratendon abnormalities of the Achilles. Tendinosis may result in expansion of the Achilles tendon as measured in the antero-posterior diameter (Fig. 8.23). Inflammation of the Achilles paratenon, termed paratenonitis, is best visualized by US at the posterior aspect of the Achilles as a thickened, hypoechoic paratenon [9]. Enthesitis is represented by erosion of the fibrocartilaginous (proximal) portion of the calcaneus and increased CPD signal in both the proximal fibrocartilage and the Achilles insertion (Fig. 8.24a, b). The significance of Achilles CPD signal within 2 mm of the calcaneus insertion or beyond of this limit in terms of true enthesitis remains uncertain, but the former has been advocated by the Outcome Measures in Rheumatology Ultrasound Task Force [33].

The fibrocartilaginous calcaneus is the site of erosions in spondyloarthropathies (SpA), and the distal calcaneus is the site of new bone formation [13]. The retrocalcaneal bursa, normally distended less than 2–3 mm [9], may become enlarged from bursitis or packed with "wet sugar" signal in urate deposition (Fig. 8.25). Active

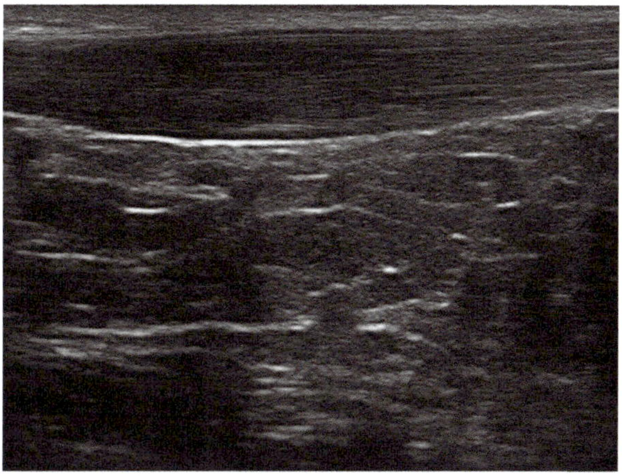

Fig. 8.23 Achilles tendinosis. Longitudinal view shows expanded and slightly hypoechoic mid-Achilles

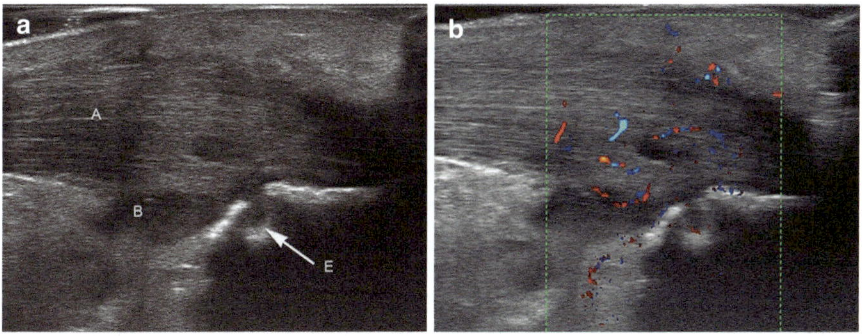

Fig. 8.24 Achilles enthesitis. (**a**) Achilles enthesitis. *A* expanded Achilles tendon, *B* enlarged retrocalcaneal bursa, *E* calcaneal erosion. (**b**) Doppler signal confirms increased blood flow to the area

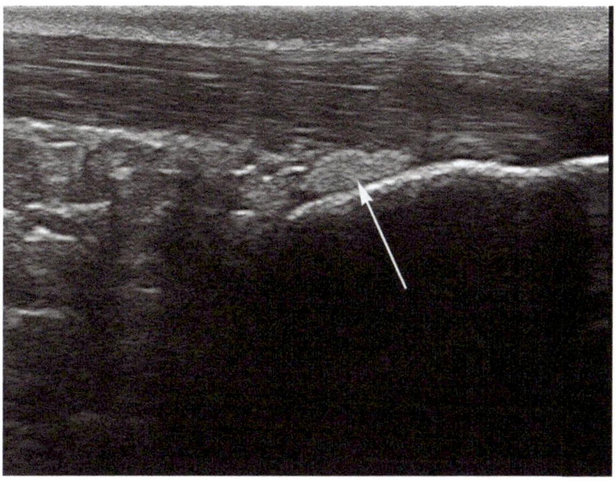

Fig. 8.25 Urate deposition in the retrocalcaneal bursa (*arrow*)

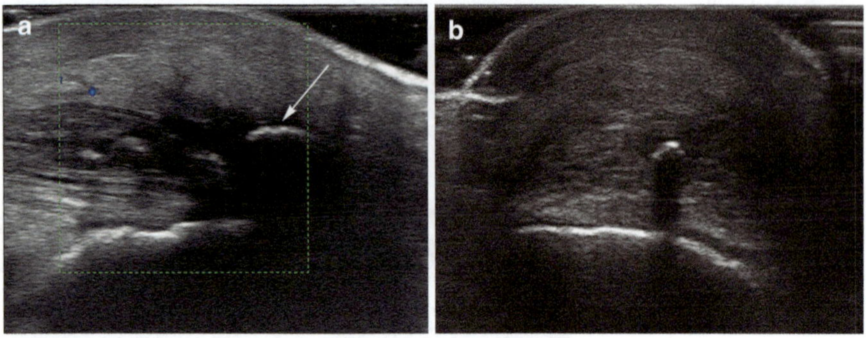

Fig. 8.26 Achilles calcifications. (**a**) Achilles tendon, posterior longitudinal view; internal calcification and large enthesophyte casting an acoustic shadow (*arrow*). No increased blood flow by Doppler signal. (**b**) Transverse view of Achilles, showing dense calcification casting acoustic shadow. A transverse view of the tip of an enthesophyte would look similar

retrocalcaneal bursitis will have increased CPD signal. The retro-Achilles bursa is not visible in the normal state but becomes visible superficial to the Achilles when enlarged [9]. A standoff view is best for imaging retro-Achilles bursitis, because it shows the skin contour and the very superficial pathology the best. New bone formation (enthesophyte) at the Achilles insertion will be represented by an elevated periosteal signal with an acoustic shadow deep to it (Fig. 8.26a). Similarly, calcifications within the Achilles tendon will be hyperechoic and, if extensive, have posterior acoustic shadowing (Fig. 8.26b). Achilles calcifications and calcaneal soft tissue inflammation have been correlated with chondrocalcinosis [14] but could also represent degenerative calcium hydroxyapatite. Dystrophic calcifications within the Achilles may become ossified, with trabeculae better seen on conventional radiography [9].

The Achilles and plantar fascia insertions were included among nine entheses in a CPD US study of enthesitis in suspected SpA [15]. Among suspected SpA with Amor criteria <6, the sensitivity and specificity of enthesitis for the development of SpA after 2 years were 90% and 77%, respectively. In a second study, however, both MRI and CPD US of the heel were not found useful for the diagnosis of SpA but did correlate with symptoms in patients with known SpA [16]. Other conditions that result in focal tendinosis at the calcaneal insertion include Haglund's syndrome, marked by prominence of the proximal posterior calcaneal tuberosity resulting in Achilles insertional tendinitis and retrocalcaneal bursitis [9]. Rheumatoid arthritis (RA) can cause both retrocalcaneal bursitis and paratenonitis [9].

Plantar Fascia

Plantar fasciitis at the calcaneal origin is readily detected by measurement of the maximum plantar fascia thickness at this location (Fig. 8.27a). Because of the broad range of plantar fascia thickness in normal, what constitutes an abnormally

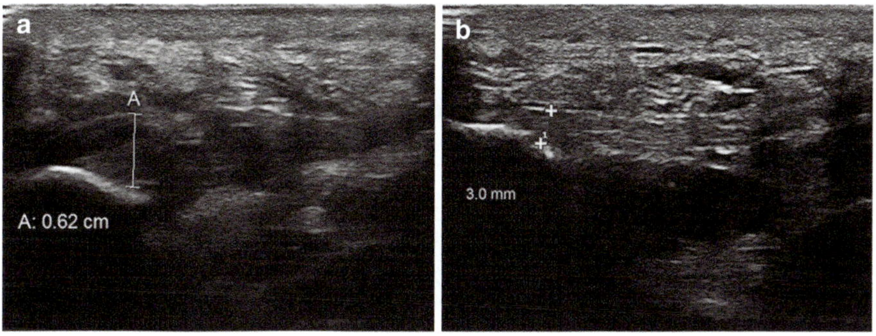

Fig. 8.27 Plantar fascia. (**a**) Plantar fascia, plantar longitudinal view, with thickening, loss of fibrillar pattern, and hypoechogenicity at the insertion. (**b**) Contralateral asymptomatic side

thickened plantar fascia is variably reported as greater than 3–4.5 mm [6, 8, 17–19]. If the contralateral foot of a patient is asymptomatic, then comparison to the symptomatic side may be useful (Fig. 8.27b). Sonopalpation (either by imaging directly over the area of palpated tenderness or by applying direct pressure of the transducer) can confirm that the identified abnormality is actually the source of symptoms.

Subtalar Joint

The subtalar joint is more obvious when an effusion protrudes from the joint lines or sinus tarsi. In one study of RA, the agreement between MRI and US for inflammation of the medial subtalar joint was 63% and for the lateral subtalar joint 73% [20].

Midfoot

Midfoot joint inflammation, especially from gout, can be identified by an expanded synovium or the appearance of "wet sugar" suggestive of urate deposits at the site of inflammation. CPD signal is not normally present in the midfoot, except for blood vessels, but may be increased in midfoot inflammatory arthritis (Fig. 8.28a, b). Dorsal nodules in the foot can be proven to be intertarsal joint osteophytes by US. Tibialis anterior or extensor digitorum tenosynovitis is identified by expansion of the synovium surrounding the tendon, with or without increased CPD signal. Ganglion cysts are common [7], usually anechoic, and are suggested if a feeder connection to a tendon can be demonstrated. Hypoechoic expansion of the subcutaneous tissue, consistent with subcutaneous edema, can be seen in the setting inflammatory arthritis or peripheral edema. A "cobblestone" appearance of the subcutaneous tissue, particularly with increased CPD signal, may represent cellulitis. Other differential diagnoses of hypoechoic lesions/masses include schwannoma and

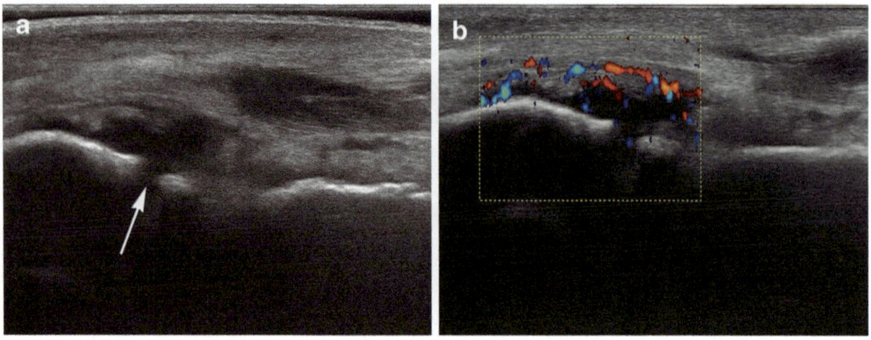

Fig. 8.28 Midfoot inflammation. (**a**) Dorsal midfoot joint inflammation. Note the hypoechoic synovium bulging from the joint. (**b**) Doppler signal is present at the site of inflammation

giant cell tumor. One percent of ankle and foot nodules in one study were soft tissue sarcomas, which required imaging modalities other than US [21].

Metatarsophalangeal Joints

The first MTP is often the target of gout. Urate deposition is suggested by the US appearance of "clumps of wet sugar" in the synovium (Fig. 8.29). The double-contour sign (Fig. 8.30) is generated by urate deposition at the surface of cartilage but is not pathognomonic of gout [22–24]. Serial follow-up of treated gout may show disappearance of the double contour after approximately 7 months [25]. Erosions of the cortical surface usually appear as discrete gaps in the periosteal surface. Isolated small erosions may be normal variants, but wet sugar clumps adjacent to erosions in the first MTP are strongly suggestive of chronic gout. CPD signal within the erosions represents increased blood flow, suggesting active inflammation in the erosion. However, increased CPD signal may also be seen in osteoarthritis of the first MTP [26].

The MTP joints, including the first MTP, may be involved in other forms of inflammatory arthritis including rheumatoid arthritis (Fig. 8.31a, b). As noted in the anatomy section, the first MTP has a normal amount of fluid, and the mean bone-capsule distance is 1.7 mm ± 0.9 standard deviation [6]. Expansion of the capsule beyond this norm or a convex contour of the fluid indicates an abnormal synovial effusion. Free-flowing fluid should be easily compressible with transducer pressure; however, during acute gout or infection, the patient may be too tender for anything but a gentle standoff view. When synovitis is present, extensor tendinitis can also occur. In addition to the joint capsule, crystalline deposition can sometimes be seen within the extensor tendon substance.

The fifth MTP is particularly useful for detecting erosions in rheumatoid arthritis (Fig. 8.32a). A true erosion should be visible in both longitudinal and transverse views and have the appearance as described earlier. CPD signal within the erosion

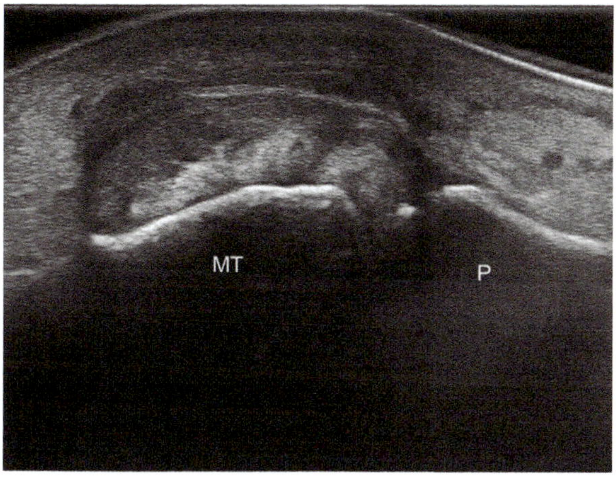

Fig. 8.29 Medial longitudinal of first MTP in gout, showing hypertrophic synovium with "clumps of wet sugar" inclusions

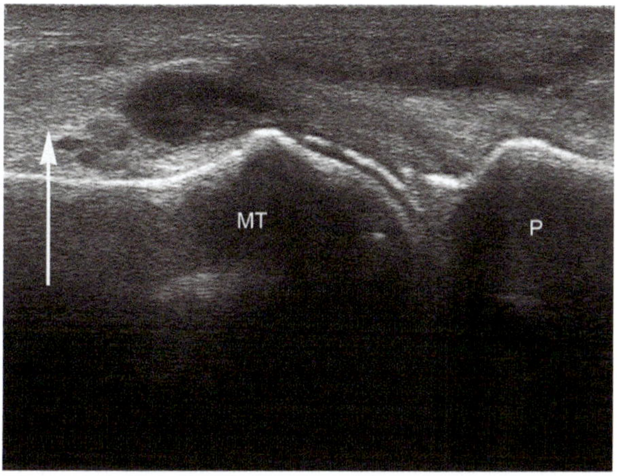

Fig. 8.30 Gout, first MTP, double-contour sign. Note also that the synovium is expanded and hyperechoic (arrow)

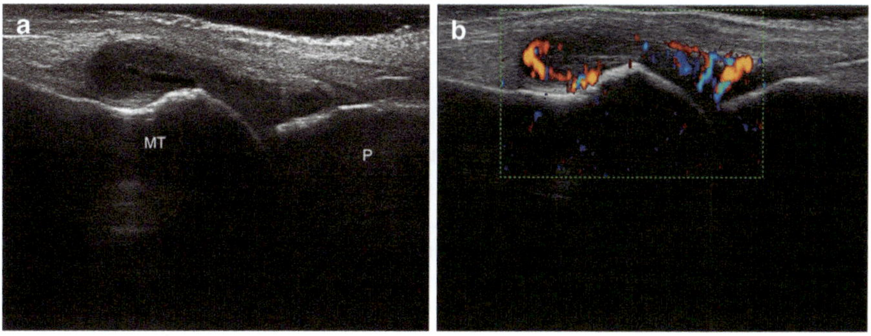

Fig. 8.31 MTP joint rheumatoid arthritis. (**a**) MTP joint rheumatoid arthritis. Note the thickened hypoechoic synovium, without inclusions as seen in gout. (**b**) Increased Doppler signal suggests active inflammation. Note that standoff view allows maximum sensitivity to blood flow

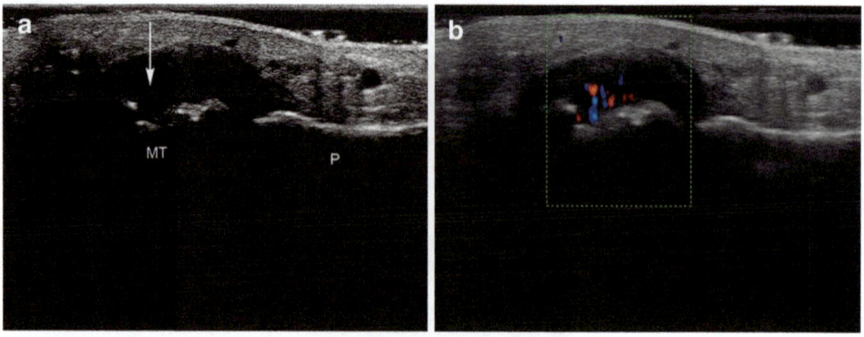

Fig. 8.32 Erosions. (**a**) Lateral view of fifth MTP from a patient with rheumatoid arthritis reveals an erosion. (**b**) Doppler study reveals increased blood flow in the erosion, suggesting active inflammation

suggests active synovitis (Fig. 8.32b). Isolated small erosions <2.5 mm may be seen in 10% of normals and may represent cortical breaks due to nutrient vessels rather than true erosions [27, 28]. Adding to the confusion, nutrient vessel cortical breaks may have increased Doppler signal due to the blood flow in the penetrating vessel. Any erosion in the fifth metatarsal head, however, has a specificity of 85% for RA, with 3.3% of normals having small cortical breaks.

In 8.6% of cases of pigmented villonodular synovitis or giant cell tumor, the toe is a primary site of involvement. The US appearance is that of hypoechoic synovial proliferation, with nodules extending from soft tissue into the joint cavity [29]. There is increased CPD signal. The US appearance of PVNS is nonspecific and requires additional evaluation. The characteristics and differential diagnosis of ganglion cysts in the forefoot (Fig. 8.33) are the same as described earlier in the midfoot.

Morton's neuroma may be imaged in either the plantar or dorsal transverse planes at the level of the metatarsal heads, with ballottement of the web space from the opposite side. Positive findings include a round or oval hypoechoic mass between the metatarsal heads [30]. Mulder's sign, whereby metatarsal compression induces symptoms and forces the neuroma in a plantar direction, can be visualized with US. The "sonographic Mulder's sign" is performed with the transducer initially exerting pressure on the plantar surface in transverse plane over the metatarsal heads. With the other hand, the examiner performs gradually increasing metatarsal compression while easing up on the transducer pressure, looking for the hypoechoic mass to be forced plantarly [31]. When compared with histopathologic confirmation in 29 cases, US was 76% sensitive for Morton's neuroma vs. 86% for MRI [30]. In this same series, the size of the neuroma (range, 3–15 mm) did not correlate with symptoms, although in other series a neuroma less than 5 mm in size was not felt to cause symptoms.

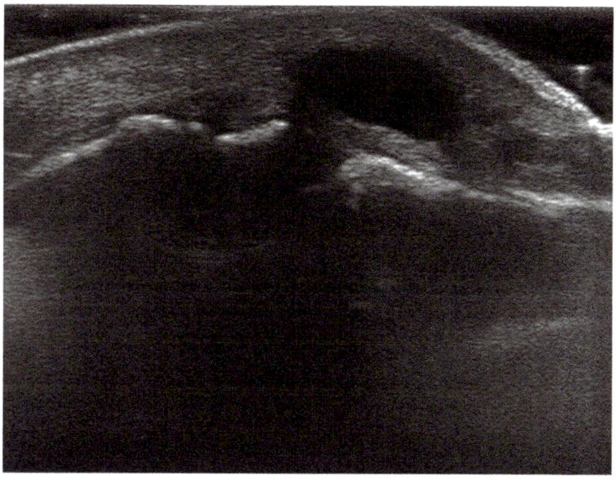

Fig. 8.33 Dorsal longitudinal scan over first IP joint nodule reveals an anechoic ganglion cyst

Conclusion

The ankle and foot are complex, both from the standpoint of normal anatomy and the myriad of rheumatic problems that affect them. MSKUS provides an additional tool to assist the rheumatologist in approaching the differential diagnosis of ankle and foot complaints. MSKUS may be used to further understand the extent of systemic inflammatory diseases as they affect the ankle and foot. Finally, MSKUS can facilitate procedures in the ankle and foot, a topic addressed in Chap. 9 "Ultrasound-Guided Injections".

Review Questions

1. Which of the following ultrasound findings are most specific for rheumatoid arthritis?
   (a) Retrocalcaneal bursitis
   (b) MTP 2 synovial thickening with increased color power Doppler signal
   (c) MTP 1 synovial fluid over 1 mm on dorsal longitudinal view
   (d) Subtalar joint effusion seen on lateral view
   (e) MTP 5 erosion <2.5 mm in diameter
2. The double-contour sign
   (a) When clearly demonstrated, is specific for urate deposition
   (b) Most often represents urate deposition on the cartilage surface
   (c) Is tapered at each end
   (d) Remains stationary when the joint is flexed and extended
   (e) Results from reverberation at the cartilage surface

3. The normal plantar fascia thickness is generally up to
   (a) 1–2 mm
   (b) 3–4 mm
   (c) 5–6 mm
   (d) 7–8 mm
   (e) 9–10 mm
4. Musculoskeletal ultrasound Achilles tendon abnormalities are marked by
   (a) Tenosynovial color power Doppler signal
   (b) Intratendinous inflammation reflected in color power Doppler signal
   (c) Narrowing of tendon diameter
   (d) Erosion at the distal calcaneal insertion
   (e) Loss of fibrillar pattern
5. The following ultrasound finding of the tibialis posterior tendon is abnormal, even if found without other findings:
   (a) 2 mm of synovial fluid at the medial malleolus
   (b) Tenosynovial thickening of 2 mm
   (c) Dense inclusion in distal aspect with acoustic shadowing
   (d) Expansion of the tendon near the navicular insertion
   (e) Enlargement twice the size of the flexor digitorum longus tendon
6. The extensor tendons as seen on the dorsal transverse view of the ankle
   (a) Are less commonly pathologic as compared to the flexors
   (b) Normally have a small amount of tenosynovial fluid in the distal aspect
   (c) Are superficial to the proximal retinaculum and deep to the distal retinaculum
   (d) Are deep to the proximal retinaculum and superficial to the distal retinaculum
   (e) Normally have a paratenon attached to the proximal retinaculum
7. The best way to determine if hypoechoic signal in a joint space is synovial fluid is
   (a) Color power Doppler signal evaluation
   (b) Look for acoustic shadowing
   (c) Measure the bone to capsule distance
   (d) Ballottement with the transducer
   (e) Recheck signal at maximum power
8. At what portion of the Achilles is paratenonitis most conspicuous?
   (a) Anterior
   (b) Posterior
   (c) Lateral
   (d) Distal
   (e) Central
9. The retro-Achilles bursa
   (a) May not be visible by US in normals
   (b) Is most often egg-shaped as visualized by US
   (c) Normally is 2 mm in maximum dimension
   (d) Lies deep to the Achilles at the proximal calcaneus
   (e) May communicate with the subtalar joint in up to 20% of normal

10. You place the probe on the dorsal longitudinal view of a swollen ankle and immediately see a normal-appearing tibiotalar joint. The next most important maneuver to perform would be
    (a) Change probe to the anterior transverse view.
    (b) Turn on color power Doppler signal using a standoff view.
    (c) Ballottement with the probe.
    (d) Look for subcutaneous edema in overlying tissue.
    (e) Move the probe laterally and medially.

Answers

1. (e) MTP 5 erosion <2.5 mm in diameter
2. (b) Most often represents urate deposition on the cartilage surface
3. (b) 3–4 mm
4. (e) Loss of fibrillar pattern
5. (b) Tenosynovial thickening of 2 mm
6. (a) Are less commonly pathologic as compared to the flexors
7. (d) Ballottement with the transducer
8. (b) Posterior
9. (a) May not be visible by US in normals
10. (e) Move the probe laterally and medially.

Disclaimer The view(s) expressed herein are those of the author(s) and do not reflect the official policy or position of Brooke Army Medical Center, the US Army Medical Department, the US Army Office of the Surgeon General, the Department of the Army, the Department of the Air Force, or the Department of Defense or the US Government.

References

1. McAlindon T, Kissin E, Nazarian L, Ranganath V, Prakash S, Taylor M, et al. American College of Rheumatology report on reasonable use of musculoskeletal ultrasonography in rheumatology clinical practice. Arthritis Care Res. 2012;64(11):1625–40.
2. D'Agostino MA. Impact of ultrasound imaging on local corticosteroid injections of symptomatic ankle, hind-, and mid-foot in chronic inflammatory diseases. Arthritis Rheum. 2005;53(2):284–92.
3. Brown AK, Roberts TE, Wakefield RJ, Karim Z, Hensor E, O'Connor PJ, et al. The challenges of integrating ultrasonography into routine rheumatology practice: addressing the needs of clinical rheumatologists. Rheumatology. 2007;46:821–9.
4. Backhaus M, Burmester GR, Gerber T, Grassi W, Machold KP, Swen WA, et al. Guidelines for musculoskeletal ultrasound in rheumatology. Ann Rheum Dis. 2001;60(7):641–9.
5. Bianchi S, Martinoli C, Gaignot C, Gautard RD, Meyer JM. Ultrasound of the ankle: anatomy of the tendons, bursae, and ligaments. Seminars Musc Rad. 2005;9(3):243–59.
6. Schmidt WA, Schmidt H, Schicke B, Gromnica-Ihle E. Standard reference values for musculoskeletal ultrasonography. Ann Rheum Dis. 2004;63(8):988–94.

7. Rawool NM, Nazarian LN. Ultrasound of the ankle and foot. Semin Ultrasound CT MRI. 2000;21(3):275–84.
8. Kotnis N, Harish S, Popowich T. Medial ankle and heel: ultrasound evaluation and sonographic appearances of conditions causing symptoms. Semin Ultrasound CT MRI. 2011;32:125–41.
9. Harris CA, Peduto AJ. Achilles tendon imaging. Australas Radiol. 2006;50:513–25.
10. Wakefield RJ, Balint PV, Szkudlarek M, Filippucci E, Backhaus M, D'Agostino MA, et al. Musculoskeletal ultrasound including definitions for ultrasonographic pathology. J Rheumatol. 2005;32(12):2485–7.
11. Premkumar A, Perry MB, Dwyer AJ, Gerber LH, Johnson D, Venzon D, et al. Sonography and MR imaging of posterior tibial tendinopathy. AJR. 2002;178:223–32.
12. Naredo E, D'Agnostino MA, Wakefield RJ, Moller I, Balint PV, Filippucci E, et al. Reliability of a consensus-based ultrasound score for tenosynovitis in rheumatoid arthritis. Ann Rheum Dis. 2013;72:1328–34.
13. McGonagle D, Wakefield RJ, Tan AL, D'Agostino MA, Toumi H, Hayashi K, et al. Distinct topography of erosion and new bone formation in Achilles tendon enthesitis. Arth Rheum. 2008;58(9):2694–9.
14. Falsetti P, Frediani B, Acciai C, Baldi F, Filippou G, Prada EP, et al. Ultrasonographic study of Achilles tendon and plantar fascia in chondrocalcinosis. J Rheumatol. 2004;31:2242–50.
15. D'Agostino MA, Aegerter P, Bechara K, Salliot C, Olivia J, Chimenti MS, et al. How to diagnose spondyloarthritis early? Accuracy of peripheral enthesitis detection by power Doppler ultrasonography. Ann Rheum Dis. 2011;70:1433–40.
16. Feydy A, Lavie-Brion MC, Gossec L, Lavie F, Guerini H, Nguyen C, et al. Comparative study of MRI and power Doppler ultrasonography of the heel in patients with spondyloarthritis with and without heel pain and in controls. Ann Rheum Dis. 2012;71:498–503.
17. Sabir N, Demirlenk S, Yagci B, Karabulut N, Cubukcu S. Clinical utility of sonography in diagnosing plantar fasciitis. J Ultrasound Med. 2005;24:1041–8.
18. Akfirata M, Senb C, Gunes T. Ultrasonographic appearance of the plantar fasciitis. J Clin Imag. 2003;27:353–7.
19. Tsai WC, Chiu MF, Wang CL, Tang FT, Wong MK. Ultrasound evaluation of plantar fasciitis. Scand J Rheumatol. 2000;29:255.
20. Wakefield RJ, Freeston JE, O'Connor P, Reay N, Budgen A, Hensor EMA, et al. The optimal assessment of the rheumatoid arthritis hindfoot: a comparative study of clinical examination, ultrasound and high field MRI. Ann Rheum Dis. 2008;67(12):1678–82.
21. Ganguly A, et al. Lumps and bumps around the foot and ankle: an assessment of frequency with ultrasound and MRI. Skelet Radiol. 2013;42:1051.
22. Thiele RG, Schlesinger N. Diagnosis of gout by ultrasound. Rheumatology. 2007;46(7):1116–21.
23. Delle Sedie A, Riente L, Iagnocco A, Filippucci E, Meenagh G, Grassi W, et al. Ultrasound imaging for the rheumatologist X. Ultrasound imaging in crystal-related arthropathies. Clin Exp Rheumatol. 2007;25(4):513–7.
24. Thiele RG. Role of ultrasound and other advanced imaging in the diagnosis and management of gout. Curr Rheumatol Rep. 2011;13(2):146–53.
25. Thiele RG, Schlesinger N. Ultrasonography shows disappearance of monosodium urate crystal deposition on hyaline cartilage after sustained normouricemia is achieved. Rheumatol Int. 2010;30(4):495–503.
26. Keen HI, Redmond A, Wakefield RJ, Freeston J, Grainger AJ, Hensor EMA, et al. An ultrasonographic study of metatarsophalangeal joint pain: synovitis, structural pathology and their relationship to symptoms and function. Ann Rheum Dis. 2011;70:2140–3.
27. Szkudlarek M, Narvestad E, Klarlund M, Court-Payen M, Thomsen HS, Østergaard M. Ultrasonography of the metatarsophalangeal joints in rheumatoid arthritis. Arth Rheum. 2004;50(7):2103–12.
28. Zayat AS, Ellegaard K, Conaghan PG, Terslev L, Hensor EM, Freeston JE, Emery P, Wakefield RJ. The specificity of ultrasound-detected bone erosions for rheumatoid arthritis. Ann Rheum Dis. 2014; https://doi.org/10.1136/annrheumdis-2013-204864.

29. Edwards C, Milner S. Pigmented villonodular synovitis of second toe interphalangeal joint: methods of imaging. Foot Ankle Surg. 2010;16:e34–6.
30. Sharp RJ, Wade CM, Hennessy MS, Saxby TS. The role of MRI and ultrasound imaging in Morton's neuroma and the effect of size of lesion on symptoms. J Bone Joint Surg. 2003;85-B:999–1005.
31. Torrian M, Kattapuram S. Dynamic sonography of the forefoot: the sonographic mulder sign. Am J Roentgen. 2003;180:1121–3.
32. Ward IM, Kissin E, Kaeley G, Scott JN, Newkirk M, Hildebrand BA, et al. Ultrasound features of the posterior tibialis tendon and peroneus brevis tendon entheses: comparison study between healthy adults and those with inflammatory arthritis. Arth Care Res. 2017;69(10):1519–25.
33. Terslev L, Naredo E, Iagnocco A, Balint PV, Wakefield RJ, Aegerter P, et al. Defining enthesitis in spondyloarthritis by ultrasound: results of a Delphi process and of a reliability reading exercise. Arthritis Care Res. 2014;66:741–8.

Ultrasound-Guided Injections 9

Wilmer L. Sibbitt Jr.

Key Points

- USG procedures are more accurate than anatomic landmark palpation-guided (ALMPAG) injections.
- USG procedures provide better outcomes than ALMPAG.
- USG procedures are less painful and traumatic than ALMPAG.
- USG procedures include: arthrocentesis, aspiration, biopsy, barbotage, lavage, and biopsy.

Introduction

With the development of relatively inexpensive ultrasound (US) units, US-guided (USG) procedures have become increasingly standard practice in rheumatology, anesthesiology, emergency medicine, pulmonary, critical care, nursing, and many other specialties. Traditionally, rheumatology, orthopedic surgery, physiatry, and sports medicine have performed anatomic landmark palpation-guided (ALMPG) needle procedures, including arthrocentesis, aspiration of cyst and abscess, intra-articular injections, injection of other musculoskeletal structures (tendon sheath, bursa, tendon/ligament insertion/origins, ganglion cyst, nodules, nerve, muscle, fascia), and biopsy of fat, muscle, parotid gland, or synovial membrane. These structures are generally superficial and characterized by palpable anatomic landmarks and are usually injected without imaging with good to excellent diagnostic and therapeutic effect. The musculoskeletal (MSK) proceduralist, even without US

W. L. Sibbitt Jr. (✉)
Division of Rheumatology, Department of Internal Medicine, University of New Mexico Health Sciences Center, University of New Mexico, Albuquerque, NM, USA
e-mail: WSibbitt@salud.unm.edu

M. J. Kohler (ed.), *Musculoskeletal Ultrasound in Rheumatology Review*,
https://doi.org/10.1007/978-3-030-73555-5_9

training, is often already adept at many ALMPG diagnostic and therapeutic procedures; thus, it is assumed before performing USG procedures, the practitioner will already be skilled with ALMPG methodology and art including differential diagnosis, indications, sterile technique, wound care, medications, equipment, anatomy, and anatomic approaches.

USG procedures have an number of advantages in that US reveals relevant deep anatomy including subtle pockets of fluid; permits acquisition of fluid diagnosis; facilitates more accurate needle placement; reduces procedural pain; improves arthrocentesis success; facilitates such procedures as USG barbotage, lavage, and biopsy; improves therapeutic outcomes, promotes procedural safety; and may improve cost-effectiveness. There are a number of excellent reviews of USG of the MSK system that provide insight into the flexibility, individual practice patterns, and potential equivalent approaches to USG procedures [1–23]. However, to use USG in an integrative way rather than the customary ALMPG, there must be an evidence base that scientifically supports the preferred use of USG.

Evidence-Based Support for US-Guided Musculoskeletal Procedures

A number of recent publications have reviewed the medical literature regarding the accuracy and effectiveness of USG versus ALMPG procedures with USG procedures predictably being more accurate and often providing better clinical outcomes and cost-effectiveness with some limitations as discussed later [15, 24].

Arthrocentesis

Kane et al., Delaunoy et al., and Ike et al. have demonstrated that US can detect small effusions and assists with successful arthrocentesis [25–27]. In a study of USG versus ALMPG, Balint et al. reported that US-guidance improved successful joint aspiration from 32% to 97% [28]. Raza et al. demonstrated that USG in 69 small joints (interphalangeal joints and metacarpophalangeal joints) improved arthrocentesis success (diagnostic samples) from 0% to 63% [29]. Wiler et al. reported that USG arthrocentesis of the knee with a palpable effusion was significantly less painful and increased fluid yield by 31% [30]. Sibbitt et al. demonstrated that in 64 knees with palpable effusions, USG for arthrocentesis of the knee resulted in statistically significant improvements in arthrocentesis including 48% less procedural pain, 183% increased aspirated synovial fluid volumes, 22% improvement in diagnostic samples, and 46% improvement in outcomes (reduced pain scores at 2 weeks) [31]. Wu et al. reviewed the data from 725 knee aspirations and concluded that USG arthrocentesis of the knee offered significantly better accuracy and clinical improvement of ALMPG knee arthrocentesis [32]. Although existing data indicate that USG arthrocentesis is clearly less painful, provides superior diagnostic samples, and provides better outcomes, there are limited cost-effectiveness data to date strictly comparing ALMPG versus USG arthrocentesis to recommend USG arthrocentesis in all joints where arthrocentesis is indicated. However, the above data do support the recommendation that USG diagnostic arthrocentesis is indicated in (1) small joints where effusion or infection is suspected, (2) in painful joints without palpable effusions where effusion or infection is suspected, (3) in deep joints where effusion is more difficult to palpate (e.g., the hip, sacroiliac joint, popliteal cyst, and flexor tendons of hand or foot), and (4) in joints with suspected effusion or infection where palpation-guided aspiration is difficult (e.g., obesity), dangerous (e.g., overlying cellulitis or proximity to an artery), or has failed to provide a necessary diagnostic sample with ALMPG aspiration [18, 20, 33].

Accuracy of US-Guided Needle Placement in Musculoskeletal Structures

Cunnington et al. demonstrated in 184 mixed joints with inflammatory arthritis that USG improved joint injection accuracy from 66% to 83% [34]. USG has been demonstrated to improve the accuracy of knee injections [35, 36]. Berkoff et al. in a review of the five studies reported that UGI improved the accuracy of intra-articular injections of the knee relative to ALMPG (95.8% vs. 77.8%, $P < 0.001$) [35]. Injections of the anserine bursa are markedly more accurate with USG (92% vs. 17%) [37]. An extensive literature review by Bloom et al. demonstrated improved accuracy of USG injections [38]. Patel et al. demonstrated that USG significantly improved posterior glenohumeral injection accuracy from 72.5% to 92.5% [39]. Amber et al. in a meta-analysis including 406 injections that USG was 93% accurate while fluoroscopy was 80% accurate [40]. Berkoff et al. reported that USG improved the accuracy in the shoulder (97.3% versus 65.4%, $P < 0.001$) [35]. USG of the acromioclavicular joint improves accuracy from 70–75% to 90–97% [41, 42]. Gazzillo et al. have found US-guidance improves injection of the bicipital tendon from 5.2% with ALMPG to 100% with USG [43]. Hashiuchi et al. demonstrated that USG of the bicipital tendon sheath improved intra-sheath injection accuracy from 26.7% to 86.7% [44]. Petscavage-Thomas et al. demonstrated that in bicipital tendon sheath injections, US-guidance was more accurate than fluoroscopic guidance [45]. Nam et al. reported that USG injections of the distal radioulnar joint were significantly more accurate than ALMPG [46]. USG wrist injections are more accurate than ALMPG [47, 48]. US-guidance of the scaphotrapeziotrapezoid joint improves accuracy from 80% to 100% [49] and of the first carpometacarpal joint from 91% to 100% [50, 51]. USG injection of stenosing tenosynovitis is more accurate than ALMPG injections [52]. US-guidance improves the accuracy of intra-sheath injections from 15% to 75% [53]. USG relative to ALMPG injections improves injection accuracy of the metacarpophalangeal joints from 80% to 100% and interphalangeal joints from 50% to 96%, [29]. Wisniewski et al. have demonstrated that US-guidance improves tibiotalar injections from 85% to 100% [54], while Khosla et al. reported that ALPG and USG were similar in accuracy [55]. Wisniewski et al. have demonstrated that USG improves subtalar joint and sinus tarsus from 35% to 90% [54]. US-guidance improves accuracy of the tarso-metatarsal joint injections from 25% to 64% [55]. Muir et al. have demonstrated that USG injections improve peroneal tendon sheath injection accuracy from 60% to 100% [56]. USG injections improve accuracy of the metacarpophalangeal joint to 100% [57] and tarsometatarsal joint injections from 25% to 64% [55]. Thus, there is a consistent finding that USG injections permit more accurate injections regardless of anatomic site over ALMPG injections.

Outcome and Cost-Effectiveness of US-Guided Procedures

Gilliland et al. demonstrated in a meta-analysis of 17 articles that USG injections were more significantly effective in 2- to 6-week outcomes compared to ALMPG especially in the shoulder and knee [58]. Sage et al. and Soh et al. reported reviews of demonstrating significant clinical improvement with USG vs. ALMPG injections [59, 60]. However, an extensive literature review by Bloom et al. demonstrated improved accuracy of USG injections, but no significant improvement in outcome [38]. Similarly, a randomized controlled trial by Dogu et al. demonstrated no difference in outcomes between USG and ALMPG injections [61].

Lee et al. demonstrated that USG injections were superior to ALMPG injections in the shoulder for adhesive capsulitis at 2 weeks [62]. Similarly, Ucuncu et al. demonstrated that USG injections were superior to ALMPG injections in the painful shoulder [63]. Hsieh et al. reported in a 145 patient study that USG injections of the subacromial bursa were more effective than ALMPG procedures [64]. Naredo et al. reported in 41 patients that USG of the subacromial bursa were more effective than ALPGI injections [65]. Ramirez reported that US-guided subacromial injection of partial thickness tears of the rotator cuff with 40 mg triamcinolone was highly effective at relieving pain and improving motion, but 17% of patients progressed to full-thickness tears [66]. A randomized controlled trial of Dogu et al. demonstrated no difference between USG and ALMPG subacromial injections [61]. Ekeberg found no difference between USG subacromial and systemic injections of corticosteroid for rotator cuff disease [67]. USG injections of the acromioclavicular (AC) joint improve outcomes [68]. Borbas et al. in a cadaver study demonstrated that US-guidance improves the accuracy of AC joint injections from 70% to 90% [41].

USG wrist injections produce better outcomes [47, 48]. In randomized control trials, Chen et al. and Tsai et al. concluded that USG injections of the plantar fascia were more effective than ALPMG injections [69, 70], confirmed in a meta-analysis by [71]. On the other hand, Ball et al. and Yucel et al. found no difference between USG injection and ALPMG injection [72, 73]. Other randomized controlled trials have reported that USG injections were superior to ALMPG injections in consecutive joints with inflammatory arthritis knees with effusions non-effusive osteoarthritic knees and carpal tunnel syndrome [31, 74–78]. However, Michell recently reported that USG did not improve outcomes of the trochanteric bursa [79]. Similarly, Moore demonstrated that USG did not improve the outcome of glenohumeral joint injections [80].

USG injections could theoretically improve cost-effectiveness due to better outcomes and less utilization of other medical resources, but cost-effectiveness, as these studies point out, are highly dependent on the costs of USG that can vary based on customary practice, insurance, reimbursement, institution, US acquisition and maintenance costs, operator training expense, operator skill, and sporadic complications. In this line, a few studies have reported improved cost-effectiveness of USG procedures relative to ALMPG injections in inflammatory arthritis, knee pain, osteoarthritis, and carpal tunnel syndrome [31, 74–78]. However, Mitchel et al. and Moore et al. have demonstrated that USG injections increase the costs of glenohumeral and trochanteric bursa without improving outcomes [79, 80].

In summary, the medical literature indicates that USG procedures generally are more accurate and may have better outcomes in certain anatomic areas compared to ALMPG procedures, but these differences in outcomes are dependent on the individual joint and US operator experience. Furthermore, based on improved outcomes, USG injections may be in certain anatomic areas more cost-effective than ALMPG injections, but improved cost-effectiveness is highly dependent on the total cost of USG, indicating that the lower the cost of US-guidance, the more cost-effective USG procedures become.

Diagnosis, Diagnostic Ultrasound, and US-Guided Procedures

Diagnostic US, as discussed in the other chapters, permits much more accurate and timely anatomic diagnosis that along with characteristic patient complaints, physical examination findings, and other clinical information can justify a subsequent USG procedure. Thus, prior to any USG procedure, a preliminary diagnostic US of the planned target area should be performed to confirm the diagnosis that justifies an USG procedure, to exclude other clinical conditions where such a needle procedure might be contraindicated, inappropriate, or dangerous (such as injection into an artery, vein, infection, tendon rupture, abscess, aneurysm, fracture, cartilage tear, tumor, foreign body, etc.) and to help determine needle choice, entry point, and tracking technique. For example, prior to performing an USG injection of the knee for knee pain, diagnostic US should be performed first to determine if effusion is present, if findings of chondrocalcinosis or gout are present in cartilage, whether ligamentous or tendinous tears, fracture, or hematoma is present, all of which may modify the approach, direction, or medications of the procedure or may prohibit the procedure entirely. Preliminary diagnostic US for planned USG injections procedures are typically included as part of USG procedure billing in the United States. However, if additional incidental findings are uncovered that are separate from indications for injection procedure, an additional diagnostic US exam study may need to be considered with appropriate documentation of findings in a complete study.

Patient Positioning

The patient should be positioned in a comfortable sitting, supine, prone, or recumbent position, but never standing. If the patient has a known history of procedural syncope, needle phobia, anxiety, or evidence of autonomic instability (sweating, paleness, hyperventilation, tachycardia), the patient should be placed in a recumbent position. If the patient has a companion or family member, that person should be queried for these same factors and, if present, should leave the room as to not have syncope and head trauma while the procedure is ongoing. Once the patient is positioned, the target area is prepared for palpation and anatomic marking.

Palpation and Identification of Local Anatomy

In most anatomic sites for USG injections, it is wise to first palpate important superficial anatomic landmarks and mark these with a surgical pen so that US images can be rapidly correlated with visible surface anatomy or area of pain without having to re-palpate the anatomy during the procedure, which might violate the sterile surface. After US gel is applied to the region, it is often difficult or impossible to mark anatomic sites with ink or surgical marker, so ideally surface markings should be completed before application of US gel. With more experience, marking with a surgical marker may not be necessary; however determining the appropriate depth and entry location of needle and its relationship to surrounding structures is still essential. Once the patient is positioned and marked, the patient should not change body positioning because with body movement in a different orientation, the surface anatomic markings no longer correspond to underlying anatomy resulting in confusion, incorrect identification, or inappropriate targeting.

Sterile Technique and Universal Precautions

All needle procedures should be performed with sterile technique. Two standard approaches are typically used: (1) conventional surgical sterility (scrubbing, gowning, hair cover, mask, gloving, draping, and local antisepsis) and local puncture site sterility also known as "no touch technique" (gloving, local antisepsis, maintenance of needle sterility, maintenance of puncture site sterility, avoidance of touch contamination). For USG injections and aspiration, both surgical sterility and local sterility have similar infection rates; thus most proceduralists utilize local puncture site sterility techniques rather than surgical sterility [81]. For the patient protection, all procedures should be performed with the operator wearing surgical gloves for both the procedural hand and the probe hand. Single-use probe cover and sterile gel have recently been included in American Institute of Ultrasound in Medicine (AIUM) transducer preparation and cleaning guidelines for any interventional percutaneous/needle procedure [82].

Antisepsis

The puncture site and surrounding tissue are prepared with povidone iodine or chlorhexidine antisepsis. Povidone iodine has the advantage of less effect on previously applied ink markings; chlorhexidine is alcohol-based and may remove the ink markings. However, some patients are allergic to povidone iodine, and such allergies should be screened prior to the procedure. To prevent the anatomic ink markings being removed with chlorhexidine, the site is blotted or dabbed with chlorhexidine rather than the conventional swirling or spiral technique, and then the excess is blotted off with a swab. Povidone iodine should be dry on the skin for full antisepsis; this is not necessary for chlorhexidine. A number of studies have suggested that chlorhexidine is more effective than povidone iodine but the use of either is acceptable [83, 84].

Ultrasound Gel

US gel is not reliably sterile especially when transversed by the probe and manipulated on the skin; thus, US gel should be kept physically away from the puncture site. If using standard US gel, it is often wise to select a longer needle and plan the puncture site further away from the planned placement of the probe so that the gel does not contaminate the puncture site. Recent AIUM guidelines recommend use of sterile gel for any percutaneous/needle procedure. Certain proceduralists use povidone iodine topical gel or chlorhexidine gel as a replacement for US gel and, thus, can more safely have antiseptic gel interact with the puncture site although there are no published outcomes studies regarding this.

Ultrasound Probe

The US probe (transducer) can be a source of infection and should be cleaned before and after each procedure; however, an US probe is considered an intermediate or low-risk of infection. After every patient exam, wipe the US gel off of the transducer, and disconnect the transducer from the system, and remove any transducer covers, biopsy guides, or tip guards. Use a soft cloth lightly dampened in a mild soap or an enzymatic cleaner (in accordance with the manufacturer's instructions) to remove any particulate matter or body fluids that remain on the transducer or cable. To remove remaining particulate and cleaning residue, rinse thoroughly with water then wipe with a dry cloth. It is wise to utilize the manufacturer's recommended cleaner for each probe. Due to changes implemented because of COVID-19, single-use probe cover and sterile gel have recently been included in American Institute of Ultrasound in Medicine (AIUM) transducer preparation and cleaning guidelines for any interventional percutaneous/needle procedure [85].

Universal Precautions

The US proceduralist should wash the hands and use bactericidal gel before the procedure and wear appropriately sized gloves throughout the procedure. Oversized gloves with redundant folds will decrease operator control: the folds will catch on instruments, and the likelihood of procedural error or operator needle stick will increase. Anti-needle stick shielded needles can be used whenever possible, but these are generally limited to 1.5 inch in length: 2 inch and longer needles are generally conventional and non-shielded [75–78]. The procedure should be planned so that whenever there is a needle extraction from the target site, the needle is either inactivated or placed where it cannot stick the operator or assistant and then disposed in an appropriate sharps container. The probe is first placed in a stable position where it cannot fall and be damaged, usually in the probe holder on the US unit. To prevent blood contamination onto the operator and a hematoma formation in the patient, as the needle is extracted, a gauze in the opposite hand simultaneously puts pressure on the puncture site as the needle is extracted so that there is no exposed blood in the procedural area. A wise proceduralist will never extract the needle or compress the wound with a gloved finger without a gauze nor extract the needle and walk away from a non-compressed wound letting the puncture site bleed into the operative area. All contaminated supplies should be disposed of properly, and the probe should be cleaned following the manufacturer's recommendations.

Prevention of Injection Site Hematoma and Hemorrhage

Since USG interventions are traumatic procedures, patients at high risk for hemorrhage (hemorrhagic diathesis, thrombocytopenia, or therapy with warfarin, clopidogrel, aspirin, and other anticoagulants) should be identified before the procedure to prevent painful and disabling hematoma, hemarthrosis, or hemorrhagic bursitis. Using a smaller needle diameter (larger gauge) and a needle technique that does not have excessive errant motion of the cutting needle tip is important, especially if the patient has a bleeding diathesis. Extremely high-risk elective procedures for hemorrhage such as barbotage, extensive hydrodissection, needle biopsy, and high-pressure injections into dense connective tissue should be delayed until the hemorrhagic condition has been corrected. For patients on warfarin or antiplatelet drugs who must have an injection procedure, typically a narrower 25 or 27 gauge needle is used. As above, after extraction of the needle, immediate compression of the puncture site is necessary to prevent bruising and hematoma. If the patient has hemorrhagic tendency, pressure should be applied for at least 5 minutes. As noted above, there is no bleeding until the needle is removed. Thus, with deep procedures, the needle is stably held by joint surfaces, connective tissue, and the tissue tract, and the patient should be instructed not to move until adequate pressure with gauze has been applied.

Prevention of Iatrogenic Corticosteroid Atrophy of Skin and Subcutaneous Fat

Corticosteroid atrophy of skin and connective tissue occurs from corticosteroid esters in the form of crystals not being injected into a constraining structure such as a synovial space (an erroneous subcutaneous or periarticular injection), from reflux of corticosteroid back the needle shaft toward the skin (if corticosteroid is injected in a constrained space, there is high pressure at the needle tip, so the corticosteroid refluxes up the side of needle shaft back into superficial tissues), from reflux up the wound tract after a high-pressure injection (typically from small joints or cysts) after the needle is removed, from using a mixture of local anesthetic and corticosteroid as local anesthesia, from test injections of corticosteroid before needle localization has been optimized, and by the use of high potency corticosteroids (usually triamcinolone) in injections that have a subcutaneous interface (epicondyle, trochanteric, and insertional injections [86–89]. Proper placement of the needle tip is critical to prevent corticosteroid atrophy; thus, US-guidance itself is a technique to reduce corticosteroid atrophy of skin [90]. Corticosteroid should not be injected until it is certain the needle is residing the target structure and intra-target flow with a neutral injectant or corticosteroid is proven without reflux or periarticular injection. A local anesthetic and corticosteroid mixture should never be used for local anesthesia in tissues superficial to the target since the corticosteroid will atrophy surrounding connective tissue. High-pressure injections should also be avoided to prevent reflux of corticosteroid up the needle tract; therefore, judicious low-pressure injectability must be maintained [88, 91]. Also, after needle extraction, pressure on the puncture wound must be immediate and prolonged to prevent reflux of corticosteroid up the tissue tract created by the needle. Finally, corticosteroids with less atrophy potential (such as methylprednisolone acetate) should be used instead of potent fluorinated corticosteroids (such as triamcinolone) for injections not constrained by membranes or a joint capsule or injections with a subcutaneous interface, such as epicondylar, trochanteric, and insertional injections. If corticosteroid atrophy is present and is causing a cosmetic or physical problem, the dermis and subcutaneous tissue can be infiltrated with normal saline, a technique that seems to disperse the crystals and permit connective tissue regeneration [89].

Needle and Syringe Selection

A needle of appropriate and sufficient length should be used with each procedure, and usually longer needles are used with an USG procedure than a corresponding ALMPG procedure to permit greater flexibility in targeting and the ability to keep the puncture site away from the US gel and probe. The length of needle required is usually typical for each procedure but if uncertain can be estimated using the depth measure or metrics of the US system. Typically 1 to 3.5 inch needles are used with most MSK USG procedures depending on obesity and approach. For needles between 5/8 inch and 1.5 inch anti-needle stick safety guarded versions should be used; these provide improved anti-needle stick operator safety as required by occupational health mandates. These needle versions may also have a larger hub to permit better gripping and more facile syringe exchanges when using one needle two syringe procedures [75–78]. Larger-diameter needles (21, 20, 19, 18 G) are rigid and thus more controllable without partial extraction in terms of alterations in direction during a procedure. Larger-diameter needles are also more US-visible than smaller-diameter needles. On the other hand, larger-diameter needles are more painful for the patient, cause more tissue trauma, are more likely to damage nerves and arteries, and are associated with increased hemorrhage and hematoma formation. Smaller-diameter needles are less painful and safer but are more difficult to visualize with US and cannot be directly moved tissues because they are flexible and bend, with potential need to partially extract and reintroduce the needle to correct targeting. Because of these characteristics, larger-diameter needles are typically used by novices who have difficulty seeing and controlling the needle with US, and smaller-diameter needles are used by experienced proceduralists. Special US-visible needles can improve needle visualization but are very expensive and because of cost are rarely used in MSK USG procedures. Specialized probes and manufacturer specific US software have recently improved needle visualization without a change in needle technology and are generally standard on modern US units. For deeper targets, spinal needles are often used. However, spinal needles are also expensive (4 to 14 US$ per needle), and with the stylet removed, the needle can become coring (that is cut a core of tissue like a biopsy needle) and become too flexible. Longer conventional needles (2, 2.75, 3.93 inch) with smaller diameters (25 G, 22 G) with non-coring tips can be obtained (HSW FINE-JECT, Germany, STERiJECT, Japan, and others) from medical supply houses, and these needles are more stable and far less expensive than spinal needles (typically 0.18–0.30 US$ per needle).

Syringe selection should be based on the amount of aspirate or injectate necessary for the procedure (typically lidocaine or saline initially), hand-control characteristics, and the injection pressure required. Typically for anesthesia and hydrodissection, 1 to 5 ml of lidocaine or saline is required; thus, for most procedures a 3 to 5 ml syringe is optimal as a needle introducer syringe. 3 ml to 5 ml syringes are also the easiest syringes to control in terms of hand dynamics during injection and aspiration and have been shown to have the best needle control characteristics and thus safety of procedure syringes [92]. 1 ml, 10 ml, 20 ml, and 60 ml syringes are physically longer than 3 and 5 ml syringes and are consequently much more difficult control [92]. High-pressure injections (used to fracture rheumatoid nodules, dilate stenosed tendon sheaths, and hydrodissect strictures and Dupuytren's nodules) are best accomplished with a 3 or 5 ml syringe because of effective thumb force-pressure generation, but high-pressure injections are almost impossible to accomplish with a 10, 20, or 60 ml syringe due to hand force – syringe area physics that generate only low pressures [91]. A 1 ml syringe can generate over 400 psi, which can hydrodissect cartilage surfaces, ligaments, and bone and must be used with caution [91]. Thus, 3 ml and 5 ml syringes are optimal for needle introduction and ease of control.

De-Bubbling the Syringe

It is important to expel all bubbles from syringes before the procedure, because injected air and bubbles will dramatically interfere with US imaging by creating US signal voids and multiple reflective surfaces that distort the image or block signal to and from deeper structures.

Relationship of the Needle to the US Beam and Probe

In-Plane Approach

The procedure needle is best observed by US when it is in-plane with the probe and at right angles (90 degrees) to the ultrasound beam (Fig. 9.1). In this orientation, the long axis of the needle can be observed (Fig. 9.2). Thus, to achieve this near 90-degree relation, the needle entry point can be quite anatomically distant from the US probe, depending on the regional anatomy. If the needle remains in-plane with the probe, but begins to move from 90 degrees to US beam to parallel to the US beam (that is the needle is angled deeper relative to the probe) (Fig. 9.3), the reflected signal becomes less until the needle becomes invisible when the needle is parallel with the US beam (Fig. 9.4). Thus, for best observable reflected US signal from the needle, the closer the shaft of the needle is to 90 degrees to the beam, the better the signal.

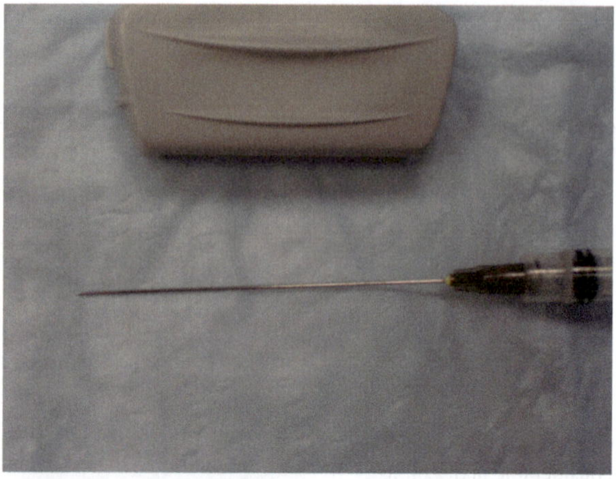

Fig. 9.1 In-plane needle. The procedure needle is best observed by US when it is in-plane with the probe and at right angles (90 degrees) to the ultrasound beam

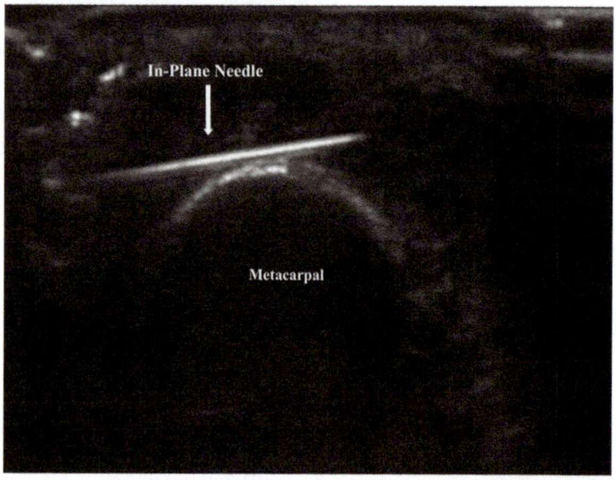

Fig. 9.2 In-plane image. US image with the needle in-plane with the probe and at right angles (90 degrees) to the ultrasound beam

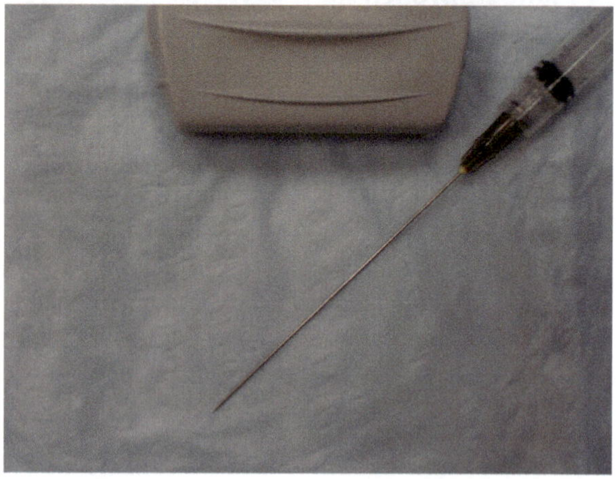

Fig. 9.3 Needle in-plane to probe but 45% to US beam. The needle remains in-plane with the probe but begins to move from 90 degrees to US beam to parallel to the US beam (that is the needle is angled deeper relative to the probe), the reflected signal becomes less until the needle becomes invisible when the needle is parallel with the ultrasound beam

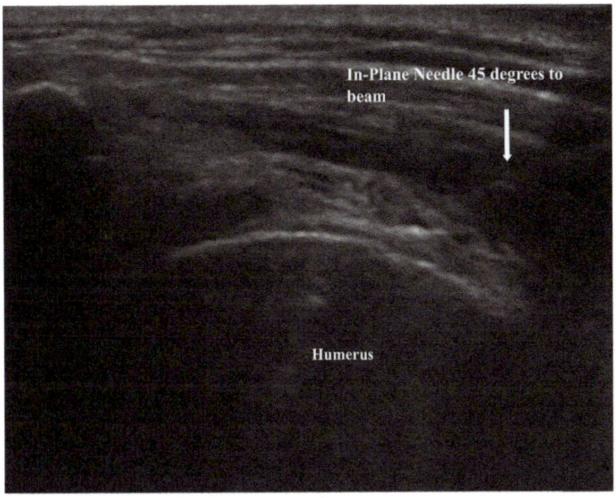

Fig. 9.4 Needle in-plane to probe but 45% to US beam. US image with the needle in-plane with the probe but 45 degrees to the US beam. The reflected signal becomes less

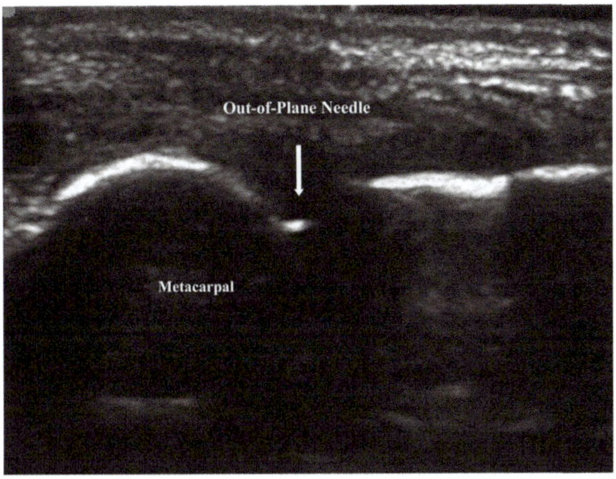

Fig. 9.5 Out-of-plane image. If the needle is out-of-plane relative to the probe but still transverses the beam, there is a cross-sectional view of the needle, usually bright echo-reflectant circle, oval, or semicircle

Out-of-Plane Approach

If the needle is out-of-plane relative to the probe but still in the beam, there is a cross-sectional view of the needle, usually bright echo-reflectant circle, oval, or semicircle (Fig. 9.5). During a procedure, the operator will often rotate the probe 90 degrees so that the needle is in-plane and then out-plane so that the proper approach can be maintained by observing anatomy in two planes, and the operator may switch between these two positions or planes to more fully understand and monitor the relationship of the needle to target and local anatomy.

Needle Visualization

The needle tip is best seen with the bevel up, because the bevel surface is echo-reflectant. If the needle cannot be observed, it may be out-of-plane of the probe and not contacting the beam, and the probe can be rotated on the skin surface until the needle is in-plane and contacting the beam. The needle may also be spatially out of the plane of the beam; in this case, the probe can be moved on the skin surface or angled until the needle is back in-plane close to 90 degrees with the beam. The probe can also be visually lined up with the needle on the skin and then the probe angled obliquely until the needle comes into view. If the needle is not at 90 degrees to the beam and the needle cannot be seen, then the one edge of the probe can be tilted into the soft tissues so that the needle and beam are closer to 90 degrees again, and the needle becomes visible. The needle can also be observed indirectly by motion of surrounding soft tissues and the tip observed by injecting small amounts of test fluid, usually anesthetic, but avoid injecting bubbles from the syringe (the syringe should be de-bubbled) that will make visualization more difficult. Needle visualization hardware and software in the US unit and US probe are well worth the investment as well.

If the needle is fully extended into the tissues but directed to the wrong target, the needle is pulled back through the tissues and redirected. This is very important to pull the needle back, particularly with a flexible needle, because it will track back along the same pathway if not pulled back about 80%, but not out of the skin. If the needle is partially extended and misdirected in soft tissues, a stiff needle (19 to 21 G) can be gently forced in the correct direction and the surrounding soft tissues will usually accommodate this correction. However, with a flexible needle (22 to 27 G) or a very long needle, with force the needle tends go in the opposite direction and then must be paradoxically directed in the opposite direction to curve it to the correct targeting or pulled back about 80% and redirected in a straight path.

Injection into potential spaces, synovial spaces, and insertions should be low-pressure; high-pressure injections can hydrodissect and disrupt tissues and can cause complications including cartilage damage, tendon rupture, and hemorrhage [91]. If the needle is correctly positioned by US-guidance but it is difficult to inject, rotate the needle to various positions on its axis without retracting, and often this will free the bevel from obstruction, and injection will become easy and low-pressure. If this is ineffective, advance or retract the needle, and attempt injection or aspiration assuring that US-observable fluid flow remains in the target. If the needle is obstructed with clogs of corticosteroid or debris during the procedure, the plunger can be pulled back to maximum vacuum, followed by injection, and this will usually unclog the needle.

Hydrodissection, Hydrodilation, Hydrodisplacement, Hydrolysis, and Hydrodisruption

USG syringe procedures have become increasingly more complex and include not only fluid aspiration and anatomically directed injection of medication but also newer procedures of syringe hydrodissection, hydrodilation, hydrodisplacement, hydrolysis, and hydrodisruption [75–96]. For hydrodissection and hydrolysis, the operator uses the syringe to inject lidocaine or saline to dissect anatomic planes and free trapped structures under US-guidance. In the case of hydrodilation, the target structure is dilated to improve intra-articular positioning and create a space for corticosteroid or hyaluronic acid, and after dilation, a syringe exchange is performed, and the selected medication is injected. In hydrodisplacement, fluid is injected to move, displace, or collapse structures that are in the needle path to the target such as veins, arteries, and ducts that the operator does not want to injure with the needle tip, so they are hydrodisplaced (pushed away) by injecting fluid, so the needle can advance. Hydrolysis and hydrodisruption are often used in barbotage and in injection and disruption of dense connective tissue lesions such as fibrosis, rheumatoid nodule, and Dupuytren's contracture [91, 97].

Common Musculoskeletal Ultrasound-Guided Interventions

Many different USG procedures can be performed. Due to the scope of this book, we focus on the following common injections that may be performed by a rheumatologist or other musculoskeletal procedurist (Table 9.1).

Knee Procedures

Needle procedures of the knee are the most common procedure in MSK medicine and, thus, are of great importance. Typical knee structures that are undergo USG interventions are the suprapatellar recess, prepatellar bursa, pes anserine bursa, and popliteal cyst. Tendon-related procedures can also be done including the quadricep and iliotibial band tendons. Injection therapy of the knee has recently been reviewed [98, 99].

In a systematic review, US-guidance has been demonstrated to improve the accuracy of knee injections [35, 36]. Berkoff et al. in a review of five studies reported that UGI improved the accuracy of intra-articular injections compared to ALMPG (95.8% versus 77.8%, $P < 0.001$) [35]. Sibbitt et al. demonstrated that US-guidance improved both arthrocentesis and outcomes of knee injections [31]. USG injection

Table 9.1 Individual procedures

Procedures	Probe positioning	Patient positioning	Access point	Target
Knee arthrocentesis	Anterior thigh proximal to patella	Supine	Lateral suprapatellar or lateral recess	Suprapatellar bursa or lateral recess
Knee injection – lateral suprapatellar	Anterior thigh proximal to patella	Supine	Lateral suprapatellar	Suprapatellar bursa
Anserine bursa	Inferomedial knee	Sitting	Inferomedial knee	Anserine bursa
Iliotibial band	Lateral proximal tibia	Lateral recumbent position	Superomedial knee	Iliotibial band insertion and lateral proximal tibial tubercle
Popliteal cyst	Medial popliteal fossa and posterior calf	Prone position	Distal to popliteal fossa	Popliteal cyst, avoid artery, vein, nerve
Glenohumeral joint, posterior approach	Inferior to the acromion and scapula	Sitting or lateral recumbent	Lateral or medial to probe	Humeral cartilage below infraspinatus
Glenohumeral joint, anterior approach	Superior and lateral to coracoid	Sitting	Lateral to coracoid and medial to humerus	Glenohumeral joint
Subacromial-subdeltoid bursa, lateral approach	Lateral deltoid below acromion	Sitting but can be supine or recumbent	Inferior or superior to probe	Subacromial-subdeltoid bursa
Acromioclavicular (AC) joint, lateral approach	Superior, on AC joint	Sitting but can be supine	Inferior to probe, anterior penetration	AC joint
Bicipital tendon sheath	Transverse or long axis	Sitting, arm externally rotated	Lateral to probe in transverse view or in axis with tendon, inferior to probe	Bicipital tendon sheath
Elbow, posterior	Transverse first, then long axis	Sitting, elbow flexed	Lateral to triceps tendon	Humeral-olecranon joint
Elbow, lateral	Transverse first to olecranon, then to humerus	Sitting, elbow flexed	Superior to olecranon	Humeral-olecranon joint
Epicondyle, medial, and lateral	In long axis of tendons over insertion	Sitting, elbow flexed for lateral, extended for medial	In axis of flexor tendons toward epicondyle	Tendinous insertions on epicondyle

Table 9.1 (continued)

Procedures	Probe positioning	Patient positioning	Access point	Target
Wrist	In long axis initially over radial tubercle	Sitting, elbow flexed palmar hand on table	Transverse axis ulnar to radius or long axis toward radius	Radiocarpal interface
Carpal tunnel	Transverse or long axis	Sitting, forearm supinated palmar hand exposed	Transverse at the level of the Pisiform-ulnar or radial approach. Longitudinal: second volar wrist crease on ulnar side of palmaris longus tendon	Carpal tunnel below the retinaculum around median nerve, avoiding contents
Small joints of the hands, fingers, feet, toes	Transverse or long axis	Sitting	Needle introduced transversely or in long axis	Joint or synovial recess
Tendon sheaths	Transverse first then long axis	As appropriate	Needle introduced in long axis	Tendon sheath, not tendon
Hip	Transverse first then long axis at femoral neck	Supine	Needle introduced laterally to medially	Proximal femoral neck
Trochanteric bursa	Over greater trochanter in long axis	Recumbent with symptomatic side up	Needle introduced distally to proximally	Trochanteric bursa and surrounding insertions
Ankle	Long axis for localization, can also visualize in transverse	Supine	Needle introduced medially, laterally, inferiorly, or superiorly	Tibiotalar joint
Tarsal tunnel	Transverse or long axis by medial malleolus	Sitting, supine, or recumbent, hip externally rotated and knee bent	Needle introduced superiorly to inferiorly	Tarsal tunnel
Plantar fascia	Long axis of foot or transverse	Supine	Needle introduced distally to proximally	Anterior calcaneus and fascial insertion

of the dry osteoarthritic knee was found to provide better outcomes and improve cost-effectiveness compared to ALMPG injections [75–78]. Gilliland et al. demonstrated in a meta-analysis of 17 articles that USG injections were more significantly effective in 2- to 6-week outcomes in the knee [58]. Recent reviews regarding the accuracy and effectiveness of USG versus ALMPG knee procedures with USG procedures are predictably being more accurate and often providing better clinical outcomes and cost-effectiveness [15, 24].

Ultrasound-Guided Arthrocentesis and Injection of the Knee

USG arthrocentesis of the knee is most often performed via lateral approach of the suprapatellar recess with the leg extended straight or mildly flexed at 30 degrees. This location is where synovial fluid preferentially collects compared to other compartments of the knee [31, 36, 93]. Techniques where the needle is directly placed in the patellofemoral joint are not recommended for arthrocentesis as the patellofemoral joint is a tight joint, the needle moves considerably during arthrocentesis, the needle tip may score the patellofemoral cartilage surfaces during maneuvers, the patellofemoral approach is more painful, fluid flow is often blocked by contact with the cartilage, and much less synovial fluid is present in the patellofemoral joint compared to the suprapatellar recess. Thus, the lateral suprapatellar or lateral recess techniques are preferred. The probe is placed in the transverse plane over the thigh just proximal to the patella (Fig. 9.6), and then the probe is moved laterally with only contact pressure (pressure from the probe will force fluid away from the lateral recess) until the effusion is identified (Fig. 9.7). The fluid will reside between the quadriceps muscle and the iliotibial band (Fig. 9.7). If synovial tissue or fibrin strands adhere to and block the needle tip, the needle and syringe are rotated slowly

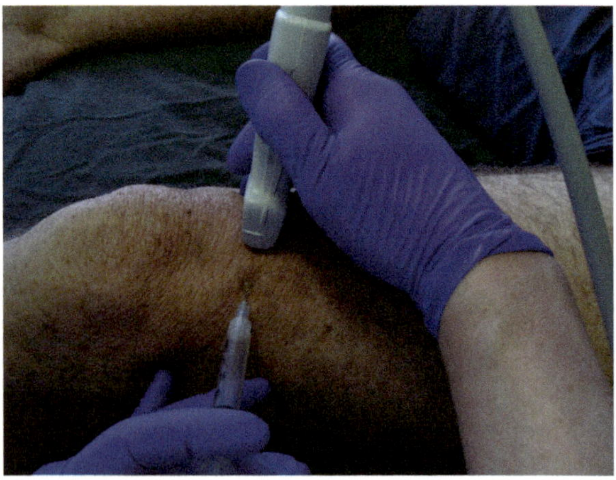

Fig. 9.6 Probe positioning for knee arthrocentesis. With the patient supine with the knee passively extended, the probe is placed in the transverse plane over the thigh just proximal to the patella and moved laterally, and the distended suprapatellar bursa or lateral recess is identified

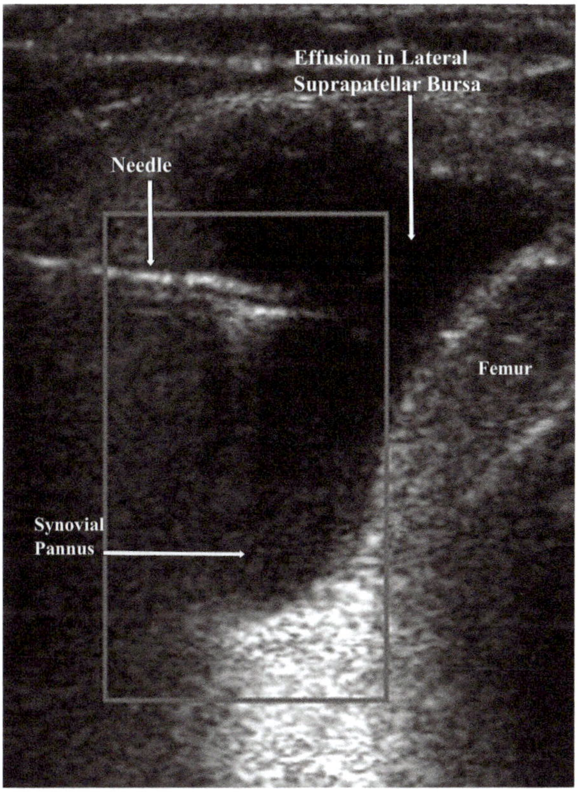

Fig. 9.7 US image of knee effusion in the lateral suprapatellar bursa. The probe is placed in the transverse plane over the thigh just proximal to the patella and moved laterally, and the distended suprapatellar bursa or lateral recess is identified

to cut through the adherent membrane until synovial fluid return is obtained, and then 5 ml synovial fluid diagnostic sample is obtained for cell count, crystal examination, gram stain, and culture and sensitivity (Fig. 9.8). This portion of the procedure can be performed by one operator. If there is more fluid present, it should be aspirated; syringe exchange can be performed with a 20 or 60 ml syringe, and the remainder of the fluid is removed. The knee can be more fully aspirated if an assistant compresses both sides of the infrapatellar knee and medial knee to force more fluid laterally. Sometimes the synovial membrane is intentionally not completely collapsed during the procedure to ensure that the needle remains within the synovial membrane, and a syringe exchange is performed and corticosteroid is injected (Fig. 9.9). US-guidance has been shown to improve the success of knee arthrocentesis, arthrocentesis fluid volume, and clinical outcomes [31, 32]. Recently Meehan et al. have demonstrated that pneumatic compression of the knee markedly increases synovial fluid available for USG aspiration [100]. Bennett et al. has demonstrated that the enhanced fluid aspiration obtained by mechanical compression of the knee improves outcomes and decreases the need for future knee procedures [101].

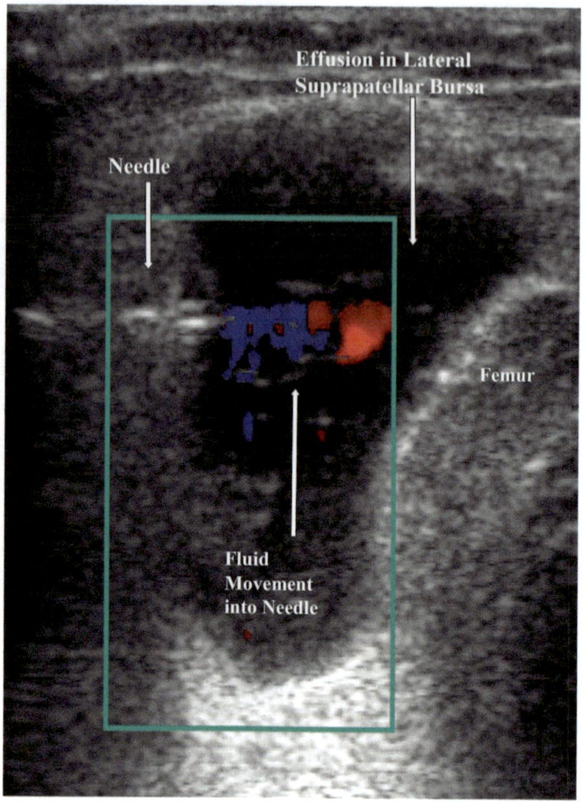

Fig. 9.8 US image of knee arthrocentesis. The needle is advanced in-plane and the fluid is aspirated

US-Guided Injection of the Knee

Injection of the non-effusive knee (dry knee) is the most common intra-articular needle procedure in medicine and thus dominates in a MSK practice. The knee can be effectively injected with US-guidance from the supine straight leg lateral suprapatellar, straight leg superolateral patellar, straight leg lateral midpatellar, or bent knee modified anterolateral infrapatellar approach [31, 36, 93]. All of the lateral approaches are more effective than the medial approaches to knee injection due to anatomy.

The most commonly used USG knee injection is performed similarly to knee arthrocentesis described above with a few modifications. With the patient supine with the knee passively extended, the probe is placed in the long axis of the thigh just proximal to the patella (Fig. 9.10), and a fluid-filled line of the synovial membrane is identified under the quadriceps tendon and muscle (Fig. 9.11). If this structure cannot be easily seen, the manual US probe pressure is reduced to eliminate synovial collapse, and the operator compresses both sides of the infrapatellar knee and medial knee to force more fluid into the synovial extension below the

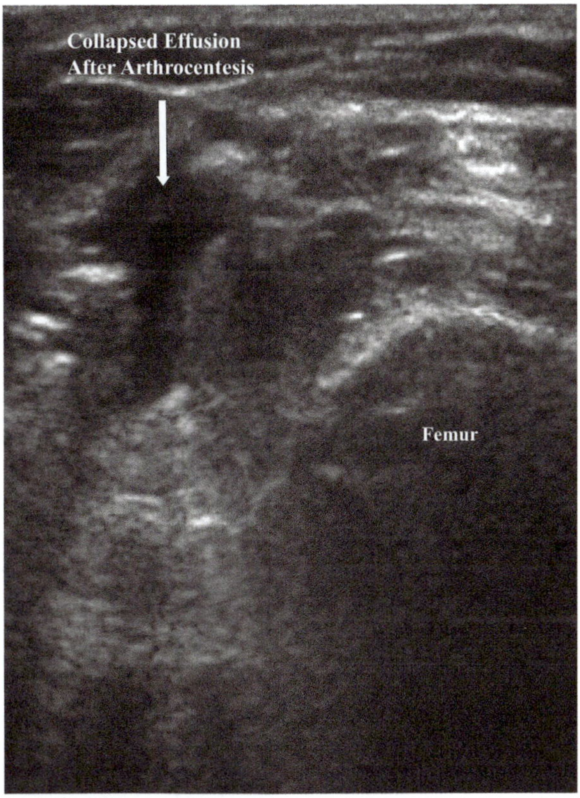

Fig. 9.9 US image of knee arthrocentesis with collapsed effusion. After the suprapatellar bursa is 90% collapsed by aspiration and assuming the fluid is not infected, a syringe exchange is performed, and the knee is injected with corticosteroid, and needle is removed with immediate compression

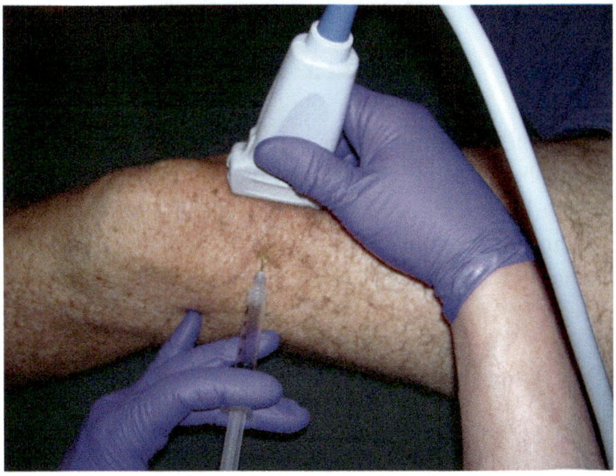

Fig. 9.10 Probe placement for knee arthrocentesis in a dry knee. With the patient supine with the knee passively extended, the probe is placed in the long axis of the thigh just proximal to the patella, the collapsed suprapatellar bursa is identified, the needle directed out-of-plane, initially toward the middle plane of the probe, and then the probe is rotated in-plane with the needle

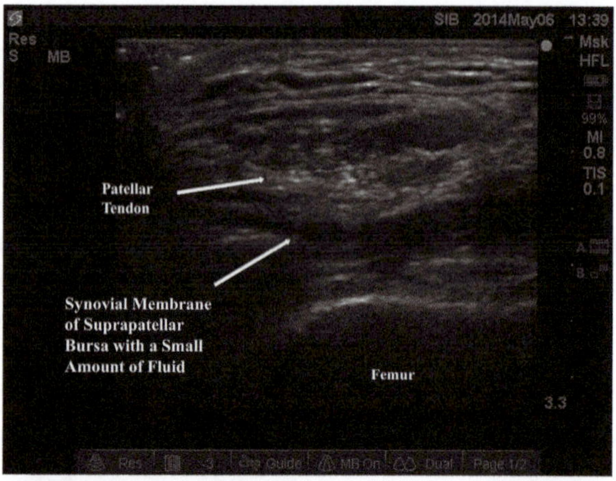

Fig. 9.11 US identification of the suprapatellar bursa. With the patient supine with the knee passively extended, the probe is placed in the long axis of the thigh just proximal to the patella and a fluid-filled or signal free line of the synovial membrane and space identified under the quadriceps tendon and muscle

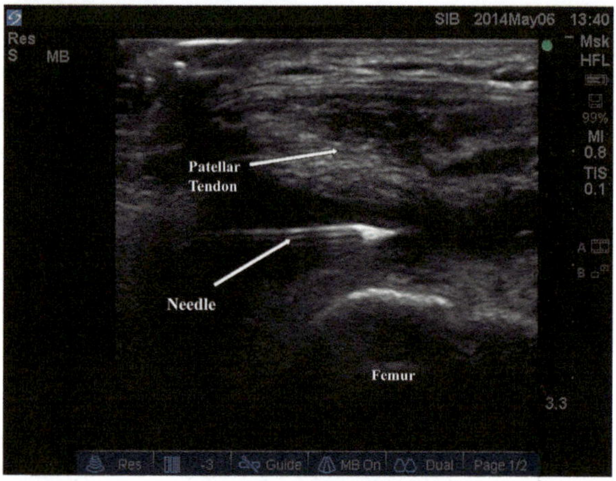

Fig. 9.12 USG injection of the suprapatellar bursa. With the patient supine with the knee passively extended, the probe is placed in the transverse plane of the thigh just proximal to the patella; the needle enters from the lateral thigh in a medial direction in-plane with the transverse probe into the synovial extension (suprapatellar bursa) under the quadriceps tendon

quadriceps tendon, and the synovial space becomes more obvious as black space of signal void. The probe is then rotated 90 degrees into the transverse plane in a positioning identical to knee arthrocentesis (Fig. 9.6), the depth is estimated, and the needle is inserted in-plane (from lateral to medial) with the transverse probe into the synovial extension under the quadriceps tendon (Fig. 9.12).

US-Guided Pes Anserine Bursa Injection

The pes anserine bursa is located distal to the joint line in close proximity and posterior to the medial collateral ligament lying between the medial collateral ligament and the sartorius, gracilis, and semitendinosus tendons. The patient is sitting or in the supine position with the knee flexed. The probe is placed in-plane over the tendinous border of the medial thigh muscles and following them from the distal medial femur across the joint line to the insertion at the pes anserine on the medial inferior knee (proximal medial tibia) (Fig. 9.13). A 25G 1 or 1.5 inch needle is inserted in-plane

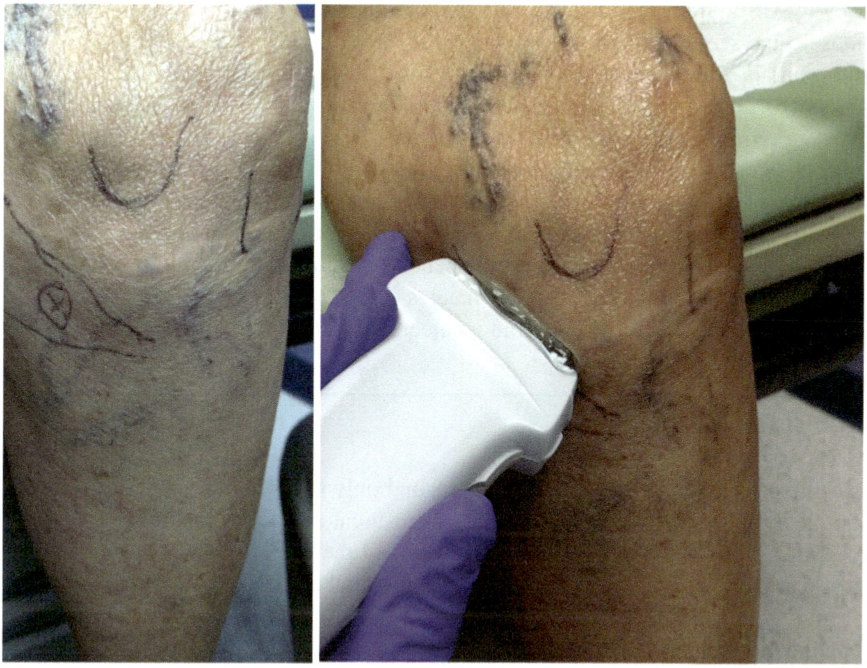

Fig. 9.13 Probe placement for anserine bursal injection. The probe is placed in-plane over the tendinous border of the medial thigh muscles and following them from the distal medial femur across the joint line to the insertion at the pes anserine on the medial inferior knee (proximal medial tibia)

under the probe over the insertional area or into the bursa if it is visible. Medication is injected over the insertional area or in the bursa. Injections of the anserine bursa are markedly more accurate with US-guidance (92% vs. 17%) [37].

US-Guided Iliotibial Band Injection

The patient is in the lateral recumbent position and the knee flexed 20 to 30 degrees. The iliotibial band originates at the lateral iliac crest and inserts on the lateral proximal tibia on Gerdy's tubercle (lateral tubercle of the tibia) that is palpated as a prominence just lateral to the distal portion of the patellar tendon. The probe is placed in the long axis of the iliotibial band, and fluid is often observe below the iliotibial band, which is the target, and the 25G 1.5 inch needle is inserted in-plane below the iliotibial band and injected. [102, 103].

US-Guided Aspiration and Injection of Popliteal Cysts

Popliteal cyst (Baker's cyst) can be effectively aspirated and injected with US-guidance [104–106]. The patient is placed in the prone position. The popliteal cyst by US in transverse view is in between the medial head of the gastrocnemius muscle and semimembranosus tendon in the posterior medial aspect of the popliteal fossa and is differentiated from an accentuated fat pad. If you visualize the popliteal artery (by observing pulsations and Doppler flow), popliteal vein (compressible and can see reflux via Doppler flow by squeezing the calf), and tibial nerve, the probe may be lateral to the popliteal cyst. Once the cyst is identified in transverse view, the probe can be turned 90 degrees to the long axis of the popliteal cyst, so that the needle can be directed in-plane from either a superior or inferior approach at a 30 to 45 degree angle (Fig. 9.14), the needle penetrates into the cyst (Fig. 9.15), and then the cyst is aspirated, with syringe exchanges if necessary until complete evacuation. After decompression, corticosteroid is injected.

Shoulder Procedures

Needle procedures of the shoulder are second only to those of the knee in terms of frequency for MSK interventions and are of great importance as upper extremity dysfunction is disabling. Common injections of the shoulder include the glenohumeral joint, subacromial bursa/rotator cuff, bicipital tendon sheath, and acromioclavicular joint. USG needle tenotomy, also known as barbotage, and lavage of calcifications can also be performed. USG interventional procedures in the shoulder have recently been reviewed [6, 16, 22, 107, 108]. When a shoulder-associated effusion is detected by US, it should be aspirated at the most visibly distended region of the structure most convenient to the operator, using similar techniques as knee arthrocentesis.

US-Guided Glenohumeral Joint Injection

In the normal joint, the glenohumeral joint is separated from the subacromial/subdeltoid bursa, but when there is rotator cuff pathology, often the two synovial

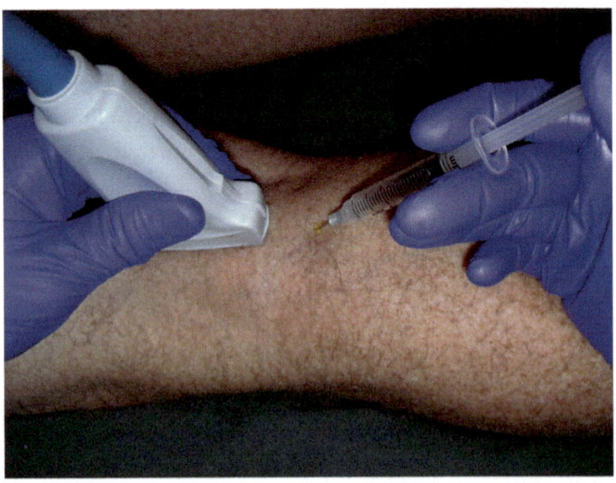

Fig. 9.14 Probe placement for popliteal cyst. The probe is held in the long axis over the popliteal fossa, the penetration point is the inferior portion of the popliteal area with the needle directed superiorly at a 30–45 degree angle in-plane with the probe, the 22 to 21 g 2 inch needle on a 10 or 20 ml syringe

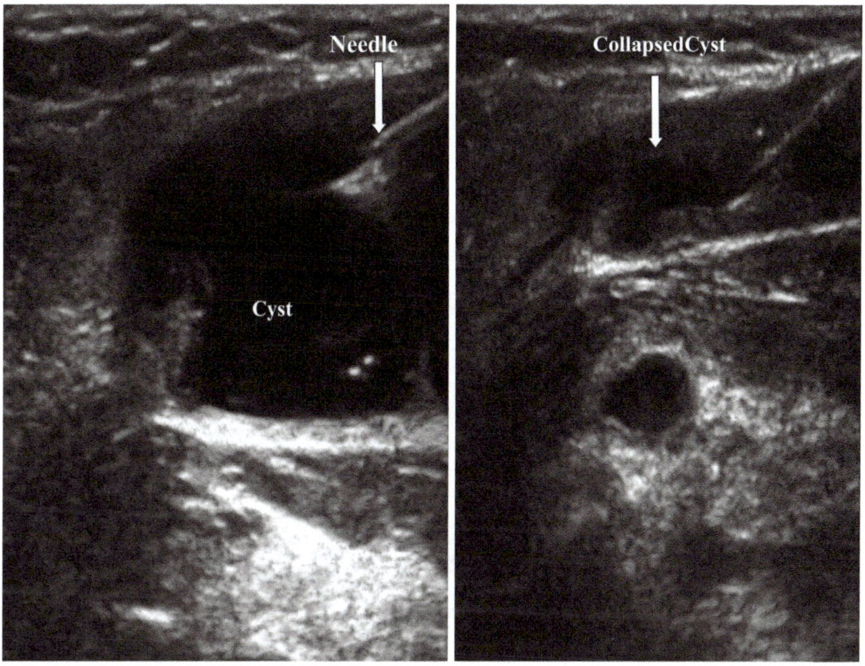

Fig. 9.15 Needle placement for popliteal cyst. The 22 to 21 g 2 inch needle on a 10 or 20 ml syringe advanced while anesthetizing with 3 ml of 1% lidocaine, the needle penetrates into the cyst, and then the cyst is aspirated almost to collapse with syringe exchanges if necessary

compartments communicate; thus, glenohumeral injections can be used to treat rotator cuff disease symptom in the abnormal shoulder. Because of this, the rheumatologist who deals with individuals with chronically pathologic shoulders often performs glenohumeral injections, while the orthopedic surgeon/sports medicine prefers subacromial bursa injections focused on rotator cuff disorders. USG glenohumeral joints can be injected with an anterior, posterior, or superior approach with equivalent accuracy, although the anterior approach appears less painful [39, 109, 110].

The posterior approach is most commonly used. The patient is sitting in a chair and the operator standing behind. The probe is placed posteriorly just inferior to the acromion and scapula (Fig. 9.16), and the infraspinatus tendon is identified. The probe is moved anteriorly in the plane of the infraspinatus until the musculotendinous junction of the infraspinatus is identified. Usually the glenoid can be observed. It is not necessary to actually put the needle into the glenoid labrum but rather only under the infraspinatus tendon at the labrum-humeral cartilage junction or actual joint surface. A 2–3.5 inch length needle may be required to reach the joint depending on body habitus. The needle is advanced in-plane either anteriorly from the posterior edge of the probe or posteriorly from the anterior edge of the probe, with the needle advancing through the infraspinatus muscle/tendon to the humeral head lateral to the glenoid labrum (Fig. 9.17). While injecting the needle, the needle tip can initially be placed against the humeral head and then rotated or slightly withdrawn until US-visible intra-articular injection occurs.

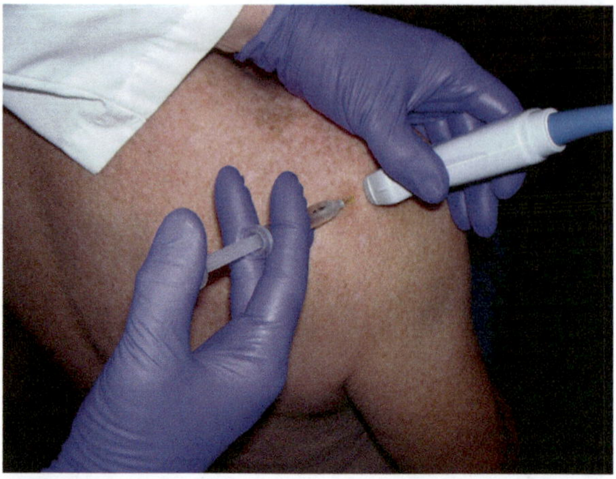

Fig. 9.16 Probe placement for a posterior glenohumeral injection. The probe is placed posteriorly just inferior to the acromion and scapula, and the infraspinatus tendon is identified

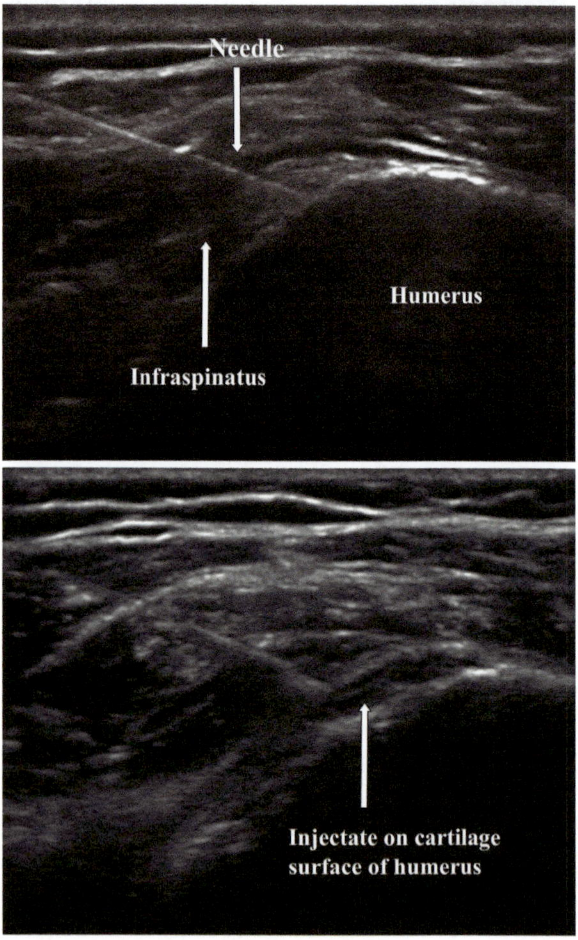

Fig. 9.17 Needle placement for a posterior glenohumeral injection A 2 inch 22 or 25 g needle is advanced in-plane either anteriorly from the posterior edge of the probe or posteriorly from the anterior edge of the probe, with the needle advancing through the infraspinatus muscle/tendon to the humeral head lateral to the glenoid labrum

Ultrasound-Guided Subacromial/Subdeltoid Bursa Injection

Subacromial injections are the most common injections for shoulder impingement syndrome due to rotator cuff tendinitis or bursitis. USG corticosteroid injection into the subacromial-subdeltoid bursa can be accomplished by the posterior, anterior, superior, and lateral approaches [111]. The patient is usually sitting but can be supine or recumbent with the pathologic side up. For the lateral injection, the probe is placed over the acromion and deltoid in the long axis, and a 2 inch, 22G needle is advanced medially in the long axis through the deltoid into the bursa between the deltoid and supraspinatus [111]. For the anterior injection, the probe is placed on the anterior shoulder with the probe in the direction of the patients ear (Fig. 9.18). The subacromial bursa is identified over the supraspinatus tendon, and the injection is performed as above (Fig. 9.19). The posterior injection is performed with the probe posterior just below the acromion, the rotator cuff is identified, and needle tip is inserted into the bursa for injection.

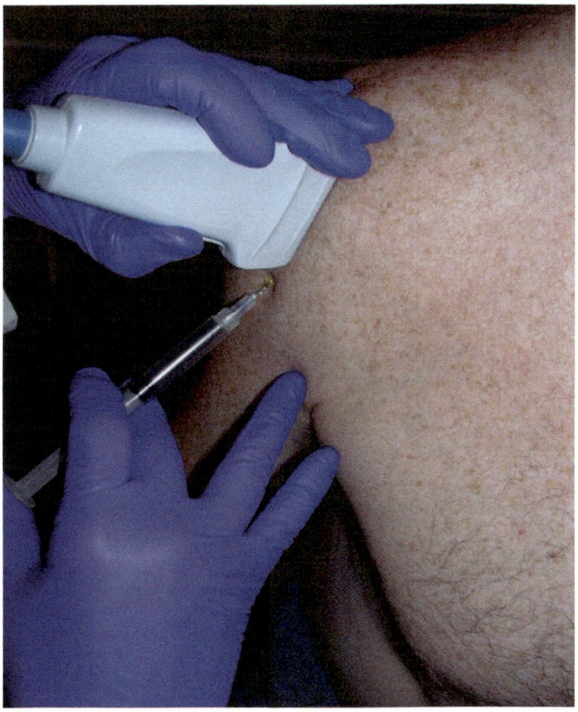

Fig. 9.18 Probe placement for lateral subacromial-subdeltoid bursa injection. For the lateral injection, the probe is placed over the acromion and deltoid in the long axis, and the 2 inch 22 g needle is advanced medially in the long axis through the deltoid into the bursa between the deltoid and supraspinatus that is expanded with lidocaine and then injected with 1 to 1.5 ml of corticosteroid

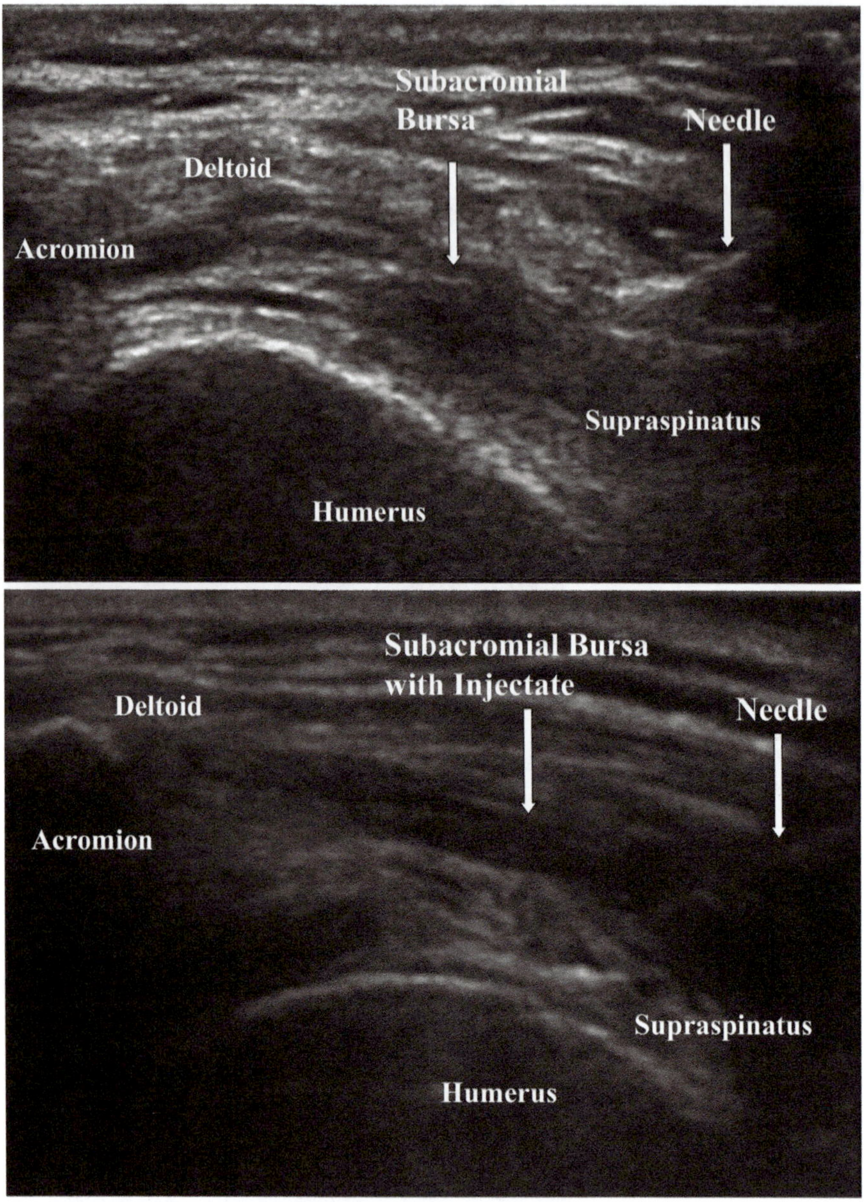

Fig. 9.19 Needle placement for lateral subacromial-subdeltoid bursa injection. The 1.5–2 inch 22 g needle is advanced medially in the long axis through the deltoid into the bursa between the deltoid and supraspinatus that is expanded with lidocaine and then injected with 1 to 1.5 ml of corticosteroid

US-Guided Acromioclavicular Joint Injection

The acromioclavicular (AC) joint can be injected anterior to posterior with the probe resting on the superior portion of the AC with the beam directed inferiorly (Fig. 9.20) or can be injected superior to inferior as the probe can be placed on the anterior AC joint with the beam directed posteriorly and the needle directed from superior AC joint inferiorly [41, 112]. The joint can usually accommodate 1–2 ml [112].

US-Guided Bicipital Tendon Sheath Injection

The patient can be sitting or supine. The bicipital tendon sheath can be injected with the shoulder in neutral position with elbow flexed at 90 degrees for an in-plane approach of the tendon in transverse view, or externally rotated with the probe placed transverse to identify the tendon, and then rotated to the long axis of the tendon (Fig. 9.21). With the probe in the long axis relative to the tendon, the needle is directed superiorly into the sheath under the probe, and care is taken to avoid dissecting or injecting the tendon itself [44].

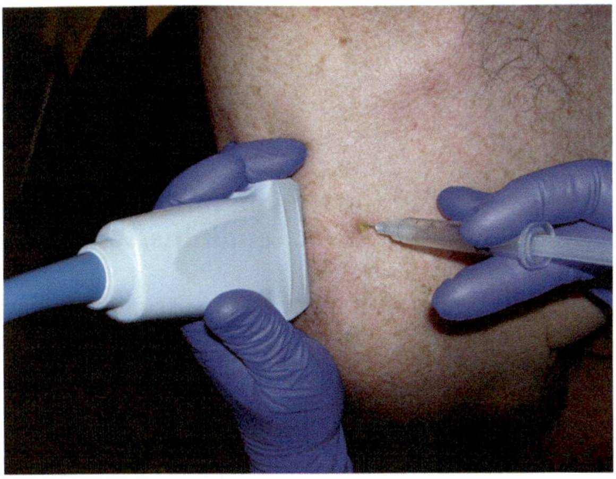

Fig. 9.20 Probe placement for acromioclavicular joint injection. The acromioclavicular (AC) joint can be injected anteriorly posterior with the probe resting on the superior portion of the AC with the beam directed inferiorly

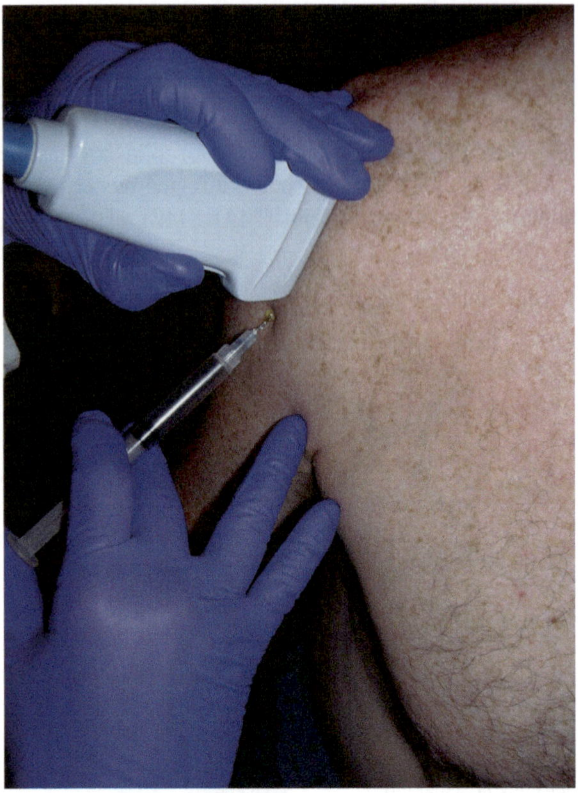

Fig. 9.21 Probe placement for bicipital tendon. The bicipital tendon sheath is injected with the shoulder externally rotated with the probe first transverse to the long axis of the arm until the tendon is identified and then the probe rotated to the long axis of the tendon

Ultrasound-Guided Needle Tenotomy (or Barbotage) and Lavage for Calcific Tendinitis/Tendinopathy

Ultrasound-Guided Needle Tenotomy, (or Barbotage)

Massive or symptomatic calcifications of the shoulder tendons, after excluding metabolic syndromes (gout, hypercalcemia), can be treated with ultrasound-guided needle tenotomy, also known as barbotage (repetitive needling), often combined with lavage and syringe aspiration of calcifications [113–115]. Since this is a traumatic procedure, patients at high risk for hemorrhage (hemorrhagic diathesis, or therapy with warfarin, clopidogrel, aspirin, and other anticoagulants) should be identified before the procedure to prevent painful and disabling hematoma, hemarthrosis, or hemorrhagic bursitis. For US-guided barbotage, the implicated tendon must be accessible; thus, the patient is usually in the sitting position or lying on the side, and the operator stands posteriorly, anteriorly, or laterally depending on the target tendon and approach. With a 20 to 21Gg 2 inch needle (which provides stiffness and enough exposed shaft) on a 5 to 10 ml syringe, the shoulder and affected tendon are anesthetized with 5 ml of 1% lidocaine. After injection of the lidocaine around the target tendon, calcifications are repeatedly impacted by the needle tip and hydrodissected by injecting lidocaine or saline, which disrupts the surface of the tendon spilling calcium hydroxyapatite or pyrophosphate crystals into the bursal structure which then can sometimes be aspirated. Some operators prefer a "surging" approach, where a small amount of lidocaine or saline is injected under pressure, and then the plunger is released or aspirated, and crystals spontaneously return in the syringe. If the needle blocks, one can forcefully and alternatively inject aspirate to clear it of crystals. When the syringe fills with cloudy fluid, a syringe exchange is performed. When the aspirate becomes clear, the surrounding bursal structure (not the tendon) can be injected with corticosteroids as in a conventional injection with a syringe exchange. Post-procedure, the area may be forcefully compressed for 5 minutes to reduce the chance of hemorrhage. The patient should rest the extremity for 3 days and perform gentle range of motion exercises, but not use the arm forcefully for at least 4–6 weeks to lessen the chance of tendon rupture.

Percutaneous needle tenotomy, high-volume lavage, and percutaneous scraping and barbotage for treatments of tendinopathy have recently been reviewed [116].

In 2004 Galletti et al. reported a series of USG needling of chronic calcific tendonitis of the rotator cuff [117]. Lee et al. have recently reviewed the technique of USG needling-barbotage-lavage of calcific tendonitis [118]. US-guided needling of chronic calcific tendinopathy of the rotator cuff appears to be safe [115], but not more effective than ultrasound-guided subacromial corticosteroid injection long-term [119]. In contrast, in a 48 patient study, de Witte et al. reported that USG needling was more effective than subacromial corticosteroid injections in terms of pain, function, and calcium deposit size up to 1 year but not at 5 years [114, 120]. The combination of both has been reported to be 71.4% effective at 6 months [121]. Housner performed US-guided needle tenotomy in 13 patients using a 22G needle and local anesthetic with reports of effectiveness at 12 weeks [122]. Jacobson et al. have also demonstrated that needle fenestration (where the needle passed completely through the tendon is effective in tendinopathies [123]. Gatt et al. have performed a systematic review of barbotage and concluded that it is indeed effective compared to conventional therapy [115]. Recently Darrieutort-Laffite et al. have demonstrated that corticosteroid injection directly after USG barbotage and lavage is superior to barbotage or lavage alone [124]. USG barbotage has also been used to remove the tophi of gout, hydroxyapatite deposition disease, and calcinosis cutis [97, 125, 126].

Lavage

Lavage, also known as tidal irrigation is another USG procedure to treat joint disease, in particular Milwaukee shoulder syndrome [127]. In this procedure, the affected shoulder compartment (usually the glenohumeral joint) is injected with 10 ml of lidocaine and then with 25 to 60 ml increments is completely dilated with normal saline, a syringe exchange is performed, and the shoulder is completely decompressed. This is repeated until the lavage fluid is clear.

Elbow Procedures

Ultrasound-Guided Elbow Joint Injection

USG injection of the elbow and epicondyles has recently been reviewed [2, 12, 128, 129]. The elbow can be aspirated and injected from a lateral or posterior approach. The patient can be sitting or supine for these procedures. In the posterior approach, with the elbow at 90 degrees, the probe is placed transversely over the triceps tendon and distal humerus to detect fluid and the joint line (Fig. 9.22), and a 22G 1.5 inch needle on a 3 ml syringe is directed in the same axis as the ulnar on the lateral side of the triceps tendon into the joint, and then the probe is rotated 90 degrees in axis with the lateral olecranon on the lateral side and in-plane with the needle. The needle is directed anteriorly into the humeroulnar joint toward the radius and injected [2, 12]. In the lateral approach, the elbow is flexed at 90 degrees, the probe is placed transversely over the lateral olecranon, and the effusion and/or joint line is identified. The needle is introduced at 90 degrees to the skin in the middle of the probe toward the joint line; once deep, the probe is moved to the distal humerus and proximal olecranon, and the needle can be observed in-plane advancing into the joint (Fig. 9.23).

Ultrasound-Guided Lateral Epicondyle Injection

The lateral epicondyle is the tendinous origin of the wrist extensor-supinator muscle group and the medial epicondyle the origin of the wrist flexor-pronator muscle group, and, thus, both are subjected to considerable physical stress. As reviewed in

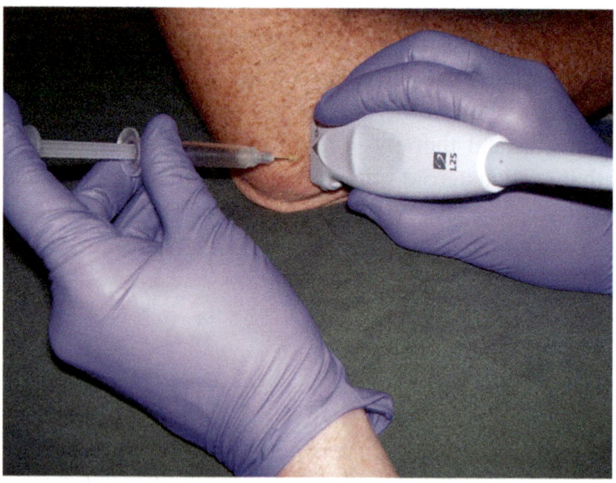

Fig. 9.22 Probe placement for posterior elbow injection. In the posterior approach, with the elbow at 90 degrees, the probe is placed transversely over the triceps tendon and distal humerus to detect fluid and the joint line, the needle is directed in the same axis as the ulnar on the lateral side of the triceps tendon into the joint, and then the probe is rotated 90 degree in axis with the lateral olecranon on the lateral side and in-plane with the needle

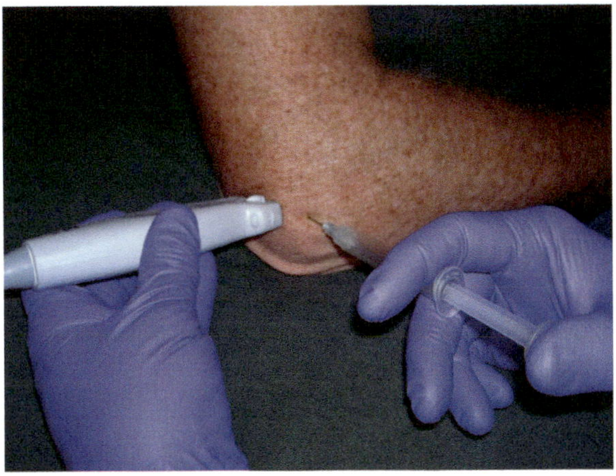

Fig. 9.23 Probe placement for lateral elbow injection. In the lateral approach, the elbow is flexed at 90 degrees, and the probe is placed transversely over the lateral olecranon, and the effusion or joint line is identified. The needle is introduced at 90 degrees to skin in the middle of the probe toward the joint line; once deep, the probe is moved to the distal humerus and proximal olecranon, and the needle can be observed in-plane advancing into the joint

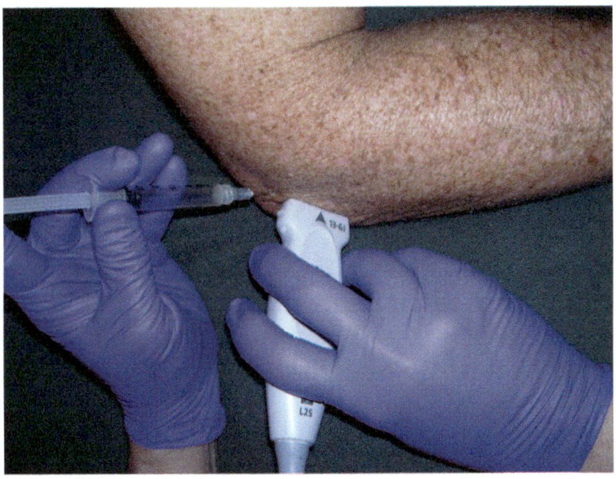

Fig. 9.24 Probe placement for lateral epicondyle. The US probe is placed in the long axis of the common extensor tendon that is inserted on the epicondyle and a 25 g 1 inch needle on a 3 ml syringe with 3 ml of lidocaine, the needle is inserted in-plane or out-of-plane

the elbow chapter earlier, lateral epicondylitis is often a tendinosis of the common extensor tendon.

USG needle tenotomy, platelet-rich plasma (PRP), and other regenerative medicine injections are being explored as treatment options given the negative long-term effects of corticosteroid injected into tendon [ref Coombes]. The patient is usually in the sitting position but can be supine. The US probe is placed in the long axis of the common extensor tendon that inserts on the epicondyle [130] (Fig. 9.24). The needle is inserted in-plane or out-of-plane; the area over the insertion is hydrodissected to lift up overlying tissues that are so narrow and particularly susceptible to

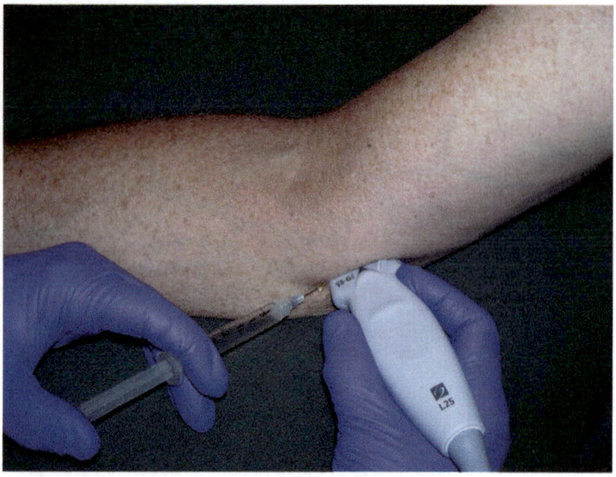

Fig. 9.25 Probe placement for medial epicondyle. The US probe is placed in the long axis of the flexor tendons that insert on the epicondyle and a 25 g 1 inch needle on a 3 ml syringe with 3 ml of lidocaine; the needle is inserted in-plane or out-of-plane

corticosteroid atrophy and to anesthetize the area. Needle tenotomy and lavage at this juncture can be performed if calcifications are present if indicated [122]. The approach to medial epicondylitis is identical to that of lateral epicondylitis (Fig. 9.25), although the operator must be cognizant that injected material may migrate to the ulnar nerve causing a temporary nerve block [131]. Zhu demonstrated that USG needling of calcifications associated with lateral epicondylitis followed by corticosteroid injection resulted in an 87% good to excellent response rate with reduction or resolution of calcifications in 74% of patients [132]. Shiple et al. found that USG corticosteroid injection of the lateral epicondyle was more effective than injection with platelet-rich plasma (PRP) or saline and clinical trials with PRP continue [133, 134]. There is little published evidence on the accuracy of USG versus ALMPG therapy of epicondylitis.

Hand and Wrist Procedures

Ultrasound-Guided Wrist (Radiocarpal) Joint Injection

USG procedures in the wrist and hand have been recently reviewed [74, 99, 135–137]. The patient is usually sitting in a chair with the forearm pronated, using the padded foot extension of the examining table as an operating platform, which is covered with a drape, and the operator sits next to the patient, or if the patient is apprehensive, the patient can be supine. Lister's tubercle (radial tubercle) is identified by palpation, the probe is placed on the radial tubercle on dorsum of the wrist in the long axis, and the radiocarpal joint space is identified by sliding the probe distally (Fig. 9.26). The needle can be directed either at 90 degrees to the skin next

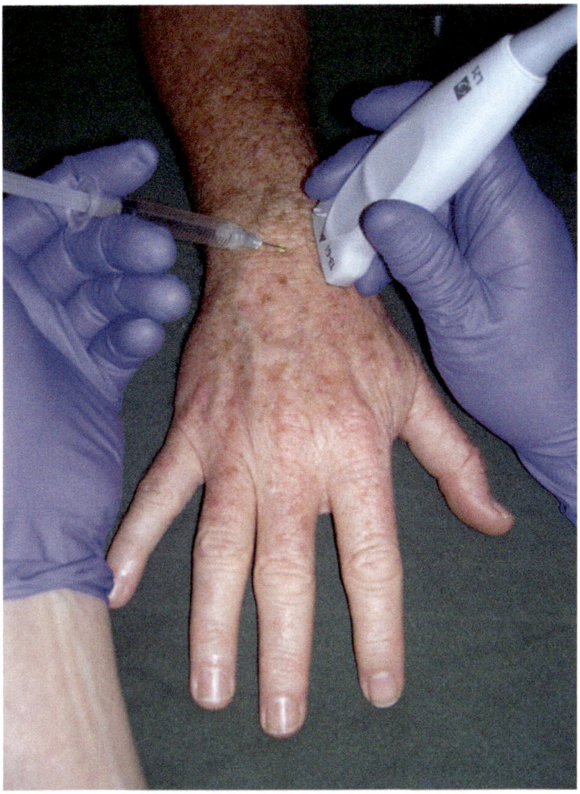

Fig. 9.26 Probe placement for wrist. The radial tubercle (Lister's tubercle) is identified by palpation, and the probe is placed on the radial tubercle on dorsum of the wrist in the long axis, and the radiocarpal joint space is identified by sliding the probe distally. The needle can be directed either at 90 degrees to the skin next to the probe or directed out-of-plane at 45 degrees to the skin from the ulnar side under the probe until the needle is visible and then the probe rotated 90 degrees so that the needle is in-plane with intra-articular positioning

to the probe or directed out-of-plane at 45 degrees to the skin from the ulnar side under the probe until the needle is visible and then the probe rotated 90 degrees so that the needle is in-plane with intra-articular positioning (Fig. 9.27).

Ultrasound-Guided Carpal Tunnel Injection

Carpal tunnel injections are generally underutilized in MSK medicine and have been shown to be as effective as surgery with less recovery time and equivalent outcomes and, unlike surgery, can be easily repeated multiple times if clinically indicated. These injections can also serve as bridging therapy until surgery eventually becomes indicated [74, 138, 139]. The patient is usually sitting in a chair with the forearm supinated, resting on an exam table, with the operator sitting next to the patient. The carpal tunnel is formed by the carpal bones dorsally and the transverse carpal ligament (flexor retinaculum) ventrally and include the vascular structures,

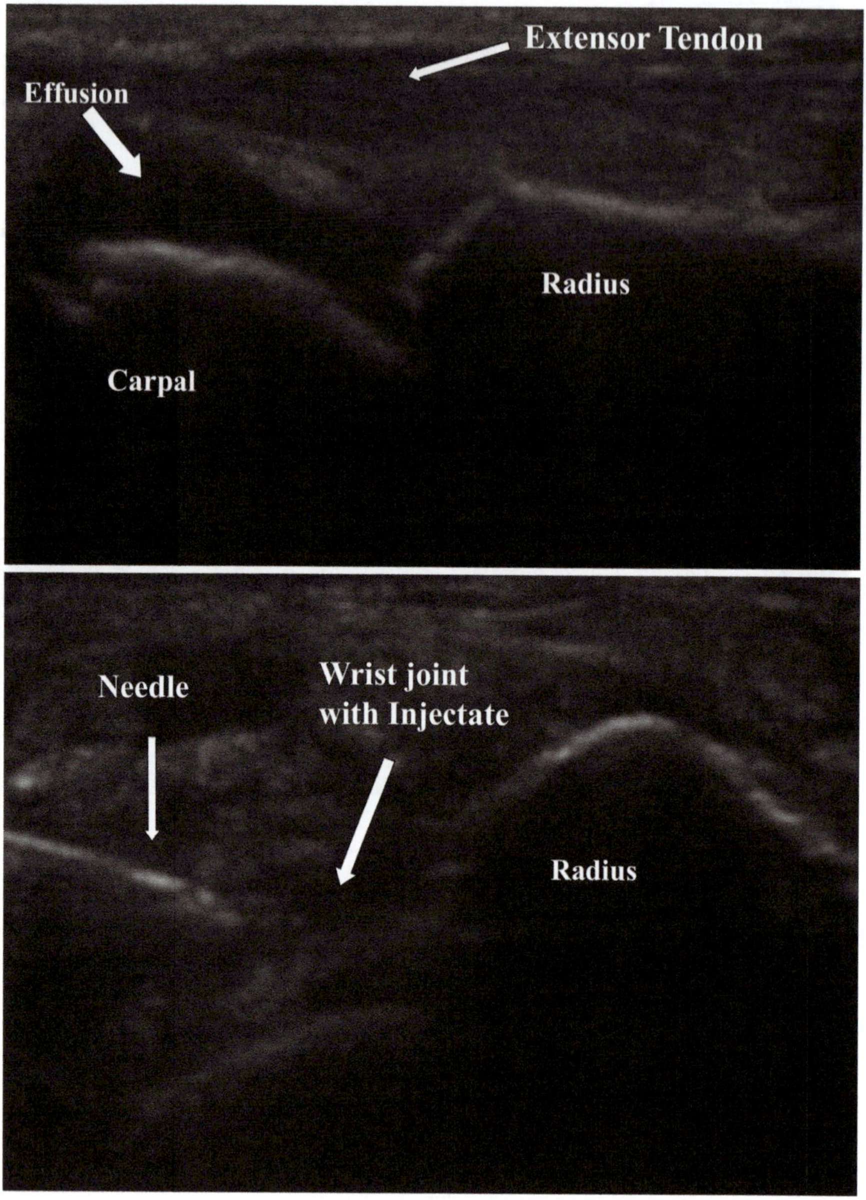

Fig. 9.27 Needle placement for wrist. The radial tubercle (Lister's tubercle) is identified by palpation, and the probe is placed on the radial tubercle on dorsum of the wrist in the long axis, and the radiocarpal joint space is identified by sliding the probe distally. The needle can be directed either at 90 degrees to the skin next to the probe or directed out-of-plane at 45 degrees to the skin from the ulnar side under the probe until the needle is visible and then the probe rotated 90 degrees so that the needle is in-plane with intra-articular positioning

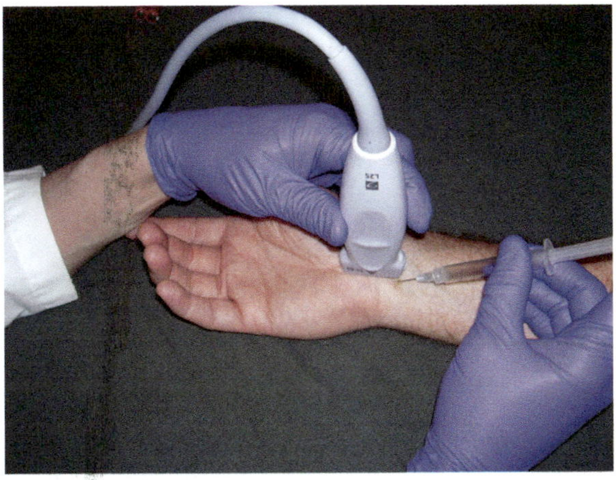

Fig. 9.28 Probe placement for carpal tunnel – long axis. After identifying the palmaris longus tendon, the median nerve, ulnar artery, and radial artery, the probe is placed in the long axis, and the needle is introduced in-plane at 30 degrees toward the ring finger

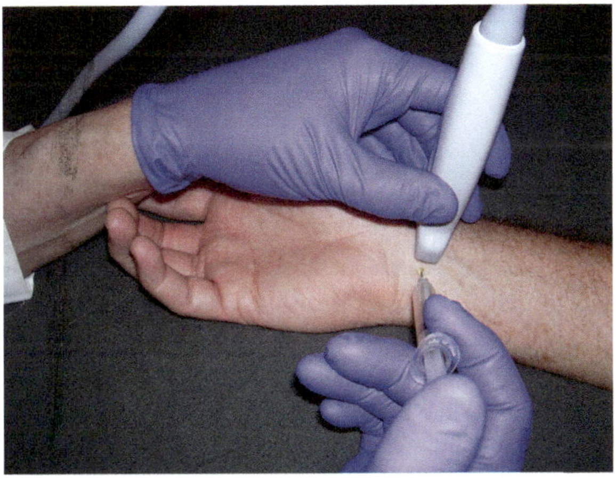

Fig. 9.29 Probe placement for carpal tunnel – transverse approach. After identifying the palmaris longus tendon and the median nerve, the probe is placed in the transverse axis, and the needle is introduced in-plane at 30 degrees toward the radial side, and lidocaine is injected to hydrodisplace the contents away from the needle tip

the median nerve, flexor digitorum profundus, and flexor pollicis longus tendons. First the ulnar border of the palmaris longus tendon is determined by having the patient oppose all the digits together while flexing the wrist – the entry target is then marked with a surgical pen on the ulnar side of the palmaris longus tendon at the second skin crease proximal to the palmar-wrist junction. This positioning is then confirmed with sonographic interrogation and identification of the median nerve, palmaris longus tendon, radial artery, and ulnar artery with Doppler imaging. USG carpal tunnel injections can be provided in various techniques: (1) in-plane ulnar approach with the probe transverse to the median nerve; (2) in-plane distal approach with the probe in long axis along the median nerve, similar to ALMPG injections; and (3) in-plane radial approach with the probe transverse to the median nerve. Out-of-plane injections around the nerve are generally not performed avoid nerve injury. With all techniques, the needle is inserted at 30 degrees (Figs. 9.28 and 9.29), and the target for corticosteroid injection is to place the needle tip below the flexor

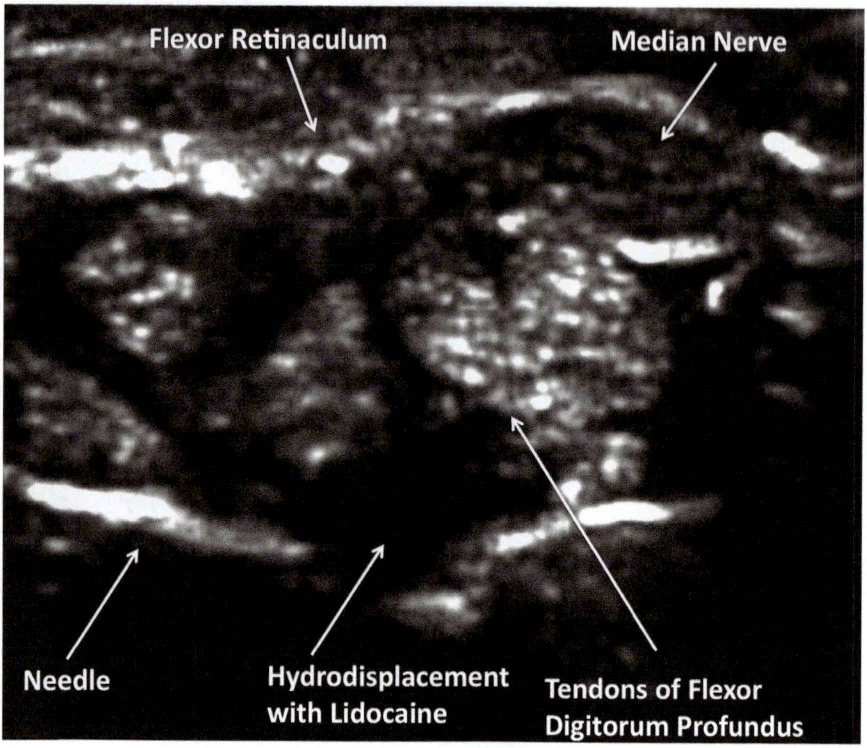

Fig. 9.30 Needle placement for carpal tunnel – transverse approach. After identifying the palmaris longus tendon and the median nerve, the probe is placed in the transverse axis, and the needle is introduced in-plane at 30 degrees toward the radial side, and lidocaine is injected to hydrodisplace the contents (nerves, tendons, and arteries) away from the needle tip

retinaculum (transverse ligament) and anatomically away from the median nerve, vascular structures, and tendon fibers. USG hydrodissection with lidocaine to move away critical structures to allow medication to surround the median nerve may be performed to further prevent needle penetration and injection injury directly into the median nerve or surrounding tendons and vascular structures [74, 140]. Once a neutral space has been created under the flexor retinaculum and the needle tip is not in a tendon sheath or tendon, corticosteroid can be injected (Fig. 9.30). USG injection of the carpal tunnel has been shown to improve accuracy, outcomes, and cost-effectiveness and can safety be repeated every 4 months as necessary [74, 141]. Recently, USG surgical release of the carpal tunnel has advanced using a number of different cutting technologies and has great promise [142, 143].

Ultrasound-Guided First Carpometacarpal (Metacarpotrapizium) Joint and Scaphotrapeziotrapezoid Joint Injections

The probe is placed over the radial aspect of the first metacarpal (thumb) in the long axis, and the probe is moved proximally until the first carpometacarpal (metacarpo-trapizium) joint is identified; the radial artery should be just dorsal to this point and the extensor pollicis tendons and should be avoided. The needle is inserted proximally in-plane with the probe and is directed to the metacarpal joint surface and then directed deeper for injection. The scaphotrapeziotrapezoid can be injected with the identical technique but with the probe in line with the index finger – great care must be taken to avoid the radial artery in a scaphotrapeziotrapezoid injection. US-guidance of the scaphotrapeziotrapezoid joint improves accuracy from 80% to 100% [49] and of the first carpometacarpal joint improves accuracy from 91% to 100%. Lack of USG injection response predicts the need for future surgery [50, 51] (Fig. 9.31).

Ultrasound-Guided First Dorsal Wrist Compartment Injection for De Quervain's Stenosing Tenosynovitis

The probe is placed transversely over the lateral side of the radius in axis with the thumb and the abductor pollicis longus (APL) and extensor pollicis brevis (EPB) tendons within the extensor compartment, and then the probe is placed in axis with the extensor compartment (Figs. 9.32 and 9.33). The needle is advanced in-plane from the distal radius into the extensor compartment avoiding the tendons themselves and then the compartments dilated with lidocaine, so that it is like a sausage when palpated. A syringe exchange can be performed and corticosteroid injected. USG injections for stenosing tenosynovitis are more accurate and more effective that ALMPG injections [52].

Ganglion Cysts and Periarticular Cysts

Masses in the wrist and periarticular structures can be diagnosed conclusively with US with dorsal wrist ganglion originating from the scapholunate joint (65% of ganglia of the wrist and hand), volar wrist ganglion originating from the distal aspect of the radius accounting for 20% to 25%, and flexor tendon sheath ganglia constituting 10% to 15% [137, 144]. If the originating joint or structure can be identified, then these structures can be directly injected using the aforementioned techniques, and when corticosteroid is injected in the originating structure, reflux of corticosteroid into the

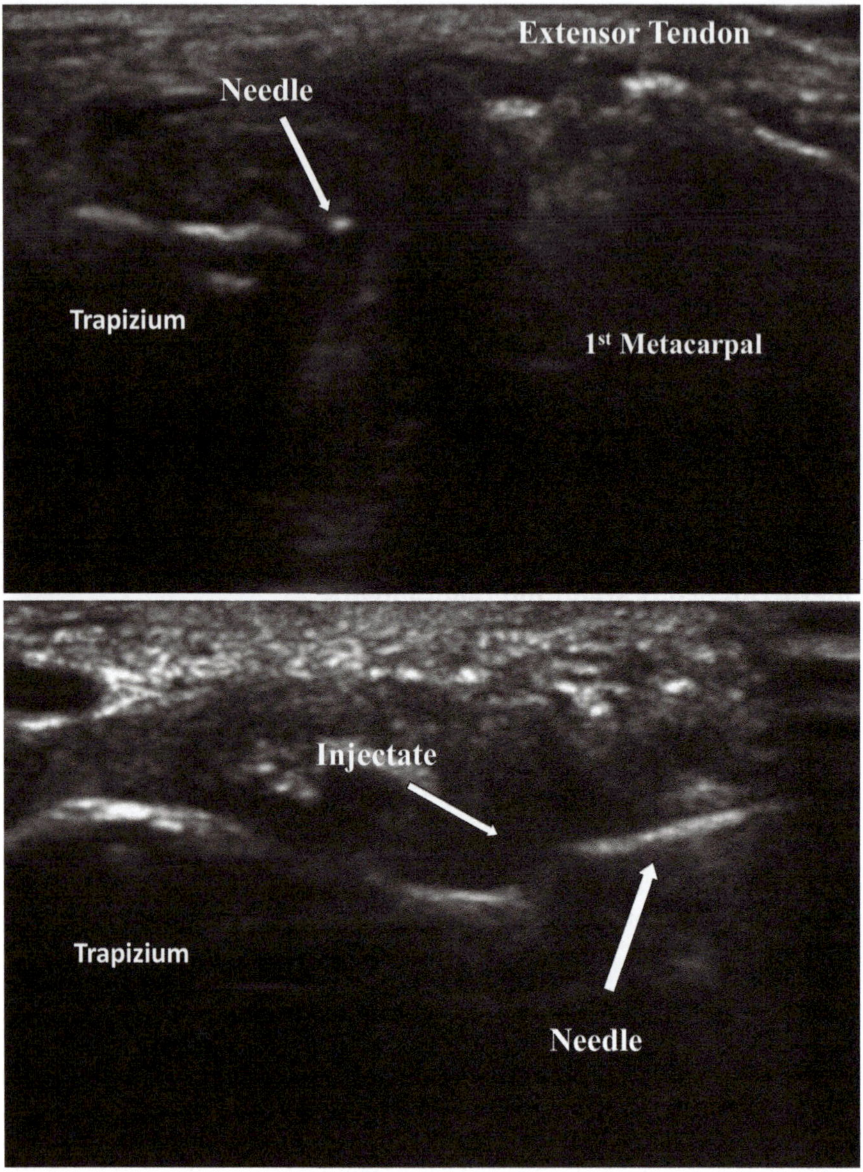

Fig. 9.31 Needle placement for carpometacarpal joint. The probe is placed over the radial aspect of the first metacarpal (thumb) in the long axis, and the probe is moved proximally until the first carpometacarpal (metacarpotrapizium) joint is identified. A 5/8–1 inch 25 gauge needle on a syringe with 1 ml of 1% lidocaine in a 3 ml syringe enters proximally in-plane with the probe and is directed to the metacarpal joint surface and then directed deeper

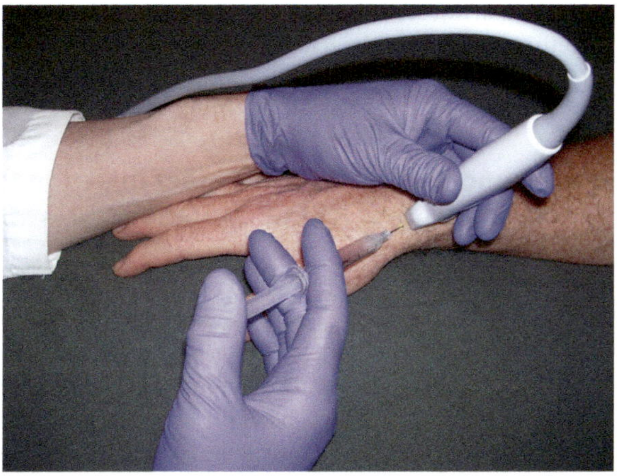

Fig. 9.32 Probe placement for de Quervain's stenosing tenosynovitis. The probe is placed transversely over the lateral side of the radius in axis with the thumb and the abductor pollicis longus and extensor pollicis brevis tendons within the extensor compartment, and then the probe is placed in the long axis with the extensor compartment

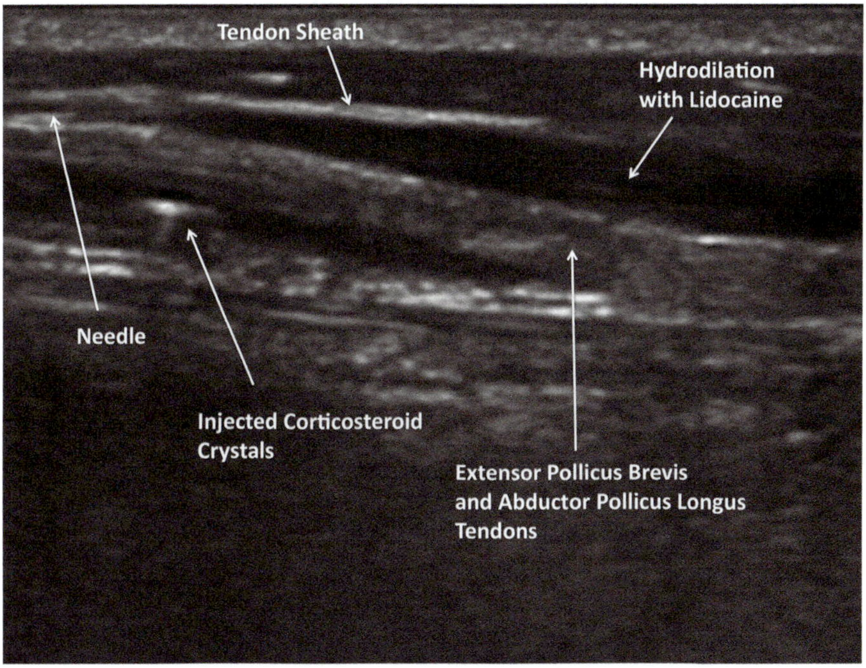

Fig. 9.33 Needle placement for de Quervain's stenosing tenosynovitis. The probe is placed transversely over the lateral side of the radius in axis with the thumb and the abductor pollicis longus and extensor pollicis brevis tendons within the extensor compartment, and then the probe is placed in the long axis with the extensor compartment

cyst is usually observed with rapid resolution. Alternatively the cystic structure can be directly aspirated and injected under US-guidance as in any joint, anesthetizing with lidocaine, followed by aspiration, syringe exchange, and corticosteroid injection.

Ultrasound-Guided Trigger Finger Injection for Digital Flexor Tenosynovitis with A1 Pulley Stenosis

Trigger finger caused by palmar flexor tenosynovitis and thickening/stenosis of the first annular (A1) pulley responds extremely well to corticosteroid injection and usually obviates hand surgery [53, 75–78, 99, 145]. The patient is positioned with the forearm supinated so that the palm is exposed, similar to positioning for a carpal tunnel injection. The US probe is placed transversely over the palmar aspect of the metacarpophalangeal joint and the flexor tendon, tendon sheath, and pulley (a thickening or squaring of the tendon sheath) for identification of structures, and then the probe is rotated in axis to the tendon (Fig. 9.34). A 5/8 to 1 inch needle is introduced proximal to the pulley in the long axis of the flexor tendon over the metacarpal hook with the needle pointing 30 degrees distally toward the affected finger and in-plane to probe. Care must be taken to inject medication to avoid dissecting tendon fibers and can be injected within the sheath (Fig. 9.35). If multiple tendon sheaths in the same hand are being injected, an USG ulnar and median nerve block with lidocaine can first be performed to decrease procedural pain [75–78]. US-guidance improves the accuracy of intra-sheath injections from 15% to 75% and reduces intratendinous

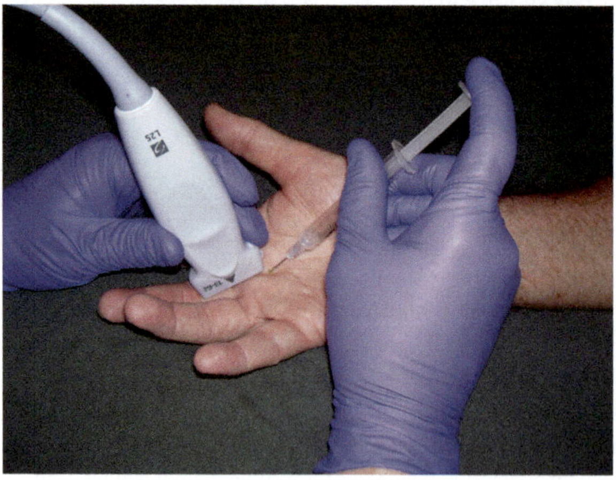

Fig. 9.34 Probe placement for digital palmar flexor tenosynovitis with A1 pulley stenosis (trigger finger). The US probe is placed transversely over palmar aspect of metacarpophalangeal joint and the flexor tendon, tendon sheath, and pulley (a thickening or squaring of the tendon sheath) identified, and then the probe is rotated in axis to the tendon. A 5/8 to 1 inch needle on a 3 ml syringe with 1.5 ml of lidocaine is introduced proximal to the pulley in the long axis of the flexor tendon over the metacarpal hook with the needle pointing 30 degrees distally toward the affected finger and in-plane to probe

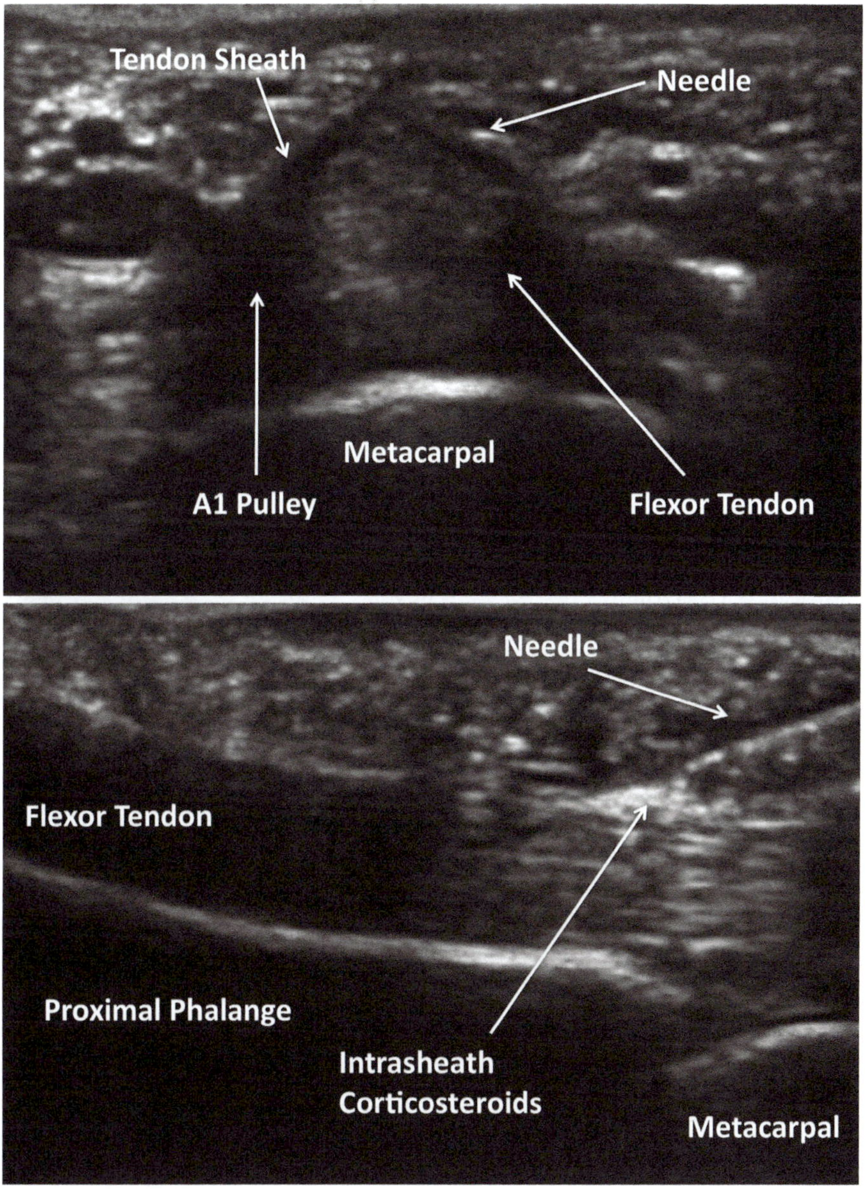

Fig. 9.35 Needle placement for digital palmar flexor tenosynovitis with A1 pulley stenosis (trigger finger). A 5/8 to 1 inch needle on a 3 ml syringe with 1.5 ml of lidocaine is introduced proximal to the pulley in the long axis of the flexor tendon over the metacarpal hook with the needle pointing 30 degrees distally toward the affected finger and in-plane to probe, and then first lidocaine and then corticosteroid are injected

injection from 30% to 0% [53]. A recent review concluded that USG injections improved the diagnosis and outcome of injections for tenosynovitis in rheumatoid arthritis [146].

Ultrasound-Guided Small Joint Injections: Metacarpophalangeal (MCP), Interphalangeal Joints (IP), and Distal Interphalangeal (DIP) Cysts

The MCP and IP joints are all similar in structure consisting of a dorsal extensor tendon apparatus superiorly, a convex proximal joint surface, a concave distal joint surface, and an interdigital nerve and artery running laterally on the palmar or flexor side. Thus, these joints are best injected on the dorsal side to avoid the artery and nerve. The probe is placed in the long axis on the extensor surface of the joint and the joint space identified (Figs. 9.36, 9.37, and 9.38). The needle can be placed

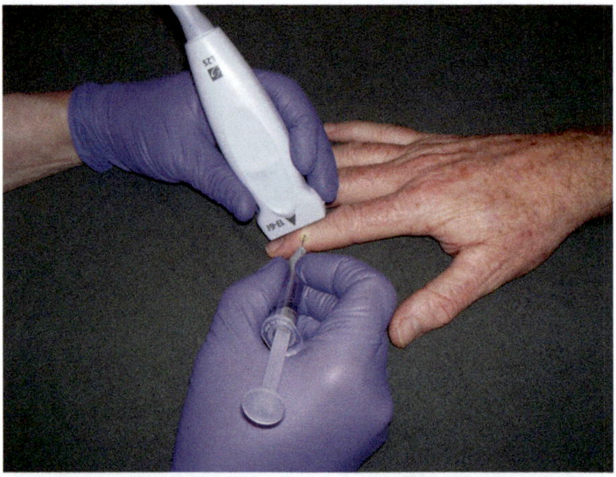

Fig. 9.36 Probe placement for distal interphalangeal joint (DIP). The probe is placed in the long axis on the extensor surface of the DIP joint and the joint space identified

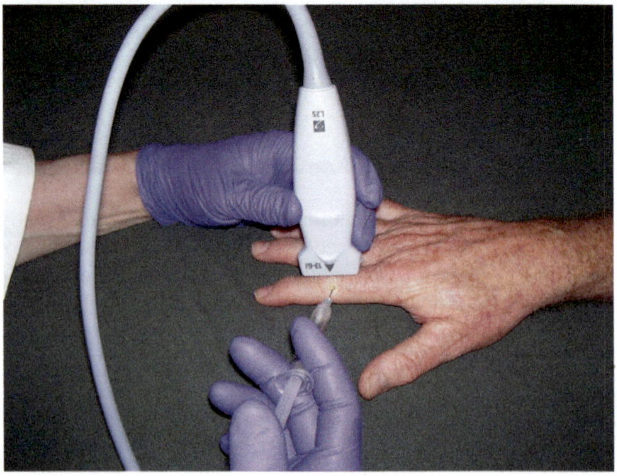

Fig. 9.37 Probe placement for proximal interphalangeal joint (PIP). The probe is placed in the long axis on the extensor surface of the DIP joint and the joint space identified

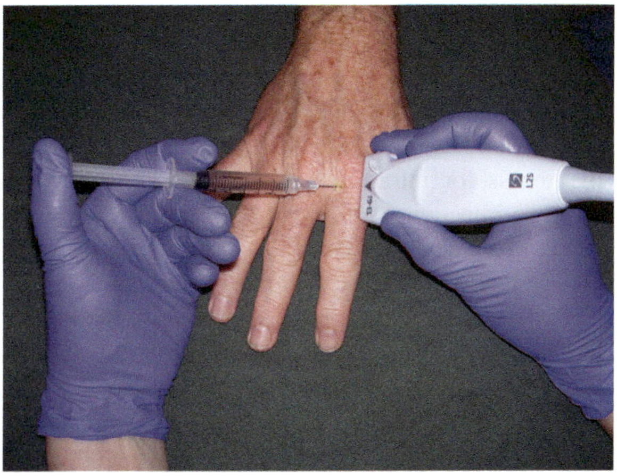

Fig. 9.38 Probe placement for metacarpophalangeal joint (MCP). The probe is placed in the long axis on the extensor surface of the MCP joint and the joint space identified

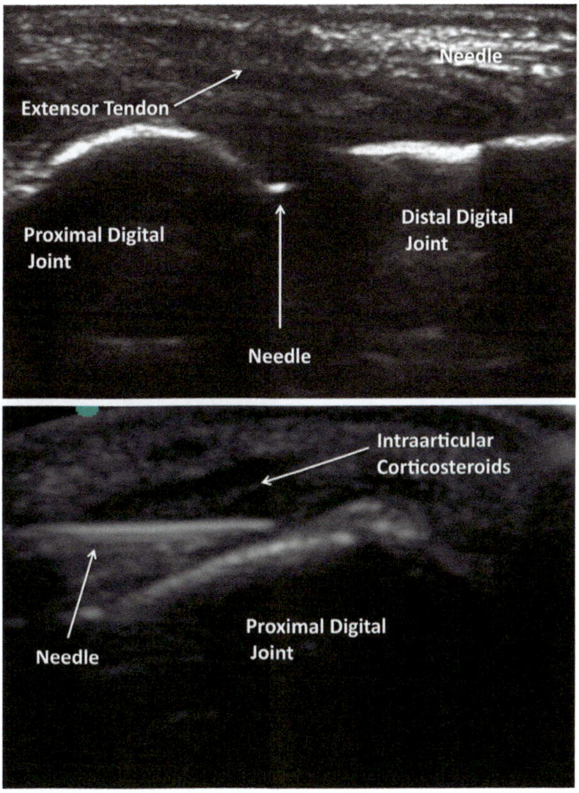

Fig. 9.39 Needle placement of small joints of the hands and feet. A 5/8–1 inch 25 or 27 g needle on a 3 ml syringe with 1 ml lidocaine is placed out-of-plane transversely about ¼ down the digit width and advanced until the tip can be seen out-of-plane in the joint and not in the tendon, and then lidocaine is injected. If the joint space does not dilate, then the needle is pulled back slightly, directed slightly deeper, and angled proximally, the probe is rotated so it is in-plane with the needle, and the needle tip is advanced to the proximal cartilage surface, and lidocaine is again injected, and if dilation of the joint space is seen, corticosteroid is injected

out-of-plane transversely about ¼ down the digit width and advanced until the tip can be seen out-of-plane in the joint and not in the tendon, and then lidocaine is injected (Fig. 9.39). If the joint space dilates, then a syringe exchange can be performed and corticosteroid is injected. If the joint space does not dilate, then the needle is pulled back slightly, directed slightly deeper, and angled proximally, the probe is rotated so it is in-plane with the needle, and the needle tip is advanced to the proximal cartilage surface and lidocaine is again injected; if dilation of the joint space is seen, corticosteroid is injected. Alternatively, the MCP and IP joints can be injected in the long axis in-plane approach where the needle is directed toward the convex surface of the proximal portion of the joint or to the distal concave surface, the recess, or intra-articular space [147]. USG injections relative to ALMPG improve injection accuracy of MCP joints from 80% to 100% and IP joints from 50% to 96% and arthrocentesis success from 0% to 63% [29].

DIP or IP cysts (so-called mucous cysts or myxoid cysts) that usually originate from the osteoarthritic joint do not usually need to be treated surgically as is traditional; rather, the affected IP joint is injected (not the cyst itself) using the same technique as above. During injection of the IP joint, the cyst will turn white with reflux of the corticosteroid crystal from the joint to the cyst (Fig. 9.40). If the cyst has ruptured or was penetrated by a needle and evacuated with external pressure before the procedure, steroid crystals will spill out of the ruptured area during the injection, but usually do not become infected. The procedure may be repeated with recurrence and surgery reserved for intractable or infected cases.

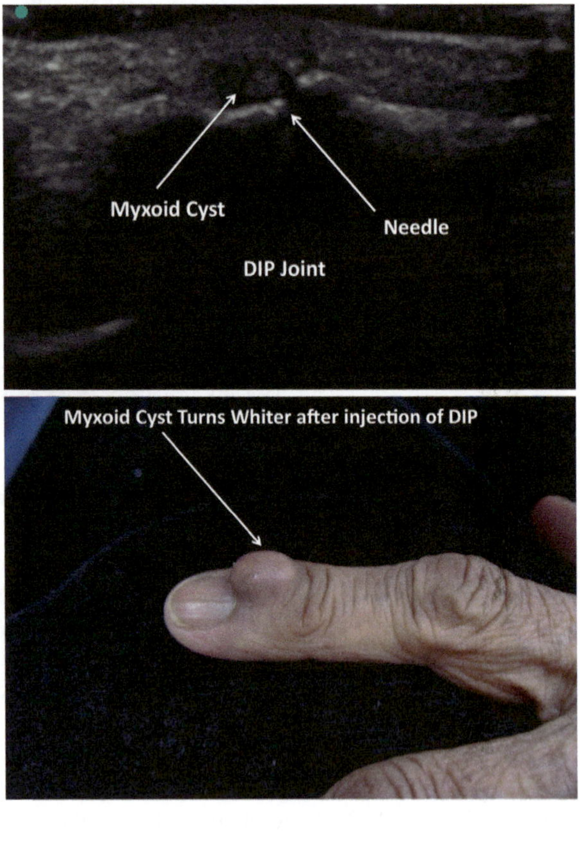

Fig. 9.40 Injection of DIP for myxoid cyst. The affected IP joint is injected (not the cyst itself) using the same technique as above. During injection of the IP joint, the cyst will turn white with reflux of the corticosteroid crystal from the joint to the cyst

Hip Procedures

Ultrasound-Guided Hip Joint Injection

USG procedures of the hip have been recently reviewed [3, 5, 7, 11, 14, 19, 148–150]. The patient is lying supine, and the anterior iliac crest, pubis, inguinal ligament, femoral artery and are identified by palpation and with US using a curvilinear probe (Fig. 9.41). After the above structures are identified, the probe is moved distally until the acetabulum and femoral head are identified. Then the probe is placed in-plane with the anterior femoral head and neck, where the anterior hip synovial recess is visualized. The proximal femoral neck is the target of the USG needle, not the acetabular-femoral joint. It is wise to use Doppler to identify any variant arteries that are in the pathway of the needle prior to the procedure. The length of needle required can be estimated by the metrics of the image or measurement software in the US unit. Usually a 3.5–4 inch length needle will access the anterior hip joint capsule, but longer needles may be necessary based on the adiposity of the patient. The needle is introduced in-plane at a 30 to 45 degree angle with the skin surface and is directed by US visualization to the femoral neck just distal to the acetabular labrum through the joint capsule (Fig. 9.42). When the needle contacts the fibrous capsule on the femoral neck, this should be observed by US, palpated through the needle as resistance, and may cause pain for the patient. USG hip injections have been reported to be 97–100% accurate [7, 49, 151]. The overall effectiveness of USG hip injections is currently being studied in controlled trials, but the safety of ALMPG hip injections is obviously suspect [152].

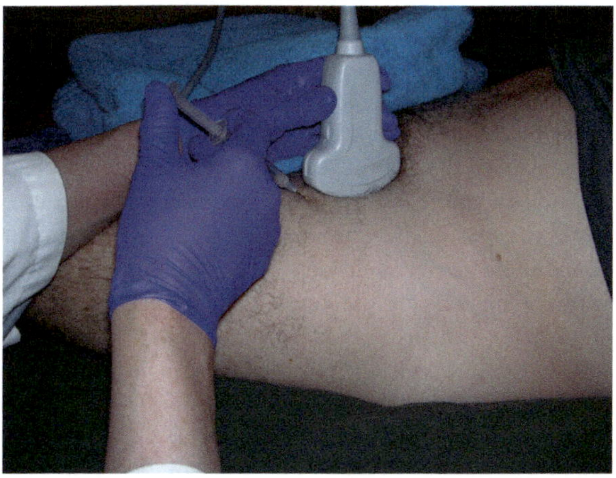

Fig. 9.41 Probe placement for the hip. The probe is placed in-plane with the femoral neck, and the anterior femoral neck adjoining the femoral head is identified as the target where the hip synovial recess resides, and the proximal femoral neck is then the target of the needle, not the acetabular-femoral joint

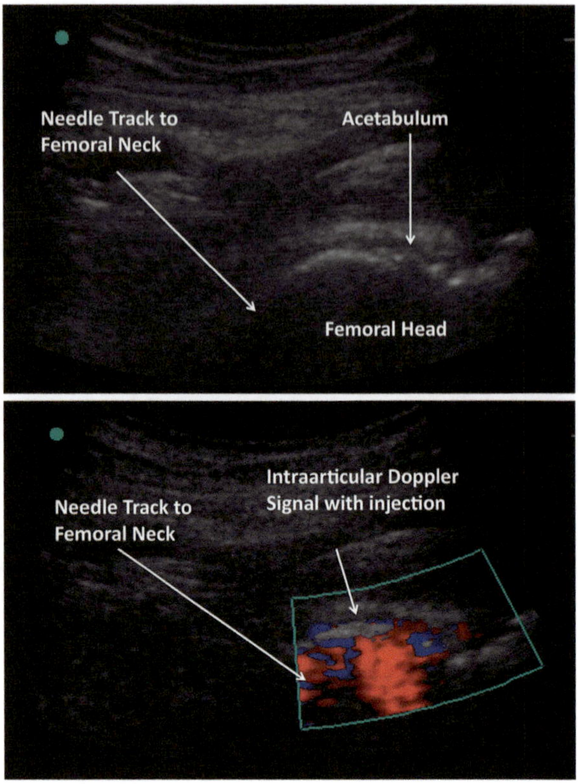

Fig. 9.42 Needle placement for the hip. The needle is introduced in-plane at a 30–45% angle with the skin surface and is directed by US visualization to the femoral neck. The needle can visualized either by US conventionally, by needle visualization software-hardware of the US unit, by indirect observation of movement of the tissues as needle passes through, and/or by observing US signal at the tip of the needle by injection of lidocaine

US-Guided Trochanteric Bursa Injections

USG injection of the trochanteric bursa has recently been reviewed [153]. The patient is placed in the lateral recumbent position with the symptomatic hip up, the hip is flexed 40 degrees, and the knee is flexed 75 degrees. The trochanteric bursa is located over the lateral aspect of the greater trochanter of the femur, and there should be tenderness in this area to justify a procedure. The superficial trochanteric bursa is superficial to the insertion of the gluteus medius tendon insertion, and the deep trochanter bursa is deep to the insertion. A linear or curvilinear probe is placed in the long axis of the femur and moved proximally to the greater trochanter (Fig. 9.43). If effusive trochanteric bursitis is present, it will be an echogenic void near the tendinous insertions; however, in most cases a heterogenous signal or thickening in the gluteal tendon and insertion or in the adjacent subcutaneous tissue is noted indicating gluteal tendinosis or painful fibroadipose tissue rather than true bursitis or inflammation [154–156] (Fig. 9.44). A 2 inch length, 25 or 22 G needle is inserted in-plane or out-of-plane with the probe, and the trochanteric bursa is injected if bursitis is present or if there is reproducible tenderness in the greater trochanter region near area of bursa is present. Forceful injection under high pressure into the insertion of the gluteus medius is not recommended and may induce rupture of the tendon and hemorrhage.

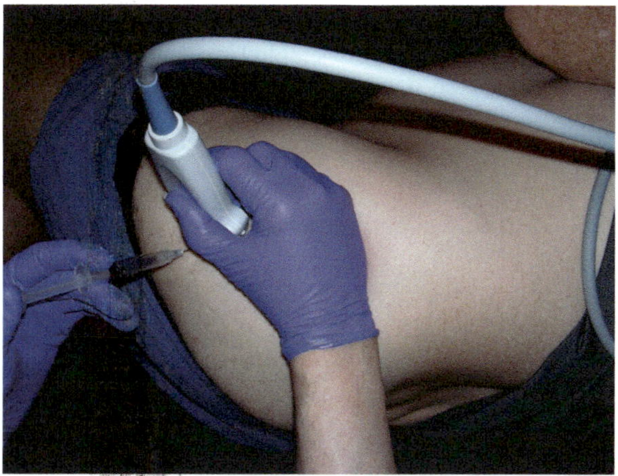

Fig. 9.43 Probe placement for the trochanteric bursa. Usually a curvilinear probe is placed in the long axis of the femur and moved proximally to the greater trochanter. The needle entry can be in-plane or out-of-plane

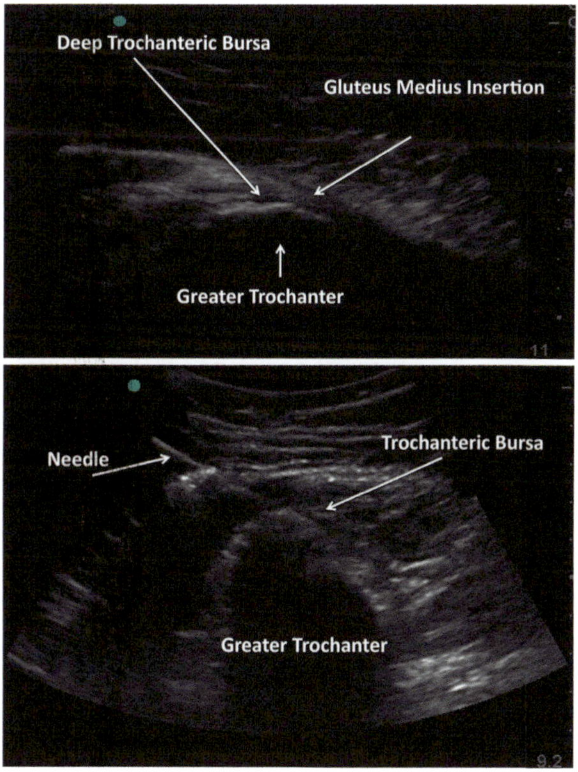

Fig. 9.44 Needle placement for the greater trochanter. If effusive trochanteric bursitis is present, it will be an echogenic void near the tendinous insertions; however, in most cases a heterogenous signal or thickening in the gluteal tendon and insertion or in the adjacent subcutaneous tissue is noted indicating gluteal tendinosis or painful fibroadipose tissue rather than true bursitis or inflammation. A 2 inch 25 or 22 gauge needle is inserted in-plane or out-of-plane with the probe, and the trochanteric bursa is injected if bursitis is present, or if bursitis is not present, the subcutaneous tissue interface with the tendinous insertion is injected

McEvoy et al. reported that true trochanteric bursal injections were more effective than subgluteus medius bursal injections [157]. Brinks et al. demonstrated that injection improves short-term, but not long-term greater trochanter pain [158]. Cohen et al. and Michell et al. demonstrated no improvement of image or USG guidance over standard ALMPG injection of the trochanteric bursa but markedly increased costs and USG should be reserved for extreme obesity and prior ALMPG failure [79, 159]. Jacobson et al. have demonstrated that USG injections of PRP and USG fenestration of the gluteal tendon are both effective for trochanteric pain [160].

US-Guided Sacroiliac Joint Injections

USG procedures of the sacroiliac (SI) joints, spine, and pelvis have been recently reviewed [3, 5, 123, 161–163]. For SI joint injections, the patient lies prone with a towel bolster placed under the upper pelvis and stomach (Fig. 9.45). The posterior superior iliac spine is palpated, and at this level, with a linear or curvilinear probe set for 7–9 cm depth, the probe is placed in the transverse orientation on the mid-dorsum spinous process of the sacrum and then moved laterally until the posterior superior iliac spine is identified, and then the probe is moved inferiorly (Fig. 9.45). The void between the posterior superior iliac crest and medial border of the plate of the sacrum is the SI joint with tracks (Fig. 9.46). A 3 to 4 inch, 22–25 G needle is advanced perpendicularly to the skin in an out-of-plane approach with the probe angled in a slightly lateral direction (if on the superior SI joint) or medial direction (if on the inferior SI joint), and slide the needle into the SI joint. And when injected, the joint capsule expands or fluid is seen tracking in the SI joint. The inferior portion of SI joint is synovial and thus can accommodate a greater volume of fluid than the upper fibrosis portion. The joint can also be injected in-plane by identifying the SI joint as above, and the needle is advanced under the probe at a 30 to 45 degree angle

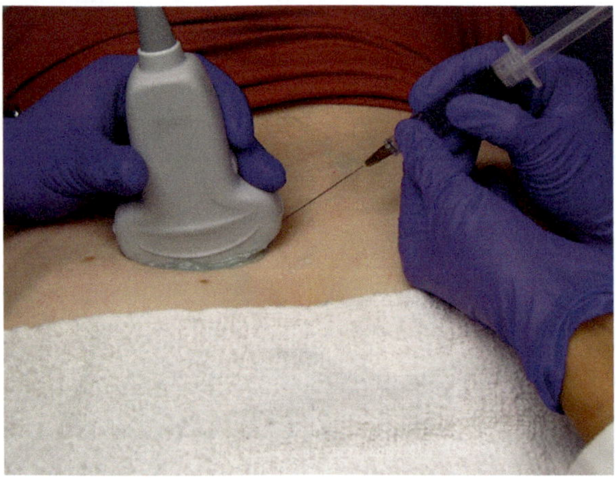

Fig. 9.45 Probe placement for the sacroiliac joints. The patient lies prone with a towel bolster placed under the upper pelvis and stomach. The posterior superior iliac spine is palpated, and at this level, with a linear or curvilinear probe set for 7–9 cm depth, probe is placed in the transverse orientation on the mid-dorsum spinous process of the sacrum and then moved laterally until the posterior superior iliac spine is identified and then the probe is moved inferiorly

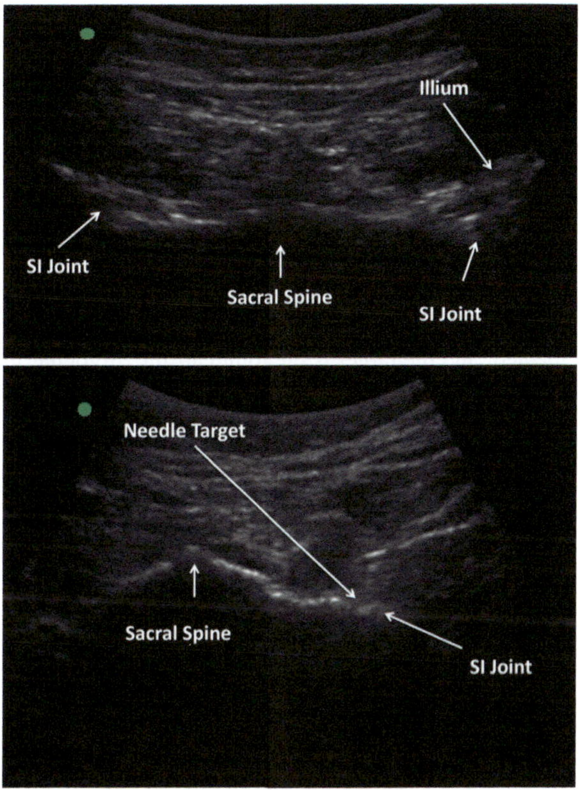

Fig. 9.46 Needle placement for the sacroiliac joints. A 3–4 inch 22–25 gauge needle on a 5 ml syringe with 1% lidocaine is advanced perpendicularly to the skin but out-of-plane probe in to a slightly lateral direction (if on the superior SI joint) or medial direction (if on the inferior SI joint), and slide the needle into the SI joint and then inject lidocaine until the joint capsule expands or fluid is seen tracking in SI joint

and can be injected once joint is confirmed. Jee et al. reported that USG SI injection had an accuracy of 83%, but this was lower than fluoroscopy (98.2%) [164]. Hartung et al. reported that USG SI injection in inflammatory arthritis was only 40% accurate but that intra-articular and periarticular injections had the same outcome [165]. Pekkafahli reported there is a flat learning curve for SI injections with 60% accuracy in the first 30 injections and 93.5% in the second 30 injections, indicating that experience is important in SI injections [166]. Other USG injections of the axial spine and pelvis including facet joints, epidural injections, pubic ramus, ischial bursa, and many other can be performed but are beyond the scope of this chapter. These injections have been recently reviewed [5, 123, 161–163, 167].

US-Guided Procedures of the Foot and Ankle

USG injections of the foot and ankle have recently been reviewed [168–172]. In general a careful history, physical examination, and conventional radiographs are performed and reviewed in addition to US examination before performing invasive procedures on the foot due to the high rate of stress fractures, neuropathic lesions, ischemic lesions, and infection of the foot. Furthermore, a skin examination should be performed inspecting the toes, toenails, periungual, interdigital, and weight-bearing areas as tinea pedis, onychomycosis, ingrown toenails, and ulcerations (ischemic, diabetic, traumatic, venous insufficiency) all predispose to infection (especially cellulitis, septic joint and tenosynovitis, and osteomyelitis), and other foot disorders and, if present, may modify or prohibit an USG needle procedure.

Ultrasound-Guided Tibiotalar Ankle Joint Injection

The patient is usually supine with the foot in the neutral position (30% plantar flexed). With the probe in the long axis of the foot, the ankle (tibiotalar) joint is located, and the target is the joint capsule, tibiotalar junction, or anterior surface of the talus between the two malleoli (Fig. 9.47). The dorsalis pedis artery (by Doppler or pulsations) and peroneal nerve and overlying veins are identified so they can be avoided, and the needle approach into the tibiotalar joint can be from either the anteromedial or anterolateral approach (Fig. 9.48). Typically in the dry joint a 25 to 22 G, 1.5 to 2 inch needle is advanced in the long or short axis with the probe in the long axis of the foot until needle tip is in the tibiotalar joint recess and the tibiotalar cartilage junction or touches the concave surface of the talus. Wisniewski et al. have demonstrated that USG improves tibiotalar injections from 85% to 100% [54], while Khosla et al. reported that ALPG and USG were similar in accuracy [55]. Peters et al. have demonstrated the USG provides improved outcomes in the foot and ankle in juvenile idiopathic arthritis [173].

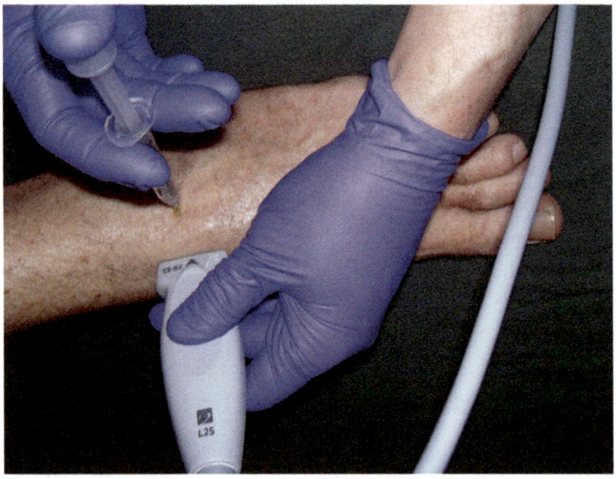

Fig. 9.47 Probe placement for the ankle. With the probe in the long axis of the foot, the ankle (tibiotalar) joint is located, and the target is the joint capsule, tibiotalar junction, or anterior surface of the talus between the two malleoli

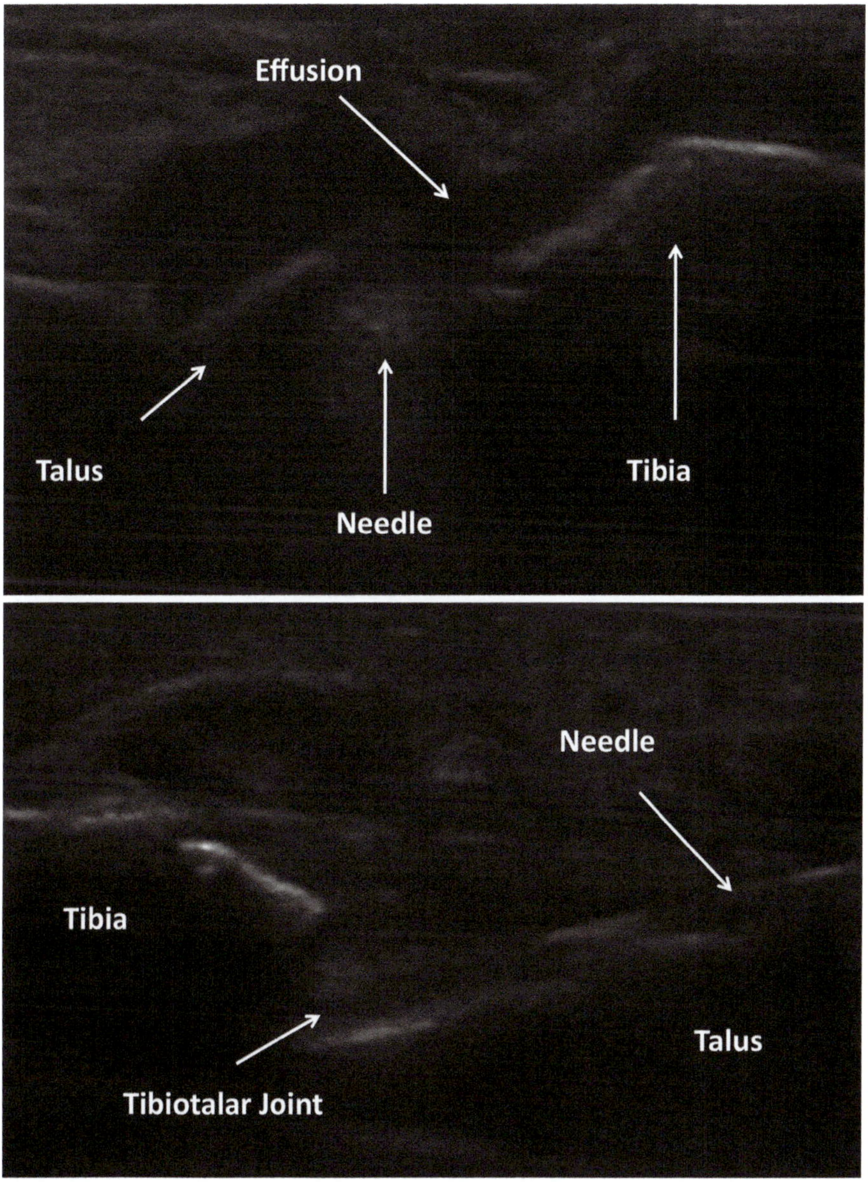

Fig. 9.48 Needle placement for the ankle. Typically in the dry joint, a 25 g to 22 g 1.5 to 2 inch needle is advanced in the long or short axis with the probe in the long axis of the foot until needle tip is in the tibiotalar joint recess, the tibiotalar cartilage junction, or touches the concave surface of the talus, and then lidocaine is injected until the synovial membrane can be seen to lift off the surface of the talus

Ultrasound-Guided Injections of the Subtalar, Tarsonavicular, and Other Midfoot Joints

USG injections of the subtalar (talocalcaneal) joint can be performed by anterolateral, posterolateral, or posterior medial approaches with similar accuracy (Smith 2009). However, the subtalar joint is usually injected anterolateral below the distal anterior fibula with the probe placed in the long axis of the foot with the needle injected in an out-of-plane approach. The talonavicular, calcaneocuboid, tarsometatarsal, naviculocuneiform, and tarsometatarsal joints are injected using an identical technique. Wisniewski et al. have demonstrated that US-guidance improves subtalar joint and sinus tarsus (recess in subtalar joint) from 35% to 90% [54, 174]. US-guidance improves accuracy of the tarsometatarsal joint injections from 25% to 64% [55].

Ultrasound-Guided Tarsal Tunnel Injection

The tarsal tunnel, analogous to the carpal tunnel, is defined by the medial malleolus and a constraining structure, the flexor retinaculum, through which the tibial artery, flexor hallucis longus, tibialis posterior and flexor digitorum longus tendons, and posterior tibial nerve passes and can be compressed, resulting in numbness, tingling, burning sensation, pain, and paresthesias in the base of the foot in the distribution of the plantar nerve worsening with weight-bearing [175]. Eliciting a positive Tinel's sign by tapping over the tarsal tunnel typically causes discomfort in the medial one third of the distal plantar foot, although the entire plantar foot surface may be affected. US should determine whether there is a cyst that should be specifically injected or the tarsal tunnel generally injected. The probe is placed posterior to the medial malleolus in the long axis or across the tarsal tunnel in the short axis so that all the anatomy is in cross section and the needle is in the long axis (Fig. 9.49). A 25 G needle is advanced in a 30 degree angle under the probe through the

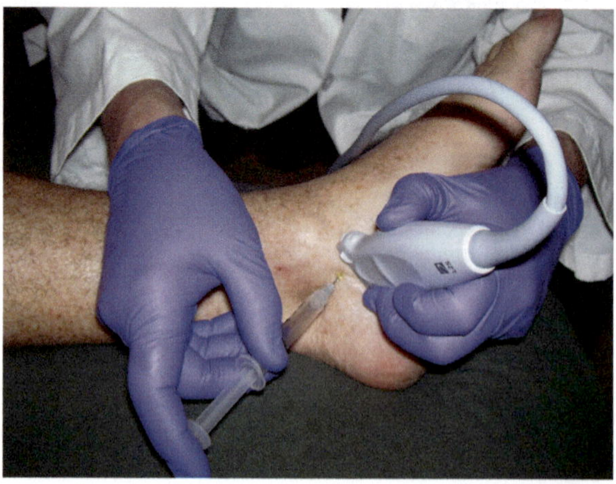

Fig. 9.49 Probe placement for the tarsal tunnel. The probe is placed posterior to the medial malleolus in the long axis or across the tarsal tunnel in the short axis so that all the anatomy is in cross section and the needle is the long axis

retinaculum, injecting lidocaine to separate the tendon sheath, expand the tarsal tunnel, and push the artery and nerve away from the needle tip and confirm that the injection is within the tunnel. Then syringe exchange is performed, and corticosteroid is injected between the tendon sheaths.

Ultrasound-Guided Peroneal Tendon Sheath Injection

The peroneal tendon sheath runs inferior to the lateral malleolus where it can be injected using a technique similar to injecting the tarsal tunnel as noted above, except from the lateral side. Muir et al. have demonstrated that US-guidance improves peroneal tendon sheath injection accuracy from 60% to 100% [56].

Ultrasound-Guided Achilles Tendon and Associated Bursae Injections

The Achilles tendon, retrocalcaneal (pre-Achilles) bursa, and subcutaneous calcaneal bursa can be diagnostically aspirated with US-guidance, but are usually not injected with corticosteroid due to the high Achilles tendon rupture rate [176]. However, high-volume (50 ml) saline mixture (HVIGI) or autologous platelet-rich plasma (APRP) is sometimes injected by sports medicine physicians into the paratenon or tendon itself without increased rupture rates [1, 177, 178]. With the patient prone with the foot hanging off the examining table, so that the foot is passively neutral, the probe is placed in the long axis of the Achilles tendon over or proximal to the calcaneus, and the needle penetrates superior to the calcaneus and is directed inferiorly under the probe in the long axis through the tendon sheath (peritendinous space) toward the area of Achilles tendinopathy (either intratendinous or insertional), and area of the tendinopathy or necrosis is hydrodissected with PRP [179]. USG injections improve the accuracy of Achilles tendon injections to 100% [174].

Ultrasound-Guided Calcaneus and Plantar Fascia Injections

The plantar fascia is best identified with the probe on the long axis of plantar foot on the distal aspect of the inferior calcaneus (Fig. 9.50). The target for injection is the perifascial area of insertion of the plantar fascia onto the calcaneus, penetrating the medial foot medial to lateral or medially but directing the needle posteriorly to the calcaneus. The goal is to *not* place the corticosteroid in the calcaneal fat pad where fat atrophy can be disabling but rather superior to the fat pad. A 25 or 27 G needle tip is best placed directly above the superior surface of the fascia, first injecting a small amount (maximum 1 ml of lidocaine) to hydrodisplace blood vessels and nerves out of the way and create a small space for the corticosteroid, and then perform a syringe exchange and a small volume (0.5–1 ml) of corticosteroid. No more than 1.5 to 2 ml total should be used to inject the plantar fascia to prevent painful dissection of the fat pad with weight bearing which can interfere with

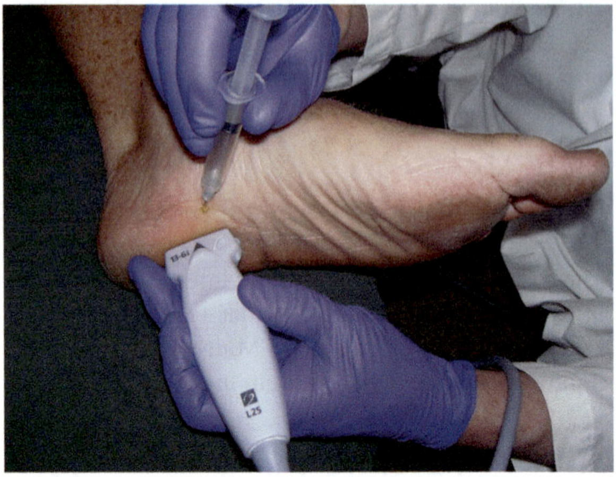

Fig. 9.50 Probe placement for the plantar fascia. The plantar fascia is best identified with the probe on the long axis of plantar foot on the distal aspect of the inferior calcaneus. The target for injection is perifascial area of insertion of the plantar fascia onto the calcaneus, penetrating the medial foot medial to lateral or medially but directing the needle posteriorly to the calcaneus

ambulation. Maida et al. demonstrated that even 1.5 ml of injectate can migrate along the fascial, tendinous, and nerve structures [180]. In a randomized control trial, Chen et al. and Tsai et al. concluded that USGI of the plantar fascia was more effective than ALPMG injection [69, 70], an observation that has been confirmed is meta-analysis by [71]. On the other hand, Ball et al. and Yucel et al. found no difference between USG injection and ALPMG injection [72, 73].

Ultrasound-Guided Morton's Neuroma Injection

Morton's neuroma appears as an anechoic or hypoechoic mass within the intermetatarsal space near the interdigital nerves in the foot. The mass can move dorsally with compression of the metatarsals (Mulder's sign) and can be injected with US-guidance with excellent effect [181]. The lesion can be visualized either plantarly or dorsally usually with the probe in the transverse plane; the 25 G, 1.5 inch needle can be advanced into the lesion either in-plane or out-of-plane, with careful attention to avoid injecting nearby neurovascular and tendon structures. Corticosteroid or sclerosing solutions are injected into the center of the neuroma [175]. Morgan et al. performed a systematic literature review and concluded that USG injections produces better short- and long-term pain relief for corticosteroid injections, reduces the need for additional procedures in a series of sclerosing alcohol injections, reduces the surgical referral rate, and adds efficacy to a single injection [182].

Ultrasound-Guided Injections of Metatarsophalangeal and Interphalangeal Joints

USG MTP and IP joints in the foot are injected in a similar way to small joints in the hands [183]. USG corticosteroid injections can be provided with either in-plane or out-of-plane approaches (Fig. 9.51a, b). Sahler et al. describes a longitudinal in-plane approach to the MTP joints [147].

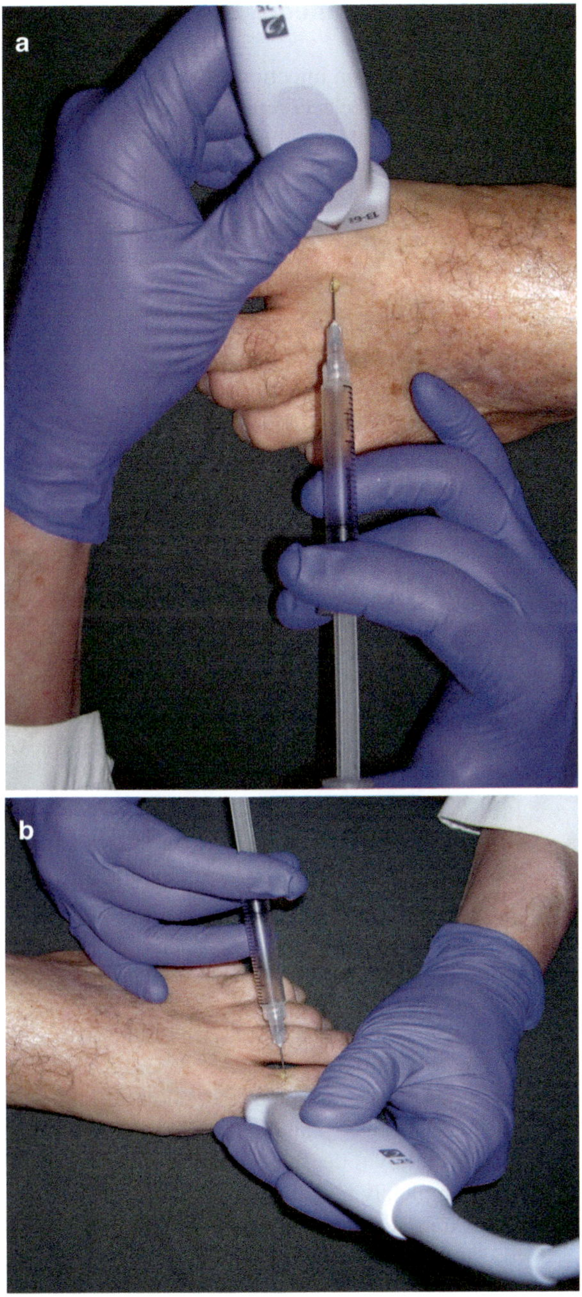

Fig. 9.51 (**a**, **b**) Probe placement for the small joints of the foot. The IP and MTP joints in the foot are injected with USG in a similar way to small joints in the hands

US-Guided Percutaneous Biopsy

Needle biopsy and/or injection of muscle, tumor, synovial tissue, parotid gland, lipoma, and fat can be accomplished in similar techniques to USG aspiration procedures but are beyond the scope of the current chapter and have been reviewed elsewhere [21, 88, 184–190].

Conclusion

USG needle procedures teach the provider anatomy, permit procedures based on a more accurate diagnosis, markedly reduce procedural pain, improve diagnostic and therapeutic arthrocentesis success, permit more accurate needle placement, improve therapeutic outcomes, improve procedural safety, and may improve cost-effectiveness, especially in more complicated cases.

Review Questions

1. The procedure needle tip and shaft is best visualized:
   (a) In-plane with the probe at 45° to the ultrasound beam
   (b) Out-of-plane with the probe at 45° to the ultrasound beam
   (c) In-plane with the probe and at right angles (90°) to the ultrasound beam
   (d) In-plane with the probe at a steep angle to the ultrasound beam
2. What safety measures can be undertaken to prevent infections in the puncture site during USG procedures?
   (a) Make certain the ultrasound gel covers the puncture site.
   (b) Use a longer needle to traverse the gel before it penetrates the skin.
   (c) Use a longer needle to keep the puncture site away from the gel.
   (d) Use a condom on the probe and then traverse the ultrasound gel with the needle.
3. In hip joint injections, the procedure needle should be directed into the:
   (a) Acetabulofemoral joint
   (b) Greater trochanter
   (c) Acetabular labrum
   (d) Synovial recess of the femoral neck
4. The needle out-of-plane of the ultrasound beam appears as:
   (a) A brightly reflective circle, crescent, or rim
   (b) Completely invisible
   (c) A long reflective shaft
   (d) A series of reflective ghosts
5. USG procedures compared to ALMPG are *not*:
   (a) More accurate
   (b) More painful
   (c) More costly per procedure
   (d) As safe

6. In an abnormal shoulder with rotator cuff pathology/tears, if you inject medication into the subacromial bursa, where else may you also see injectate?
   (a) Bicipital tendon sheath
   (b) Glenohumeral joint
   (c) Medication stays only in the subacromial bursa
   (d) Supraspinatus tendon
7. Which USG needle approach method is *not* recommended for carpal tunnel injections?
   (a) Probe in transverse view of the median nerve, needle in-plane ulnar approach
   (b) Probe in transverse view of the median nerve, needle in-plane radial approach
   (c) Probe in transverse view of the median nerve, needle out-of-plane approach
   (d) Probe in longitudinal view of the median nerve, needle in-plane approach
8. For aspiration procedures, the best reimbursable indication to use ultrasound guidance is to:
   (a) Enhance standard anatomic palpation-guided approaches to joint aspiration.
   (b) Visualize the needle in normal anatomic structures for accuracy.
   (c) Make the aspiration less painful.
   (d) Confirm fluid to be aspirated and direct the needle into the fluid, in a previously failed anatomic palpation-guided aspiration.
9. If a flexible procedure needle on a syringe is angling away from the intended forward target, the best technique to redirect it is:
   (a) Forcefully point the syringe in the direction of the target.
   (b) Forcefully point the syringe in direction of the angling needle.
   (c) Pull back slightly, and point the syringe in the direction of the target.
   (d) Pull back slightly, and point the syringe in the direction of the angling needle.
10. In USG needle procedures, bubbles in the fluid in the syringe are:
   (a) Useful as US contrast to see where the needle tip is.
   (b) A dangerous source of infection.
   (c) Indicate contamination of the lidocaine or corticosteroid.
   (d) Should be expelled before the procedure because injected bubbles interfere with US imaging.

Answers

1. (c) In-plane with the probe and at right angles (90°) to the ultrasound beam
2. (c) Use a longer needle to keep the puncture site away from the gel.
3. (d) Synovial recess of the femoral neck
4. (a) A brightly reflective circle, crescent, or rim
5. (b) More painful.
6. (b) Glenohumeral joint
7. (c) Probe in transverse view of the median nerve, needle out-of-plane approach.

8. (d) Confirm fluid to be aspirated and direct the needle into the fluid, in a previously failed anatomic palpation-guided aspiration.
9. (d) Pull back slightly, and point the syringe in the direction of the angling needle.
10. (d) Should be expelled before the procedure because injected bubbles interfere with US imaging

References

1. Barile A, La Marra A, Arrigoni F, Mariani S, Zugaro L, Splendiani A, Di Cesare E, Reginelli A, Zappia M, Brunese L, Duka E, Carrafiello G, Masciocchi C. Anaesthetics, steroids and platelet-rich plasma (PRP) in ultrasound-guided musculoskeletalprocedures. Br J Radiol. 2016;89(1065):20150355. https://doi.org/10.1259/bjr.20150355. Epub 2016 Jul 7
2. Boniface KS, Ajmera K, Cohen JS, Liu YT, Shokoohi H. Ultrasound-guided arthrocentesis of the elbow: a posterior approach. J Emerg Med. 2013;45(5):698–701.
3. Chang KV, Wu WT, Lew HL, Özçakar L. Ultrasound imaging and guided injection for the lateral and posterior hip. Am J Phys Med Rehabil. 2018;97(4):285–91.
4. Chianca V, Orlandi D, Messina C, Albano D, Corazza A, Rapisarda S, Pozzi G, Cazzato RL, Mauri G, Silvestri E, Sconfienza LM. Interventional therapeutic procedures to treat degenerative and inflammatory musculoskeletal conditions: state of the art. Radiol Med. 2019; https://doi.org/10.1007/s11547-019-01018-8. [Epub ahead of print]
5. Chen CP, Lew HL, Tsai WC, Hung YT, Hsu CC. Ultrasound-guided injection techniques for the low back and hip joint. Am J Phys Med Rehabil. 2011;90(10):860–7.
6. Delle Sedie A, Riente L, Iagnocco A, Carli L, Ceccarelli F, Di Geso L, Filippucci E, Sakellariou G, Bombardieri S. Ultrasound imaging for the rheumatologist XLVI. Ultrasound guided injection in the shoulder: a descriptive literature review. Clin Exp Rheumatol. 2013;31(4):477–83. Epub 2013 Jul 29
7. Epis O, Bruschi E. Interventional ultrasound: a critical overview on ultrasound-guided injections and biopsies. Clin Exp Rheumatol. 2014;32(1 Suppl 80):S78–84.
8. Finnoff JT. The evolution of diagnostic and interventional ultrasound in sports medicine. PM R. 2016;8(3 Suppl):S133–8.
9. Finnoff JT, Hall MM, Adams E, Berkoff D, Concoff AL, Dexter W, Smith J, American Medical Society for Sports Medicine. American Medical Society for Sports Medicine position statement: interventional musculoskeletal ultrasound in sports medicine. Clin J Sport Med. 2015a;25(1):6–22.
10. Finnoff JT, Hall MM, Adams E, Berkoff D, Concoff AL, Dexter W, Smith J. American Medical Society for Sports Medicine (AMSSM) position statement: interventional musculoskeletal ultrasound in sports medicine. Br J Sports Med. 2015b;49(3):145–50.
11. Jacobson JA, Bedi A, Sekiya JK, Blankenbaker DG. Evaluation of the painful athletic hip: imaging options and imaging-guided injections. AJR Am J Roentgenol. 2012;199(3):516–24.
12. Kim TK, Lee JH, Park KD, Lee SC, Ahn J, Park Y. Ultrasound versus palpation guidance for intra-articular injections in patients with degenerative osteoarthritis of the elbow. J Clin Ultrasound. 2013b;41(8):479–85.
13. Kumar Sahu A, Rath P, Aggarwal B. Ultrasound-guided injections in musculo-skeletal system – an overview. J Clin Orthop Trauma. 2019;10(4):669–73.
14. Nestorova R, Vlad V, Petranova T, Porta F, Radunovic G, Micu MC, Iagnocco A. Ultrasonography of the hip. Med Ultrason. 2012;14(3):217–24.
15. Nwawka OK. Update in musculoskeletal ultrasound research. Sports Health. 2016;8(5):429–37.
16. Peng PW, Cheng P. Ultrasound-guided interventional procedures in pain medicine: a review of anatomy, sonoanatomy, and procedures. Part III: shoulder. Reg Anesth Pain Med. 2011;36(6):592–605.

17. Rand E, Welbel R, Visco CJ. Fundamental considerations for ultrasound-guided musculoskeletal interventions. Phys Med Rehabil Clin N Am. 2016;27(3):539–53.
18. Robotti G, Canepa MG, Bortolotto C, Draghi F. Interventional musculoskeletal US: an update on materials and methods. J Ultrasound. 2013;16(2):45–55.
19. Rowbotham EL, Grainger AJ. Ultrasound-guided intervention around the hip joint. AJR Am J Roentgenol. 2011;197(1):W122–7.
20. Royall NA, Farrin E, Bahner DP, Stawicki SP. Ultrasound-assisted musculoskeletal procedures: a practical overview of current literature. World J Orthop. 2011;2(7):57–66.
21. Sperandeo M, Trovato FM, Melillo N, Dimitri L, Musumeci G, Guglielmi G. The role of ultrasound-guided fine needle aspiration biopsy in musculoskeletal diseases. Eur J Radiol. 2017;90:234–44.
22. Tagliafico A, Russo G, Boccalini S, Michaud J, Klauser A, Serafini G, Martinoli C. Ultrasound-guided interventional procedures around the shoulder. Radiol Med. 2014;119(5):318–26. https://doi.org/10.1007/s11547-013-0351-2. Epub 2013 Dec 3. PMID: 24297588.
23. Smith J, Finnoff JT. Diagnostic and interventional musculoskeletal ultrasound: part 1. Fundamentals. PM R. 2009a Jan;1(1):64-75. https://doi.org/10.1016/j.pmrj.2008.09.001. PMID: 19627875.
24. Kane D, Koski J. Musculoskeletal interventional procedures: with or without imaging guidance? Best Pract Res Clin Rheumatol. 2016;30(4):736–50.
25. Delaunoy I, Feipel V, Appelboom T, Hauzeur JP. Sonography detection threshold for knee effusion. Clin Rheumatol. 2003;22:391–2.
26. Ike RW, Somers EC, Arnold EL, Arnold WJ. Ultrasound of the knee during voluntary quadriceps contraction: a technique for detecting otherwise occult effusions. Arthritis Care Res (Hoboken). 2010;62(5):725–9.
27. Kane D, Balint PV, Sturrock RD. Ultrasonography is superior to clinical examination in the detection and localization of knee joint effusion in rheumatoid arthritis. J Rheumatol. 2003;30:966–71.
28. Balint PV, Kane D, Hunter J, McInnes IB, Field M, Sturrock RD. Ultrasound guided versus conventional joint and soft tissue fluid aspiration in rheumatology practice: a pilot study. J Rheumatol. 2002;29:2209–13.
29. Raza K, Lee CY, Pilling D, Heaton S, Situnayake RD, Carruthers DM, Buckley CD, Gordon C, Salmon M. Ultrasound guidance allows accurate needle placement and aspiration from small joints in patients with early inflammatory arthritis. Rheumatology (Oxford). 2003;42(8):976–9.
30. Wiler JL, Costantino TG, Filippone L, Satz W. Comparison of ultrasound-guided and standard landmark techniques for knee arthrocentesis. J Emerg Med. 2010;39(1):76–82.
31. Sibbitt WL Jr, Kettwich LG, Band PA, Chavez-Chiang NR, DeLea SL, Haseler LJ, Bankhurst AD. Does ultrasound guidance improve the outcomes of arthrocentesis and corticosteroid injection of the knee? Scand J Rheumatol. 2012;41(1):66–72.
32. Wu T, Dong Y, Song HX, Fu Y, Li JH. Ultrasound-guided versus landmark in knee arthrocentesis: a systematic review. Semin Arthritis Rheum. 2016;45(5):627–32.
33. D'Agostino MA, Schmidt WA. Ultrasound-guided injections in rheumatology: actual knowledge on efficacy and procedures. Best Pract Res Clin Rheumatol. 2013;27(2):283–94. https://doi.org/10.1016/j.berh.2013.04.001. PMID: 23731936.
34. Cunnington J, Marshall N, Hide G, Bracewell C, Isaacs J, Platt P, Kane D. A randomized, double-blind, controlled study of ultrasound-guided corticosteroid injection into the joint of patients with inflammatory arthritis. Arthritis Rheum. 2010;62(7):1862–9.
35. Berkoff DJ, Miller LE, Block JE. Clinical utility of ultrasound guidance for intra-articular knee injections: a review. Clin Interv Aging. 2012;7:89–95. https://doi.org/10.2147/CIA.S29265.
36. Maricar N, Parkes MJ, Callaghan MJ, Felson DT, O'Neill TW. Where and how to inject the knee--a systematic review. Semin Arthritis Rheum. 2013;43(2):195–203.
37. Finnoff JT, Nutz DJ, Henning PT, Hollman JH, Smith J. Accuracy of ultrasound-guided versus unguided pes anserinus bursa injections. PM R. 2010;2(8):732–9.

38. Bloom JE, Rischin A, Johnston RV, Buchbinder R. Image-guided versus blind glucocorticoid injection for shoulder pain. Cochrane Database Syst Rev. 2012;8:CD009147.
39. Patel DN, Nayyar S, Hasan S, Khatib O, Sidash S, Jazrawi LM. Comparison of ultrasound-guided versus blind glenohumeral injections: a cadaveric study. J Shoulder Elb Surg. 2012;21(12):1664–8.
40. Amber KT, Landy DC, Amber I, Knopf D, Guerra J. Comparing the accuracy of ultrasound versus fluoroscopy in glenohumeral injections: a systematic review and meta-analysis. J Clin Ultrasound. 2014;42(7):411–6.
41. Borbas P, Kraus T, Clement H, Grechenig S, Weinberg AM, Heidari N. The influence of ultrasound guidance in the rate of success of acromioclavicular joint injection: an experimental study on human cadavers. J Shoulder Elb Surg. 2012;21(12):1694–7.
42. Sabeti-Aschraf M, Lemmerhofer B, Lang S, Schmidt M, Funovics PT, Ziai P, Frenzel S, Kolb A, Graf A, Schueller-Weidekamm C. Ultrasound guidance improves the accuracy of the acromioclavicular joint infiltration: a prospective randomized study. Knee Surg Sports Traumatol Arthrosc. 2011;19(2):292–5.
43. Gazzillo GP, Finnoff JT, Hall MM, Sayeed YA, Smith J. Accuracy of palpating the long head of the biceps tendon: an ultrasonographic study. PM R. 2011;3(11):1035–40.
44. Hashiuchi T, Sakurai G, Morimoto M, Komei T, Takakura Y, Tanaka Y. Accuracy of the biceps tendon sheath injection: ultrasound-guided or unguided injection? A randomized controlled trial. J Shoulder Elb Surg. 2011;20(7):1069–73.
45. Petscavage-Thomas J, Gustas C. Comparison of ultrasound-guided to fluoroscopy-guided biceps tendon sheath therapeutic injection. J Ultrasound Med. 2016;35(10):2217–21.
46. Nam SH, Kim J, Lee JH, Ahn J, Kim YJ, Park Y. Palpation versus ultrasound-guided corticosteroid injections and short-term effect in the distal radioulnar joint disorder: a randomized, prospective single-blinded study. Clin Rheumatol. 2013;33:1807–14. [Epub ahead of print]
47. Dubreuil M, Greger S, LaValley M, Cunnington J, Sibbitt WL Jr, Kissin EY. Improvement in wrist pain with ultrasound-guided glucocorticoid injections: a meta-analysis of individual patient data. Semin Arthritis Rheum. 2013;42(5):492–7.
48. Lohman M, Vasenius J, Nieminen O. Ultrasound guidance for puncture and injection in the radiocarpal joint. Acta Radiol. 2007;48(7):744–7.
49. Smith J, Brault JS, Rizzo M, Sayeed YA, Finnoff JT. Accuracy of sonographically guided and palpation guided scaphotrapeziotrapezoid joint injections. J Ultrasound Med. 2011;30(11):1509–15. https://doi.org/10.7863/jum.2011.30.11.1509. PMID: 22039023.
50. Mandl LA, Hotchkiss RN, Adler RS, Ariola LA, Katz JN. Can the carpometacarpal joint be injected accurately in the office setting? Implications for therapy. J Rheumatol. 2006;33(6):1137–9.
51. McCann PA, Wakeley CJ, Amirfeyz R. The effect of ultrasound guided steroid injection on progression to surgery in thumb CMC arthritis. Hand Surg. 2014;19(1):49–52.
52. Kume K, Amano K, Yamada S, Amano K, Kuwaba N, Ohta H. In de Quervain's with a separate EPB compartment, ultrasound-guided steroid injection is more effective than a clinical injection technique: a prospective open-label study. J Hand Surg Eur Vol. 2012;37(6):523–7.
53. Lee DH, Han SB, Park JW, Lee SH, Kim KW, Jeong WK. Sonographically guided tendon sheath injections are more accurate than blind injections: implications for trigger finger treatment. J Ultrasound Med. 2011;30(2):197–203.
54. Wisniewski SJ, Smith J, Patterson DG, Carmichael SW, Pawlina W. Ultrasound-guided versus nonguided tibiotalar joint and sinus tarsi injections: a cadaveric study. PM R. 2010;2(4):277–81.
55. Khosla S, Thiele R, Baumhauer JF. Ultrasound guidance for intra-articular injections of the foot and ankle. Foot Ankle Int. 2009;30(9):886–90.
56. Muir JJ, Curtiss HM, Hollman J, Smith J, Finnoff JT. The accuracy of ultrasound-guided and palpation-guided peroneal tendon sheath injections. Am J Phys Med Rehabil. 2011;90(7):564–71.
57. Wempe MK, Sellon JL, Sayeed YA, Smith J. Feasibility of first metatarsophalangeal joint injections for sesamoid disorders: a cadaveric investigation. PM R. 2012;4(8):556–60.

58. Gilliland CA, Salazar LD, Borchers JR. Ultrasound versus anatomic guidance for intra-articular and periarticular injection: a systematic review. Phys Sportsmed. 2011;39(3):121–31. https://doi.org/10.3810/psm.2011.09.1928. PMID: 22030948.
59. Sage W, Pickup L, Smith TO, Denton ER, Toms AP. The clinical and functional outcomes of ultrasound-guided vs landmark-guided injections for adults with shoulder pathology–a systematic review and meta-analysis. Rheumatology (Oxford). 2013;52(4):743–51.
60. Soh E, Li W, Ong KO, Chen W, Bautista D. Image-guided versus blind corticosteroid injections in adults with shoulder pain: a systematic review. BMC Musculoskelet Disord. 2011;12:137.
61. Dogu B, Yucel SD, Sag SY, Bankaoglu M, Kuran B. Blind or ultrasound-guided corticosteroid injections and short-term response in subacromial impingement syndrome: a randomized, double-blind, prospective study. Am J Phys Med Rehabil. 2012;91(8):658–65.
62. Lee HJ, Lim KB, Kim DY, Lee KT. Randomized controlled trial for efficacy of intra-articular injection for adhesive capsulitis: ultrasonography-guided versus blind technique. Arch Phys Med Rehabil. 2009;90(12):1997–2002.
63. Ucuncu F, Capkin E, Karkucak M, Ozden G, Cakirbay H, Tosun M, Guler M. A comparison of the effectiveness of landmark-guided injections and ultrasonography guided injections for shoulder pain. Clin J Pain. 2009;25(9):786–9.
64. Hsieh LF, Hsu WC, Lin YJ, Wu SH, Chang KC, Chang HL. Is ultrasound-guided injection more effective in chronic subacromial bursitis? Med Sci Sports Exerc. 2013;45(12):2205–13.
65. Naredo E, Cabero F, Beneyto P, Cruz A, Mondéjar B, Uson J, Palop MJ, Crespo M. A randomized comparative study of short term response to blind injection versus sonographic-guided injection of local corticosteroids in patients with painful shoulder. J Rheumatol. 2004;31(2):308–14.
66. Ramírez J, Pomés I, Cabrera S, Pomés J, Sanmartí R, Cañete JD. Incidence of full-thickness rotator cuff tear after subacromial corticosteroid injection: a 12-week prospective study. Mod Rheumatol. 2014;24(4):667–70.
67. Ekeberg OM, Bautz-Holter E, Tveitå EK, Juel NG, Kvalheim S, Brox JI. Subacromial ultrasound guided or systemic steroid injection for rotator cuff disease: randomised double blind study. BMJ. 2009;338:a3112.
68. Sabeti-Aschraf M, Stotter C, Thaler C, Kristen K, Schmidt M, Krifter RM, Hexel M, Ostermann R, Hofstaedter T, Graf A, Windhager R. Intra-articular versus periarticular acromioclavicular joint injection: a multicenter, prospective, randomized, controlled trial. Arthroscopy. 2013;29(12):1903–10.
69. Chen CM, Chen JS, Tsai WC, Hsu HC, Chen KH, Lin CH. Effectiveness of device-assisted ultrasound-guided steroid injection for treating plantar fasciitis. Am J Phys Med Rehabil. 2013;92(7):597–605.
70. Tsai WC, Hsu CC, Chen CP, Chen MJ, Yu TY, Chen YJ. Plantar fasciitis treated with local steroid injection: comparison between sonographic and palpation guidance. J Clin Ultrasound. 2006;34(1):12–6.
71. Li Z, Xia C, Yu A, Qi B. Ultrasound- versus palpation-guided injection of corticosteroid for plantar fasciitis: a meta-analysis. PLoS One. 2014;21;9(3):e92671. https://doi.org/10.1371/journal.pone.0092671. PMID: 24658102; PMCID: PMC3962443.
72. Ball EM, McKeeman HM, Patterson C, Burns J, Yau WH, Moore OA, Benson C, Foo J, Wright GD, Taggart AJ. Steroid injection for inferior heel pain: a randomised controlled trial. Ann Rheum Dis. 2013;72(6):996–1002.
73. Yucel I, Yazici B, Degirmenci E, Erdogmus B, Dogan S. Comparison of ultrasound-, palpation-, and scintigraphy-guided steroid injections in the treatment of plantar fasciitis. Arch Orthop Trauma Surg. 2009;129(5):695–701. https://doi.org/10.1007/s00402-008-0760-1. Epub 2008 Oct 7. PMID: 18839190.
74. Makhlouf T, Emil NS, Sibbitt WL Jr, Fields RA, Bankhurst AD. Outcomes and cost-effectiveness of carpal tunnel injections using sonographic needle guidance. Clin Rheumatol. 2014;33(6):849–58.

75. Sibbitt WL Jr, Band PA, Kettwich LG, Chavez-Chiang NR, Delea SL, Bankhurst AD. A randomized controlled trial evaluating the cost-effectiveness of sonographic guidance for intra-articular injection of the osteoarthritic knee. Sibbitt WL Jr, Band PA. J Clin Rheumatol. 2011a;17(8):409–15.
76. Sibbitt WL Jr, Band PA, Kettwich LG, Sibbitt CR, Sibbitt LJ, Bankhurst AD. Safety syringes and anti-needlestick devices in orthopaedic surgery. J Bone Joint Surg Am. 2011b;93(17):1641–9.
77. Sibbitt WL Jr, Michael AA, Poole JL, Chavez-Chiang NR, Delea SL, Bankhurst AD. Nerve blocks at the wrist for painful injections of the palm. J Clin Rheumatol. 2011c;17(4):173–8.
78. Sibbitt WL Jr, Band PA, Chavez-Chiang NR, Delea SL, Norton HE, Bankhurst AD. A randomized controlled trial of the cost-effectiveness of ultrasound-guided intraarticular injection of inflammatory arthritis. J Rheumatol. 2011d;38(2):252–63.
79. Mitchell WG, Kettwich SC, Sibbitt WL Jr, Sibbitt RR, Muruganandam M, Rolle NA, Hayward WA, Fields RA, Roldan LP, Emil NS, Fangtham M, Bankhurst AD. Outcomes and cost-effectiveness of ultrasound-guided injection of the trochanteric bursa. Rheumatol Int. 2018;38(3):393–401.
80. Moore TS, Paffett CL, Sibbitt WL Jr, Hayward WA, Gibb JI, Kettwich SD, Fields RA, Emil NS, Fangtham M, Bankhurst AD. Glenohumeral injection using anatomic landmark versus sonographic needle guidance. bioRxiv. 2018:389973. https://doi.org/10.1101/395293.
81. Jaradat S, Muruganandam M, Rolle NA, Sibbitt WL Jr, Hayward WA, Emil NS, Fangtham M, Fields RA, Bankhurst AD. Safety of ultrasound-guided injections using local puncture site sterility. Arthritis Rheumatol. 2018;70(suppl):Abstract ID: 75138.
82. American Institute of Ultrasound in Medicine. AIUM practice guidelines for selected ultrasound-guided procedures. 2014. aium.org/resources/guidelines/usguidedprocedures.pdf.
83. Dumville JC, McFarlane E, Edwards P, Lipp A, Holmes A. Preoperative skin antiseptics for preventing surgical wound infections after clean surgery. Cochrane Database Syst Rev. 2013;3:CD003949.
84. Yamamoto N, Kimura H, Misao H, Matsumoto H, Imafuku Y, Watanabe A, Mori H, Yoshida A, Miura S, Abe Y, Toba M, Suzuki H, Ogawa K, Kanemitsu K. Efficacy of 1.0% chlorhexidine-gluconate ethanol compared with 10% povidone-iodine for long-term central venous catheter care in hematology departments: a prospective study. Am J Infect Control. 2014;42(5):574–6.
85. American Institute of Ultrasound in Medicine. AIUM practice guidelines for cleaning and preparing external- and internal-use ultrasound transducers and equipment between patients as well as safe handling and use of ultrasound coupling gel. Reapproved 2020. aium.org/officialstatements/57.
86. Guidelli GM, Menza L, Selvi E. Clinical image: linear branching depigmentation of the leg. Arthritis Rheum. 2013;65(12):3318.
87. Habib GS, Saliba W, Nashashibi M. Local effects of intra-articular corticosteroids. Clin Rheumatol. 2010;29(4):347–56.
88. Hayward WA, Sibbitt WL Jr, Sibbitt RR, Muruganandam M, Rolle NA, Fangtham M, Emil NS, Kettwich SK. Intralesional injection of triamcinolone Acetonide for subcutaneous lipoma causing musculoskeletal or neurological symptoms. J Clin Aesthet Dermatol. 2018;11(5):38–42. Epub 2018 May 1. PMID: 29785238
89. Shumaker PR, Rao J, Goldman MP. Treatment of local, persistent cutaneous atrophy following corticosteroid injection with normal saline infiltration. Dermatol Surg. 2005;31(10):1340–3. https://doi.org/10.1111/j.1524-4725.2005.31216. PMID: 16188192.
90. Young CM, Shiels WE 2nd, Coley BD, Hogan MJ, Murakami JW, Jones K, Higgins GC, Rennebohm RM. Ultrasound-guided corticosteroid injection therapy for juvenile idiopathic arthritis: 12-year care experience. Pediatr Radiol. 2012;42(12):1481–9.
91. Hayward WA, Haseler LJ, Kettwich LG, Michael AA, Sibbitt WL Jr, Bankhurst AD. Pressure generated by syringes: implications for hydrodissection and injection of dense connective tissue lesions. Scand J Rheumatol. 2011;40(5):379–82.

92. Michael AA, Moorjani GR, Peisajovich A, Park KS, Sibbitt WL Jr, Bankhurst AD. Syringe size: does it matter in physician-performed procedures? J Clin Rheumatol. 2009;15(2):56–60.
93. Chavez-Chiang CE, Sibbitt WL Jr, Band PA, Chavez-Chiang NR, Delea SL, Bankhurst AD. The highly accurate anterolateral portal for injecting the knee. Sports Med Arthrosc Rehabil Ther Technol. 2011;3(1):6.
94. DeLea SL, Chavez-Chiang NR, Poole JL, Norton HE, Sibbitt WL Jr, Bankhurst AD. Sonographically guided hydrodissection and corticosteroid injection for scleroderma hand. Clin Rheumatol. 2011;30(6):805–13.
95. Gimbel HV. Hydrodissection and hydrodelineation. Int Ophthalmol Clin. 1994;34:73–90.
96. Sibbitt WL Jr, Peisajovich A, Michael AA, Park KS, Sibbitt RR, Band PA, Bankhurst AD. Does sonographic needle guidance affect the clinical outcome of intraarticular injections? J Rheumatol. 2009;36(9):1892–902.
97. Colberg RE, Henderson RG. Diagnosis and treatment of gouty tophi in the patellar tendon using ultrasound-Guided Needle Barbotage: a case presentation. PM R. 2017;9(9):938–42.
98. Lueders DR, Smith J, Sellon JL. Ultrasound-guided knee procedures. Phys Med Rehabil Clin N Am. 2016;27(3):631–48.
99. Orlandi D, Corazza A, Silvestri E, Serafini G, Savarino EV, Garlaschi G, Mauri G, Cimmino MA, Sconfienza LM. Ultrasound-guided procedures around the wrist and hand: how to do. Eur J Radiol. 2014;83(7):1231–8.
100. Meehan R, Wilson C, Hoffman E, Altimier L, Kaessner M, Regan EA. Ultrasound measurement of knee synovial fluid during external pneumatic compression. J Orthop Res. 2019;37(3):601–8.
101. Bennett JF, Sibbitt WL Jr, Band PA, Yaqub S, Emil NS, Fangtham M, Fields RA, Hayward WA, Kettwich SD, Bankhurst AD. Compression-assisted arthrocentesis as a quality improvement intervention. bioRxiv. 2018:395376. https://doi.org/10.1101/395376
102. Hong JH, Kim JS. Diagnosis of iliotibial band friction syndrome and ultrasound guided steroid injection. Korean J Pain. 2013;26(4):387–91.
103. Jelsing EJ, Finnoff JT, Cheville AL, Levy BA, Smith J. Sonographic evaluation of the iliotibial band at the lateral femoral epicondyle: does the iliotibial band move? J Ultrasound Med. 2013;32(7):1199–206.
104. Bandinelli F, Fedi R, Generini S, Porta F, Candelieri A, Mannoni A, Innocenti M, Matucci CM. Longitudinal ultrasound and clinical follow-up of Baker's cysts injection with steroids in knee osteoarthritis. Clin Rheumatol. 2012;31(4):727–31.
105. Di Sante L, Paoloni M, Ioppolo F, Dimaggio M, Di Renzo S, Santilli V. Ultrasound-guided aspiration and corticosteroid injection of Baker's cysts in knee osteoarthritis: a prospective observational study. Am J Phys Med Rehabil. 2010;89(12):970–5.
106. Smith MK, Lesniak B, Baraga MG, Kaplan L, Jose J. Treatment of Popliteal (Baker) Cysts With Ultrasound-Guided Aspiration, Fenestration, and Injection: Longterm Follow-up. Sports Health. 2015;7(5):409–14. https://doi.org/10.1177/1941738115585520. Epub 2015 May 5. PMID: 26502415; PMCID: PMC4547114.
107. Pourcho AM, Colio SW, Hall MM. Ultrasound-guided interventional procedures about the shoulder: anatomy, indications, and techniques. Phys Med Rehabil Clin N Am. 2016;27(3):555–72.
108. Wilson DJ, Scully WF, Rawlings JM. Evolving role of ultrasound in therapeutic injections of the upper extremity. Orthopedics. 2015;38(11):e1017–24.
109. Kim JS, Kim MW, Park DY. Indirect ultrasound guidance increased accuracy of the glenohumeral injection using the superior approach: a cadaveric study of injection accuracy. Ann Rehabil Med. 2013a;37(2):202–7.
110. Rutten MJ, Collins JM, Maresch BJ, Smeets JH, Janssen CM, Kiemeney LA, Jager GJ. Glenohumeral joint injection: a comparative study of ultrasound and fluoroscopically guided techniques before MR arthrography. Eur Radiol. 2009;19(3):722–30. https://doi.org/10.1007/s00330-008-1200-x. Epub 2008 Oct 29. PMID: 18958474; PMCID: PMC2816243.

111. Molini L, Mariacher S, Bianchi S. US guided corticosteroid injection into the subacromial-subdeltoid bursa: technique and approach. J Ultrasound. 2012;15(1):61–8.
112. Edelson G, Saffuri H, Obid E, Lipovsky E, Ben-David D. Successful injection of the acromioclavicular joint with use of ultrasound: anatomy, technique, and follow-up. J Shoulder Elb Surg. 2014;23(10):e243–50. pii: S1058-2746
113. Davidson J, Jayaraman S. Guided interventions in musculoskeletal ultrasound: what's the evidence? Clin Radiol. 2011;66(2):140–52.
114. de Witte PB, Selten JW, Navas A, Nagels J, Visser CP, Nelissen RG, Reijnierse M. Calcific tendinitis of the rotator cuff: a randomized controlled trial of ultrasound-guided needling and lavage versus subacromial corticosteroids. Am J Sports Med. 2013;41(7):1665–73.
115. Gatt DL, Charalambous CP. Ultrasound-Guided Barbotage for calcific tendonitis of the shoulder: a systematic review including 908 patients. Arthroscopy. 2014;30(9):1166–72. pii: S0749-8063(14)00237-0
116. Peck E, Jelsing E, Onishi K. Advanced ultrasound-guided interventions for tendinopathy. Phys Med Rehabil Clin N Am. 2016;27(3):733–48.
117. Galletti S, Magnani M, Rotini R, Mignani G, Affinito D, Pelotti P, Battaglia M, Rollo G. The echo-guided treatment of calcific tendinitis of the shoulder. Chir Organi Mov. 2004;89(4):319–23.
118. Lee KS, Rosas HG. Musculoskeletal ultrasound: how to treat calcific tendinitis of the rotator cuff by ultrasound -guided single-needle lavage technique. AJR Am J Roentgenol. 2010;195(3):638.
119. Louwerens JK, Sierevelt IN, van Noort A, van den Bekerom MP. Evidence for minimally invasive therapies in the management of chronic calcific tendinopathy of the rotator cuff: a systematic review and meta-analysis. J Shoulder Elb Surg. 2014;23(8):1240–9. pii: S1058-2746
120. de Witte PB, Kolk A, Overes F, Nelissen RGHH, Reijnierse M. Rotator cuff calcific tendinitis: ultrasound-guided needling and lavage versus subacromial corticosteroids: five-year outcomes of a randomized controlled trial. Am J Sports Med. 2017;45(14):3305–14.
121. Yoo JC, Koh KH, Park WH, Park JC, Kim SM, Yoon YC. The outcome of ultrasound-guided needle decompression and steroid injection in calcific tendinitis. J Shoulder Elb Surg. 2010;19(4):596–600.
122. Housner JA, Jacobson JA, Misko R. Sonographically guided percutaneous needle tenotomy for the treatment of chronic tendinosis. J Ultrasound Med. 2009;28(9):1187–92.
123. Jacobson JA, Rubin J, Yablon CM, Kim SM, Kalume-Brigido M, Parameswaran A. Ultrasound-guided fenestration of tendons about the hip and pelvis: clinical outcomes. J Ultrasound Med. 2015;34(11):2029–35.
124. Darrieutort-Laffite C, Varin S, Coiffier G, Albert JD, Planche L, Maugars Y, Cormier G, Le Goff B. Are corticosteroid injections needed after needling and lavage of calcific tendinitis? Randomised, double-blind, non-inferiority trial. Ann Rheum Dis. 2019;78(6):837–43.
125. Klontzas ME, Vassalou EE, Zibis AH, Karantanas AH. Hydroxyapatite deposition disease around the hip: outcomes of CT-guided treatment. Diagn Interv Radiol. 2016;22(5):466–70.
126. Reiter N, El-Shabrawi L, Leinweber B, Berghold A, Aberer E. Calcinosis cutis: part II. Treatment options. J Am Acad Dermatol. 2011;65(1):15–22.
127. Epis O, Caporali R, Scirè CA, Bruschi E, Bonacci E, Montecucco C. Efficacy of tidal irrigation in Milwaukee shoulder syndrome. J Rheumatol. 2007;34(7):1545–50.
128. Bodor M, Fullerton B. Ultrasonography of the hand, wrist, and elbow. Phys Med Rehabil Clin N Am. 2010;21(3):509–31.
129. Sussman WI, Williams CJ, Mautner K. Ultrasound-guided elbow procedures. Phys Med Rehabil Clin N Am. 2016;27(3):573–87.
130. Chaudhury S, de La Lama M, Adler RS, Gulotta LV, Skonieczki B, Chang A, Moley P, Cordasco F, Hannafin J, Fealy S. Chaudhury S, de La Lama M, Adler RS, Gulotta LV, Skonieczki B, Chang A, Moley P, Cordasco F, Hannafin J, Fealy S. Platelet-rich plasma for the treatment of lateral epicondylitis: sonographic assessment of tendon morphology and vascularity (pilot study). Skelet Radiol. 2013;42(1):91–7.
131. Suresh SP, Ali KE, Jones H, Connell DA. Medial epicondylitis: is ultrasound guided autologous blood injection an effective treatment? Br J Sports Med. 2006;40(11):935–9.

132. Zhu J, Hu B, Xing C, Li J. Ultrasound-guided, minimally invasive, percutaneous needle puncture treatment for tennis elbow. Adv Ther. 2008;25(10):1031–6.
133. Chiavaras MM, Jacobson JA, Carlos R, Maida E, Bentley T, Simunovic N, Swinton M, Bhandari M. IMpact of Platelet Rich plasma OVer alternative therapies in patients with lateral Epicondylitis (IMPROVE): protocol for a multicenter randomized controlled study: a multicenter, randomized trial comparing autologous platelet-rich plasma, autologous whole blood, dry needle tendon fenestration, and physical therapy exercises alone on pain and quality of life in patients with lateral epicondylitis. Acad Radiol. 2014;21(9):1144–55.
134. Shiple BJ. How effective are injection treatments for lateral epicondylitis? Clin J Sport Med. 2013;23(6):502–3.
135. Colio SW, Smith J, Pourcho AM. Ultrasound-guided interventional procedures of the wrist and hand: anatomy, indications, and techniques. Phys Med Rehabil Clin N Am. 2016;27(3):589–605.
136. Vuillemin V, Guerini H, Morvan G. Musculoskeletal interventional ultrasonography: the upper limb. Diagn Interv Imaging. 2012;93(9):665–73. https://doi.org/10.1016/j.diii.2012.07.013. Epub 2012 Aug 21. PMID: 22921692.
137. Louis LJ. Musculoskeletal ultrasound intervention: principles and advances. Radiol Clin N Am. 2008;46(3):515–33.
138. Hui AC, Wong S, Leung CH, Tong P, Mok V, Poon D, Li-Tsang CW, Wong LK, Boet R. A randomized controlled trial of surgery vs steroid injection for carpal tunnel syndrome. Neurology. 2005;64:2074–8.
139. Ly-Pen D, Andreu JL, de Blas G, Sanchez-Olaso A, Millan I. Surgical decompression versus local steroid injection in carpal tunnel syndrome: a one-year, prospective, randomized, open, controlled clinical trial. Arthritis Rheum. 2005;52:612–9.
140. Smith J, Wisniewski SJ, Finnoff JT, Payne JM. Sonographically guided carpal tunnel injections: the ulnar approach. J Ultrasound Med. 2008;27(10):1485–90. https://doi.org/10.7863/jum.2008.27.10.1485. PMID: 18809959.
141. Goldberg G, Wollstein R, Chimes GP. Carpal tunnel injection: with or without ultrasound guidance? PM R. 2011;3(10):976–81.
142. Apard T, Candelier G. Surgical ultrasound-guided carpal tunnel release. Hand Surg Rehabil. 2017;36(5):333–7.
143. Hebbard PD, Hebbard AIT, Tomka J, Appleyard R. Ultrasound-guided microinvasive carpal tunnel release using a novel retractable needle-mounted blade: a cadaveric study. J Ultrasound Med. 2018;37(8):2075–81.
144. Freire V, Guérini H, Campagna R, Moutounet L, Dumontier C, Feydy A, Drapé JL. Imaging of hand and wrist cysts: a clinical approach. AJR Am J Roentgenol. 2012;199(5):W618–28.
145. Sibbitt WL Jr, Eaton RP. Corticosteroid responsive tenosynovitis is a common pathway for limited joint mobility in the diabetic hand. J Rheumatol. 1997;24(5):931–6.
146. Danielsen MA. Ultrasonography for diagnosis, monitoring and treatment of tenosynovitis in patients with rheumatoid arthritis. Dan Med J. 2018;65(3):pii: B5474.
147. Sahler CS, Spinner DA, Kirschner JS. Ultrasound-guided first metatarsophalangeal joint injections: description of an in-plane, gel standoff technique in a cadaveric study. Foot Ankle Spec. 2013;6(4):303–6.
148. Dodré E, Lefebvre G, Cockenpot E, Chastanet P, Cotten A. Interventional MSK procedures: the hip. Br J Radiol. 2016;89(1057):20150408. https://doi.org/10.1259/bjr.20150408. Epub 2015 Sep 23
149. McCarthy E, Hegazi TM, Zoga AC, Morrison WB, Meyers WC, Poor AE, Nevalainen MT, Roedl JB. Ultrasound-guided interventions for core and hip injuries in athletes. Radiol Clin N Am. 2016;54(5):875–92.
150. Peng PW. Ultrasound-guided interventional procedures in pain medicine: a review of anatomy, sonoanatomy, and procedures. Part IV: hip. Reg Anesth Pain Med. 2013;38(4):264–73.
151. Levi DS. Intra-articular hip injections using ultrasound guidance: accuracy using a linear array transducer. PM R. 2013;5(2):129–34.

152. Paskins Z, Hughes G, Myers H, Hughes E, Hennings S, Cherrington A, Evans A, Holden M, Stevenson K, Menon A, Bromley K, Roberts P, Hall A, Peat G, Jinks C, Oppong R, Lewis M, Foster NE, Mallen C, Roddy E. A randomised controlled trial of the clinical and cost-effectiveness of ultrasound-guided intra-articular corticosteroid and local anaesthetic injections: the hip injection trial (HIT) protocol. BMC Musculoskelet Disord. 2018;19(1):218.
153. Mallow M, Nazarian LN. Greater trochanteric pain syndrome diagnosis and treatment. Phys Med Rehabil Clin N Am. 2014;25(2):279–89.
154. Klauser AS, Martinoli C, Tagliafico A, Bellmann-Weiler R, Feuchtner GM, Wick M, Jaschke WR. Greater trochanteric pain syndrome. Semin Musculoskelet Radiol. 2013;17(1):43–8.
155. Silva F, Adams T, Feinstein J, Arroyo RA. Trochanteric bursitis: refuting the myth of inflammation. J Clin Rheumatol. 2008;14(2):82–6.
156. Wilson SA, Shanahan EM, Smith MD. Greater trochanteric pain syndrome: does imaging-identified pathology influence the outcome of interventions? Int J Rheum Dis. 2013;17(6):621–7.
157. McEvoy JR, Lee KS, Blankenbaker DG, del Rio AM, Keene JS. Ultrasound-guided corticosteroid injections for treatment of greater trochanteric pain syndrome: greater trochanter bursa versus subgluteus medius bursa. AJR Am J Roentgenol. 2013;201(2):W313–7.
158. Brinks A, van Rijn RM, Willemsen SP, Bohnen AM, Verhaar JA, Koes BW, Bierma-Zeinstra SM. Corticosteroid injections for greater trochanteric pain syndrome: a randomized controlled trial in primary care. Ann Fam Med. 2011;9(3):226–34.
159. Cohen SP, Strassels SA, Foster L, Marvel J, Williams K, Crooks M, Gross A, Kurihara C, Nguyen C, Williams N. Comparison of fluoroscopically guided and blind corticosteroid injections for greater trochanteric pain syndrome: multicentre randomised controlled trial. BMJ. 2009;338:b1088.
160. Jacobson JA, Yablon CM, Henning PT, Kazmers IS, Urquhart A, Hallstrom B, Bedi A, Parameswaran A. Greater trochanteric pain syndrome: percutaneous tendon fenestration versus platelet-rich plasma injection for treatment of gluteal tendinosis. J Ultrasound Med. 2016;35(11):2413–20.
161. Hurdle MF. Ultrasound-guided spinal procedures for pain: a review. Phys Med Rehabil Clin N Am. 2016;27(3):673–86.
162. Narouze S, Peng PW. Ultrasound-guided interventional procedures in pain medicine: a review of anatomy, sonoanatomy, and procedures. Part II: axial structures. Reg Anesth Pain Med. 2010;35(4):386–96.
163. Provenzano DA, Narouze S. Sonographically guided lumbar spine procedures. J Ultrasound Med. 2013;32(7):1109–16.
164. Jee H, Lee JH, Park KD, Ahn J, Park Y. Ultrasound -guided versus fluoroscopy-guided sacroiliac joint intra-articular injections in the noninflammatory sacroiliac joint dysfunction: a prospective, randomized, single-blinded study. Arch Phys Med Rehabil. 2014;95(2):330–7.
165. Hartung W, Ross CJ, Straub R, Feuerbach S, Schölmerich J, Fleck M, Herold T. Ultrasound-guided sacroiliac joint injection in patients with established sacroiliitis: precise IA injection verified by MRI scanning does not predict clinical outcome. Rheumatology (Oxford). 2010;49(8):1479–82.
166. Pekkafahli MZ, Kiralp MZ, Başekim CC, Silit E, Mutlu H, Oztürk E, Kizilkaya E, Dursun H. Sacroiliac joint injections performed with sonographic guidance. J Ultrasound Med. 2003;22(6):553–9.
167. Chan BY, Lee KS. Ultrasound intervention of the lower extremity/pelvis. Radiol Clin N Am. 2018;56(6):1035–46. https://doi.org/10.1016/j.rcl.2018.06.011.
168. Beard NM, Gousse RP. Current ultrasound application in the foot and ankle. Orthop Clin North Am. 2018;49(1):109–21.
169. Masala S, Fiori R, Bartolucci DA, Mammucari M, Angelopoulos G, Massari F, Simonetti G. Diagnostic and therapeutic joint injections. Semin Intervent Radiol. 2010;27(2):160–71.
170. Morvan G, Vuillemin V, Guerini H. Interventional musculoskeletal ultrasonography of the lower limb. Diagn Interv Imaging. 2012;93(9):652–64.
171. Walter WR, Burke CJ, Adler RS. Ultrasound-guided therapeutic injections for neural pathology about the foot and ankle: a 4 year retrospective review. Skelet Radiol. 2017;46(6):795–803.

172. Yablon CM. Ultrasound-guided interventions of the foot and ankle. Semin Musculoskelet Radiol. 2013;17(1):60–8.
173. Peters SE, Laxer RM, Connolly BL, Parra DA. Ultrasound-guided steroid tendon sheath injections in juvenile idiopathic arthritis: a 10-year single-center retrospective study. Pediatr Rheumatol Online J. 2017;15(1):22. https://doi.org/10.1186/s12969-017-0155-3.
174. Reach JS, Easley ME, Chuckpaiwong B, Nunley JA 2nd. Accuracy of ultrasound guided injections in the foot and ankle. Foot Ankle Int. 2009;30(3):239–42.
175. Sofka CM, Adler RS. Ultrasound-guided interventions in the foot and ankle. Semin Musculoskelet Radiol. 2002;6(2):163–8.
176. Vallone G, Vittorio T. Complete Achilles tendon rupture after local infiltration of corticosteroids in the treatment of deep retrocalcaneal bursitis. J Ultrasound. 2014;17(2):165–7.
177. Dallaudière B, Pesquer L, Meyer P, Silvestre A, Perozziello A, Peuchant A, D'Agostino MA, Schmidt WA. Ultrasound-guided injections in rheumatology: actual knowledge on efficacy and procedures. Best Pract Res Clin Rheumatol. 2013;27(2):283–94.
178. Filardo G, Kon E, Di Matteo B, Di Martino A, Tesei G, Pelotti P, Cenacchi A, Marcacci M. Platelet-rich plasma injections for the treatment of refractory Achilles tendinopathy: results at 4 years. Blood Transfus. 2014;19:1–8.
179. Ferrero G, Fabbro E, Orlandi D, Martini C, Lacelli F, Serafini G, Silvestri E, Sconfienza LM. Ultrasound-guided injection of platelet-rich plasma in chronic Achilles and patellar tendinopathy. J Ultrasound. 2012;15(4):260–6.
180. Maida E, Presley JC, Murthy N, Pawlina W, Smith J. Sonographically guided deep plantar fascia injections: where does the injectate go? J Ultrasound Med. 2013;32(8):1451–9.
181. Markovic M, Crichton K, Read JW, Lam P, Slater HK. Effectiveness of ultrasound-guided corticosteroid injection in the treatment of Morton's neuroma. Foot Ankle Int. 2008;29(5):483–7. https://doi.org/10.3113/FAI.2008.0483.
182. Morgan PA, Monaghan GA, Richards S. A systematic review of ultrasound-guided and non ultrasound-guided therapeutic injections to treat Morton's neuroma. J Am Podiatr Med Assoc. 2014;104(4):337–48.
183. Fredberg U, van Overeem Hansen G, Bolvig L. Placement of intra-articular injections verified by ultrasonography and injected air as contrast medium. Ann Rheum Dis. 2001;60(5):542.
184. Coiffier G, Ferreyra M, Albert JD, Stock N, Jolivet-Gougeon A, Perdriger A, Guggenbuhl P. Ultrasound-guided synovial biopsy improves diagnosis of septic arthritis in acute arthritis without enough analyzable synovial fluid: a retrospective analysis of 176 arthritis from a French rheumatology department. Clin Rheumatol. 2018;37(8):2241–9.
185. Kim SY, Chung HW. Small musculoskeletal soft-tissue lesions: US-guided core needle biopsy–comparative study of diagnostic yields according to lesion size. Radiology. 2016;278(1):156–63.
186. Lazarou I, Kelly SG, Meric de Bellefon L. Ultrasound-guided synovial biopsies of wrists, metacarpophalangeal, metatarsophalangeal, interphalangeal joints, and tendon sheaths. Front Med (Lausanne). 2019;6:2. https://doi.org/10.3389/fmed.2019.00002. eCollection 2019
187. Meric De Bellefon L, Lazarou I. US-guided biopsies: overarching principles. Front Med (Lausanne). 2019;6:1. https://doi.org/10.3389/fmed.2019.00001. eCollection 2019
188. Micheroli R, Wagner U, Mueller-Gerbl M, Toranelli M, Marx C, Bruyn GAW, Jousse-Joulin S, Tamborrini G. Minimally invasive ultrasound-guided parotid gland biopsy in cadavers performed by rheumatologists. J Ultrason. 2019;19(77):125–7.
189. Polido-Pereira J. Ultrasound-guided biopsies: medium and large joints. Front Med (Lausanne). 2019;6:95. https://doi.org/10.3389/fmed.2019.00095. eCollection 2019
190. Smits M, van de Groes S, Thurlings RM. Synovial tissue biopsy collection by rheumatologists: ready for clinical implementation? Front Med (Lausanne). 2019;6:138. https://doi.org/10.3389/fmed.2019.00138. eCollection 2019
191. Smith J, Finnoff JT. Diagnostic and interventional musculoskeletal ultrasound: part 2. Clinical applications. PM R. 2009b Feb;1(2):162–77. https://doi.org/10.1016/j.pmrj.2008.09.002. PMID: 19627890.

Pediatric Musculoskeletal Ultrasonography

10

Johannes Roth

Key Points

- The assessment of the pediatric joint often presents a challenge by clinical exam alone. Ultrasonography can aid in the exact assessment of joint disease activity, which is especially important in pediatrics, as it can directly impact long-term outcomes in preventing joint damage and disability.
- Knowledge of entheseal development as well as bone maturation is essential in the interpretation of ultrasound images in children of various ages.
- In children and adolescents, significant physiologic blood flow manifesting as Doppler signals might be present in various structures forming the joint, including the synovial recess. The recognition of physiologic blood flow is important in order to differentiate pathologic from normal findings.

Introduction

The main objective of this chapter is to explain the principles that will be relevant in assessing musculoskeletal structures with ultrasonography (US) in children. Taking into account these principles will enable the sonographer to obtain reliable and useful information through US that will be an important addition to the history and physical exam.

The exact assessment of joint disease activity is especially important in the pediatric field as it will directly impact on the long-term outcomes including prevention of joint damage and disability. With new treatments, the induction of permanent

J. Roth (✉)
Division of Pediatric Dermatology and Rheumatology, Children's Hospital of Eastern Ontario, Ottawa, ON, Canada

University of Ottawa, Ottawa, ON, Canada
e-mail: jroth@cheo.on.ca

M. J. Kohler (ed.), *Musculoskeletal Ultrasound in Rheumatology Review*,
https://doi.org/10.1007/978-3-030-73555-5_10

remission is possible for an increasing percentage of children but cannot always be reliably demonstrated on clinical exam alone [1–3]. In addition, the exact determination of remission status will be helpful for the decision to taper medication, thereby preventing side effects from long-term use.

While most physicians fairly regularly order imaging studies on their pediatric patients, the interpretation is often challenging due to the unique aspects of the growing skeleton. The meaningful application of any imaging method in children and adolescents is impossible without a basic understanding of the musculoskeletal (MSK) anatomy.

Comparing the different imaging technologies, radiographs have been the traditional method of choice. They are readily available but will mainly provide information on structural changes (joint space narrowing, erosions) which are usually a consequence of insufficiently controlled disease. They do not allow assessment of active inflammation. Especially with modern approaches to treatment, their value is limited. Additional challenges in the interpretation result from the fact that the growing skeleton displays a variable amount of hyaline cartilage in the epiphyseal regions, which is not always readily visible on radiographs.

Magnetic resonance imaging (MRI) is potentially very useful but is time-consuming, expensive, and not widely available for routine clinical use in many places. It also frequently requires sedation especially in younger children, who unfortunately are among the most commonly affected by juvenile idiopathic arthritis (JIA). MRI does not usually allow a functional exam of the joint in question, and the standardization for pediatric MSK imaging is still in its infancy [4–7].

In contrast, US is relatively cheap, fast, and virtually free of side effects. It does not require sedation, and all peripheral joints can be examined as many times as required at the time of consultation, improving the accuracy of clinical evaluation [7]. From the patient's perspective, many children will enjoy US scanning of their joints as they can directly see images that help to explain their disease.

Diagnostic US clearly has the potential to be the most important imaging technique in pediatric rheumatology. In order to use the technique reliably, a solid evidence base is necessary. An increasing literature has emerged over the past decade including the description of physiologic findings, standardization of the scanning technique, normative data acquisition, definitions for pathology, and documenting the responsiveness to change [8–25].

Technical Requirements

The technical requirements for scanning children are no different than for scanning adults. US technology has been advancing greatly over the past years, and even entry-level machines now provide very high-quality images especially in B-mode. The biggest difference still exists in terms of Doppler imaging capabilities.

At least as important as the technical standard of the machine itself is the quality of the probe. Essentially, a linear, multifrequency probe will be able to cover most scans. Even the hip joint can often be documented very well with such a probe especially in younger children. A curved array probe might be helpful for the hip in older or obese children. Generally, due to smaller dimensions in children, higher frequencies might be used improving the resolution of the images. Therefore, investing in a very high-quality linear probe will pay back immensely with excellent images.

It is almost never a problem to get children to cooperate with the scans. It might be interesting to use a gel warmer to avoid exposure to cold gel, but this will on the other hand result in a more fluid gel which can be a disadvantage. In addition, the examiner might have to be prepared to scan the child in other positions than just lying on an exam bed. For example, it might be necessary to scan while the child is sitting on the parent's lap. It is nevertheless important to not produce suboptimal images due to this approach. No clinical conclusions should be drawn from suboptimal images.

Normal Ultrasound Anatomy in Children

Bony anatomy is important in US imaging as the articulating bones or attachment sites of tendons and ligaments will usually serve as the reference point, whereas the skeleton of an adult person is completely ossified except for the articular cartilage portion, a varying degree of hyaline cartilage, and in some locations, fibrocartilage is present in addition to articular cartilage in children [8].

Two main processes of ossification exist in humans: (1) enchondral ossification, in which bone forms on the background of a cartilaginous matrix, and (2) intramembranous ossification, where bone is derived from mesenchymal cells. All of the long bones as well as most of the short bones develop through enchondral ossification (Fig. 10.1). Most of the bones of the skull, including the maxilla as well as the mandible, develop through intramembranous ossification. The condyle of the mandible nevertheless develops through enchondral ossification [27]. In the tibial tuberosity on the other hand, areas of membranous bone formation are present adjacent to areas of enchondral ossification. This is especially the case in the distal tibial tuberosity where some limited intramembranous bone formation occurs. In addition to hyaline cartilage, fibrocartilage is present in these same entheseal/apophyseal regions [28], not only in the tibial tuberosity but also, for example, at the insertion of the Achilles tendon into the calcaneus.

The histologic presence of ossification centers will not always correlate precisely with detection on imaging, and the various imaging methods might differ in their sensitivity to show the first signs of ossification. Any reference to the presence of ossification in this chapter will therefore need to be interpreted in the context of the imaging method used to describe it.

At birth, cortical bone is present in most long bone diaphyses representing the primary ossification center. Many ossification centers in short bones (e.g., the wrist) are not present yet, and hardly, any epiphyseal bone is present on imaging with radiographs. The secondary ossification centers will only subsequently become apparent. The progress of ossification varies significantly between the anatomical

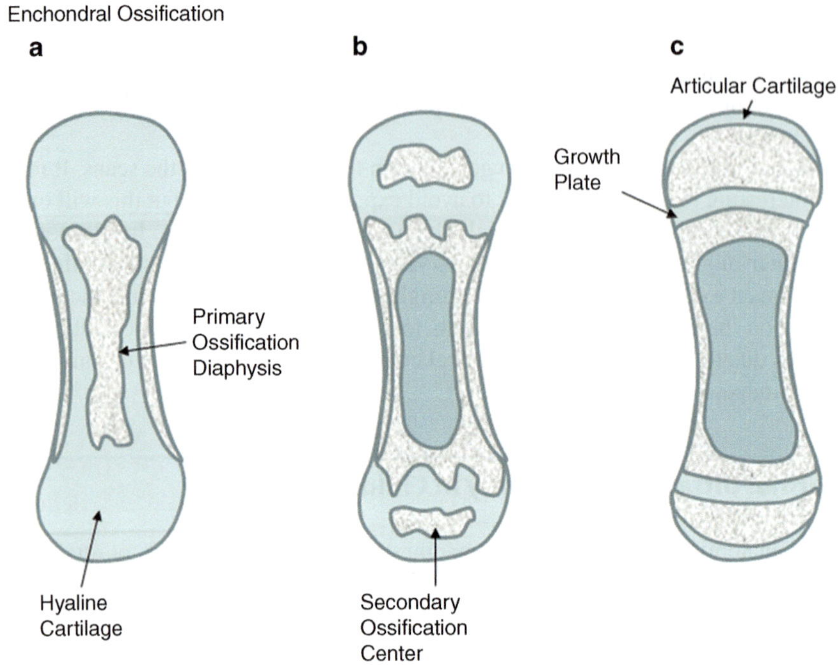

Fig. 10.1 Stages of enchondral ossification in a long bone. (**a**) At birth, with no epiphyseal bone present. (**b**) Subsequently, secondary ossification centers will appear in the epiphysis. (**c**) Finally, an almost fully ossified skeleton with growth plates still open

sites and is also dependent on gender and within the same gender on the degree of maturation, i.e., the pubertal stages. An excellent example where this can be used clinically is the bone age determination on wrist radiographs. It has to be noted though that especially inflammatory diseases like JIA can lead to a significant alteration of these time points, often in fact an acceleration of maturation of an affected skeletal area.

As further discussed later, some bones will have several secondary ossification centers, and the number might vary among different children. This will be important, for example, in the imaging of apophysitis and the determination whether pathologic fragmentation of the secondary ossification center is present.

The specific time points for the progress of postnatal ossification in all anatomical areas cannot be discussed in detail in this chapter, and for many areas, only limited data is available. A significant amount of work combining radiographic and histologic analysis has been provided by JA Ogden who published a whole series describing ossification for various anatomical areas [28–34].

Generally, radiographs have limited value in the depiction of epiphyseal cartilage, and this represents unique challenges in the interpretation especially in younger children with regard to fractures and other pathology [4]. US, however, can usually show the outline of the cartilage portion very well and is therefore a very

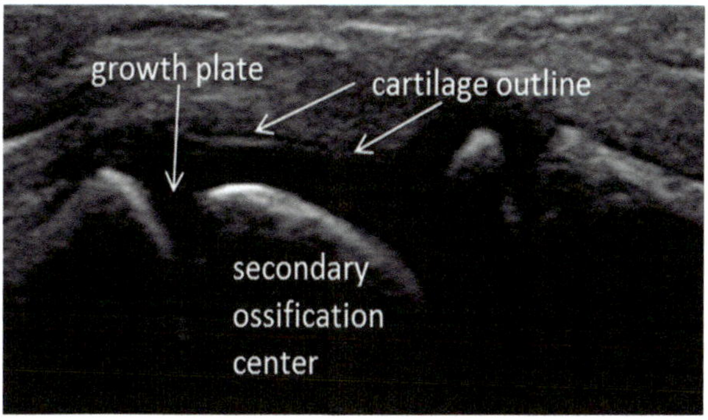

Fig. 10.2 Dorsal view of the MCP joint in a 10-year-old child

suitable technique for the depiction of the growing skeleton [8]. Enchondral ossification with development of a cartilaginous matrix and subsequent ossification is the most relevant process in the joints commonly imaged. The major implication for MSK ultrasonography is that depending on the age of the child, anechoic or hypoechoic cartilage will be defining the bone contour in a joint as opposed to the hyperechoic outline with fully ossified bone usually seen on imaging in adults (Fig. 10.2).

Joint

When imaging a joint with US, it is always important to clearly show the bone contour of the bones adjacent to the joint and the cartilage lining the bone. Especially in those areas of the cartilage where it is hit perpendicular by the US beam, the top border of the cartilage will be visible clearly, and often a thin white line will appear [8]. This is also called the cartilage interface sign and is not to be confused with the especially prominent double contour sign in gout, where the entire cartilage surface will appear very hyperechoic. When scanning children, it is important to show not only the articular cartilage directly adjacent to the joint but also the hyaline cartilage in the metaphyseal and epiphyseal part of the bone, which has not ossified yet. As shown in Fig. 10.2, the hyaline cartilage will appear anechoic or slightly hypoechoic with the ossification center present depending on the age. The growth plate (physis) is also seen as a hypoechoic or anechoic line separating the epiphyseal from the meta-/diaphyseal part of the bone.

Cartilage can be identified and differentiated from pathology (e.g., effusion) by showing the form which outlines the future bone as in Figs. 10.3 and 10.4.

Finally, cartilage might exhibit hyperechoic areas which likely represent vascular channels and are not pathologic as in Fig. 10.5.

It is important to distinguish cartilage from effusions in children. In the presence of a joint effusion, the cartilage interface sign will often be more prominent as the physical properties of fluid vs. cartilage differ more than soft tissue vs. cartilage. In addition, the phenomenon of posterior enhancement of tissues positioned behind fluid also contributes to stronger reflections of the US beam. Cartilage will not be

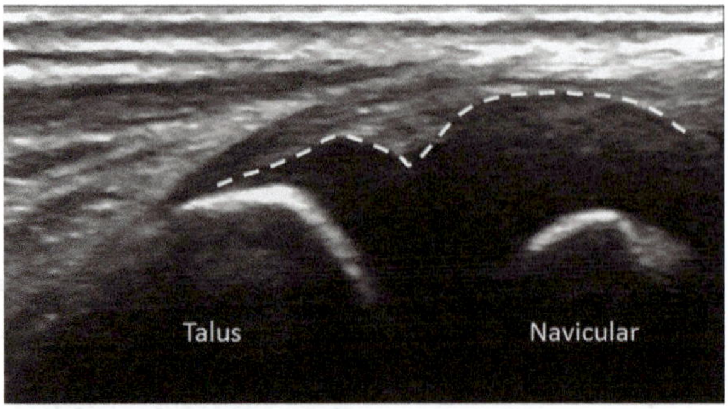

Fig. 10.3 Partly ossified talonavicular joint in a 5-year-old girl: the an-/hypoechoic outline of the cartilage portion of the distal talus and the navicular bone can be differentiated from the more hyperechoic connective tissues above it

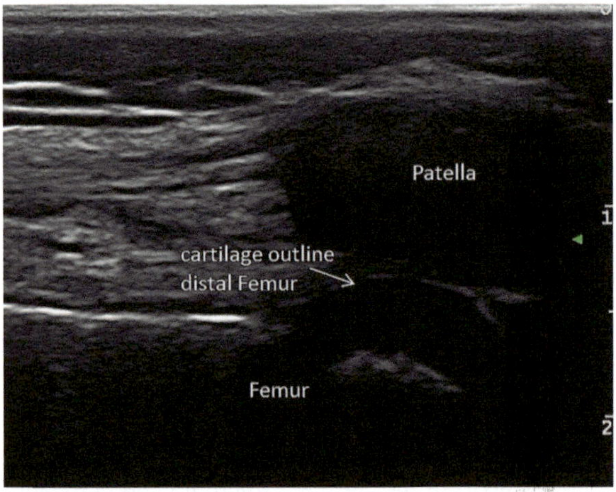

Fig. 10.4 Knee joint in a 3-year-old boy, the outline of the largely unossified patella as well as the distal femur can be seen as a *thin white line*

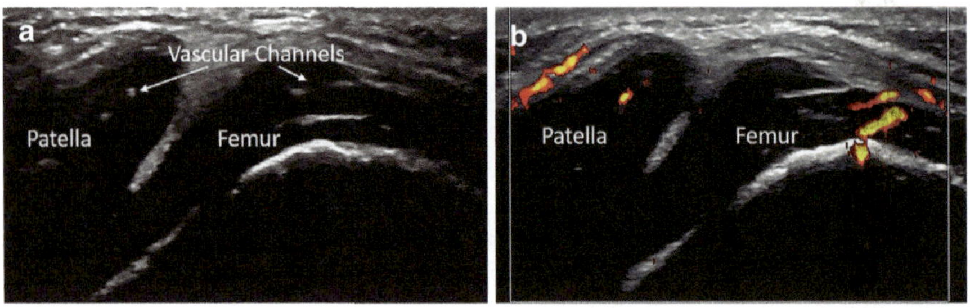

Fig. 10.5 Vascular channels within the cartilage. (**a**) B-mode image and (**b**) corresponding Doppler image

displaceable by the US probe whereas fluid is. The anatomical location of the anechoic area will also help to differentiate cartilage vs. fluid (Figs. 10.6 and 10.7). Finally, movement of the joint can clarify findings, where cartilage will keep the same shape throughout movement, but fluid will change its shape.

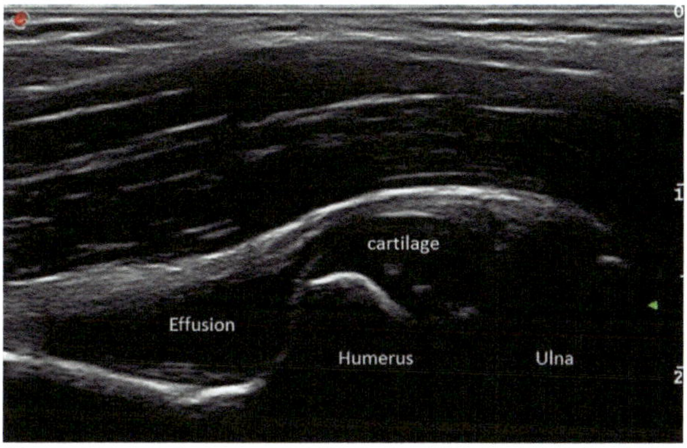

Fig. 10.6 Effusion in the humeroulnar joint of the elbow. The anechoic structure in the coronoid fossa represents an effusion, whereas the anechoic structure around the epiphysis represents cartilage. Note the hyperechoic dots indicating vascular channels within the cartilage

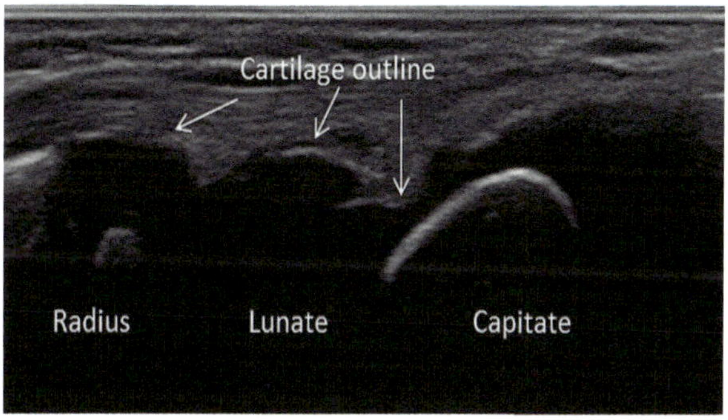

Fig. 10.7 Image of a healthy wrist in a 4-year-old with growth plate, hyaline cartilage at the epiphysis and secondary ossification center in the distal radius, a completely unossified lunate bone, and a partly ossified capitate bone as well as the cartilage interface sign

Cartilage Assessment

Joint damage and especially cartilage loss is one of the most important outcome parameters in inflammatory arthritis. Given the excellent imaging capabilities of cartilage by US, this technology might play an important role in the monitoring of patients with chronic arthritis. The clinical utility of MSK US in cartilage assessments is likely to be at least as important in pediatric rheumatology as it is in adult rheumatology.

Traditionally, cartilage assessment is done by measuring cartilage thickness [35], but it is yet to be determined whether this is the best method to assess damage.

Even in adults, the measurement of cartilage thickness is not easy, and careful scanning technique as well as knowledge of US physics in order to obtain precise measurements is essential [36].

Measurements in children might be even more challenging given the presence of the hyaline cartilage of the epiphysis, which cannot necessarily be distinguished from the articular cartilage depending on the age of the child. As the secondary ossification centers in the epiphysis can be very irregular, measurements of cartilage thickness can be challenging. In JIA, the acceleration of maturation in affected joints introduces further variability in the thickness of the remaining cartilage. Finally, edema of the cartilage with increased thickness as opposed to loss of cartilage thickness has been described especially in the earlier stages of inflammation [4, 37]. Several authors have therefore suggested that the assessment of the cartilage contour might be more discriminative between pathologic changes and healthy cartilage than the measurement of cartilage thickness [4, 37].

This is further supported by the fact that only limited data for cartilage thickness in children are available so far. One publication has studied cartilage thickness in the knee joint, wrist, and fingers [23]. The data are provided according to age but not according to pubertal stage, which will limit the applicability. In addition, fairly high variability among observers has been documented for some of the joints, which is probably not surprising given the irregular shape of the secondary ossification centers in the epiphyses. The measurement of cartilage thickness might therefore prove challenging in pediatric rheumatology, and special care should be taken when applying normative data scales to assess a given patient's results.

It might indeed be more promising to investigate the possibility of reliably grading the cartilage contour in certain locations.

Tendon and Enthesis/Apophysis

Tendons do not differ significantly from the imaging in adults, but the anatomical references in terms of bone contours can be slightly different in children. This is again related to the cartilage that is not ossified yet depending on the age of the child. Figures 10.8, 10.9, and 10.10 illustrate this for various anatomic regions.

Knowledge of entheseal development in children as well as consideration of vascularization is important in order to differentiate pathologic from normal findings. From an imaging point of view, it is also important to remember that depending on the age of the child, a significant part of what later becomes the osseous insertion is still composed of hyaline cartilage as well as fibrocartilage and will therefore appear hypoechoic or anechoic on US. The details of the enthesis, which is really

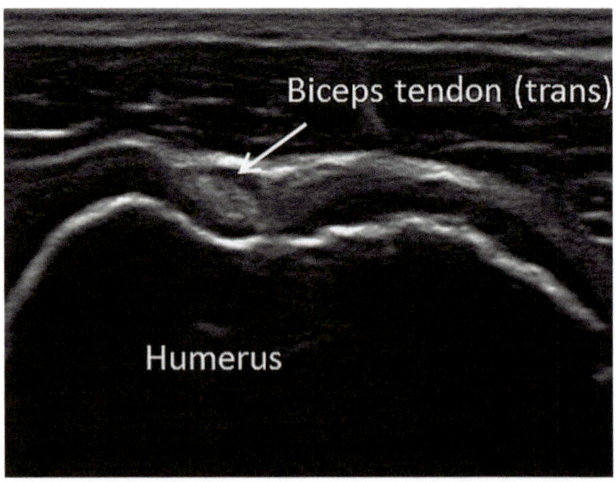

Fig. 10.8 Biceps tendon in transverse view at the bicipital groove

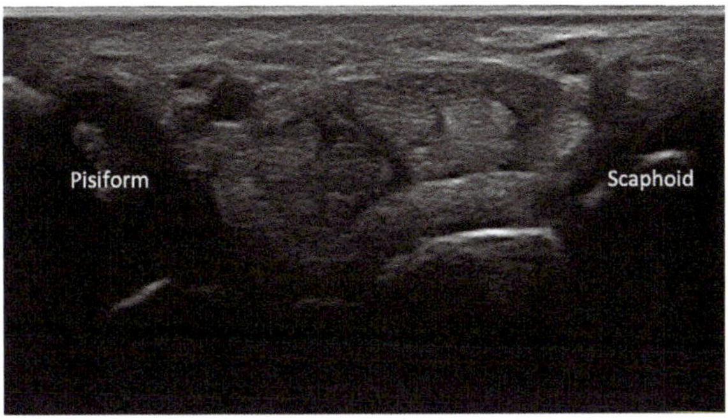

Fig. 10.9 Carpal tunnel at the level of scaphoid and pisiform bones

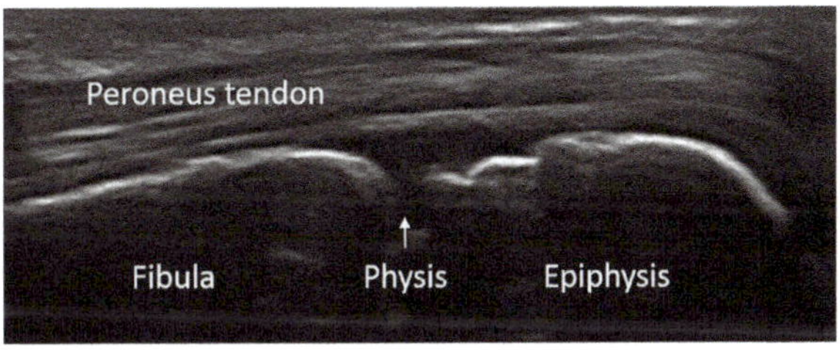

Fig. 10.10 Peroneus tendons along the fibula

considered an entheseal organ including bone, hyaline cartilage, fibrocartilage, fat, bursae, and the tendon, cannot be covered in detail in this chapter [38]. It is nevertheless fascinating to see how the development of these various tissues changes the imaging properties of a given anatomic region throughout childhood and adolescence. This is especially true for apophyseal regions like the tibial tuberosity as well as the Achilles tendon insertion [28–31, 39, 40].

Entheses development has nicely been described for the Achilles tendon. Fornage and Grechenig described the progress and change of the sono-anatomy as follows: (1) From 2 months to 3 years, no ossification of the secondary center of calcaneus is visible; (2) from 4 to 6 years, early signs of the secondary ossification center appear; (3) from 7 to 11 years, the posterior bony contour of the primary ossification center of the calcaneus has got a wavy appearance; (4) from 12 to 18 years, the secondary ossification center then appears, and full ossification of the apophyseal cartilage occurs [39, 40] (Fig. 10.11a–d).

Ligaments

There is no principal difference in the ultrasonographic appearance of ligaments in children vs. adults. If anything, the appearance of ligaments in children might be more echogenic and easier to demonstrate given the smaller geometric dimensions with less subcutaneous tissue and better penetration of the US beam. As with the

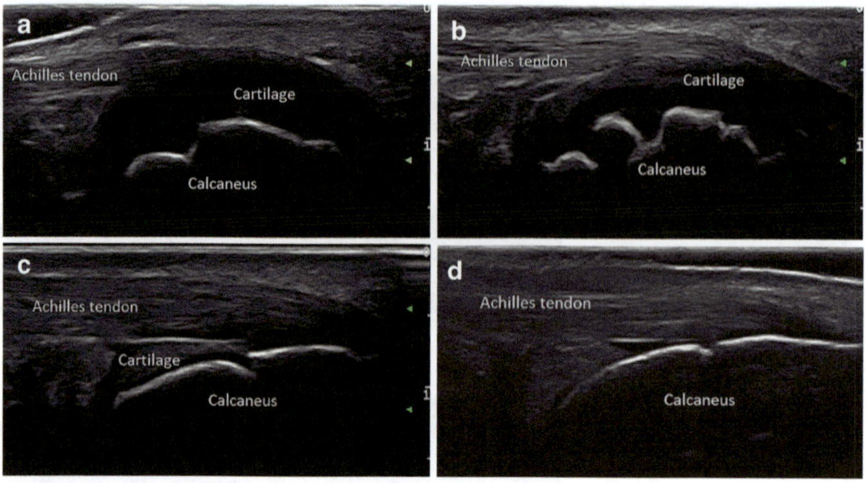

Fig. 10.11 (**a–d**) Achilles tendon insertion in a healthy child at various ages. Note the different echogenicity of various aspects of the cartilage of the calcaneus. Whereas parts of it are anechoic, the posterior part directly adjacent to the Achilles tendon can have a different, rather hypoechoic echogenicity. This should not be confused with the retrocalcaneal bursa. (**a**) 3 years, (**b**) 7 years, (**c**) 11 years and (**d**) 16 years

enthesis, the insertion might still be cartilaginous and therefore might appear hypoechoic or anechoic.

Joint Capsule

In many publications on MSK US, the terms joint capsule and synovium are used interchangeably, i.e., the same anatomical location will be called intracapsular or intrasynovial. The term joint space will also be applied to both locations without differentiation.

While the synovial membrane is directly lining the inside of the joint capsule of the hip, other joints like the elbow or ankle joints have intracapsular fat which is extrasynovial, i.e., going from superficial to deep, the joint capsule comes first, followed by intracapsular fat and connective tissue, followed by the synovial membrane defining the intrasynovial space. In the presence of a joint effusion, this intracapsular fat/connective tissue might be displaced and even appear thinned out. The clear differentiation of intracapsular vs. intrasynovial areas of the joint is important in order to not misinterpret findings that are intra-articular/intracapsular but extrasynovial as synovitis.

In children (but also adults), the joint capsule itself can often be shown very nicely as a fibrillar structure. In the following image examples, the hip joint capsule is visualized with its anterior and posterior layer directly lined by the synovial membrane (Fig. 10.12) as well as in the ankle joint where the synovial space itself is separated from the joint capsule by intracapsular fat/connective tissue (Fig. 10.13).

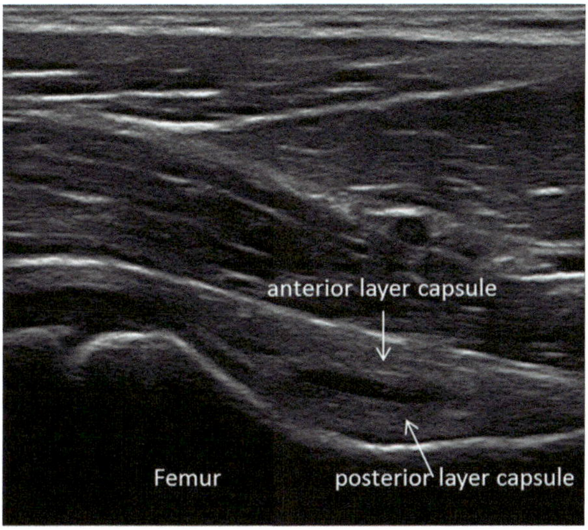

Fig. 10.12 Hip joint capsule. The anterior and posterior layer of the capsule can usually be shown nicely in children. The synovial membrane lines the capsule directly as a thin layer which cannot be distinguished. A *white interface line* separating the two layers of the joint capsule might be seen

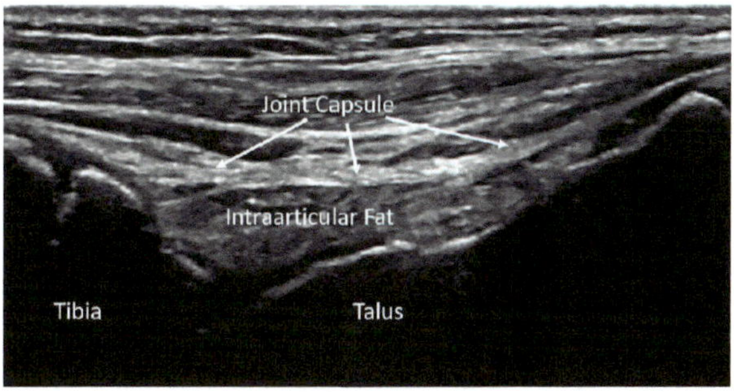

Fig. 10.13 Longitudinal view of the ankle joint with the joint capsule

Doppler

Structural abnormalities found on B-mode US such as joint effusions or synovial thickening can be residual findings and may not necessarily represent ongoing active disease. Both color Doppler and power Doppler US techniques detect synovial blood flow, which is a sign of increased synovial vascularization [41]. Doppler US is therefore considered superior in distinguishing active synovitis from inactive intra-articular synovial thickening compared to the B-mode technique alone [42–47].

It is important to note though that healthy joints may also show Doppler flow within the joint space, and classifications which consider any Doppler flow within a joint as a sign of synovitis are therefore problematic. This is even more relevant for children and adolescents as significant Doppler flow may be present both within the intracapsular but extrasynovial joint space as well as in areas of tendon insertions. To simply apply adult rheumatology scoring systems and consider the presence of any Doppler signal as a sign of synovitis is therefore not possible and cannot be done in order to compare clinical and US assessment in JIA. One important finding in children is the presence of feeding vessels, i.e., the very clear visibility of blood vessels entering the bone at the meta-epiphyseal junction of long bones but also in many long bones [12] which are physiologic and need to be distinguished from pathologic Doppler signals. Until a better understanding of the normal anatomy is available, Doppler signals may be especially helpful if found in areas of synovial hypertrophy/enlarged joint recesses but need to be interpreted with caution otherwise. The same is true for the enthesis, where a completely normal tendon structure with Doppler flow might be physiologic as opposed to a pathologic tendon structure (edema, thickening) with Doppler flow that might not be. Only the latter may be indicative of an enthesitis. Several publications have suggested that it is unusual to find Doppler signals in the enthesis of healthy children [24, 48] or that at least only very low-grade signals would be present [24]. There is nevertheless some variability in the US machines and their Doppler abilities that have been used for these studies as well as the definitions for the grading of the Doppler signals which raise questions about the true absence of these Doppler signals in the entheses of healthy children. Recent studies have indicated a more significant presence of physiologic Doppler signals at the enthesis [25], but interestingly, the presence of these Doppler signals has not been associated with any other abnormalities of the enthesis like thickening or disruption of the fibrillar pattern. This would suggest that these Doppler signals are reflective of physiologic blood flow but not a pathologic inflammatory process. It might be necessary to distinguish pathology from physiologic findings in children based on a combination of B-mode and Doppler findings, but data on this are currently not available for the enthesis. It is also interesting to ask whether all the entheses would be equally sensitive, but even more important, specific for the detection of pathologic Doppler signals. A recent publication looking into the lower extremity entheses of healthy children at the peak growth spurt has found a presence of significant Doppler signal at the insertion of the quadriceps tendon and the distal patellar tendon but not the proximal patellar tendon and the Achilles tendon, suggesting that the presence of Doppler signals at the proximal patellar tendon as well as the Achilles tendon might be much more specific for pathology than at the other two sites [25]. See image examples for the presence of Doppler signals (Figs. 10.14, 10.15, 10.16, and 10.17).

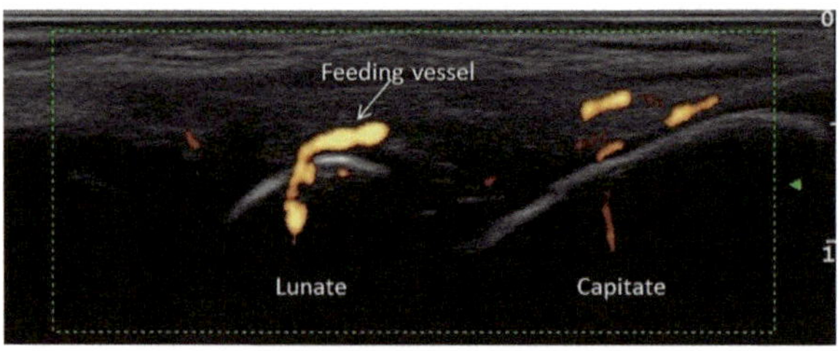

Fig. 10.14 A typical feeding vessel entering the lunate bone in the wrist is shown. In addition, there is a small feeding vessel entering the capitate bone. These vessels do have a physiologic role and are not indicative of synovitis

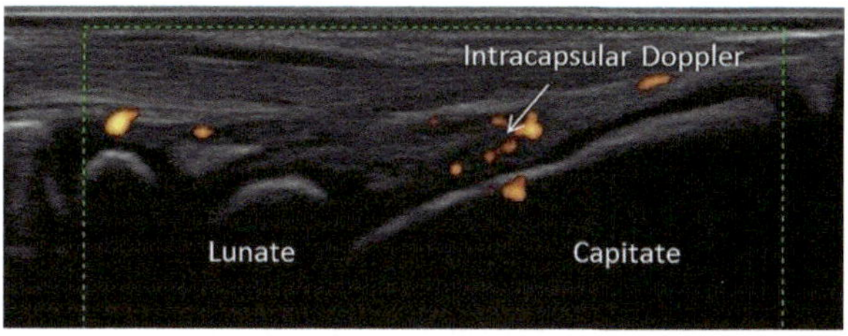

Fig. 10.15 Normal wrist joint in a 9-year-old

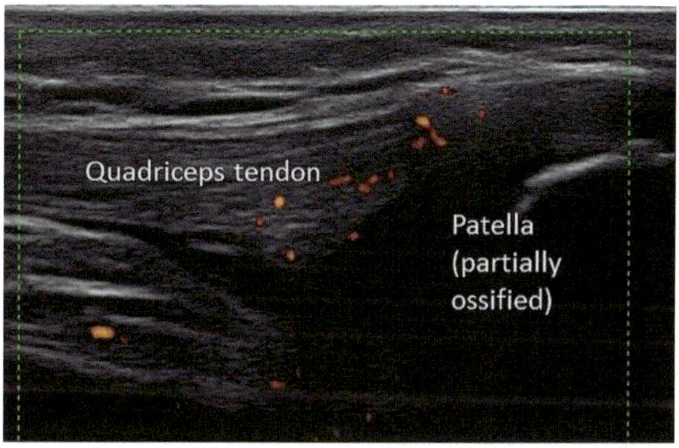

Fig. 10.16 Knee joint and quadriceps tendon in a healthy 10-year-old boy. Note the significant Doppler flow in the quadriceps tendon and the suprapatellar fat pad

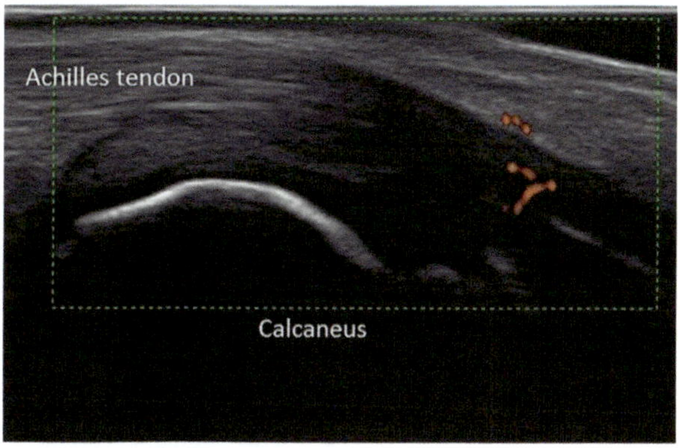

Fig. 10.17 Achilles tendon insertion in a healthy 10-year-old boy. Note the Doppler flow within the tendon insertion

Traction Apophysitis

Traction apophysitis is a term used to describe the occurrence of an insertional tendinopathy at an apophyseal site and possible avulsion of osteochondral fragments. The most common examples are Osgood–Schlatter's disease at the site of the patellar tendon's insertion into the proximal tibia and Sever's disease at the insertion of the Achilles tendon into the calcaneus. The inflammation and injury result from chronic repetitive traction exceeding the resistance to tensile forces at the insertion site of the tendon. It will typically occur during a period of rapid growth, especially in physically very active children. This period coincides with the ossification of the previously cartilaginous insertion of the tendon. In the case of the patellar tendon insertion into the tibial tuberosity, the secondary ossification center forming the tibial tuberosity has not completely united with the other ossification centers of the tibia. In addition, the area of hyaline cartilage, which then transforms into bone, is expanding and replacing to some extent the fibrocartilage that is present at earlier stages of development. This area of cartilage–bone transformation, which is not fully united with the other ossification centers and at the same time exposed to very high tensile forces through the patellar tendon, is therefore prone to injury including avulsion of cartilage and bone fragments [28, 29, 31]. As mentioned earlier, in addition to the avulsion of osteochondral fragments, inflammation of the tendon as well as the cartilage insertion site can also be demonstrated including adjacent bursitis. This might often be present without evidence of bone fragmentation. From this perspective, it is then clear that US is much better situated than radiographs to diagnose and follow this disease process as US can demonstrate and differentiate all involved structures very well.

In the case of bone fragmentation, the examiner has to be careful to clearly distinguish physiological irregularities of the ossification centers from pathologic fragmentation. One also needs to be aware that a variable number of ossification centers (e.g., the calcaneus) can be present and mimic fragmentation. Publications have nevertheless shown that with an increasing number of fragments, the presence of an avulsion fracture is much more likely than the physiologic presence of several ossification centers [49]. In addition, the presence of increased Doppler signals, changes in tendon echogenicity, and associated pathologies, like bursitis, will help to support the diagnosis. Figures 10.18 and 10.19 show images of Osgood–Schlatter's disease.

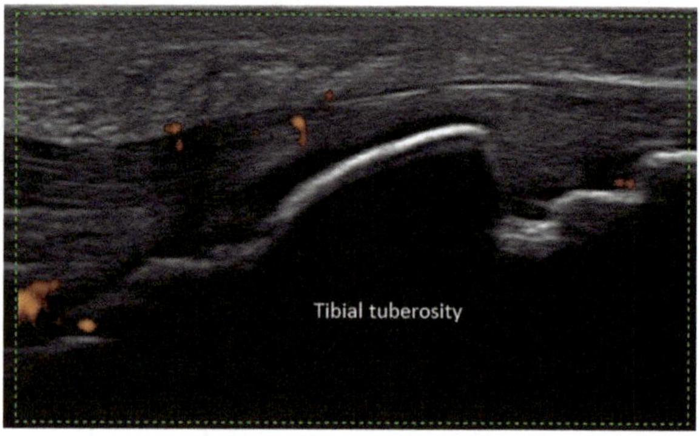

Fig. 10.18 US images of Osgood–Schlatter's disease showing the unaffected side in a 13-year-old boy

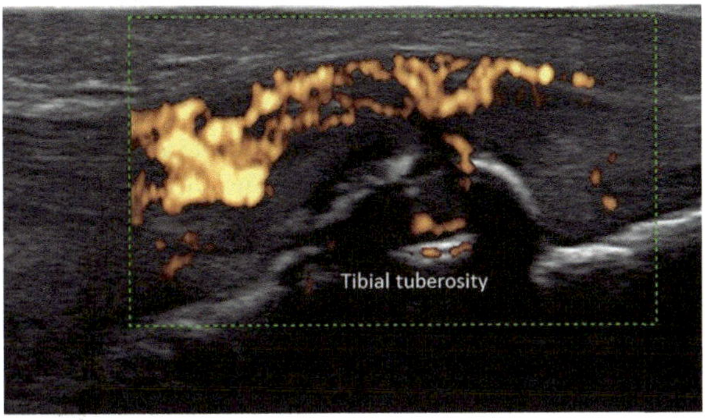

Fig. 10.19 Affected side in Osgood–Schlatter's disease in a 13-year-old with fragmentation of the ossification center, thickening of the tendon insertion, and increased Doppler signals

Reactive Arthritis: Transient Synovitis of the Hip

The principles and examples of an inflamed joint that will be outlined in the upcoming section "Juvenile Idiopathic Arthritis" will also apply to a large extent to the imaging of reactive arthritis. It has to be noted that the author will use the term "reactive arthritis" for arthritis following any infection, which is not a septic arthritis, i.e., where no live organism is present in the synovial tissue or fluid. The difference to the imaging of a chronic arthritis is that the sonographer can expect less of the structural alterations including possibly less synovial hypertrophy and cartilage thinning as well as erosions, although this might not be true in all cases.

Robben et al. [50] have very nicely illustrated this in their study, assessing the thickness of the joint capsule as well as the overall joint space in children suffering from transient synovitis of the hip, a very frequent condition affecting an estimated 1.1 in 1000 children.

They were able to show that whereas the overall thickness of the joint space increases during the acute phase, this increase is entirely due to the accumulation of fluid, whereas the anterior and posterior joint capsule thickness remains the same, and therefore, no significant degree of synovial hypertrophy is present.

It is important to note though that *a hip effusion is not specific for transient synovitis of the hip* and can also occur as part of other pathology including osteonecrosis, slipped capital epiphysis, osteomyelitis, and chronic types of arthritis.

While US is capable of showing abnormalities of the femoral head occurring in Perthes disease and slipped capital epiphysis, it is not the imaging modality of choice, and a suspected diagnosis should be confirmed or ruled out by other imaging modalities including MRI. The same applies to acute or chronic osteomyelitis where US is able to show cortical abnormalities, but diagnosis should not be made solely on the basis of the US exam.

Juvenile Idiopathic Arthritis

Juvenile idiopathic arthritis (JIA), which used to be called juvenile rheumatoid arthritis in North America and juvenile chronic arthritis in Europe, is a chronic arthritis of at least 6 weeks duration without specific cause that begins before the patient is 16 years old [51]. The now accepted international classification for arthritis divides JIA into seven subtypes. It is a relatively frequent disease with an estimated incidence of 1:1000 children. New treatment modalities have greatly improved possible outcomes, including the possibility for long-term remissions. The reliable diagnosis of the presence of synovitis, as well as remission, is of utmost importance, increasing the need to employ imaging modalities like US to refine the clinical assessment. US can be very helpful in demonstrating subclinical synovitis in children suffering from JIA [1, 15, 16, 26, 52]. Some of the earlier studies had limitations including the lack of information on normal US anatomy in children, absence of consensus-based definitions for pathology on US, and the use of scoring and grading systems that had not been validated for children. These methodological deficiencies might also explain why some of the existing literature has yielded conflicting results, including the inability of the presence of US findings to predict disease flares in earlier studies [52]. More recent studies have nevertheless demonstrated subclinical findings both cross-sectionally and longitudinally [1, 15, 16, 26] and also demonstrated that subclinical findings are predictive of flares [16].

No standard scanning protocols have been collectively defined for pediatric rheumatology applications, but they are now available for several anatomic regions, including the knee [13, 17]. It is also reasonable to apply standard MSK scanning protocols that have been developed for adults [53]. While some of these views might not be as relevant for the pediatric patient as they are for adults (e.g., rotator cuff pathology), they will still provide a complete assessment of the joint and surrounding soft tissue structures.

Synovitis

Synovial fluid has been defined by OMERACT as an abnormally anechoic joint space, which is displaceable. This needs to be differentiated from synovial hypertrophy, which is an abnormal hypoechoic joint space which cannot be displaced (or at least hardly displaced). The presence of one or both of these findings on US does not necessarily indicate active inflammation, and therefore, Doppler US can be helpful in demonstrating the increased blood flow in true synovitis. OMERACT has also issued pediatric definitions for synovitis [11], and these have stressed the need to detect Doppler signals within an area of synovial hypertrophy in order to qualify as a sign of synovitis. At the same time, the definition also stresses the fact that physiologic blood flow, for example, in the form of feeding vessels can be present in any part of the joint including, for example, crossing synovial recesses. Examples of feeding vessels and physiologic intra-articular Doppler flow have already been given in Figs. 10.14 and 10.15. Figure 10.20 illustrates abnormalities indicative of

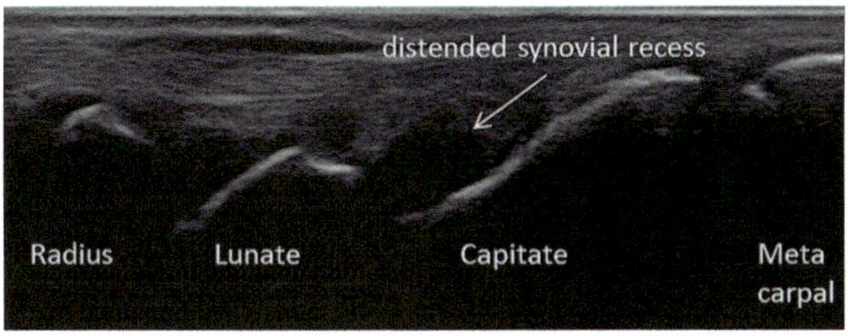

Fig. 10.20 B-mode image of a wrist showing distension of the midcarpal joint recess

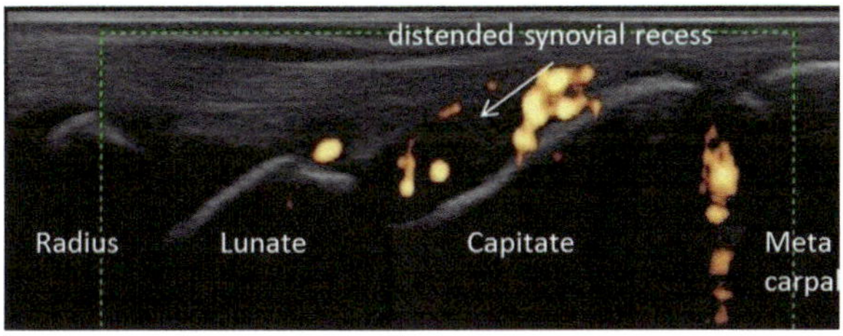

Fig. 10.21 Corresponding color power Doppler image to Fig. 10.20 showing increased intrasynovial Doppler signals in the midcarpal and carpometacarpal joint

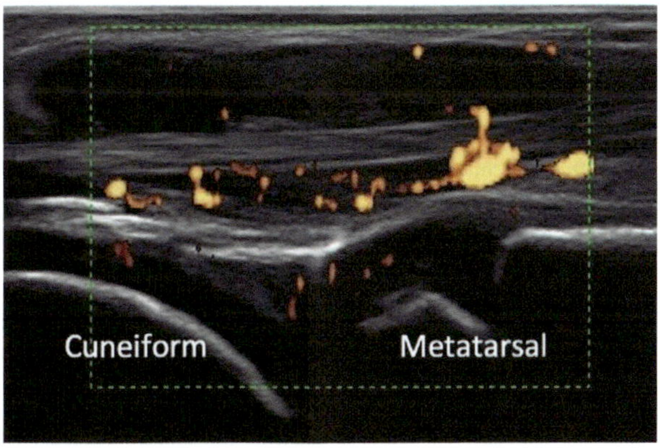

Fig. 10.22 Tenosynovitis in the midfoot of a 9-year-old boy

synovitis in B-mode, and Fig. 10.21 the corresponding Doppler image showing convoluted intrasynovial signals in an area of B-mode abnormalities which are indicative of synovitis.

Tenosynovitis is a frequent finding in children as well, and it is often difficult to differentiate synovitis from tenosynovitis clinically. Especially when planning a joint injection, this differentiation might be important for a more targeted approach. Figure 10.22 shows an example of tenosynovitis of the midfoot in a 9-year-old boy.

Enthesitis

Detection of hyperemia right at the insertion of the tendon into the cortical bone may be an indication for inflammatory enthesitis in adults although not an exclusive finding [54]. In addition, the tendon may appear more hypoechoic and also thickened close to its insertion. In the later stages, calcifications as well as enthesophytes can become visible. Few publications have addressed enthesitis in children [48, 55], suggesting that there may be a significant percentage of subclinical entheseal inflammation in children. As shown in Fig. 10.23 and also demonstrated in the literature [24, 25], physiologic Doppler signals may not be so uncommon even close to the enthesis in children and adolescents. The diagnosis of enthesitis based on the presence of Doppler signals alone must be made with caution, and the coexistence of B-mode abnormalities may be important. Figure 10.24 is showing structural abnormalities of the enthesis in B-mode with coexisting Doppler signals, and Fig. 10.25 is showing US findings at diagnosis and with resolution on treatment.

Synovial Cysts

The classic synovial cyst (e.g., Baker's cyst) is most commonly found as fluid accumulation in the gastrocnemius and/or semimembranosus bursa. In fact, the first publication on the use of diagnostic US in rheumatology reported the differentiation of Baker's cyst from thrombophlebitis [56]. In children, synovial cysts can also be commonly found in other locations, originating not only from bursae but also along tendons. The biceps tendon in such a location and children with the systemic type

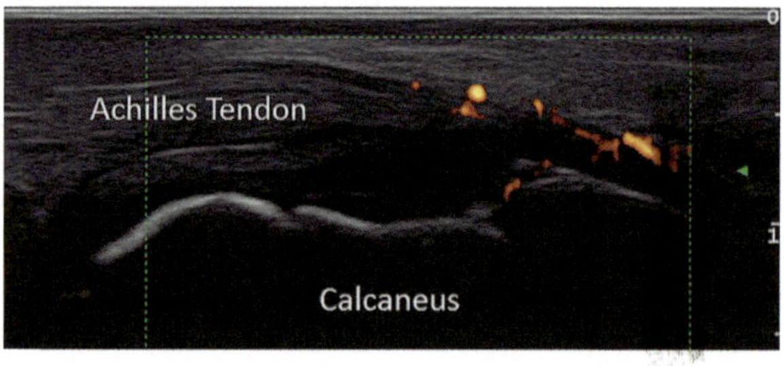

Fig. 10.23 Achilles tendon insertion with Doppler signals in a healthy 14-year-old male

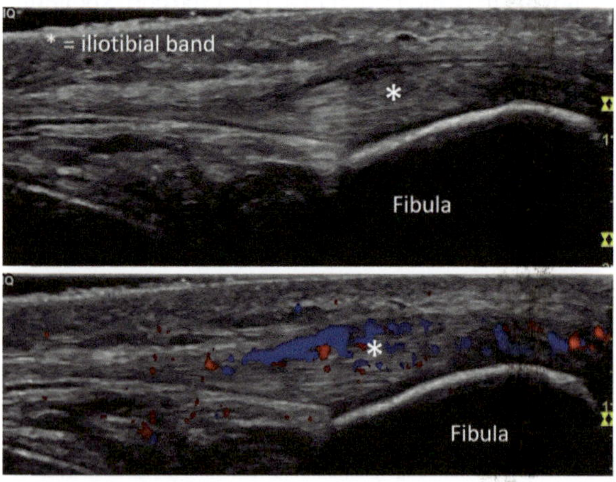

Fig. 10.24 Iliotibial band showing anechoic thickened areas on B-mode and increased Doppler signals

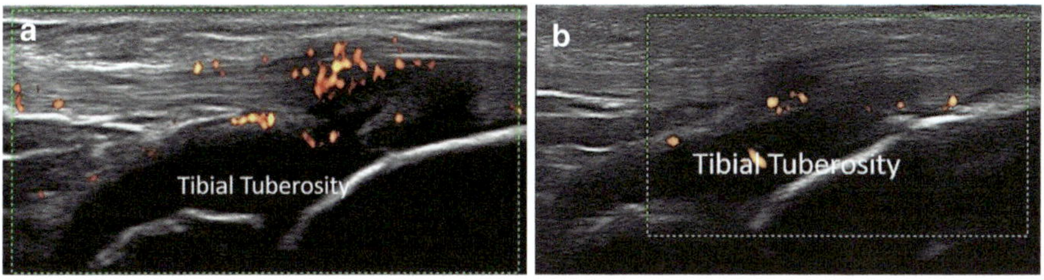

Fig. 10.25 Tibial tuberosity (unossified) in a 10-year-old showing (**a**) enthesitis of the distal patella tendon and (**b**) almost complete resolution of findings on treatment

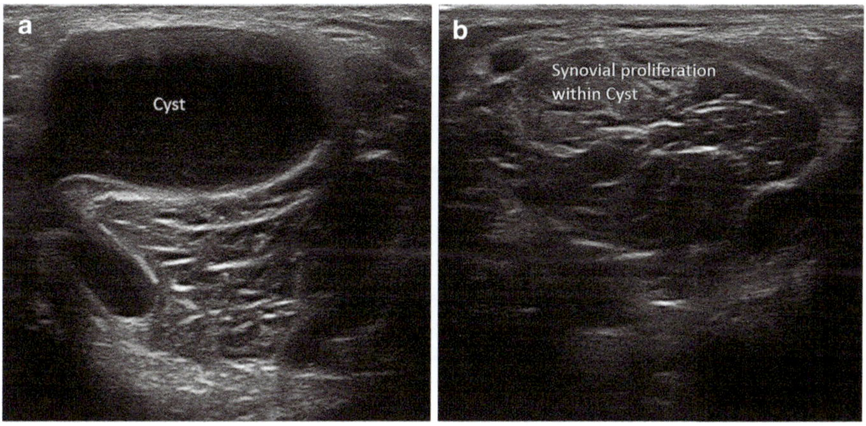

Fig. 10.26 Baker's cyst in the knee (**a**) before and (**b**) after aspiration

of JIA might be particularly prone to the development of synovial cysts originating, for example, from the biceps tendon sheath [57]. US can be very helpful in differentiating a synovial cyst from other pathology like a soft tissue mass or hemorrhage. It will often be able to demonstrate the communication of the cyst with the joint space. Figure 10.24 shows a Baker's cyst before and after aspiration (Fig. 10.26).

Erosions

US has been shown to be more sensitive than radiographs and, depending on the location, equally sensitive as MRI for the demonstration of erosions. Whereas bone erosions might overall be less common in JIA than RA, they still occur and are an important sign of joint damage. Not many publications have studied the appearance of bone erosions in JIA with US. It does seem however that the location can be more epiphyseal than in adults where the location might be more commonly meta-epiphyseal [58]. This is likely due to the fact that the epiphyseal cartilage, especially in younger children, is vascularized and allows inflammatory cells and lytic factors to invade more easily and cause destruction. A recent publication has demonstrated that these erosions can be reliably demonstrated in children also [14].

Cartilage

The imaging and assessment of cartilage have been discussed in the normal ultrasound anatomy in children section. Careful imaging technique is essential to show the cartilage well. Rather than cartilage thickness measurements, assessments of the cartilage contour might prove to be more reliable. Especially in the earlier phases of arthritis, cartilage swelling might be observed. Finally, damage to the subchondral bone can sometimes be observed without loss of thickness of the overlying cartilage. This might be due to the fact that the cartilage is much more vascularized than in an adult.

Point-of-Care US in Pediatric Rheumatology

Point-of-care (POC) US is defined as an US exam performed and interpreted by the clinician in the office or at the bedside. This also implies that it will often be a more targeted exam looking at specific aspects of a joint, for example, the presence of synovitis in a given joint and not necessarily assessing every single component of the joint. It might be particularly helpful with serial assessments to monitor therapeutic responses.

The advantages of POCUS are:

- Quick diagnosis
- Direct correlation with patient presentation (signs and symptoms)
- The possibility to do a functional or dynamic exam
- Easily repeatable (condition of patient changes/therapeutic response)

US performed by the rheumatologist or other MSK provider will therefore improve the standard of clinical care by refining the clinical assessment. If provided in a POC setting during the clinic visit, it will be more time efficient for both the patient and the physician, who has the information available immediately compared to booking an US exam separately. In most cases, it will also save resources and cost less than separate referrals. As such, POCUS is an extremely important addition to a modern pediatric rheumatology practice.

Interventions

US can be extremely helpful in guiding procedures, and data in adult rheumatology have clearly demonstrated higher accuracy in needle placement for US-guided vs. palpation-guided injections. In pediatric rheumatology, the same can be expected. US-guided injections also alleviate the need to follow a standard approach to the injection and instead allow the most convenient approach to the synovial recess. At the same time, contact with structures like blood vessels, nerves, cartilage, or bone can be avoided. Often, this may reduce the procedural pain, a very important aspect of pediatric care. In some patients, this may even allow procedures to be done without sedation which otherwise would have required the involvement of the anesthetist (Fig. 10.27).

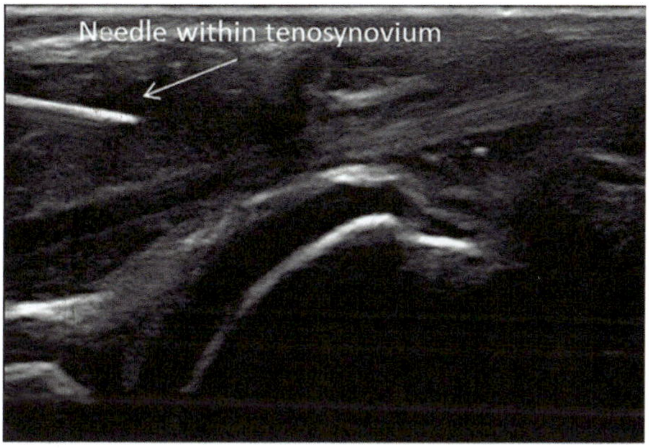

Fig. 10.27 US-guided injection for tenosynovitis of a 9-year-old boy with systemic JIA

Conclusion

MSK US of pediatric patients provides many advantages when compared to other imaging modalities, including imaging without sedation, no radiation exposure, and the ability to visualize structures dynamically. It allows for diagnostic and monitoring capabilities that have the potential to expedite diagnosis, improve medical decision-making in regard to treatment plans, and additionally provide guided/targeted injections that are associated with reduced procedural pain. In the growing skeleton, care must be taken to avoid interpreting normal physiologic blood flow in pediatric images vs. images reflecting true pathologic disease.

Review Questions

1. In this longitudinal scan along the distal femur of a 3-year-old girl with juvenile idiopathic arthritis, the arrows are pointing to a hypoechoic area with hyperechoic signals. This represents:

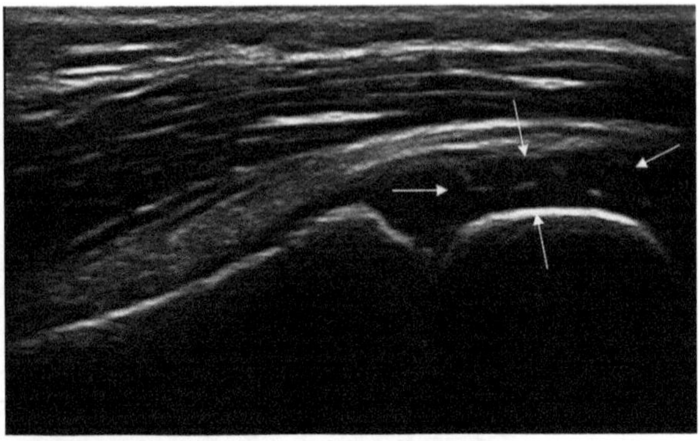

   (a) A joint effusion in the knee joint with hyperechoic signals
   (b) Osteochondrosis of the cartilage of the femur
   (c) Hyaline cartilage in the femur epiphysis with normal cartilage signals likely representing vascular channels
   (d) Chronic damage to the cartilage from the juvenile arthritis

2. This longitudinal scan along the humeroradial joint in a 3-year-old girl shows:

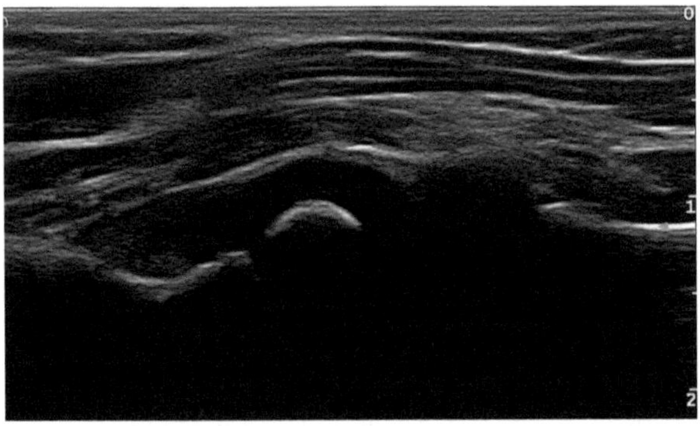

   (a) A hypoechoic area representing an effusion extending from the radial fossa up to the radial head
   (b) An effusion in the radial fossa and hyaline cartilage in the epiphysis of humerus and radius
   (c) A normal humeroradial joint with incomplete ossification of the hyaline cartilage
   (d) A subluxation of the humeroulnar joint

3. This suprapatellar longitudinal scan in a 3-year-old girl shows:

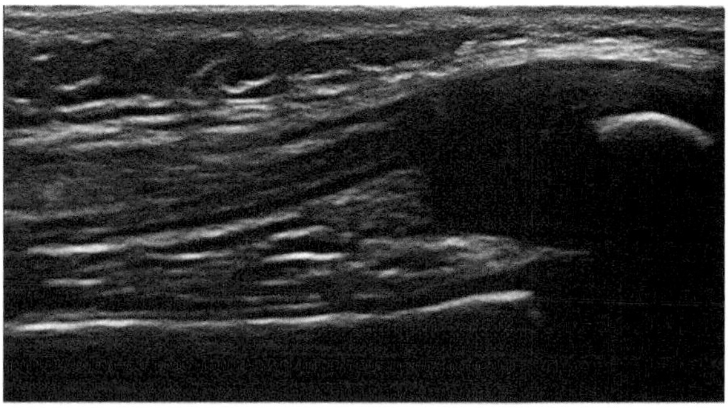

   (a) An effusion of the suprapatellar recess
   (b) The cartilage of the developing patella but no fluid in the suprapatellar recess
   (c) Quadriceps tendinopathy
   (d) None of the above
4. This longitudinal scan of the hip shows:

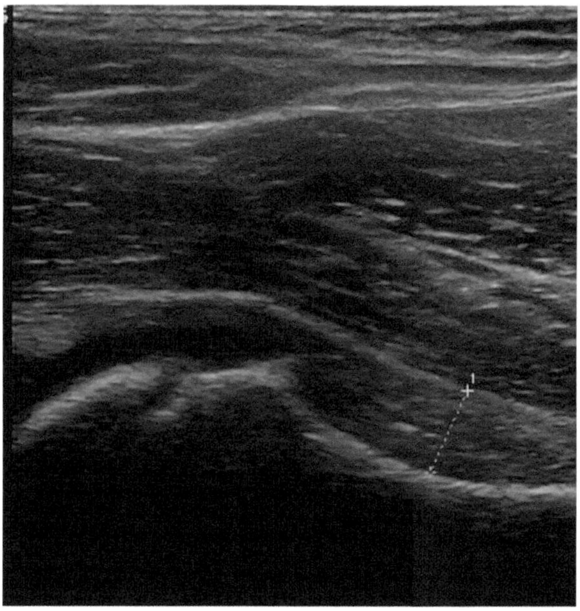

   (a) Thickening of the joint capsule of the hip with a double contour sign
   (b) The two layers of the joint capsule of the hip
   (c) A fracture of the femoral head
   (d) None of the above

5. Which of the following statements is correct with regard to ultrasound findings of the hip joint?
   (a) In transient synovitis, fluid accumulates between the anterior and posterior layer of the joint capsule without thickening of the capsule itself.
   (b) The demonstration of synovial thickening without Doppler signals is suggestive of transient synovitis.
   (c) A hypoechogenic distension of the intra-articular space is suggestive of septic arthritis (high cell count within the intra-articular fluid).
   (d) Changes of the morphology of the femoral head in advanced Perthes disease can be seen on radiographs but not ultrasonography which can only demonstrate soft tissue abnormalities involving the joint space.
6. For TMJ ultrasound, which statement is correct?
   (a) Diagnostic ultrasound of the temporomandibular joint (TMJ) is not possible for technical reasons.
   (b) MSK ultrasound cannot reliably demonstrate synovitis of the TMJ.
   (c) MRI and ultrasonography are equally sensitive for demonstration of synovitis in the TMJ.
   (d) Synovitis in the TMJ can be reliably demonstrated, but the disc position cannot be fully assessed.
7. When examining clinically swollen ankles in children suffering from JIA with ultrasonography, the ultrasound exam will typically demonstrate the following:
   (a) Children with polyarticular disease are more likely to have complex involvement including synovitis as well as tenosynovitis than those with oligoarticular JIA.
   (b) More than 50% of children with oligoarticular JIA have tibiotalar joint synovitis.
   (c) The highest percentage of any pathology in oligo JIA is lateral tenosynovitis.
   (d) 1/3 to 1/2 of children had tenosynovitis only.

8. This longitudinal midline scan of the wrist with power Doppler in a 10-year-old boy shows:

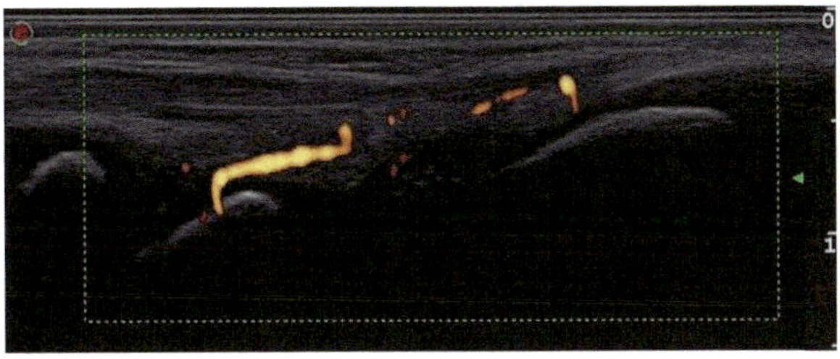

   (a) Synovitis of the radiocarpal joint with a pathologic Doppler signal at the site of an early erosion of the lunate bone
   (b) A feeding vessel entering the lunate bone
   (c) A pathologic shunt between the extra- and intra-articular space
   (d) None of the above
9. This longitudinal scan of the posterior calcaneus and Achilles tendon demonstrates:

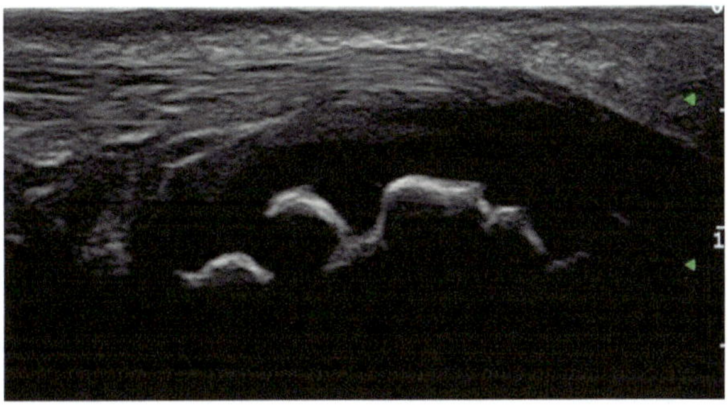

   (a) The normal appearance of a calcaneus in a 1-year-old child
   (b) Erosive disease of the posterior calcaneus
   (c) The normal appearance of a calcaneus in a 7-year-old child
   (d) An advanced Achilles tendinopathy
10. Which of the following statements with regard to erosions in the small joints of the fingers is true?
    (a) Erosions in the MCP joints cannot be shown with ultrasonography.
    (b) In children, erosions of the small finger joints can be expected in a more epiphyseal location than in adults.
    (c) Erosions of the MCP joints in children cannot be visualized due to the cartilage in the epiphyseal areas.
    (d) Erosions only occur in a mature skeleton with full ossification.

Answers

1. (c) Hyaline cartilage in the femur epiphysis with normal cartilage signals likely representing vascular channels
2. (b) An effusion in the radial fossa and hyaline cartilage in the epiphysis of humerus and radius
3. (b) The cartilage of the developing patella but no fluid in the suprapatellar recess
4. (b) The two layers of the joint capsule of the hip
5. (a) In transient synovitis, fluid accumulates between the anterior and posterior layer of the joint capsule without thickening of the capsule itself.
6. (a) Diagnostic ultrasound of the temporomandibular joint (TMJ) is not possible for technical reasons.
7. (d) 1/3 to 1/2 of children had tenosynovitis only.
8. (b) A feeding vessel entering the lunate bone
9. (c) The normal appearance of a calcaneus in a 7-year-old child
10. (b) In children, erosions of the small finger joints can be expected in a more epiphyseal location than in adults.

References

1. Haslam KE, McCann LJ, Wyatt S, Wakefield RJ. The detection of subclinical synovitis by ultrasound in oligoarticular juvenile idiopathic arthritis: a pilot study. Rheumatology (Oxford). 2010;49(1):123–7.
2. Rooney ME, McAllister C, Burns JF. Ankle disease in juvenile idiopathic arthritis: ultrasound findings in clinically swollen ankles. J Rheumatol. 2009;36(8):1725–9.
3. Nistala K, Babar J, Johnson K, Campbell-Stokes P, Foster K, Ryder C, McDonagh JE. Clinical assessment and core outcome variables are poor predictors of hip arthritis diagnosed by MRI in juvenile idiopathic arthritis. Rheumatology (Oxford). 2007;46(4):699–702.
4. Chauvin NA, Khwaja A. Imaging of inflammatory arthritis in children: status and perspectives on the use of ultrasound, radiographs, and magnetic resonance imaging. Rheum Dis Clin N Am. 2016;42:587–606.
5. Malattia C, Tzaribachev N, van den Berg M, Magni-Manzoni S. Juvenile idiopathic arthritis – the role of imaging from a rheumatologist's perspective. Pediatr Radiol. 2018;48:785–91.
6. Lanni S, Martini A, Malattia C. Heading toward a modern imaging approach in juvenile idiopathic arthritis. Curr Rheumatol Rep. 2014;16:416.
7. Malattia C, Rinaldi M, Martini A. The role of imaging in juvenile idiopathic arthritis. Expert Rev Clin Immunol. 2018;20:1–14.
8. Roth J, Jousse-Joulin S, Magni-Manzoni S, Rodriguez A, Tzaribachev N, Iagnocco A, Naredo E, D'Agostino MA, Collado P. Omeract definitions for the sonographic features of the normal pediatric joint. Arthritis Care Res (Hoboken). 2015;67(1):136–42.
9. Weiss PF, Chauvin NA, Roth J. Imaging in juvenile spondyloarthritis. Curr Rheumatol Rep. 2016;18:75.
10. Collado P, Naredo E, Calvo C, et al; ECO-JIA Study Group. Reduced joint assessment vs comprehensive assessment for ultrasound detection of synovitis in juvenile idiopathic arthritis. Rheumatology (Oxford). 2013;52:1477–84.
11. Roth J, Ravagnani V, Backhaus M, Balint P, Bruns A, Bruyn GA, Collado P, De la Cruz L, Guillaume-Czitrom S, Herlin T, Hernandez C, Iagnocco A, Jousse-Joulin S, Lanni S, Lilleby

V, Malattia C, Magni-Manzoni S, Modesto C, Rodriguez A, Nieto JC, Ohrndorf S, Rossi-Semerano L, Selvaag AM, Swen N, Ting TV, Tzaribachev N, Vega-Fernandez P, Vojinovic J, Windschall D, D'Agostino MA, Naredo E, OMERACT Ultrasound Group. Preliminary Definitions for the Sonographic Features of Synovitis in Children. Arthritis Care Res. 2017;69:1217–23.
12. Windschall D, Collado P, Vojinovic J, Magni-Manzoni S, Balint P, Bruyn GAW, Hernandez-Diaz C, Nieto JC, Ravagnani V, Tzaribachev N, Iagnocco A, D'Agostino MA, Naredo E, OMERACT paediatric ultrasound subtask force. Age-related vascularization and ossification of joints in children: an international pilot study to test multi-observer ultrasound reliability. Arthritis Care Res (Hoboken). 2020;72(4):498–506. https://doi.org/10.1002/acr.23335.
13. Ting TV, Vega-Fernandez P, Oberle EJ, De Ranieri D, Bukulmez H, Lin C, Moser D, Barrowman NJ, Zhao Y, Benham HM, Tasan L, Thatayatikom A, Roth J, CARRA JIA Ultrasound Workgroup. A novel ultrasound image acquisition protocol and scoring system for the pediatric knee. Arthritis Care Res. 2019;71(7):977–85.
14. Ventura-Rios L, Faugier E, Barzola L, De la Cruz Becerra LB, Sanchez-Bringas G, Rodriguez Garcia A, Maldonado R, Roth J, Hernandez C. Reliability of ultrasonography to detect inflammatory lesions and structural damage in juvenile idiopathic arthritis. Pediatr Rheumatol. 2018;16:58.
15. Lanni S, van Dijkhuizen EHP, Vanoni F, Viola S, Magnaguagno F, Magnano GM, Gandolfo C, Ravelli A, Malattia C. Ultrasound changes in synovial abnormalities induced by treatment in juvenile idiopathic arthritis. Clin Exp Rheumatol. 2018;36(2):329–34.
16. De Lucia O, Ravagnani V, Pregnolato F, Hila A, Pontikaki I, Gattinara M, Romano M, Gerloni V, Pieropan S, Murgo A, Rossini M, Cimaz R, Meroni PL. Baseline ultrasound examination as possible predictor of relapse in patients affected by juvenile idiopathic arthritis (JIA). Ann Rheum Dis. 2018;77(10):1426–31.
17. Collado P, Vojinovic J, Nieto JC, et al. Toward standardized musculoskeletal ultrasound in pediatric rheumatology: normal age-related ultrasound findings. Arthritis Care Res (Hoboken). 2016;68:348–56.
18. Rohrschneider WK, Fuchs G, Tröger J. Ultrasonographic evaluation of the anterior recess in the normal hip: a prospective study on 166 asymptomatic children. Pediatr Radiol. 1996;26:629–34.
19. Windschall D, Trauzeddel R, Haller M, Krumrey-Langkammerer M, Nimtz-Talaska A, Berendes R, Ganser G, Nirschl C, Schoof P, Trauzeddel RF, Palm-Beden K, Lehmann H, Imaging Working Group of the German Society of Rheumatology in Childhood and Adolescence (GKJR). Pediatric musculoskeletal ultrasound: age- and sex-related normal B-mode findings of the knee. Rheumatol Int. 2016;36(11):1569–77.
20. Trauzeddel R, Lehman H, Trauzeddel RF, Haller M, Palm-Beden K, Ganser G, Berendes R, Nirschl C, Nimtz-Talaska A, Krumrey-Langkammerer M, Schoof P, Windschall D. Age dependent ultrasound B-mode findings of the elbow joint in healthy children and adolescents. Rheumatol Int. 2019;39(6):1007–18.
21. Trauzeddel R, Windschall D, Trauzeddel RF, Nirschl C, Ganser G, Palm-Beden K, Berendes R, Haller M, Krumrey-Langkammerer M, Nimtz-Talaska A, Schoof P, Lehmann H. Arthrosonographic reference values of the shoulder joint in healthy children and adolescents: a cross-sectional multicentre ultrasound study. Klin Padiatr. 2017;229(5):293–301. https://doi.org/10.1055/s-0043-111596. Epub 2017 Aug 24
22. Trauzeddel RF, Lehmann H, Windschall D, Ganser G, Berendes R, Haller M, Krumrey-Langkammerer M, Palm-Beden K, Nimtz-Talaska A, Nirschl C, Schoof P, Trauzeddel R. Age-dependent arthrosonographic reference values of the hip joint in healthy children and adolescents – a cross-sectional multicenter ultrasound study. Pediatr Radiol. 2017;47(10):1329–36.
23. Spannow AH, Pfeiffer-Jensen M, Andersen NT, Herlin T, Stenbög E. Ultrasonographic measurements of joint cartilage thickness in healthy children: age- and sex-related standard reference values. J Rheumatol. 2010;37:2595–601.

24. Chauvin NA, Ho-Fung V, Jaramillo D, Edgar JC, Weiss PF. Ultrasound of the joints and entheses in healthy children. Pediatr Radiol. 2015;45(9):1344–54.
25. Roth J, Stinson SE, Chan J, Barrowman N, DiGeso L. Differential pattern of Doppler signals at lower-extremity entheses of healthy children. Pediatr Radiol. 2019; https://doi.org/10.1007/s00247-019-04464-8.
26. Rebollo-Polo M, Koujok K, Weisser C, et al. Ultrasound findings on patients with juvenile idiopathic arthritis in clinical remission. Arthritis Care Res (Hoboken). 2011;63:10131019.
27. Lee SK, Kim YS, Oh HS, Yang KH, Kim EC, Chi JG. Prenatal development of the human mandible. Anat Rec. 2001;263:314–25.
28. Ogden JA, Hempton RF, Southwick WO. Development of the tibial tuberosity. Anat Rec. 1974;182:431–46.
29. Ogden JA, Southwick WO. Osgood-Schlatter's disease and tibial tuberosity development. Clin Orthop Relat Res. 1976;116:180–9.
30. Ogden JA. Radiology of postnatal skeletal development IX. Proximal tibia and fibula. Skelet Radiol. 1984;11(4):169–77.
31. Ogden JA. Radiology of postnatal skeletal development. X. Patella and tibial tuberosity. Skelet Radiol. 1984;11(4):246–57.
32. Ogden JA, McCarthy SM. Radiology of postnatal skeletal development. VIII. Distal tibia and fibula. Skelet Radiol. 1983;10(4):209–20.
33. McCarthy SM, Ogden JA. Radiology of postnatal skeletal development. VI. Elbow joint, proximal radius, and ulna. Skelet Radiol. 1982;9(1):17–26.
34. McCarthy SM, Ogden JA. Radiology of postnatal skeletal development. V. Distal humerus. Skeletal Radiol. 1982;7(4):239–49.
35. Miller B, Bonel H, Rotzetter M, Villiger PM, Ziswiler HR. Measuring finger joint cartilage by ultrasound as a promising alternative to conventional radiograph imaging. Arthritis Rheum. 2009;61:435–41.
36. Torp-Pedersen S, Bartels EM, Wilhjelm J, Bliddal H. Articular cartilage thickness measured with US is not as easy as it appears: a systematic review of measurement techniques and image interpretation. Ultraschall Med. 2011;32(1):54–61. Epub 2010 May 28
37. Sureda D, Quiroga S, Arnal C, Boronat M, Andreu J, Casas L. Juvenile rheumatoid arthritis of the knee: evaluation with US. Radiology. 1994;190(2):403–6.
38. Benjamin M, Moriggl B, Brenner E, Emery P, McGonagle D, Redman S. The "enthesis organ" concept: why enthesopathies may not present as focal insertional disorders. Arthritis Rheum. 2004;50:3306–13.
39. Fornage BD. Achilles tendon: US examination. Radiology. 1986;159:759–64.
40. Grechenig W, Mayr JM, Peicha G, Hammerl R, Schatz B, Grechenig S. Sonoanatomy of the Achilles tendon insertion in children. J Clin Ultrasound. 2004;32:338–43.
41. Murphy KJ, Rubin JM. Power Doppler: it's a good thing. Semin Ultrasound CT MR. 1997;18(1):13–21.
42. Terslev L, Torp-Pedersen S, Savnik A, von der Recke P, Quvistgard E, Danneskiold-Samsoe B, Bliddal H. Doppler ultrasound and magnetic resonance imaging of synovial inflammation of the hand in rheumatoid arthritis: a comparative study. Arthritis Rheum. 2003;48(9):2434–41.
43. Szkudlarek M, Court-Payen M, Strandberg C, Klarlund M, Klausen T, Ostergaard M. Power Doppler ultrasonography for assessment of synovitis in the metacarpophalangeal joints of patients with rheumatoid arthritis: a comparison with dynamic magnetic resonance imaging. Arthritis Rheum. 2001;44(9):2018–23.
44. Schmidt WA, Volker L, Zacher J, Schlafke M, Ruhnke M, Gromnica-Ihle E. Colour Doppler ultrasonography to detect pannus in knee joint synovitis. Clin Exp Rheumatol. 2000;18(4):439–44.
45. Walther M, Harms H, Krenn V, Radke S, Faehndrich TP, Gohlke F. Correlation of power Doppler sonography with vascularity of the synovial tissue of the knee joint in patients with osteoarthritis and rheumatoid arthritis. Arthritis Rheum. 2001;44(2):331–8.

46. Walther M, Harms H, Krenn V, Radke S, Kirschner S, Gohlke F. Synovial tissue of the hip at power Doppler US: correlation between vascularity and power Doppler US signal. Radiology. 2002;225(1):225–31.
47. Albrecht K, Muller-Ladner U, Strunk J. Quantification of the synovial perfusion in rheumatoid arthritis using Doppler ultrasonography. Clin Exp Rheumatol. 2007;25(4):630–8.
48. Jousse-Joulin S, Breton S, Cangemi C, Fenoll B, Bressolette L, de Parscau L, Saraux A, Devauchelle-Pensec V. Ultrasonography for detecting enthesitis in juvenile idiopathic arthritis. Arthritis Care Res (Hoboken). 2011;63(6):849–55.
49. Volpon JB, de Carvalho Filho G. Calcaneal apophysitis: a quantitative radiographic evaluation of the secondary ossification center. Arch Orthop Trauma Surg. 2002;122:338–41.
50. Robben SG, Lequin MH, Diepstraten AF, den Hollander JC, Entius CA, Meradji M. Anterior joint capsule of the normal hip and in children with transient synovitis: US study with anatomic and histologic correlation. Radiology. 1999;210(2):499–507.
51. Petty RE, Southwood TR, Manners P, International League of Associations for Rheumatology, et al. International League of Associations for Rheumatology classification of juvenile idiopathic arthritis, 2nd revision, Edmonton, 2001. J Rheumatol. 2004;31:390–2.
52. Magni-Manzoni S, Scirè CA, Ravelli A, Klersy C, Rossi S, Muratore V, et al. Ultrasound-detected synovial abnormalities are frequent in clinically inactive juvenile idiopathic arthritis, but do not predict a flare of synovitis. Ann Rheum Dis. 2013;72(2):223–8. Epub 2012 Jun 26
53. Möller I, Janta I, Backhaus M, Ohrndorf S, Bong DA, Martinoli C, Filippucci E, Sconfienza LM, Terslev L, Damjanov N, Hammer HB, Sudol-Szopinska I, Grassi W, Balint P, Bruyn GAW, D'Agostino MA, Hollander D, Siddle HJ, Supp G, Schmidt WA, Iagnocco A, Koski J, Kane D, Fodor D, Bruns A, Mandl P, Kaeley GS, Micu M, Ho C, Vlad V, Chávez-López M, Filippou G, Cerón CE, Nestorova R, Quintero M, Wakefield R, Carmona L, Naredo E. The 2017 EULAR standardised procedures for ultrasound imaging in rheumatology. Ann Rheum Dis. 2017;76(12):1974–9.
54. D'Agostino MA, Said-Nahal R, Hacquard-Bouder C, Brasseur JL, Dougados M, Breban M. Assessment of peripheral enthesitis in the spondylarthropathies by ultrasonography combined with power Doppler. Arthritis Rheum. 2003;48:523–33.
55. Weiss PF, Chauvin NA, Klink AJ, Localio R, Feudtner C, Jaramillo D. Detection of enthesitis in children with enthesitis-related arthritis: dolorimetry compared to ultrasonography. Arthritis Rheum. 2014;66(1):218–27.
56. Moore CP, Sarti DA, Louie JS. Ultrasonographic demonstration of popliteal cysts in rheumatoid arthritis. A noninvasive technique. Arthritis Rheum. 1975;18(6):577–80.
57. Roth J, Scheer I, Kraft S, Keitzer R, Riebel T. Uncommon synovial cysts in children. Eur J Pediatr. 2006;165(3):178–81.
58. Karmazyn B, Bowyer SL, Schmidt KM, Ballinger SH, Buckwalter K, Beam TT, Ying J. US findings of metacarpophalangeal joints in children with idiopathic juvenile arthritis. Pediatr Radiol. 2007;37(5):475–82. Epub 2007 Mar 20

Part I

Rheumatic Diseases

Ultrasound in Rheumatoid Arthritis

11

Hilde Berner Hammer and Lene Terslev

Key Points

- Synovitis in joints and tendons can be scored semiquantitatively for both grayscale synovitis and power Doppler activity to assess hypervascularity.
- Several scoring systems for evaluating inflammation in rheumatoid arthritis patients have been validated and shown to be reliable and responsive to treatment.
- Appropriate adjustment of ultrasound equipment settings is critical in accurately assessing power Doppler activity.
- Too much pressure on the probe can result in displacement of effusion and compression of blood vessels, leading to inadequate and inaccurate imaging of the joint.

Introduction

The history and physical exam are vital to the rheumatologist in evaluating patients for suspected inflammatory arthritis. Musculoskeletal ultrasound allows for extension of the physical examination, often revealing pathology in difficult-to-examine

H. B. Hammer (✉)
Department of Rheumatology, Diakonhjemmet Hospital, Oslo, Norway
e-mail: h-hammer@diakonsyk.no

L. Terslev
Center for Rheumatology and Spine Diseases, Rigshospitalet-Glostrup, Copenhagen, Denmark
e-mail: lene.terslev.01@regionh.dk

M. J. Kohler (ed.), *Musculoskeletal Ultrasound in Rheumatology Review*,
https://doi.org/10.1007/978-3-030-73555-5_11

patients, as well as patients with subclinical inflammation. This chapter provides further details on how to assess your patient for synovitis by ultrasound. Several scoring systems have been shown to be responsive to treatment, but the optimal joint/tendon score is yet to be explored. Doppler activity may be quantified by use of pixel counts and flow may be examined by use of resistive index.

How to Obtain Good Images for Evaluation of Synovitis in Joints and Tendons

As discussed in Chap. 1 "Introduction: Musculoskeletal Ultrasound Indications and Fundamentals," a good working position is of utmost importance. It is recommended to have an adjustable examination bed and a chair that allows free movement of the legs to allow for proper positioning of both the patient and examiner [1]. For the patient, this means that the joint examined must be in a relaxed and comfortable position. For the lower extremities, this often means having the patient lying in prone position on the examination bed whereas the upper extremities may be examined with the patient sitting opposite the examiner with the arm resting on a small table or the examination bed.

For the examiner, the height of the examination bed is important together with optional armrest. The transducer grip should be light and relaxed. This may be obtained by holding the probe close to the sole of the probe using the ulnar fingers for support. It is important to avoid pull of the probe while scanning, and some sonographers prefer to have the cable around their neck, while others would choose another way to avoid the pull of the cable. Whatever method is used, it is necessary to have a relaxed grip and keep the surface (footplate) of the probe in contact with the skin. A good transducer grip, as well as plenty of ultrasound (US) gel, will also prevent putting too much pressure on the probe, which would result in displacement of effusion and during Doppler examination compression of vessels both resulting in inadequate results (see Fig. 11.1). In addition, during Doppler examinations, it is necessary to keep the probe still since movements of the probe or of the patient during scanning will cause motion artifacts, making it difficult to interpret the Doppler signals. During all US examinations, it is important to hold the probe perpendicular on the tissues being examined to obtain good US images.

Temperature and vasodilating agents can also potentially affect the degree of hyperemia of the tissue being scanned.

Ultrasound Evaluation of Inflammation

Joint and tendon inflammation may be evaluated clinically. However, several studies have found US to be more sensitive in detecting joint inflammation [2–5]. In addition, US gives the clinician additional information by evaluation of the degree

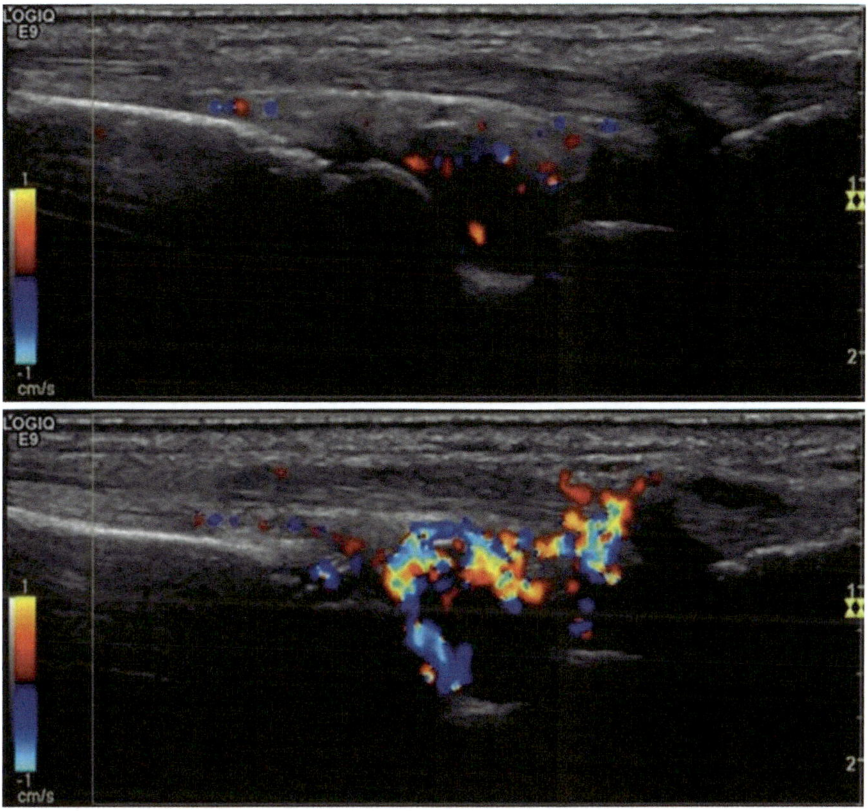

Fig. 11.1 Pressure. The *top* image shows the Doppler findings in a wrist joint when applying too much pressure on the probe. Flow information is lost. The *bottom* image shows Doppler flow in the same wrist when applying only light probe pressure

of synovitis by use of grayscale US (GS). Inflammation of the synovial lining is a key feature of rheumatoid arthritis (RA), and the hyperemia during active inflammation can be visualized by use of power (PD) or color (CD) Doppler. PD displays the energy of the moving erythrocytes, while CD displays the velocity and direction of moving erythrocytes. Changes in Doppler activity reflect changes in disease activity [6–8], and the presence of PD has been associated with later development of erosions [9, 10].

Most joints tendons are quite superficial, and thus high frequencies (i.e., 10–18 MHz) are chosen to get optimal grayscale images. However, for deeper structures like the hip and glenohumeral joint, low frequencies are necessary to reach the joints (i.e., 5–10 MHz). Usually, the working depth for most superficial joints will be 2.5–3 cm, which will be sufficient for evaluating most peripheral joints. However, it will be necessary to adjust the focus to be in plane with the synovitis to be evaluated.

Doppler Ultrasound

When applying Doppler to the US examination, it becomes possible to visualize the hyperemic part of the inflammatory process as Doppler depicts flow because of the Doppler shift. The submitted wavelength (frequency) is changed when it is reflected by an object in motion which for all practical purposes are the erythrocytes. The difference between the submitted and received frequency is then translated into color information which is superimposed on the grayscale image, and the depicted reflection of erythrocytes is the actual flow. Only flow moving toward or away from the transducer is detected, which means that if the flow runs parallel to the probe (the insonation angle being 90°), then no flow can be detected. In every pixel inside the Doppler box, the returned frequencies are analyzed and represented as color data on the screen. The reflected frequencies have different velocities because the erythrocytes travel with different velocities, and every velocity has its individual energy. This results in two Doppler options: power Doppler (PD) and color Doppler (CD). Both PD and CD are used extensively to evaluate hyperemia as they both show the reflections of the moving erythrocytes, however in different ways. PD is showing the *energy* from all the moving erythrocytes and is therefore an image of the detected blood pool, whereas CD is displaying the *mean velocity* of the moving erythrocytes and is therefore an image of the blood velocity [11]. PD has always been perceived as the most sensitive Doppler modality; however, software has advanced tremendously within the last 12 years, and CD has now been shown to be more sensitive than PD on some machines though no obvious explanation has been put forth to explain this. In evaluation of synovitis, the main issue when choosing Doppler modality is its sensitivity for slow flow. It is therefore recommended to choose the modality which is most sensitive to slow flow, and the choice between PD and CD depends on the equipment [12]. On most portable, compact US machines, PD is the most sensitive choice.

Optimization of Doppler Settings

Since high Doppler sensitivity is important in rheumatology, it is necessary to optimize the settings of the machine. The settings to adjust for Doppler evaluation include frequency, gain, wall filter, pulse repetitive frequency (PRF), color priority (or threshold), and color box size [11].

- *Doppler frequency* is independent of the grayscale frequency. Lower Doppler frequency will allow more penetration but also a more grainy Doppler image (larger color pixels). Higher Doppler frequency gives a more detailed image of the vessels but at the expense of penetration. As most of the structures of interest are fairly superficial, a high frequency is often optimal.
- *Doppler gain* is independent of the grayscale gain. On some US machines, the Doppler gain knob/button differs from the grayscale gain, while on other machines, the grayscale and Doppler gain knob/button are the same and will

automatically change over when the color or power Doppler knob/button is turned on. The gain setting determines the sensitivity of the system to flow. By lowering the gain, noise and motion artifacts may be prevented, but weak flow signals will go undetected. The gain should therefore be adjusted correctly by increasing it until a lot of noise pixels are seen in the Doppler box and then lowering the gain until only very few noise pixels are visible [11]. Gain will then be most sensitive to slow flow (see Fig. 11.2).

- *Wall filter* is to prevent arterial wall motion from interfering with detection of blood flow. Low blood flow states, as seen in flow of synovium, have no significant wall motion, whereas larger blood vessels such as the axillary artery will have more wall motion. Minimizing wall filter may increase tissue motion artifact.
- *Pulse repetition frequency (PRF)* is the frequency of the emitted pulses (in Hz) and determines the sensitivity for slow flow because of linked control with the wall filters. The two cannot be adjusted independently of each other though the filters may be fine-tuned for every PRF. A high PRF will *always* have a higher wall filter than a low PRF. The wall filters are there to remove noise from surrounding tissue and moving vessels walls. Unfortunately, the Doppler shifts from noise and slow flow are very close. When working with fast flow, a high PRF is important, but with a high PRF, the high wall filters will eliminate both noise and slow flow. When examining synovitis, slow flow is important, and therefore, the PRF should be kept as low as possible to keep the wall filters low, thereby allowing slow flow to be shown. With some portable US machines, adjustment of PRF may be limited to high, medium, and low.
- *Color priority (threshold)* is a function that determines what has the highest priority in the US image: color or grayscale. To avoid the grayscale overriding the color information and thereby hiding flow information, color priority should be kept as high as possible (100%). Some portable US machines automatically adjust this.
- *Color box size* is an adjustable box which should be large enough to cover the area of interest and extend to the top of the screen to recognize the possibility of mirror artifact, which may occur from a more superficially located vessel. A larger box will reduce Doppler sensitivity, so care should be taken to appropriately adjust the size.

Table 11.1 shows the optimal settings of Doppler [13].

Doppler optimization may need to be carried out at every examination although higher-end US machines will allow saving a preset setting for optimal settings for slow flow that can be used for every examination. It is imperative to use the same settings and the same machine for follow-up of patients in order for the findings of Doppler activity in synovitis to be comparable. Additionally, for all Doppler assessments, it is important that the examination is carried out on a joint, tendon, or enthesis in the neutral position without any muscle strain in order to obtain optimal flow information [14–16].

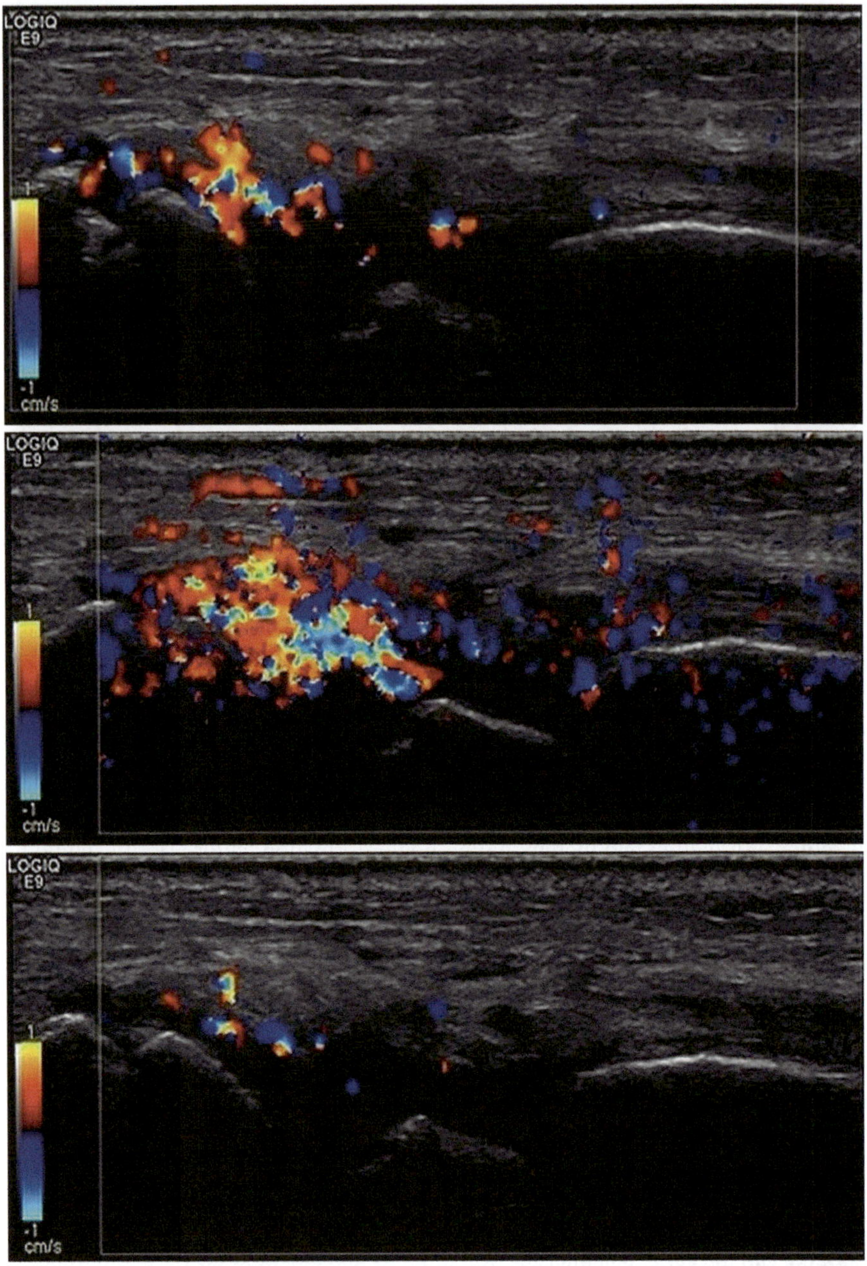

Fig. 11.2 Gain. The image shows the wrist with correctly adjusted gain in the *top* image, a too high-gain setting in the *middle* image with lots of noise pixels visible, and a too low-gain setting at the *bottom* image where flow information is lost

Table 11.1 Optimal settings for Doppler [13]

Function	How to adjust
Doppler frequency	Choose the frequency that gives the best penetration in the joint. It depends on the machine and may be in either highest or lowest frequency area.
PRF and wall filter	Choose the lowest possible PRF (and the lowest possible wall filter) without motion artifacts.
Gain	Adjust until there is hardly any noise pixel visible in the image.
Focus	Adjust the focus to the level of the region of interest to obtain highest sensitivity.
Color priority (threshold)	Not readily available on all machines Set the color priority to 100% to get all flow displayed

Scoring of Synovitis

Synovitis is defined as hypoechoic synovial hypertrophy with or without Doppler activity [17]. To be able to monitor the efficacy of medical treatment, it is necessary both in clinical practice and in research to assess the changes in grayscale (GS) and Doppler over time, and different scoring systems have been developed. GS synovial hypertrophy—especially minimal degrees —is often perceived as having limited ability to change, especially in the feet [18]. However, a recent study has shown both components respond to treatment—even synovial hypertrophy without Doppler activity [19] and low-grade synovial hypertrophy. Furthermore, both components predict erosive progression over time in conventional DMARD-treated patients [20]. This highlights that both components are relevant for monitoring purposes.

US is sensitive for detection of synovitis in joints and tendons during follow-up of rheumatoid arthritis (RA) patients initiating effective antirheumatic treatment [21]. However, recent studies have not found US or MRI to have added value to clinical examination in treat-to-target follow-up of early or established RA [22–24].

Semiquantitative Synovitis Scoring Systems

For scoring GS synovial hypertrophy, a semiquantitative scale from 0 to 3 reflecting the size of the synovial hypertrophy is applied (0 = normal, 1 = minor, 2 = moderate, and 3 = major amount of synovial hypertrophy), as shown in Fig. 11.3.

For power or color Doppler, there are two main scoring systems. The first scoring system was proposed by Szkudlarek et al. [2] and is a semiquantitative scoring system 0–3; 0 = no doppler signals, 1 = single vessel signals, 2 = confluent vessel signals in less than half of the area of the synovium, and 3 = vessel signals in more than 50% of the area of the synovium (see Fig. 11.4).

It is, however, difficult to make a division between the scores of Doppler signals covering less/more than 50% of the synovitis area. In addition, a recent study including pixel counts to objectively evaluate the degree of power Doppler activity has

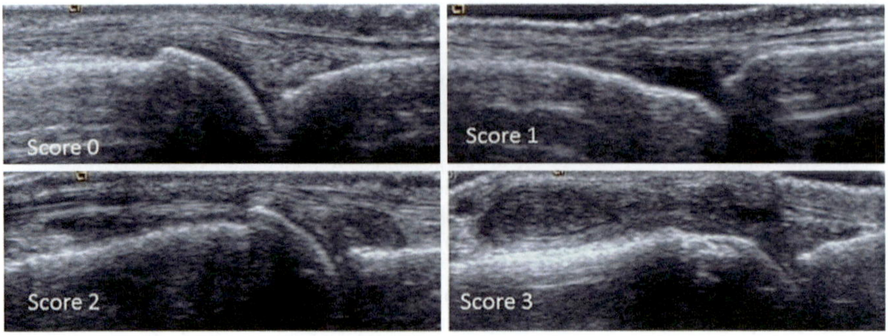

Fig. 11.3 US Scoring MCP synovial hypertrophy in grayscale

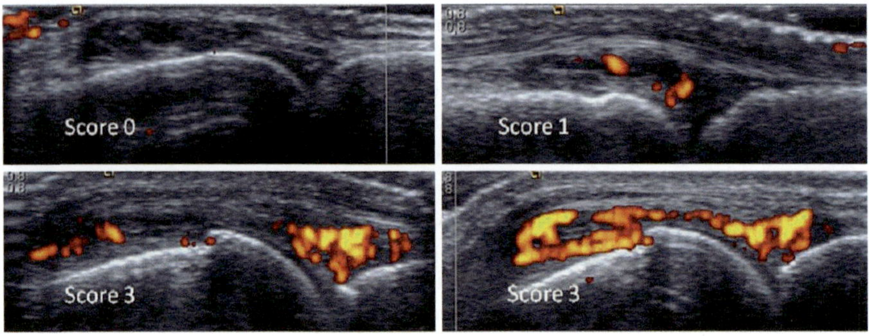

Fig. 11.4 US Scoring MCP power Doppler. US scoring of MCP joints. Power Doppler scored on a semiquantitative scoring system: 0 = normal, 1 = minor, 2 = moderate, and 3 = major pathology

shown that power Doppler pixels covering more than 50% is very seldom, and by using this scoring system, most of the synovitis would be scored as 2 [25].

Another scoring system is built on a semiquantitative scoring 0–3 where the degree of PD activity is divided into scoring levels dependent on the amount of PD activity, with the scoring of 0 = none, 1 = minor, 2 = moderate, and 3 = major degree of PD activity relative to what is known as maximal degree of PD activity in that joint. The basis for this scoring system is a reference atlas that is published, including four examples of each score in a large number of joints (Fig. 11.4). A study has shown that use of this atlas resulted in excellent intra- and interobserver reliability for scoring of synovitis in a large number of joints in RA patients [26]. Figure 11.5 illustrates representative scores in MCP joints. The concordance of scoring by use of two scoring systems has been explored, finding almost similar scoring by use of the two methods [27].

A validated consensus-based EULAR-OMERACT scoring system (Table 11.2) has been developed in which GS and Doppler are scored semiquantitatively 0–3 as shown in Fig. 11.3 and can be used for a combined score of the joint choosing the highest score of the two components as the final score [17, 30]. The scoring system is validated for both small and larger joints and has been applied in clinical trials [28].

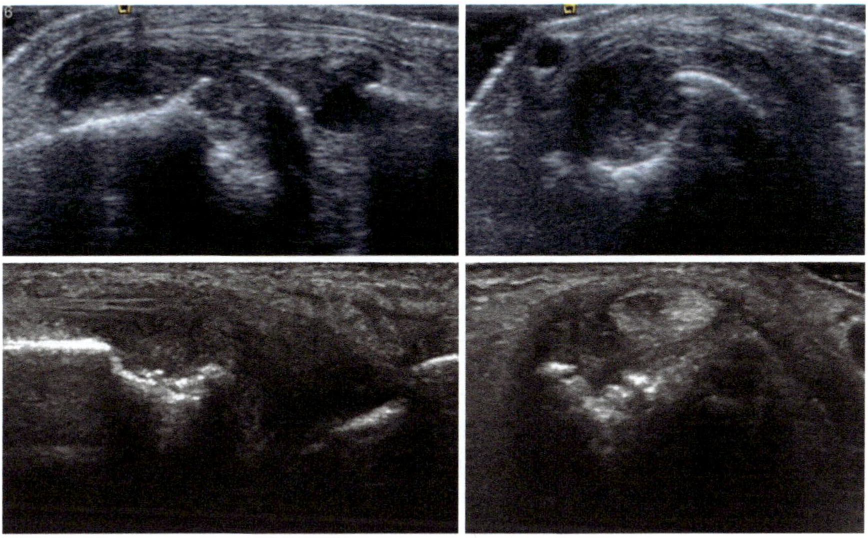

Fig. 11.5 US Scoring MCP bony erosions and grayscale. Grayscale scored on a semiquantitative scoring system: 0 = normal, 1 = minor, 2 = moderate, and 3 = major pathology. Grade 3 synovial hypertrophy and erosions present in 2 orthogonal planes

Table 11.2 The EULAR OMERACT scoring system

Grade	Description	Grayscale score	Doppler score	Combined score
Grade 0	None	No synovial hypertrophy independent of the presence of effusion	No Doppler activity	No grayscale-detected synovial hypertrophy and no Doppler signal (within the synovium)
Grade 1	Minimal	Synovial hypertrophy with or without effusion up to level of horizontal line connecting bone surfaces of the metacarpal head and the proximal phalanx	Up to 3 single Doppler spots OR up to 1 confluent spot and 2 single spots OR up to 2 confluent spots	Grade 1 synovial hypertrophy and ≤ grade 1 Doppler signal
Grade 2	Moderate	Synovial hypertrophy with or without effusion extending beyond joint line but with upper surface convex (curved downward) or hypertrophy extending beyond joint line but with upper surface flat	Greater than grade 1 but <50% Doppler signals in the total grayscale background	Grade 2 synovial hypertrophy and ≤ grade 2 Doppler signal or grade 1 synovial hypertrophy *and* a grade 2 Doppler signal
Grade 3	Severe	Synovial hypertrophy with or without effusion extending beyond joint line but with upper surface flat or concave (curved upward)	Greater than grade 2 (>50% of the background gray scale)	Grade 3 synovial hypertrophy and ≤ grade 3 Doppler signal or grade 1 or 2 synovial hypertrophy *and* a grade 3 Doppler signal

Quantitative Synovitis Scoring

Another way of scoring vascularization in synovitis is by quantitative scoring, which is not an operator-dependent system for the evaluation of Doppler activity. The automatic calculation of pixel counts applies both CD or PD and will give a number reflecting the amount of colored pixels in the synovium [13]—either in the longitudinal plane alone or as a sum for both the longitudinal and transverse plane for each joint [7]. A new technique is now available allowing the calculation of pixels to be carried out on the US machine instead of the more time-consuming transfer of US images from the US machine to a computer for post-processing. This scoring method has the potential of being an objective and possibly more sensitive evaluation of pathology and monitoring of treatment response (see Fig. 11.6).

A direct comparison between a semiquantitative scoring system and a quantitative scoring system has shown high reliability of both scoring systems (highest for the quantitative scoring). High association between the two scoring systems was also found when applied to the same patient population, indicating that studies using different scoring systems reflect the same disease activity [27, 31].

The resistive index (RI) is another method for quantitative scoring. This technique uses spectral Doppler where the inflammation is characterized by the flow pattern in the inflamed tissues. The spectral Doppler modality shows the flow profile of the perfusion in the region of interest, and based on the flow curve, the RI is automatically calculated. The RI is defined as peak systolic velocity minus the end diastolic velocity divided with the peak systolic velocity, and the maximum value of RI is 1.00 when there is no diastolic flow, indicating a normal vessel with no inflammation. However, when there is inflammatory activity with release of a large

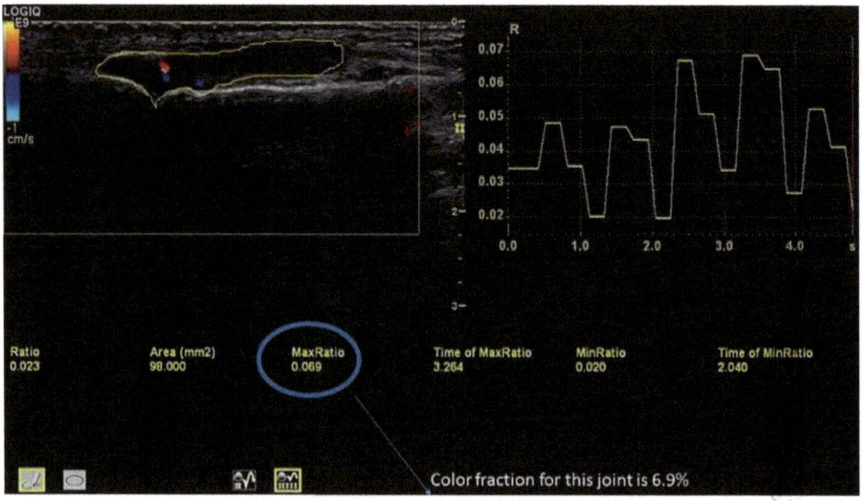

Fig. 11.6 Pixel calculation. The image shows how pixel calculation may be performed on a US machine with dedicated software. The region of interest is traced, and the color fraction is automatically calculated—for this MCP joint, it is 6.9%

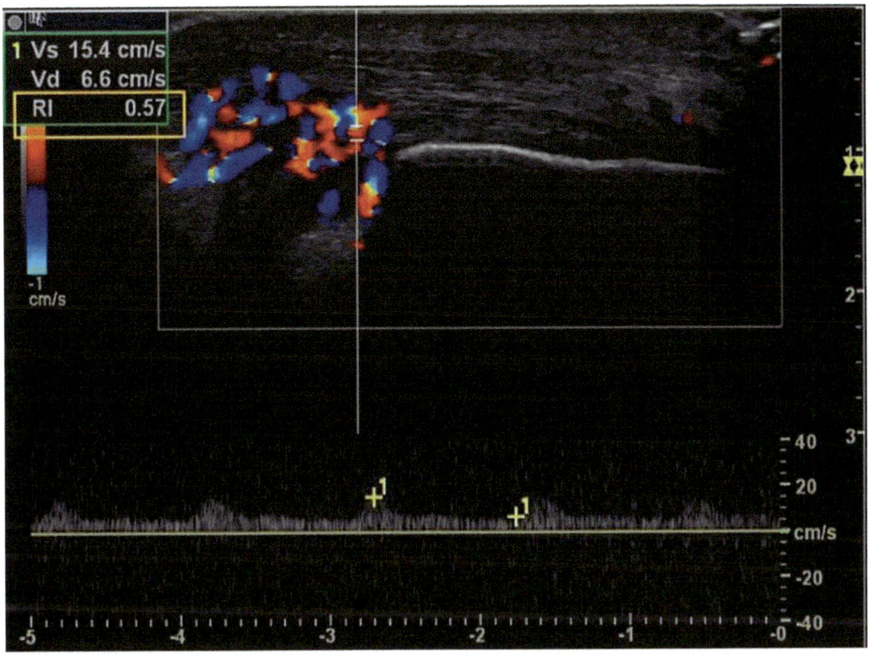

Fig. 11.7 RI calculation. The RI for the inflamed Achilles tendon with bursitis is 0.57 for the traced vessel. The gate is put over a vessel, the flow curve for that vessel is shown at the *bottom*, and the resistive index is calculated automatically as the peak systolic value minus the end diastolic value divided by the peak systolic value

number of cytokines and molecules causing dilatation of vessels, the RI will be lower, depending on the degree of inflammation. There are not many studies using spectral Doppler even if it has been shown that RI correlates with the degree of inflammation and is sensitive to change [32, 33] as well as being validated with MRI as gold standard [34]. Two studies have evaluated RI in healthy volunteers and RA patients with active disease, and a cutoff value of 0.84–0.86 was established with lower values defining inflammation [33, 35]. Use of spectral Doppler is more time-consuming than semiquantitative scores, but by immediately obtaining the inflammatory index, it is possible to differentiate a normal from abnormal joint perfusion. However, the finding of different RI values inside the same joint may reduce the reliability of this method, even if it is usual to measure the RI in several vessels inside the inflamed synovium and calculate a mean value. Figure 11.7 shows the measurement of RI in an inflamed joint.

Number of Joints to Be Examined

There is no consensus on the number of joints to be examined by US for diagnostic purpose or during follow-up of RA patients. However, the number will depend on the clinical situation. When the purpose of an US examination is to assess the extent of disease activity in a patient with arthritis for evaluation of indication for medical treatment, it may be necessary to examine a high number of joints. On the other hand, if the purpose is to follow the response to medical treatment in an RA patient, a reduced number of joints may be sufficient. Even if there is no agreement on which joints should be included in a standard follow-up protocol for US joint examination, several reduced joint scores have been proposed [36–39]. However, in a longitudinal study of RA patients where 78 joints were examined, almost all the examined joints were inflamed in at least one patient during the study [39, 40]. Even so, examination of only one joint (the most affected wrist) was found to be a valid measure of disease activity in RA patients [38]. From a 12-joint score, a reduced set including six joints (bilateral wrist, MCP 2, and knee) was found to give a valid and sensitive US score [39]. A joint score including seven joints (metacarpophalangeal (MCP) joint 2 and 3, wrist (maximum of the radiocarpal, midcarpal, and radioulnar joints), and metatarsophalangeal (MTP) joint 2 and 5 (at the clinically dominant side)) has been found to be a practical tool for examining patients with arthritis in daily rheumatologic practice because it significantly reflected the response to medical treatment [36]. A 44-joint score (glenohumeral joint, elbow, wrist, MCP 1–5, proximal interphalangeal (PIP) 1–5, hip, knee, ankle, midtarsal joints, and MTP 1–5 joints bilaterally) was shown to improve during biological treatment [37], and from this score, a reduced 12-joint score was explored (bilateral elbow, wrist, MCP 2 and 3, knee, ankle, medial and lateral ankle tendon compartments). Also, this reduced score was found to be sensitive to change during medical treatment of RA patients [37]. A study exploring the responsiveness of different joint scores including 7 to 44 joints found similar responsiveness as in the total joint score including 78 joints in RA patients during anti-TNF treatment [40]. A recent study used a data-driven approach to reach a reduced number of joints (seven or nine joints bilaterally) to give almost the same information as a more comprehensive examination [29, 41].

Table 11.3 gives an overview of the joints included in several published joint scores. The clinical experience is that hands (finger joints), wrist (radiocarpal, midcarpal, and radioulnar joints), and feet (MTPs) are regularly involved in RA patients, and it may turn out that these joints will be the most important to include in a US joint score. However, further studies are necessary to conclude on the optimal joints to assess in follow-up of patients with inflammatory joint diseases [10, 35, 36, 38, 42].

Evaluation of Tenosynovitis

Many arthritis conditions are associated with tenosynovitis especially in the wrist and ankles, which may result in degeneration and rupture of the tendon. Tenosynovitis contributes to joint deformities and loss of functional capacity especially in RA patients. Clinically, it can be difficult to diagnose tenosynovitis, and both US and MRI are more sensitive than clinical examination for the detection of tenosynovitis [43–46]. There is growing evidence that the presence of tenosynovitis may have both diagnostic and predictive value especially in

Table 11.3 Joints and tendons included in several published reduced joint scores [2]

Reduced joint score	Joints and tendons included
6-joint score [39]	Bilateral examination of: *Joints*: Wrist, MCP 2, and knee
7-joint score [36]	On the clinically dominant side: *Joints*: Wrist, MCP 2 and 3, PIP 2 and 3, and MTP 2 and 5 *Tendons*: Dorsal, ulnar, and palmar tendon sheaths of the wrist and flexor tendon sheaths of 2 and 3 fingers
9-joint score [41]	Uni- and bilateral examination of: *Joints:* MCP1-3, PIP 2-3, radiocarpal joint, and MTP 2-3 *Tendons:* Extensor carpi ulnaris
12-joint score [37]	Bilateral examination of: *Joints*: Elbow, wrist, MCP 2 and 3, knee, and ankle *Tendons*: Medial and lateral tendon sheaths of the ankle
28-joint score [10]	Bilateral examination of: *Joints*: Shoulder (glenohumeral), elbow, wrist, MCP 1–5, PIP 1–5, and knee
44-joint score [42]	Bilateral examination of: *Joints*: Shoulder (glenohumeral), elbow, wrist, MCP 1–5, PIP 1–5, hip, knee, ankle, midtarsal, and MTP 1–5 *Tendons*: Biceps tendon sheath; extensor and flexor tendons sheaths of the wrist; flexor tendons sheaths of the fingers; and anterior, medial, and lateral tendon sheaths of the ankle. In addition: the subdeltoid bursa

RA. Extensor carpi ulnaris (ECU) tenosynovitis in grayscale have been shown to be associated with erosive progression at 1-year follow-up at the distal ulna [48] and was a statistically significant univariate predictor of 3-year erosive progression on MR erosion score [47]. Likewise, a high score of wrist synovitis and flexor tenosynovitis in a cohort of recent-onset polyarthritis was a strong predictor for developing RA [49].

Tendon involvement may differ between early and late RA though only a few studies have addressed this. In early RA with a disease duration of less than 12 months, flexor and extensor tendon disease was more frequent in the second and third fingers than fourth and fifth fingers [49, 50]. In more established disease with a disease duration of at least 7 years, the ECU tendon in the wrist and posterior tibialis tendon in the ankle are involved, but there are reports that involvement of the flexor digitorum longus and peroneal tendons also is frequent [51, 52].

Tenosynovitis is defined as a peritendinous widening of the synovial sheath and must be seen in two perpendicular planes. Tenosynovitis can be seen using both GS and Doppler, and as with synovitis changes in the joint, the synovial swelling and Doppler activity is believed to reflect changes in disease activity. To be able to monitor changes during treatment, different scoring systems have been developed to assess the changes in both GS and Doppler over time. For tenosynovitis, there are two main scoring systems, and both are semiquantitative: (1) the subjective scoring system where the assessor grades both GS and PD on a four-point scale (0 = none, 1 = minor, 2 = moderate, or 3 = major presence) [50, 52], and (2) the more detailed OMERACT scoring system by Naredo et al. [53] in which the GS scoring is still subjective on a four-point scale (0 = none, 1 = minor, 2 = moderate, or 3 = major

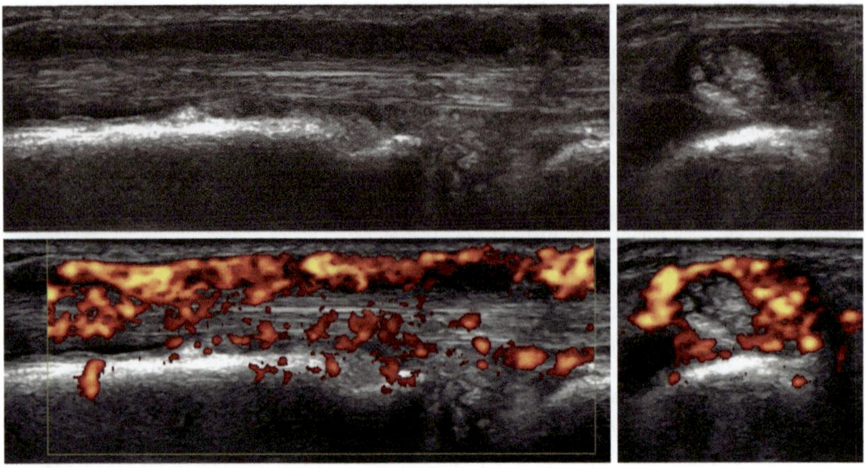

Fig. 11.8 Longitudinal and cross-sectional scan of the extensor carpi ulnaris tendon in an RA patient with tenosynovitis. Grayscale score 3, power Doppler score 3

presence), but where the Doppler scoring is scored according to the distribution of flow: grade 0 = no signal within the widened synovial sheath, grade 1 = only focal signal within the widened synovial sheath, grade 2 = multifocal signal within the widened synovial sheath, and grade 3 = diffuse signal within the widened synovial sheath (filling most of the widened sheath). This scoring system also takes into account possible affection of the tendon so that if there is an abnormal intratendinous Doppler signal in addition to an abnormal peritendinous Doppler signal, then grades 1 and 2 would be increased by one point [53]. Figure 11.8 illustrates inflammation in the ECU tendon with GS and PD scores.

In the OMERACT scoring system by Naredo et al. [53] the intra-observer reliability for tenosynovitis varied from moderate for GS to good for Doppler signal. The overall interobserver reliability for tenosynovitis was excellent for both GS and Doppler and has also been tested in single and multicenter trials during treatment [54, 55].

The subjective scoring system by Hammer et al. [52] has been shown to be able to detect changes during systemic treatment with anti-TNF alpha treatment, whereas the scoring system from Naredo et al. still needs to be tested in clinical trials.

Special Considerations When Performing Ultrasound of RA Patients

Assessment of the Wrist

Several studies examine the wrist as one joint even though it is actually composed of many joints. The three largest joints are (1) the radiocarpal joint, (2) the midcarpal joint, and (3) the radioulnar joint; each joint may be scored separately. The

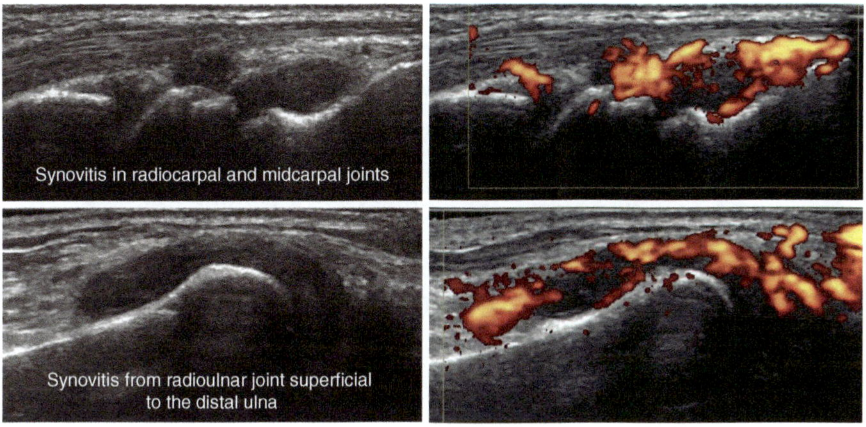

Fig. 11.9 RA patient with synovitis in the wrist, including radiocarpal joint, midcarpal joint and radioulnar joint (with synovitis located superficial to the distal ulna)

radioulnar joint is located between the distal radius and distal ulna. When it is inflamed, the synovitis will be seen with increasing size at both dorsal and palmar sides of the distal ulna. The most feasible location for assessing synovitis from the radioulnar joint is a longitudinal scan of the distal ulna. Figure 11.9 shows synovitis in the three main wrist joints.

Paratenonitis

At the dorsal part of MCP joints, there may be a hypoechoic swelling surrounding the extensor digitorum tendon which may have Doppler signals. This is a special form of tenosynovitis since these extensor tendons do not have any tendon sheath. No general definition has been given, but it is usually called paratenonitis. This form of synovitis is often in combination with intra-articular synovitis in the joints. It has been described as typical for swollen MCP joints in patients with psoriatic arthritis [56], but this pathology is also often found in patients with RA (Fig. 11.10). Thus, the sonographers should be aware of this special phenotype especially when assessing patients with undifferentiated arthritis since it may indicate psoriatic or rheumatoid arthritis [56].

Intermetatarsal Bursitis

Patients with RA may have intermetatarsal bursitis, which are easily detected by use of longitudinal scanning over the spaces between the MTPs (intermetatarsal spaces). The bursitis is also seen on transverse scans. Figure 11.11 illustrates an inflamed intermetatarsal bursitis. This may cause pain in the forefoot and must be addressed during US examination of patients with foot pain. Intermetatarsal bursitis typically

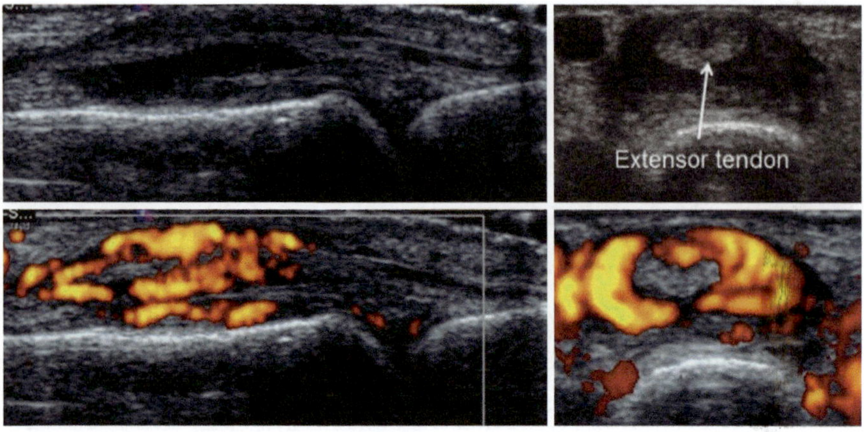

Fig. 11.10 Paratenonitis with grade 3 power Doppler activity

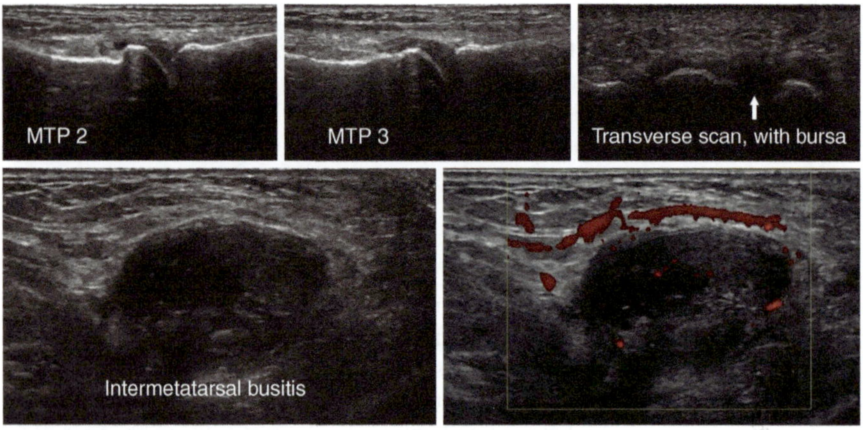

Fig. 11.11 Intermetatarsal bursitis, longitudinal scan between MTP 2 and MTP 3, Grayscale and power Doppler

responds well to steroid injections (can be performed US guided in plane between the two neighboring MTPs by use of dorsal longitudinal scan).

Baker's Cyst (Popliteal Cyst)

RA patients with synovitis in the knee joint may experience posterior knee pain and swelling due to fluid moving posteriorly between the gastrocnemius and semitendinosus/semimembranosus. Large amounts of fluid or bursal thickening contributing to popliteal pain are amenable to US-guided aspiration and corticosteroid injection. In some cases, the bursa may rupture, causing acute pain and

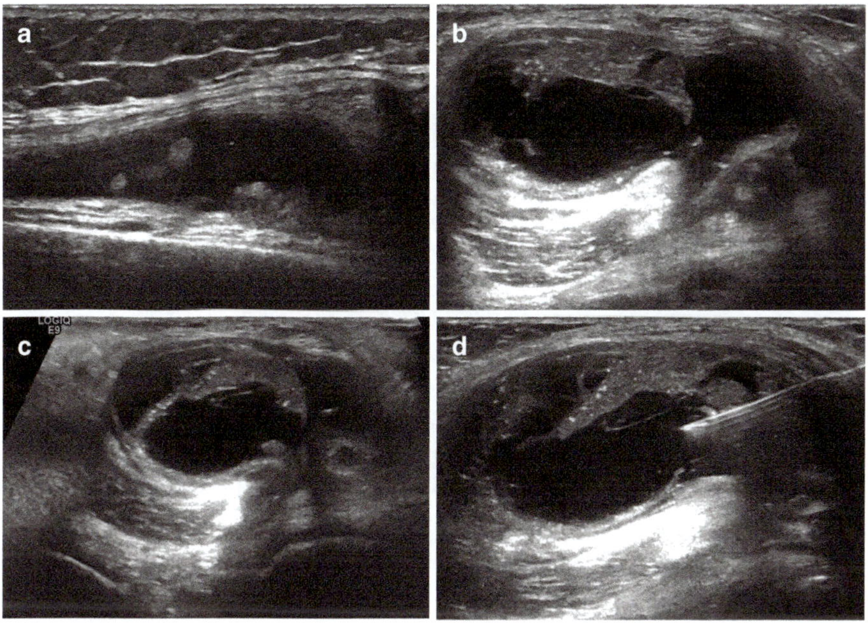

Fig. 11.12 Knee joint with synovitis and Baker cyst. (**a**) Anterior longitudinal scan: suprapatellar recess. (**b**) Posterior longitudinal scan: Bakers cyst with fluid and hypoechoic tissue thickening. (**c**) Posterior transverse scan with femoral condyles seen in the deep part of the image. (**d**) Ultrasound-guided aspiration of fluid

swelling of the calf, mimicking deep venous thrombosis. Figure 11.12 shows a typical Baker's cyst.

Erosions

Arthritis may cause erosions, which can be detected by use of US with a better sensitivity than x-ray [57]. Long-lasting clinical experience indicates that the medial side of MCP 2 and the lateral side of MTP 5 are predilection sites for early erosions in RA. US is however not as sensitive as MRI or CT for bone erosions as there are areas of the joint where US has no access. In the US accessible areas, the joint surfaces may be examined for erosions with a high sensitivity, specificity, and accuracy when compared to CT [58]. Several studies have scored erosions, and different systems have been used, usually a semiquantitative score dependent on the size of the erosion [48]; however, scoring erosions are rarely used in the clinic (see Fig. 11.13).

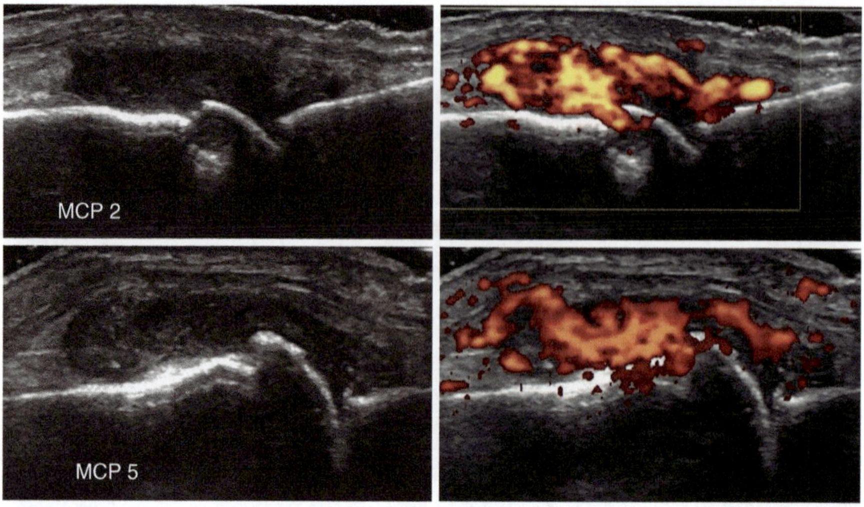

Fig. 11.13 Erosive disease in two RA patients with grade 3 synovial hypertrophy, grade 3 power Doppler activity, and erosions of the distal metacarpal with power Doppler activity inside the erosion

Conclusion

Grayscale and Doppler assessment of synovitis in rheumatoid arthritis allows for evaluation of subclinical inflammation in joints and tendons as well as monitoring treatment. Learning how to use the probe with minimal pressure and motion and optimizing US machine settings are critical in distinguishing true hyperemic inflammation versus artifacts. Semiquantitative synovitis scoring is most widely used for reporting the degree of synovitis present, but quantitative synovitis scoring has potential for more precise depiction of activity.

Review Questions

1. What is the main difference between power and color Doppler?
   (a) Power Doppler is more sensitive than color Doppler.
   (b) Power Doppler works with the energy and color Doppler with the velocity of the moving erythrocytes.
   (c) The Doppler shift only applies to color Doppler.
   (d) Color Doppler is gain dependent, but power Doppler is not.
2. How would you adjust the pulse repetitive frequency (PRF) when you want to evaluate flow in joint synovitis?
   (a) Increase the PRF and wall filter to increase sensitivity.
   (b) Increase the PRF but lower the wall filter to increase the sensitivity.
   (c) Decrease PRF and wall filter to increase the sensitivity.
   (d) Decrease PRF but increase the wall filter to increase sensitivity.

3. How do you adjust the Doppler gain when scanning a joint with synovitis?
   (a) Increase the gain until just below the level of noise.
   (b) Increase the gain to just above the level of noise.
   (c) Decrease the gain until only superficial vessels are visible.
   (d) Decrease the gain until only flow in the synovium is visible.
4. How should you adjust grayscale settings on the US machine when changing scanning from superficial to deep joints? You need to:
   (a) Increase the gain.
   (b) Decrease the frequency of the probe.
   (c) Increase the frequency of the probe.
   (d) Increase the wall filters.
5. What is the optimal method for evaluation of synovitis?
   (a) Scoring the Doppler from 0 to 3
   (b) Calculating the Doppler pixels
   (c) Measuring RI using the spectral Doppler
   (d) No consensus exists on the optimal method to score synovitis.
6. Please select the correct statement. Evaluating tenosynovitis in rheumatoid arthritis___.
   (a) Has no clinical relevance and should only be evaluated if symptomatic
   (b) Has predictive value for diagnosis and erosive progression
   (c) Is only relevant when compared to MRI of the same tendon
   (d) Should be dichotomous as no validated scoring system exists
7. What is the optimal number of joints to evaluate in scoring synovitis for rheumatoid arthritis?
   (a) 28 joints; it gives the best evaluation of the patient
   (b) 12 joints as it gives the best evaluation of the patient
   (c) One joint; it can be used as a target joint.
   (d) No consensus exists on the optimal joint count for synovitis.
8. The optimal technique to assess Doppler activity is to:
   (a) Use firm pressure for obtaining a good image.
   (b) Be light-handed, and use rich amounts of gel.
   (c) Use little gel as not to disturb the Doppler activity.
   (d) Always use power Doppler.
9. The optimal positioning for assessing Doppler activity in joints and tendons is to:
   (a) Actively stretch out the joint.
   (b) Always to use a pillow when performing examinations.
   (c) Be supine when performing all Doppler examinations.
   (d) Always have a relaxed joint/tendon when performing Doppler examination.
10. When doing follow-up examinations of Doppler activity of patients with joint inflammation for treatment response monitoring, it is important to:
   (a) Use the same machine and the same Doppler settings.
   (b) Increase the gain to increase the sensitivity.
   (c) Examine the joints in similar order each time.
   (d) Ask the patient to rest for 10 min before the examination.

Answers

1. (b) Power Doppler works with the energy and color Doppler with the velocity of the moving erythrocytes.
2. (c) Decrease PRF and wall filter to increase the sensitivity.
3. (a) Increase the gain until just below the level of noise.
4. (b) Decrease the frequency of the probe.
5. (d) No consensus exists on the optimal method to score synovitis.
6. (b) Has predictive value for diagnosis and erosive progression.
7. (d) No consensus exists on the optimal joint count for synovitis.
8. (b) Be light-handed, and use rich amounts of gel.
9. (d) Always have a relaxed joint/tendon when performing Doppler examination.
10. (a) Use the same machine and the same Doppler settings.

References

1. Jaeger KA, Imfeld S. The damaging effect of ultrasound – to the examiner. Ultraschall Med. 2006;27(2):131–3.
2. Szkudlarek M, Court-Payen M, Jacobsen S, Klarlund M, Thomsen HS, Østergaard M. Interobserver agreement in ultrasonography of the finger and toe joints in rheumatoid arthritis. Arthritis Rheum. 2003;48:955–62.
3. Brown AK, Quinn MA, Karim Z, Conaghan PG, Peterfy CG, Hensor E, et al. Presence of significant synovitis in rheumatoid arthritis patients with disease-modifying antirheumatic drug-induced clinical remission: evidence from an imaging study may explain structural progression. Arthritis Rheum. 2006;54(12):3761–73.
4. Wakefield RJ, Green MJ, Marzo-Ortega H, Conaghan PG, Gibbon WW, McGonagle D, et al. Should oligoarthritis be reclassified? Ultrasound reveals a high prevalence of subclinical disease. Ann Rheum Dis. 2004;63(4):382–5.
5. Hammer HB, Michelsen B, Sexton J, Haugen IK, Provan SA, Haavardsholm EA, Uhlig T, Kvien TK. Swollen, but not tender joints, are independently associated with ultrasound synovitis: results from a longitudinal observational study of patients with established rheumatoid arthritis. Ann Rheum Dis. 2019;78(9):1179–85. https://doi.org/10.1136/annrheumdis-2019-215321.
6. Terslev L, Torp-Pedersen S, Qvistgaard E, Danneskiold-Samsoe B, Bliddal H. Estimation of inflammation by Doppler ultrasound: quantitative changes after intra-articular treatment in rheumatoid arthritis. Ann Rheum Dis. 2003;62(11):1049–53.
7. Taylor PC, Steuer A, Gruber J, Cosgrove DO, Blomley MJ, Marsters PA, et al. Comparison of ultrasonographic assessment of synovitis and joint vascularity with radiographic evaluation in a randomized, placebo-controlled study of infliximab therapy in early rheumatoid arthritis. Arthritis Rheum. 2004;50:1107–16.
8. Hammer HB, Sveinsson M, Kongtorp AK, Kvien TK. A 78-joints ultrasonographic assessment is associated with clinical assessments and is highly responsive to improvement in a longitudinal study of patients with rheumatoid arthritis starting adalimumab treatment. Ann Rheum Dis. 2010;69:1349–51.
9. Brown AK, Conaghan PG, Karim Z, Quinn MA, Ikeda K, Peterfy CG, et al. An explanation for the apparent dissociation between clinical remission and continued structural deterioration in rheumatoid arthritis. Arthritis Rheum. 2008;58(10):2958–67.
10. Naredo E, Möller I, Cruz A, Carmona L, Garrido J. Power Doppler ultrasonographic monitoring of response to anti-tumor necrosis factor therapy in patients with rheumatoid arthritis. Arthritis Rheum. 2008;58:2248–56.

11. Torp-Pedersen ST, Terslev L. Settings and artefacts relevant in colour/power Doppler ultrasound in rheumatology. Ann Rheum Dis. 2008;67:143–9.
12. Torp-Pedersen S, Christensen R, Szkudlarek M, Ellegaard K, D'Agostino MA, Iagnocco A, et al. Power and color Doppler ultrasound settings for inflammatory flow: impact on scoring of disease activity in patients with rheumatoid arthritis. Arthritis Rheumatol. 2015;67(2):386–95.
13. Qvistgaard E, Røgind H, Torp-Pedersen S, Terslev L, Danneskiold-Samsøe B, Bliddal H. Quantitative ultrasonography in rheumatoid arthritis: evaluation of inflammation by Doppler technique. Ann Rheum Dis. 2001;60:690–3.
14. Gutierrez M, Filippucci E, Grassi W, Rosemffet M. Intratendinous power Doppler changes related to patient position in seronegative spondyloarthritis. J Rheumatol. 2010;37(5):1057–9.
15. Lee V, Zayat A, Wakefield RJ. The effect of joint position on Doppler flow in finger synovitis. Ann Rheum Dis. 2009;68(4):603–4.
16. Koenig MJ, Torp-Pedersen ST, Christensen R, Boesen MI, Terslev L, Hartkopp A, et al. Effect of knee position on ultrasound Doppler findings in patients with patellar tendon hyperaemia (jumper's knee). Ultraschall Med. 2007;28(5):479–83.
17. D'Agostino MA, Terslev L, Aegerter P, Backhaus M, Balint P, Bruyn GA, Filippucci E, Grassi W, Iagnocco A, Jousse-Joulin S, Kane D, Naredo E, Schmidt W, Szkudlarek M, Conaghan PG, Wakefield RJ. Scoring ultrasound synovitis in rheumatoid arthritis: a EULAR-OMERACT ultrasound taskforce-part 1: definition and development of a standardised, consensus-based scoring system. RMD Open. 2017;3(1):e000428.
18. Witt M, Mueller F, Nigg A, Reindl C, Leipe J, Proft F, Stein N, Hammitzsch A, Mayer S, Dechant C, Schulze-Koops H, Grunke M. Relevance of grade 1 gray-scale ultrasound findings in wrists and small joints to the assessment of subclinical synovitis in rheumatoid arthritis. Arthritis Rheum. 2013;65(7):1694–701.
19. Terslev L, Østergaard M, Sexton J, Hammer HB. Synovial hypertrophy without Doppler activity sensitive to change? Post-hoc analysis from a rheumatoid arthritis ultrasound study. Arthritis Res Ther. 2018;20(1):224.
20. Brown AK, Conaghan PG, Karim Z, Quinn MA, Ikeda K, Peterfy CG, Hensor E, Wakefield RJ, O'Connor PJ, Emery P. An explanation for the apparent dissociation between clinical remission and continued structural deterioration in rheumatoid arthritis. Arthritis Rheum. 2008;58(10):2958–67.
21. Naredo E, Möller I, Cruz A, Carmona L, Garrido J. Power Doppler ultrasonographic monitoring of response to anti-tumor necrosis factor therapy in patients with rheumatoid arthritis. Arthritis Rheum. 2008;58(8):2248–56.
22. Haavardsholm EA, Aga AB, Olsen IC, Lillegraven S, Hammer HB, Uhlig T, Fremstad H, Madland TM, Lexberg ÅS, Haukeland H, Rødevand E, Høili C, Stray H, Noraas A, Hansen IJ, Bakland G, Nordberg LB, van der Heijde D, Kvien TK. Ultrasound in management of rheumatoid arthritis: ARCTIC randomised controlled strategy trial. BMJ. 2016;354:i4205.
23. Dale J, Stirling A, Zhang R, Purves D, Foley J, Sambrook M, Conaghan PG, van der Heijde D, McConnachie A, McInnes IB, Porter D. Targeting ultrasound remission in early rheumatoid arthritis: the results of the TaSER study, a randomised clinical trial. Ann Rheum Dis. 2016;75(6):1043–50.
24. Møller-Bisgaard S, Hørslev-Petersen K, Ejbjerg B, Hetland ML, Ørnbjerg LM, Glinatsi D, Møller J, Boesen M, Christensen R, Stengaard-Pedersen K, Madsen OR, Jensen B, Villadsen JA, Hauge EM, Bennett P, Hendricks O, Asmussen K, Kowalski M, Lindegaard H, Nielsen SM, Bliddal H, Krogh NS, Ellingsen T, Nielsen AH, Balding L, Jurik AG, Thomsen HS, Østergaard M. Effect of magnetic resonance imaging vs conventional treat-to-target strategies on disease activity remission and radiographic progression in rheumatoid arthritis: the IMAGINE-RA randomized clinical trial. JAMA. 2019;321(5):461–72.
25. Schmidt WA, Schönau V, Reiche BE, Oberdorfer PD, Ohrndorf S, Backhaus M. Grading of ultrasound Doppler signals in synovitis: does it need an update? Rheumatology (Oxford). 2015;54(10):1897–903.
26. Hammer HB, Bolton-King P, Bakkeheim V, Berg TH, Sundt E, Kongtorp AK, et al. Examination of intra and interrater reliability with a new ultrasonographic reference atlas for scoring of synovitis in patients with rheumatoid arthritis. Ann Rheum Dis. 2011;70:1995–8.

27. Rezaei H, Af Klint E, Hammer HB, Terslev L, D'Agostino MA, Kisten Y, Arnaud L. Analysis of correlation and causes for discrepancy between quantitative and semi-quantitative Doppler scores in synovitis in rheumatoid arthritis. Rheumatology (Oxford). 2017;56(2):255–62.
28. D'Agostino MA, Boers M, Wakefield RJ, Berner Hammer H, Vittecoq O, Filippou G, Balint P, Möller I, Iagnocco A, Naredo E, Østergaard M, Gaillez C, Le Bars M. Exploring a new ultrasound score as a clinical predictive tool in patients with rheumatoid arthritis starting abatacept: results from the APPRAISE study. RMD Open. 2016;2(1):e000237.
29. Aga AB, Hammer HB, Olsen IC, Uhlig T, Kvien TK, van der Heijde D, Fremstad H, Madland TM, Lexberg ÅS, Haukeland H, Rødevand E. Development of a feasible and responsive ultrasound inflammation score for rheumatoid arthritis through a data-driven approach. RMD Open. 2016;2:e000325.
30. Terslev L, Naredo E, Aegerter P, Wakefield RJ, Backhaus M, Balint P, Bruyn GAW, Iagnocco A, Jousse-Joulin S, Schmidt WA, Szkudlarek M, Conaghan PG, Filippucci E, D'Agostino MA. Scoring ultrasound synovitis in rheumatoid arthritis: a EULAR-OMERACT ultrasound taskforce-part 2: reliability and application to multiple joints of a standardised consensus-based scoring system. RMD Open. 2017;3(1):e000427.
31. Terslev L, Ellegaard K, Christensen R, Szkudlarek M, Schmidt WA, Jensen PS, et al. Head-to-head comparison of quantitative and semi-quantitative ultrasound scoring systems for rheumatoid arthritis: reliability, agreement and construct validity. Rheumatology (Oxford). 2012;51(11):2034–8.
32. Terslev L, Torp-Pedersen S, Qvistgaard E, Bliddal H. Spectral Doppler and resistive index. A promising tool in ultrasonographic evaluation of inflammation in rheumatoid arthritis. Acta Radiol. 2003;44:645–52.
33. Carotti M, Salaffi F, Morbiducci J, Ciapetti A, Bartolucci L, Gasparini S, et al. Colour Doppler ultrasonography evaluation of vascularization in the wrist and finger joints in rheumatoid arthritis patients and healthy subjects. Eur J Radiol. 2012;81:1834–8.
34. Terslev L, Torp-Pedersen S, Savnik A, von der Recke P, Qvistgaard E, Danneskiold-Samsøe B, et al. Doppler ultrasound and magnetic resonance imaging of synovial inflammation of the hand in rheumatoid arthritis: a comparative study. Arthritis Rheum. 2003;48:2434–41.
35. Terslev L, von der Recke P, Torp-Pedersen S, Koenig MJ, Bliddal H. Diagnostic sensitivity and specificity of Doppler ultrasound in rheumatoid arthritis. J Rheumatol. 2008;35(1):49–53.
36. Backhaus M, Ohrndorf S, Kellner H, Strunk J, Backhaus TM, Hartung W, et al. Evaluation of a novel 7-joint ultrasound score in daily rheumatologic practice: a pilot project. Arthritis Rheum. 2009;61:1194–201.
37. Naredo E, Rodríguez M, Campos C, Rodríguez-Heredia JM, Medina JA, Giner E, et al. Validity, reproducibility, and responsiveness of a twelve-joint simplified power Doppler ultrasonographic assessment of joint inflammation in rheumatoid arthritis. Arthritis Rheum. 2008;59:515–22.
38. Ellegaard K, Torp-Pedersen S, Terslev L, Danneskiold-Samsøe B, Henriksen M, Bliddal H. Ultrasound colour Doppler measurements in a single joint as measure of disease activity in patients with rheumatoid arthritis – assessment of concurrent validity. Rheumatology. 2009;48:254–7.
39. Perricone C, Ceccarelli F, Modesti M, Vavala C, Di Franco M, Valesini G, et al. The 6-joint ultrasonographic assessment: a valid, sensitive-to-change and feasible method for evaluating joint inflammation in RA. Rheumatology (Oxford). 2012;51(5):866–73.
40. Hammer HB, Kvien TK. Comparisons of 7- to 78-joint ultrasonography scores: all different joint combinations show equal response to adalimumab treatment in patients with rheumatoid arthritis. Arthritis Res Ther. 2011;13:R78.
41. Aga AB, Hammer HB, Olsen IC, Uhlig T, Kvien TK, van der Heijde D, et al. First step in the development of an ultrasound joint inflammation score for rheumatoid arthritis using a data-driven approach. Ann Rheum Dis. 2015;75(8):1444–51.
42. Scirè CA, Montecucco C, Codullo V, Epis O, Todoerti M, Caporali R. Utrasonographic evaluation of joint involvement in early rheumatoid arthritis in clinical remission: power Doppler signal predicts short-term relapse. Rheumatology (Oxford). 2009;48(9):1092–7.

43. Lehtinen A, Paimela L, Kreula J, Leirisalo-Repo M, Taavitsainen M. Painful ankle region in rheumatoid arthritis. Analysis of soft-tissue changes with ultrasonography and MR imaging. Acta Radiol. 1996;37(4):572–7.
44. Maillefert JF, Dardel P, Cherasse A, Mistrih R, Krause D, Tavernier C. Magnetic resonance imaging in the assessment of synovial inflammation of the hindfoot in patients with rheumatoid arthritis and other polyarthritis. Eur J Radiol. 2003;47(1):1–5.
45. McQueen F, Beckley V, Crabbe J, Robinson E, Yeoman S, Stewart N. Magnetic resonance imaging evidence of tendinopathy in early rheumatoid arthritis predicts tendon rupture at six years. Arthritis Rheum. 2005;52(3):744–51.
46. Micu MC, Serra S, Fodor D, Crespo M, Naredo E. Inter-observer reliability of ultrasound detection of tendon abnormalities at the wrist and ankle in patients with rheumatoid arthritis. Rheumatology (Oxford). 2011;50(6):1120–4.
47. Bøyesen P, Haavardsholm EA, van der Heijde D, Østergaard M, Hammer HB, Sesseng S, et al. Prediction of MRI erosive progression: a comparison of modern imaging modalities in early rheumatoid arthritis patients. Ann Rheum Dis. 2011;70:176–9.
48. Hammer HB, Haavardsholm EA, Bøyesen P, Kvien TK. Bone erosions at the distal ulna detected by ultrasonography are associated with structural damage assessed by conventional radiography and MRI: a study of patients with recent onset rheumatoid arthritis. Rheumatology. 2009;48:1530–2.
49. Navalho M, Resende C, Rodrigues AM, Pereira da Silva JA, Fonseca JE, Campos J, et al. Bilateral evaluation of the hand and wrist in untreated early inflammatory arthritis: a comparative study of ultrasonography and magnetic resonance imaging. J Rheumatol. 2013;40(8):1282–92.
50. Wakefield RJ, O'Connor PJ, Conaghan PG, McGonagle D, Hensor EM, Gibbon WW, et al. Finger tendon disease in untreated early rheumatoid arthritis: a comparison of ultrasound and magnetic resonance imaging. Arthritis Rheum. 2007;57(7):1158–64.
51. Wakefield RJ, Freeston JE, O'Connor P, Reay N, Budgen A, Hensor EM, et al. The optimal assessment of the rheumatoid arthritis hindfoot: a comparative study of clinical examination, ultrasound and high field MRI. Ann Rheum Dis. 2008;67(12):1678–82.
52. Hammer HB, Kvien TK. Ultrasonography shows significant improvement in wrist and ankle tenosynovitis in rheumatoid arthritis patients treated with adalimumab. Scand J Rheumatol. 2011;40(3):178–82.
53. Naredo E, D'Agostino MA, Wakefield RJ, Möller I, Balint PV, Filippucci E, OMERACT Ultrasound Task Force, et al. Reliability of a consensus-based ultrasound score for tenosynovitis in rheumatoid arthritis. Ann Rheum Dis. 2013;72(8):1328–34.
54. Ammitzbøll-Danielsen M, Østergaard M, Naredo E, Terslev L. Validity and sensitivity to change of the semi-quantitative OMERACT ultrasound scoring system for tenosynovitis in patients with rheumatoid arthritis. Rheumatology (Oxford). 2016;55(12):2156–66.
55. Ammitzbøll-Danielsen M, Østergaard M, Fana V, Glinatsi D, Døhn UM, Ørnbjerg LM, Naredo E, Terslev L. Intramuscular versus ultrasound-guided intratenosynovial glucocorticoid injection for tenosynovitis in patients with rheumatoid arthritis: a randomised, double-blind, controlled study. Ann Rheum Dis. 2017;76(4):666–72.
56. Gutierrez M, Filippucci E, Salaffi F, Di Geso L, Grassi W. Differential diagnosis between rheumatoid arthritis and psoriatic arthritis: the value of ultrasound findings at metacarpophalangeal joints level. Ann Rheum Dis. 2011;70(6):1111–4.
57. Wakefield RJ, et al. The value of sonography in the detection of bone erosions in patients with rheumatoid arthritis: a comparison with conventional radiography. Arthritis Rheum. 2000;43(12):2762–70.
58. Døhn UM, Terslev L, Szkudlarek M, Hansen MS, Hetland ML, Hansen A, Madsen OR, Hasselquist M, Møller J, Ostergaard M. Detection, scoring and volume assessment of bone erosions by ultrasonography in rheumatoid arthritis: comparison with CT. Ann Rheum Dis. 2013;72(4):530–4.

Ultrasound in Psoriatic Arthritis

12

Gurjit Singh Kaeley

Key Points

- Enthesitis is a crucial pathological finding in psoriatic arthritis (PsA).
- Ultrasound can depict reversible and irreversible changes at the entheses.
- Biomechanical confounders influence sonographic entheseal findings.
- Ultrasound can depict inflammation of multiple digital structures in an active dactylitic digit.
- Sonography detects synovitis as well as bony changes in joints of PsA subjects.

Introduction

The modern concept of psoriatic disease emphasizes that patients with this condition have more than skin and joint involvement. It recognizes the domains of enthesitis, dactylitis, and nail disease. These concepts are increasingly becoming important, as highlighted in the Group for Research and Assessment of Psoriasis and Psoriatic Arthritis (GRAPPA) treatment guidelines [1]. In the advent of an ever-increasing armamentarium of targeted therapies, it is essential to focus therapies on the worst domains affected. Clinical evaluation of some of the manifestations may underestimate the burden of inflammation in the different areas affected. Ultrasound

G. S. Kaeley (✉)
Division of Rheumatology, University of Florida College of Medicine, Jacksonville, FL, USA
e-mail: Gurjit.Kaeley@jax.ufl.edu

M. J. Kohler (ed.), *Musculoskeletal Ultrasound in Rheumatology Review*,
https://doi.org/10.1007/978-3-030-73555-5_12

can be used at the point-of-care to efficiently evaluate for evidence of subclinical inflammation at the entheses, joints, digits, and nail entheses. This chapter will discuss the following topics: (1) enthesitis, (2) dactylitis, (3) the involvement of multiple structures of the digit in dactylitis, and (4) the evaluation of peripheral joints affected by enthesitis.

Enthesitis

Traditionally, entheses were regarded as ligament or tendon attachments to bone. Clinically, these are detected by palpation of entheseal sites. The prevalence of enthesitis in psoriatic arthritis (PsA) ranges from 35% to 50% in cross-sectional studies and 56–83% in clinical trials [2, 3]. The Classification Criteria for Psoriatic Arthritis (CASPAR) criteria include enthesitis as one of its requirements for the classification of psoriatic arthritis [4]. Enthesitis is associated with increased levels of radiologic damage in PsA subjects as well as impaired function, work impairment, and pain [5–7]. Treatment of enthesitis has been reported to improve physical function [8]. Enthesitis is therefore an important manifestation of PsA that needs to be recognized and treated. Clinical examination underestimates the presence of enthesitis and correlates best when large entheses have chronic structural changes [9, 10]. Ultrasound is an excellent tool to detect enthesitis. In the next section, an outline of the newer pathoanatomical concepts of entheses will enable a better understanding of sonographic imaging.

Pathoanatomical Definitions of Entheses

The traditional view of entheses encompasses direct attachment of the ligament or tendon to the bone. There are two types of attachments – fibrous and fibrocartilaginous attachments. Fibrous attachments are where the collagen fibers are directly encased into the bone. Examples of fibrous attachments include the deltoid insertion at the deltoid tuberosity, as well as the anterior and posterior origins of the deltoid muscle. Metabolic enthesopathies occur at fibrous entheses. In contrast, enthesitis occurs solely at fibrocartilaginous entheses. Fibrocartilaginous entheses are where there is a fibrocartilaginous transitional layer proximal to the bone [11]. Fibrocartilaginous entheses include the Achilles, patellar ligament, quadriceps, and triceps entheses. The primary purpose of the fibrocartilage transition is to aid in force dissipation. Fibrocartilage is present at bone adjacent to the enthesis, such as at the superior pole of the calcaneus, as well as the inner portion of the Achilles tendon. Other structures about the entheses such as bursae lined with synovial cells, fat pads, also contribute to the dissipation of mechanical energy. On magnetic resonance imaging (MRI) and ultrasound imaging, inflammation of these structures may be seen, which has led to the concept of the "synovial entheseal complex" or "enthesis organ" [12].

Sonopathology of Enthesitis

Structural changes at the enthesis and adjoining tendon or ligament that may be potentially reversible include entheseal thickening, hypoechogenicity, and bursitis. Enthesophyte formation, intratendinous calcification, erosions, osteoproliferation, and tendon thinning or tears are considered indications of damage [3, 13] (Table 12.1). Sonographic indices of enthesitis incorporate some or all of these lesions (see next section). Of note, the Outcome Measures in Rheumatology (OMERACT) Ultrasound (US) working group definition calls for the elementary lesions to be within 2 mm of the bone. This requirement is problematic since entheses are not of equal size, and some structures such as collateral ligaments of the finger are 2 mm in length in their entirety. Furthermore, the current concepts of triggering of innate immunity do not artificially occur within 2 mm of the entheseal attachments. Finally, imaging changes occur in continuity of the entheses and surrounding structures, in keeping with the enthesis organ concept.

Table 12.1 Important entheseal B-mode elementary lesions and their definitions

Lesion	Definition	Example
Reversible		
Entheseal hypoechogenicity	Entheseal loss of fibrillar echotexture defined as loss of dense parallel echogenic lines despite correcting for anisotropy	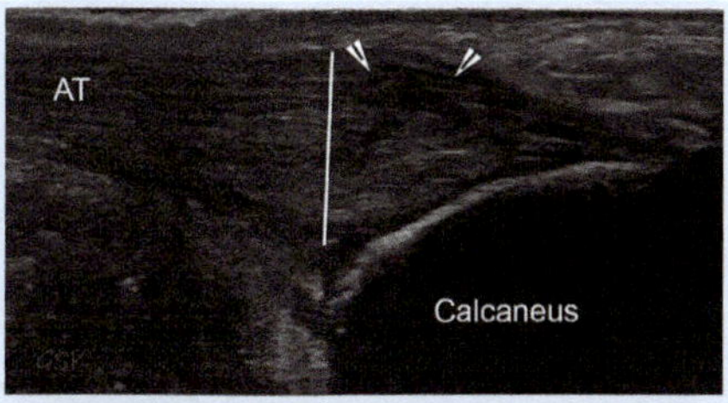 Long axis scan of distal Achilles tendon (AT) and enthesis. The enthesis is thickened (white band). Loss of fibrillar echotexture indicated by arrowheads
Entheseal thickening	Entheseal thickening adjacent to the bone when compared to proximal tendon or normative values	
Bursitis	Well-demarcated anechoic or hypoechoic distension of the bursa adjacent to enthesis	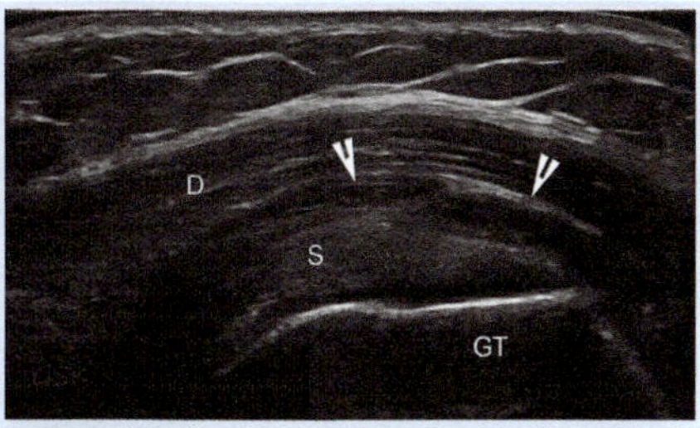 Modified crass view of the supraspinatus (S) attachment at the greater tuberosity (GT) in a patient with active PsA. Bursal distension is seen underneath the deltoid muscle (D) and above the supraspinatus (arrowheads).

(continued)

Table 12.1 (continued)

Lesion	Definition	Example
Irreversible or indicators of damage		
Enthesophyte	Step-up bony prominence in continuity with entheseal bone attachment	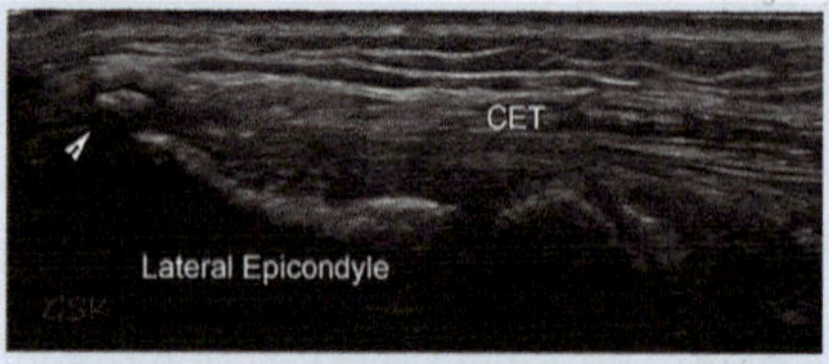 Long axis scan of common extensor tendon (CET) origin. Arrowhead indicates enthesophyte.
Calcification	Independent intrasubstance hyperechoic foci, with or without posterior acoustic shadowing	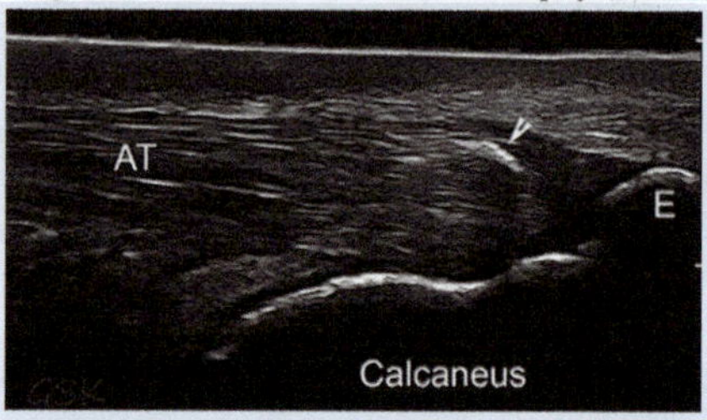 Long axis scan of distal Achilles tendon (AT) and enthesis. Intratendinous calcification (arrowhead) which is distinct and separate from enthesophyte (E)
Erosions	Cortical break seen in orthogonal planes	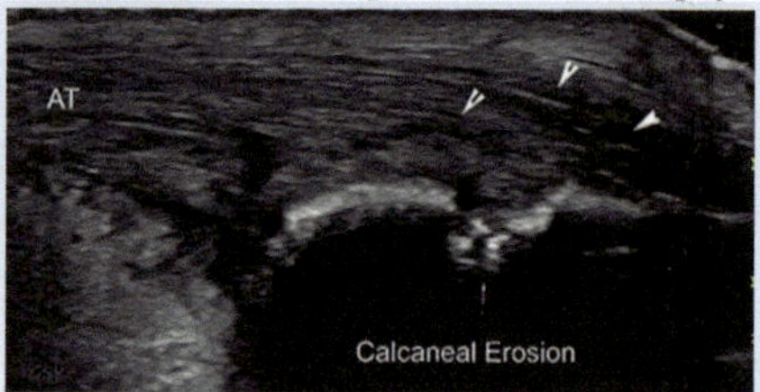 Long axis scan of distal Achilles tendon (AT) and enthesis. The enthesis is thickened. Loss of fibrillar echotexture indicated by arrowheads. Erosion at the calcaneus is labelled.
Bone irregularity/ periosteal reaction	Step-up bony prominence in the bone adjacent to entheses	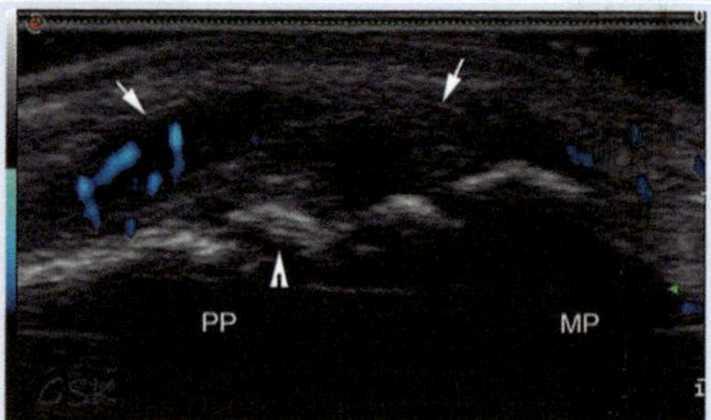 Long axis scan over the radial aspect of the third proximal interphalangeal joint. Step-up deformity (arrowhead) seen at the head of the proximal phalange (PP). The collateral ligament is thickened (arrowheads) between the base of the middle phalange (MP) and proximal metacarpal head. Power Doppler is noted at the hypoechoic areas consistent with collateral ligament enthesitis.

Derived from Ref. [13]

Doppler may detect increased vascularity of entheseal and adjacent structures. Doppler signal within the tendon or enthesis has to be interpreted with care since it may be due to neovascularity due to healing or inflammation. Doppler signal sensitivity may decrease when the enthesis is under tension with collapsing low-resistance blood vessels. It is essential to place the enthesis in a relaxed posture [14]. For example, the Doppler signal detection is more sensitive at the Achilles enthesis when the ankle is relaxed while flexed; with ankle dorsiflexion, resulting in tightening of the tendon and entheses, the Doppler signal decreases. Similar to the B-mode definitions, the OMERACT US working group has strictly defined the presence of Doppler signal to be within 2 mm of the bone attachment despite acknowledging that Doppler signal in proximal regions is more prevalent [13]. The Madrid group, as well as the GRAPPA US working group, classify Doppler at <2 mm of the entheseal bone and >2 mm of the entheseal margin, as well as in the bursa. The Madrid group also included non-nutrient vessels at the paratenon and cortical bone [15, 16]. In a cross-sectional study of 27 PsA patients, Macia-Villa et al. studied the prevalence of Doppler by anatomical site in 27 patients with metacarpophalangeal joint (MCP) swelling. Global B-mode entheseal abnormality prevalence ranged from 19% to 36% of entheses; 81.5% of the subjects had enthesis Doppler signal. The knee and Achilles tendon entheses had the highest prevalence of Doppler signal, while the plantar fascia had none. The Madrid definition of Doppler compared to the OMERACT definition was most sensitive, but both were reliable [15]. The greatest discordance of the Madrid Doppler compared to the OMERACT definition was at the quadriceps and distal patellar ligament entheses. Bursitis was only seen at the Achilles enthesis, and Doppler prevalence was low at 1.2%.

Entheseal Indices and the Choice of Entheseal Sites

Entheseal indices aim to serve as a sonographic imaging outcome measure which can be used to follow change after therapeutic intervention or as diagnostic tools. Several indices primarily based on mixed populations of spondyloarthritis (SpA) subjects are available (Table 12.2). The first index was the Glasgow Ultrasound Enthesis Scoring System (GUESS) [17], which evaluated five lower extremity entheses. Entheseal

Table 12.2 Contemporary ultrasound entheseal indices

Entheseal site	US-GRAPPA	US-OMERACT	MASEI	GUESS
Shoulder – Supraspinatus	+	–	+	–
Elbow – Triceps enthesis	+	–	+	–
Elbow – Lateral epicondyle	+	+	–	–
Knee – Quadriceps	+	+	+	+
Knee – Proximal patellar ligament	+	+	+	+
Knee – Distal patellar ligament	+	–	+	+
Ankle – Achilles tendon	+	+	+	+
Ankle – Plantar fascia	+	–	+	+

US-GRAPPA proposed entheseal sites by GRAPPA US working group, *US-OMERACT* proposed entheseal sites by OMERACT US enthesitis working group, *MASEI* Madrid Sonography Enthesitis Index, *GUESS* Glasgow Ultrasound Enthesitis Score thickness, enthesophyte formation, adjacent bone erosions, and presence of bursitis were assessed. Of note, this system did not incorporate the use of power Doppler. Predominantly long-standing axial SpA subjects were included in the validation study. This publication is important in demonstrating that clinical examination is insensitive and nonspecific compared to the ultrasonographic survey of enthesitis.

Next, the Madrid sonography enthesitis index (MASEI) aimed to discriminate predominantly long-standing axial SpA subjects from healthy controls [18]. In addition to elements included in the GUESS index, structural evaluation of the enthesis, as well as Doppler examination, was added. Entheseal loss of fibrillar echotexture, as well as hypoechoic or fusiform thickening, constituted the elementary lesions for entheseal structure. The candidate set of entheses include the triceps enthesis and the five lower extremity entheses used in the GUESS index. Interestingly, the sole upper extremity enthesis was added to mitigate possible mechanical confounding of lower extremity entheses. The maximum MASEI total sum score for 12 entheses is 136. There were interesting observations from the validation study. First, there was an overlap of the sum scores between healthy volunteers and SpA subjects; indeed, one healthy control had the highest MASEI score. Healthy women had less enthesitis than control men, but in subjects with SpA, sex differences were not observed. A cutoff score of 18 differentiated healthy controls from SpA patients. Of note, Doppler had good sensitivity and specificity in the global score, but the prevalence was low, and 60% had Doppler in at least one entheseal area. Doppler was seen in healthy controls but was less prevalent. Reliability statistics among six readers indicated good to excellent inter-reader reliability.

More recently, the OMERACT US working group have proposed a five-region consensus-based enthesitis index. (Table 12.2) [13]. The enthesis is strictly defined as tendon within 2 mm of the bone. While this may improve specificity, limitations of this approach have been discussed in the previous section. This group and others have agreed that "inflammatory" or potentially reversible elementary lesions include entheseal Doppler signal, hypoechogenicity, and thickness. Consensus-based structural lesions unlikely to improve include entheseal calcification or enthesophytes and erosion at the enthesis.

All the aforementioned indices heavily weight the lower extremity entheses. Obesity and physical activity can cause similar inflammatory and degenerative changes at the entheses. In a study comparing 60 psoriatic arthritis (PsA) compared to 66 psoriasis and 66 healthy controls, Eder et al. reported that the MASEI instrument could not distinguish between the three groups when the body mass index (BMI) was higher than thirty [19]. Wervers et al. reported that the MASEI score did not differentiate PsA subjects from young, healthy controls [20]. When the thickness of knee entheses was excluded, and power Doppler scoring was expanded from three to four scores, differences within groups could be discerned. In a study of 80 healthy subjects, Bakirci et al. reported that approximately 20% of the population had entheseal abnormalities [21]. The most frequent findings were entheseal thickening and enthesophyte formation. Regression analysis indicated that age, male sex, BMI, and high physical activity were independent predictors of sonographic entheseal scores.

Psoriatic arthritis subjects tend to have higher BMI. The GRAPPA US working group is developing an enthesitis tool that minimizes these confounders. A pilot study of 50 PsA subjects and 50 controls used logistic regression modeling to eliminate candidate entheses [16]. Eight entheses were selected, out of which three are in the upper extremity (Table 12.2). The proposed GRAPPA US enthesis index will be tested in the upcoming international GRAPPA-DUET study.

Dactylitis

Dactylitis is a characteristic manifestation of PsA. Its prevalence ranges from 16% to 49% of PsA patients and is associated with higher disease severity, enthesitis, and erosive joint disease [22, 23]. Dactylitis can be asymmetric and affects the toes more than the fingers. Acute dactylitis presents as a uniformly swollen, painful digit. After the acute phase has resolved, the digit may not resume normal thickness. In an MRI study of symptomatic and non-tender dactylitis digits, Healy et al. found widespread inflammation of the soft tissues and bone in symptomatic digits [24]. Of note, asymptomatic digits had similar fewer but similar qualitative findings.

Early MRI and US studies of dactylitis suggested that tenosynovitis was the predominant finding with occasional signs of synovitis [25–28]. Recent reviews have highlighted the involvement of multiple compartments in the digit, supporting a concept of "polyenthesitis" [29, 30] (Fig. 12.1). Interestingly, acute and chronic residual involvement of the digital pulleys has been reported with imaging studies [31, 32]. In summary, subjects with PsA suffering from dactylitis have the involvement of multiple structures of the digit, which may persist in the asymptomatic phase. Table 12.3 summarizes the structures documented to be involved in dactylitis.

Ultrasound of the Peripheral Joints in Psoriatic Arthritis

Joint involvement in psoriatic arthritis (PsA) has traditionally been categorized by Moll and Wright into an oligoarticular pattern, polyarticular pattern, and arthritis mutilans [33]. Publications over the last two decades have indicated that the polyarticular pattern is most frequent and tends to be symmetrical [34, 23]. The following topics will be discussed in the next sections: (1) unique features of joint

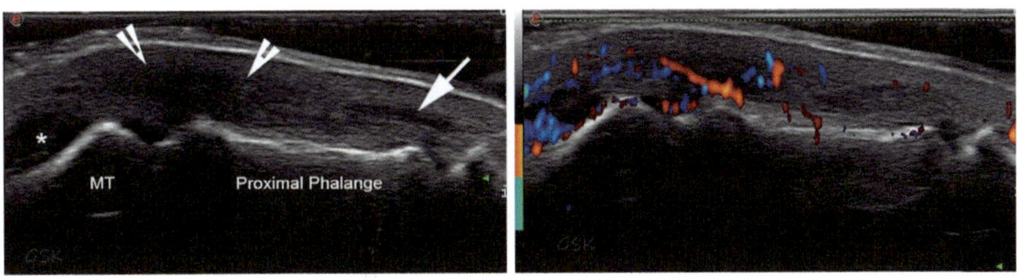

Fig. 12.1 Ultrasound of the dorsum of a dactylitic second toe. Dorsal long B-mode and power Doppler scans of a dactylitic second toe. Synovial hypertrophy (*) at the metatarsophalangeal joint is seen above the metatarsal head (MT). Arrowheads point to soft tissue edema which seems to be in continuity with the extensor hallucis tendon. The tendon is seen more distinctly distally but is edematous (long arrow)

involvement in PsA, (2) use of US for earlier diagnosis of PsA, and (3) US findings to differentiate PsA from other inflammatory arthritides.

Ultrasound Features of Joint Involvement in Psoriatic Arthritis

It has long been recognized that PsA is not just rheumatoid arthritis (RA) with the coexistence of psoriasis. PsA may affect all the digital joints, including the distal interphalangeal joints, and is associated with both erosive changes and periarticular new bone formation [35, 36]. Abnormalities of the extra-synovial tissues characterize ultrasound examination of small joints at the hands or feet. Dactylitis also may coexist in which case more extensive soft tissue involvement can be seen.

Erosive synovitis and tenosynovitis can be detected with US in PsA as in RA patients [37] (Fig. 12.2). Histologically, the pattern of vascularity in the synovium of PsA subjects is seen as multiple interconnecting loops, while in RA, the vessels macroscopically tend to be linear. By ultrasound, these differences cannot be discerned. The main difference is that extracapsular structures are more commonly affected in PsA. In one of the earliest sonographic comparisons of PsA vs. RA fingers, Fournie et al. reported that 84% of PsA fingers had extra-synovial changes and none in RA subjects. The most prevalent extra-synovial changes reported were periosteal reaction, capsular enthesophyte, and soft tissue thickening [37]. Subsequent studies have reported inflammation affecting the extensor tendons of the hands as frequently as synovitis [38, 39].

Table 12.3 Structures involved in dactylitis by MRI or ultrasound

Structures
Soft tissues – thickening or edema
Extensor tendon enthesitis
Collateral ligament enthesitis
Volar or plantar plate inflammation
Flexor tendon tenosynovitis
Volar pulley inflammation/thickening
Synovitis
Erosions
Osteoproliferation

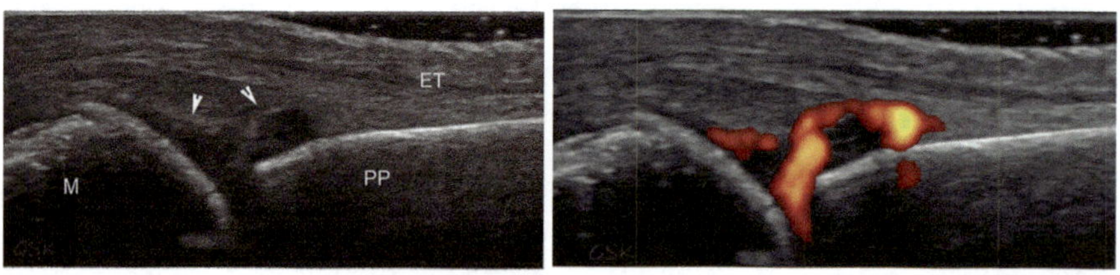

Fig. 12.2 Synovitis at the metacarpophalangeal joint. Top picture is long axis B-mode scan of the distal portion of the metacarpophalangeal joint. Synovial hypertrophy (arrowheads) is seen between the metacarpal head (M) and proximal phalange (PP). The extensor tendon (ET) is normal in appearance. The bottom picture shows power Doppler signal overlying synovial hypertrophy

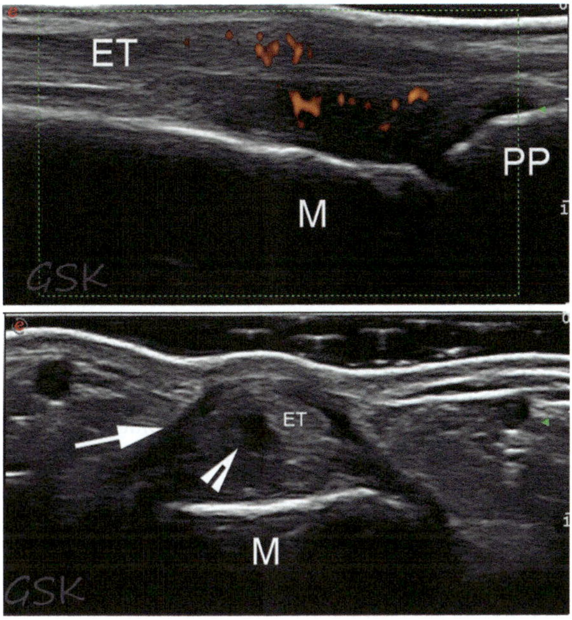

Fig. 12.3 Paratenonitis at the metacarpophalangeal joint. Top picture demonstrating thickening of the extensor tendon (ET) with hypoechoic material adjacent to it, with active power Doppler signal. On short axis, at the level of the metacarpal neck (M), the extensor tendon (ET) is seen with an anechoic rim (arrow). Large arrow points to the annual apparatus. PP – proximal phalange

One of the common extra-articular features seen at metacarpophalangeal (MCP) joints is inflammation of the extensor tendon and is variably termed as paratenonitis or paratendinitis (Fig. 12.3). Of note, the extensor tendon at this level does not have a sheath. On long axis views, the tendon may be thickened, with loss of fibrillar echotexture, and may have adjoining hypoechoic material. On short axis, an anechoic rim around the extensor tendon is characteristic. Power Doppler may be seen within the tendon as well as adjacent tissues (Fig. 12.3). At the level of the metacarpal neck, the annular apparatus may appear mildly thickened and may also display the Doppler signal. In a case series of 18 RA patients, compared with 20 PsA subjects, paratenonitis about the MCP joints was seen in 66% of PsA patients while none was seen in RA subjects [40]. Paratenonitis about the MCP joint may be more prevalent in PsA but also occurs in RA [41, 42]. Widespread involvement of extracapsular structures such as the palmar plates, collateral ligaments, and extensor tendons may help differentiate PsA from RA [43].

At the dorsal proximal interphalangeal (PIP) joints, analogous changes may be noted [44]. Synovitis may be present at the same time as central slip thickening and vascularity. Care has to be undertaken in evaluating power Doppler at this site since the signal from overlying veins may bleed into inferior structures. One way to mitigate this is to examine the joint in the short axis where the veins are readily identified.

Sonography and Diagnosis of PsA

One of the areas where ultrasound aids in the diagnosis of inflammatory arthritis is when patients present with sparse clinical signs. Ultrasound is more sensitive than clinically swollen or tender joint counts in detecting synovitis. It is of value to diagnose PsA early and initiate second-line agents to achieve low disease activity. Freeston et al. studied 49 patients of recent-onset PsA who were disease-modifying antirheumatic drug (DMARD) naïve [45]. Ultrasound of 40 joints was compared to 68/66 clinical joint count. Active US synovitis was defined as a grayscale score of ≥2, and/or a power Doppler score of ≥1.75% of the subjects were found to have subclinical synovitis with a median of three joints involved. The most common areas for subclinical synovitis were the wrist, knee, and metatarsophalangeal (MTP) joints. Of the 12 patients that were classified as oligoarthritis, eight were reclassified as polyarthritis.

In patients with undifferentiated inflammatory arthritis, ultrasound of the hand may be able to appreciate extracapsular manifestations of PsA, as discussed above, to allow more accurate diagnosis and classification [43]. However, if predominantly PIP and distal interphalangeal (DIP) joints are involved, it may be challenging to differentiate PsA from osteoarthritis or erosive osteoarthritis [46]. Careful correlation with plain X-rays may help distinguish these conditions if erosions are present. In erosive osteoarthritis, erosions predominantly occur in the subchondral area, whereas in PsA, "bare areas" are afflicted [35].

Finally, patients with PsA share risk factors for tophaceous gout [47]. Psoriasis itself is a risk factor for gout. It may be clinically challenging to distinguish PsA from gout. One clinical scenario is when PsA may not seem to respond to DMARD escalation if the active underlying pathology was due to gout. Ultrasound is eminently suited to elicit sonographic manifestations of gout in joints, ligaments, and tendons and may help target therapy appropriately [48].

Sonographic Outcome Measures for Joint Involvement

There are no formal sonographic outcome measures for joint involvement solely. Two groups have included sonographic articular measures in their composite tool. Gutierrez et al. included wrist, MCP, and MTP joints in a composite measure that spanned 60 anatomical sites [49]. Joints were scored according to the OMERACT methodology. The authors reported that the maximum time it took to scan 60 sites was 16 min. Data on the joints were not reported separately. Husic et al. and Ficjan et al. reported on a more extensive set of articular scans which formed part of the PsASon composite score [50, 51]. Using a reductive approach, and after scanning 68 joints, and 14 entheses, two scores were finalized. The PsASon22 scans structures bilaterally and includes 22 joints and four entheses, while the unilateral PsASon13 comprises of 13 joints and two entheses [51]. Of note, extensor tendon paratenonitis about the MCP joint was scored dichotomously as well as semiquantitative synovitis scoring. Tenosynovitis was scored 0–3, and enthesophyte formation and erosions were scored dichotomously. Analysis of the value of palmar/plantar scans revealed that at the wrists and MTP joints, these added little additional value. In contrast, more than 20% of the pathologies at the PIP and DIP joints were identified at palmar or dorsal scans only. At the knees, bilateral parapatellar scans and suprapatellar recess scans were required in order not to miss any patients with power Doppler signal at this site. The maximum reported time to complete the bilateral and unilateral scans was 26 and 13 min respectively. Thus, there is an ongoing need to develop a feasible articular index in PsA that is feasible and which can contend with the heterogeneous nature of synovitis and periarticular tissue involvement.

Conclusion

Psoriatic arthritis can affect many musculoskeletal targets, and many times, the heterogeneity can be appreciated in the same limb. Clinical examination is insensitive and does not inform of the underlying spectrum of pathology. Ultrasound has evolved to evaluate the diverse musculoskeletal pathology – from large and small entheses to joints and dactylitis. Imaging is shedding new insights into the pathophysiology of PsA such as the periarticular soft tissue involvement around involved joints. It is also highlighting the link between biomechanical factors and the expression of musculoskeletal manifestations of the disease. With the advent of an ever-expanding therapeutic armamentarium, it is indeed an exciting time to apply point-of-care imaging to understanding the underlying pathophysiology and making better decisions for our patients.

Review Questions

1. Which of the following is *not* a typical location for enthesitis?
   (a) Membranous entheses
   (b) Fibrocartilaginous entheses
   (c) Functional entheses such as fingers
   (d) Bone pulley enthesis, such as the posterior tibial tendon at medial malleolus
2. Which of the following has *the least sensitivity for detecting the entheseal Doppler signal*?
   (a) Knee positioned in extension
   (b) Examination of the Achilles tendon with the foot in 90 degrees dorsiflexion
   (c) Examination of the Achilles tendon with the foot in plantar flexion
   (d) Common extensor origin with the elbow at 90 degrees flexion
3. The Glasgow Ultrasound Enthesis Scoring System (GUESS) evaluates the following *except?*
   (a) Quadriceps, patellar ligament, Achilles tendon, and plantar fascia entheses
   (b) Entheseal thickness
   (c) Presence of erosions adjacent to the enthesis
   (d) Presence of bursitis
   (e) Doppler signal at the entheses and bursa
4. The Madrid sonography enthesitis index (MASEI) includes the following *except?*
   (a) Quadriceps, patellar ligament, Achilles tendon, and plantar fascia entheses
   (b) Common extensor origin enthesis
   (c) Triceps enthesis

   (d) Utilization of Doppler to detect vascularity at the entheses
5. The Outcome Measures in Rheumatology (OMERACT) Ultrasound Working Group have defined the enthesis as one of the following:
   (a) Bone pulley enthesis
   (b) Functional enthesis, such as the finger
   (c) Inclusion of the proximal tendon and bursa
   (d) The 2 mm zone proximal to the bony attachment
6. Entheseal inflammatory lesions include the following *except?*
   (a) Enthesophyte formation
   (b) Thickening of the enthesis
   (c) Hypoechogenicity of the enthesis
   (d) Doppler signal in the enthesis
7. Studies have shown that the following factors are associated with higher severity in entheseal scores, *except*?
   (a) Male sex
   (b) Female sex
   (c) Body mass index above 30
   (d) Moderate to high physical activity
8. Compared to rheumatoid arthritis, psoriatic arthritis displays which of the following unique feature?
   (a) Intra-articular hypoechogenicity
   (b) Doppler signal within the joint
   (c) Erosions
   (d) Extra-articular inflammation
9. In the study of early PsA by Freeston et al., active joints by ultrasound were defined by which of the following definitions?
   (a) Grayscale >1
   (b) Grayscale >1 and Doppler >1
   (c) Grayscale >2 and Doppler >1
   (d) Grayscale >2 and Doppler >2
10. Imaging studies of dactylitis have demonstrated inflammatory involvement of the following *except one of the following*?
   (a) Digital pulleys
   (b) Soft tissue inflammation or polyenthesitis
   (c) Synovitis
   (d) Nails

Answers

1. (a) Inflammatory enthesitis generally does not occur at membranous entheses.
2. (b) The foot in 90 degrees dorsiflexion will tighten the enthesis and collapse the vessels and hence lowering Doppler sensitivity.
3. (e) The GUESS system does not utilize Doppler.
4. (b) The MASEI does not include the common extensor origin enthesis.
5. (d) The OMERACT group strictly defines an enthesis within 2 mm of its attachment. Proximal and adjacent structures are not included.

6. (a) Enthesophyte is not a reversible lesion and hence is not considered an "inflammatory" lesion.
7. (e) Female sex
8. (d) Extra-articular inflammation
9. (c) Grayscale >2 and Doppler >1
10. (d) Nails. The literature of imaging of the nail in subjects with dactylitis is sparse. Polyenthesitis refers to dactylitis affecting numerous structures in the finger.

References

1. Coates LC, Kavanaugh A, Mease PJ, Soriano ER, Acosta-Felquer ML, Armstrong AW, et al. Group for research and assessment of psoriasis and psoriatic arthritis 2015 treatment recommendations for psoriatic arthritis. Arthritis Rheumatol. 2016;68(5):1060–71.
2. Polachek A, Li S, Chandran V, Gladman D. Clinical enthesitis in a prospective longitudinal psoriatic arthritis cohort: incidence, prevalence, characteristics and outcome. Arthritis Care Res (Hoboken). 2016;69(11):1685–91.
3. Kaeley GS, Eder L, Aydin SZ, Gutierrez M, Bakewell C. Enthesitis: a hallmark of psoriatic arthritis. Semin Arthritis Rheum. 2018;48(1):35–43.
4. Taylor W, Gladman D, Helliwell P, Marchesoni A, Mease P, Mielants H, et al. Classification criteria for psoriatic arthritis: development of new criteria from a large international study. Arthritis Rheum. 2006;54(8):2665–73.
5. Polachek A, Cook R, Chandran V, Gladman DD, Eder L. The association between sonographic enthesitis and radiographic damage in psoriatic arthritis. Arthritis Res Ther. 2017;19(1):189.
6. Mease PJ, Karki C, Palmer JB, Etzel CJ, Kavanaugh A, Ritchlin CT, et al. Clinical characteristics, disease activity, and patient-reported outcomes in psoriatic arthritis patients with dactylitis or enthesitis: results from the corrona psoriatic arthritis/spondyloarthritis registry. Arthritis Care Res. 2017;69(11):1692–9.
7. Sunar I, Ataman S, Nas K, Kilic E, Sargin B, Kasman SA, et al. Enthesitis and its relationship with disease activity, functional status, and quality of life in psoriatic arthritis: a multi-center study. Rheumatol Int. 2019;40(2):283–94.
8. McInnes IB, Puig L, Gottlieb AB, Ritchlin C, Song M, You Y, et al. Association between enthesitis and health-related quality of life in psoriatic arthritis in anti-TNF-naïve patients from two phase 3 ustekinumab trials. J Rheumatol. 2019;46(11):1458–61. https://doi.org/10.3899/jrheum.180792.
9. McGonagle D, Khan M, Marzo-Ortega H, O'Connor P, Gibbon W, Emery P. Enthesitis in spondyloarthropathy. Curr Opin Rheumatol. 1999;11(4):244–50.
10. Aydin SZ, Bakirci S, Kasapoglu E, Castillo-Gallego C, Alhussain FA, Ash ZR, et al. The relationship between physical examination and ultrasonography for large entheses is best for the Achilles tendon and patellar tendon origin. J Rheumatol. 2019;47(7):1026–30.
11. Benjamin M, McGonagle D. The anatomical basis for disease localisation in seronegative spondyloarthropathy at entheses and related sites. J Anat. 2001;199(Pt 5):503–26.
12. McGonagle D, Lories RJ, Tan AL, Benjamin M. The concept of a "synovio-entheseal complex" and its implications for understanding joint inflammation and damage in psoriatic arthritis and beyond. Arthritis Rheum. 2007;56(8):2482–91.
13. Balint PV, Terslev L, Aegerter P, Bruyn GAW, Chary-Valckenaere I, Gandjbakhch F, et al. Reliability of a consensus-based ultrasound definition and scoring for enthesitis in spondyloarthritis and psoriatic arthritis: an OMERACT US initiative. Ann Rheum Dis. 2018;77(12):1730–5.

14. Gutierrez M, Filippucci E, Grassi W, Rosemffet M. Intratendinous power doppler changes related to patient position in seronegative spondyloarthritis. J Rheumatol. 2010;37(5):1057–9.
15. Macía-Villa C, Falcao S, Medina J, Miguel ED. Ultrasonography of enthesis in psoriatic arthritis: a descriptive and reliability analysis of elemental lesions and power Doppler subtypes. Scand J Rheumatol. 2019;48(6):454–9.
16. Tom S, Zhong Y, Cook R, Aydin SZ, Kaeley G, Eder L. Development of a preliminary ultrasonographic enthesitis score in psoriatic arthritis – GRAPPA ultrasound working group. J Rheumatol. 2019;46(4):384–90.
17. Balint PV, Kane D, Wilson H, McInnes IB, Sturrock RD. Ultrasonography of entheseal insertions in the lower limb in spondyloarthropathy. Ann Rheum Dis. 2002;61(10):905–10.
18. de Miguel E, Cobo T, Munoz-Fernandez S, Naredo E, Uson J, Acebes JC, et al. Validity of enthesis ultrasound assessment in spondylarthropathy. Ann Rheum Dis. 2008;68(2):169–74.
19. Eder L, Jayakar J, Thavaneswaran A, Haddad A, Chandran V, Salonen D, et al. Is the MAdrid Sonographic Enthesitis index useful for differentiating psoriatic arthritis from psoriasis alone and healthy controls? J Rheumatol. 2014;41(3):466–72.
20. Wervers K, Vis M, Rasappu N, van der Ven M, Tchetverikov I, Kok MR, et al. Modification of a sonographic enthesitis score to differentiate between psoriatic arthritis and young healthy volunteers. Scand J Rheumatol. 2018;47(4):291–4.
21. Bakirci S, Solmaz D, Stephenson W, Eder L, Roth J, Aydin SZ. Entheseal changes in response to age, body mass index and physical activity: an ultrasound study in healthy people. J Rheumatol. 2020;47(7):968–72. Available from: http://www.jrheum.org/content/early/2020/01/27/jrheum.190540
22. Brockbank JE, Stein M, Schentag CT, Gladman DD. Dactylitis in psoriatic arthritis: a marker for disease severity? Ann Rheum Dis. 2005;64(2):188–90.
23. Helliwell PS. Established psoriatic arthritis: clinical aspects. J Rheumatol Suppl. 2009;83:21–3.
24. Healy PJ, Groves C, Chandramohan M, Helliwell PS. MRI changes in psoriatic dactylitis–extent of pathology, relationship to tenderness and correlation with clinical indices. Rheumatology (Oxford). 2008;47(1):92–5.
25. Kane D, Greaney T, Bresnihan B, Gibney R, FitzGerald O. Ultrasonography in the diagnosis and management of psoriatic dactylitis. J Rheumatol. 1999;26(8):1746–51.
26. Olivieri I, Scarano E, Padula A, Giasi V. Dactylitis involving most of the fingers. Clin Exp Rheumatol. 2003;21(3):406.
27. Olivieri I, Padula A, Scarano E, Scarpa R. Dactylitis or "sausage-shaped" digit. J Rheumatol. 2007;34(6):1217–22.
28. Olivieri I, Scarano E, Padula A, D'Angelo S, Salvarani C, Cantini F, et al. Fast spin echo-T2-weighted sequences with fat saturation in toe dactylitis of spondyloarthritis. Clin Rheumatol. 2008;27(9):1141–5.
29. Bakewell CJ, Olivieri I, Aydin SZ, Dejaco C, Ikeda K, Gutierrez M, et al. Ultrasound and magnetic resonance imaging in the evaluation of psoriatic dactylitis: status and perspectives. J Rheumatol. 2013;40(12):1951–7.
30. Kaeley GS, Eder L, Aydin SZ, Gutierrez M, Bakewell C. Dactylitis: a hallmark of psoriatic arthritis. Semin Arthritis Rheum. 2018;48(2):263–73.
31. Tan AL, Fukuba E, Halliday NA, Tanner SF, Emery P, McGonagle D. High-resolution MRI assessment of dactylitis in psoriatic arthritis shows flexor tendon pulley and sheath-related enthesitis. Ann Rheum Dis. 2015;74(1):185–9.
32. Tinazzi I, McGonagle D, Aydin SZ, Chessa D, Marchetta A, Macchioni P. 'Deep Koebner' phenomenon of the flexor tendon-associated accessory pulleys as a novel factor in tenosynovitis and dactylitis in psoriatic arthritis. Ann Rheum Dis. 2018;77(6):922–5.
33. Moll JMH, Wright V. Psoriatic arthritis. Semin Arthritis Rheum. 1973;3(1):55–78.
34. Helliwell PS, Porter G, Taylor WJ, Group CS. Polyarticular psoriatic arthritis is more like oligoarticular psoriatic arthritis, than rheumatoid arthritis. Ann Rheum Dis. 2007;66(1):113–7.
35. Martel W, Stuck K, Dworin A, Hylland R. Erosive osteoarthritis and psoriatic arthritis: a radiologic comparison in the hand, wrist, and foot. Am J Roentgenol. 1980;134(1):125–35.

36. Tan AL, McGonagle D. Psoriatic arthritis: correlation between imaging and pathology. Joint Bone Spine. 2010;77(3):206–11.
37. Fournie B, Margarit-Coll N, Champetier de Ribes TL, Zabraniecki L, Jouan A, Vincent V, et al. Extrasynovial ultrasound abnormalities in the psoriatic finger. Prospective comparative power-doppler study versus rheumatoid arthritis. Joint Bone Spine. 2006;73(5):527–31.
38. Wiell C, Szkudlarek M, Hasselquist M, Moller JM, Vestergaard A, Norregaard J, et al. Ultrasonography, magnetic resonance imaging, radiography, and clinical assessment of inflammatory and destructive changes in fingers and toes of patients with psoriatic arthritis. Arthritis Res Ther. 2007;9:R119.
39. Macía-Villa C, Falcao S, Gutierrez M, Medina J, Hammer HB, De Miguel E. What is metacarpophalangeal joint swelling in psoriatic arthritis? Ultrasound findings and reliability assessment. Clin Exp Rheumatol. 2018;36(5):896–9.
40. Gutierrez M, Filippucci E, Salaffi F, Di Geso L, Grassi W. Differential diagnosis between rheumatoid arthritis and psoriatic arthritis: the value of ultrasound findings at metacarpophalangeal joints level. Ann Rheum Dis. 2011;70(6):1111–4.
41. Ramrattan L, Kaeley G. Ultrasound characteristics of extensor tendon abnormalities and peritendinous fluid in rheumatoid arthritis. Arthritis Rheum. 2013;65(Suppl. 10):S2686.
42. Backhaus M, Ohrndorf S, Kellner H, Strunk J, Backhaus TM, Hartung W, et al. Evaluation of a novel 7-joint ultrasound score in daily rheumatologic practice: a pilot project. Arthritis Rheum. 2009;61(9):1194–201.
43. Kaeley GS, Bakewell C, Deodhar A. The importance of ultrasound in identifying and differentiating patients with early inflammatory arthritis: a narrative review. Arthritis Res Ther. 2020;22(1):1.
44. Filippou G, Di Sabatino V, Adinolfi A, Bertoldi I, Picerno V, Biasi G, et al. No enthesis should be overlooked when psoriatic arthritis is suspected: enthesitis of the extensor digitorum tendons. J Rheumatol. 2013;40(3):335.
45. Freeston J, Coates L, Nam J, Moverley A, Hensor E, Wakefield R, et al. Is there sub-clinical synovitis in early psoriatic arthritis? A clinical comparison with grey scale and power Doppler ultrasound. Arthritis Care Res. 2013;66(3):432–9.
46. Tan AL, Grainger AJ, Tanner SF, Emery P, McGonagle D. A high-resolution magnetic resonance imaging study of distal interphalangeal joint arthropathy in psoriatic arthritis and osteoarthritis: are they the same? Arthritis Rheum. 2006;54(4):1328–33.
47. Felten R, Duret P-M, Gottenberg J-E, Spielmann L, Messer L. At the crossroads of gout and psoriatic arthritis: "psout". Clin Rheumatol. 2020;39(5):1405–13. https://doi.org/10.1007/s10067-020-04981-0.
48. O'Connor PJ. Crystal deposition disease and psoriatic arthritis. Semin Musculoskelet Radiol. 2013;17(1):74–9.
49. Gutierrez M, Di Geso L, Salaffi F, Bertolazzi C, Tardella M, Filosa G, et al. Development of a preliminary US power Doppler composite score for monitoring treatment in PsA. Rheumatology (Oxford). 2012;51(7):1261–8.
50. Husic R, Gretler J, Felber A, Graninger WB, Duftner C, Hermann J, et al. Disparity between ultrasound and clinical findings in psoriatic arthritis. Ann Rheum Dis. 2013;73(8):1529–36.
51. Ficjan A, Husic R, Gretler J, Lackner A, Graninger WB, Gutierrez M, et al. Ultrasound composite scores for the assessment of inflammatory and structural pathologies in Psoriatic Arthritis (PsASon-Score). Arthritis Res Ther. 2014;16(5):476.

Ultrasound in Crystalline Diseases: Gout and Calcium-Associated Arthritis 13

Ralf G. Thiele

Introduction

Crystalline deposits in human tissues are strong reflectors of ultrasound waves, and the sonographic appearance and characteristics of their distribution allow the examiner to identify crystalline arthropathies. Ultrasonography has been used to detect crystalline deposits since the early 1960s when US was used to identify kidney stones [1, 2]. Combining ultrasound with conventional radiography has allowed distinguishing calcium containing kidney stones (visible on US and radiography) from urate stones (visible on US but not on x-rays). The same principles hold true for crystal deposition in and around joints.

Crystalline arthropathies represent the most common forms of arthritis and are associated with higher health-care expenditures than other arthritides combined. While rheumatoid arthritis (RA) and spondyloarthritis (SpA) affect 1.3 and 2.4 million Americans, respectively, gout affects 9.2 and osteoarthritis 26.9 million [3–5]. In the United States, hospitalization rates for a principal diagnosis of gout have doubled over the past two decades, whereas those for RA have decreased by 67% [6].

The current gold standard for the identification of crystals includes fluid aspiration from an affected joint, with subsequent polarizing microscopy. However, in a primary care setting, joint aspiration is not always performed. Aspiration would also require the presence of joint fluid containing crystals. An attack of gout or pseudogout may affect extra-articular tissues such as tendon insertions or bursae or may involve hyperemia of fibrovascular tissue associated with a tophus with development of subcutaneous edema, and no fluid could be aspirated. If a joint aspiration is attempted, it may be successful less than 50% of the time. Once fluid is sent to the lab, correct identification of monosodium urate crystals is accomplished in 43–79%

R. G. Thiele (✉)
Division of Allergy/Immunology & Rheumatology, Department of Medicine, University of Rochester School of Medicine and Dentistry, Rochester, NY, USA
e-mail: ralf_thiele@urmc.rochester.edu

M. J. Kohler (ed.), *Musculoskeletal Ultrasound in Rheumatology Review*,
https://doi.org/10.1007/978-3-030-73555-5_13

of the cases, and up to 24% may yield false positives [7–11]. Ultrasonography can improve detection and management of crystal-induced arthritis.

Calcium-Associated Arthritis: Basic Calcium Phosphate Disease and Calcium Pyrophosphate Deposition Disease

Basic Calcium Phosphate

Basic calcium phosphate (BCP) may represent by far the most common arthropathy. Calcium containing crystals including BCP but also calcium pyrophosphate seems to be closely involved in the pathogenesis of osteoarthritis [12]. BCP crystals can typically not be seen on polarizing microscopy, and CPPD crystals are weakly birefringent [11]. Both can be detected by ultrasound.

Commonly found BCP crystals in arthropathy include hydroxyapatite and carbonate apatite, characterized by a hydroxy group or carbonate group, respectively.

- *Hydroxyapatite* $Ca_{10}(PO_4)_6(OH)_2$
- *Carbonate apatite* $Ca_{10}(PO_4)_6CO_3$

In osteoarthritis (OA), BCP is present in the synovial fluid of up to 60% of patients. At the time of joint replacement, BCP is present in the cartilage of up to 100% percent of patients [13, 14]. Calcific tendinitis is another example of BCP deposition. Carbonite apatite or hydroxyapatite can be aspirated from affected tendons.

Sonographic features of OA include periarticular bone spur formation, small hyperechoic "bubbles" of calcium crystal that can be seen "floating" within synovial fluid, and aggregates of BCP crystals that can assume a conformation of grape-like clusters or "balloons on a string" (Fig. 13.1). Typical joints affected by OA that

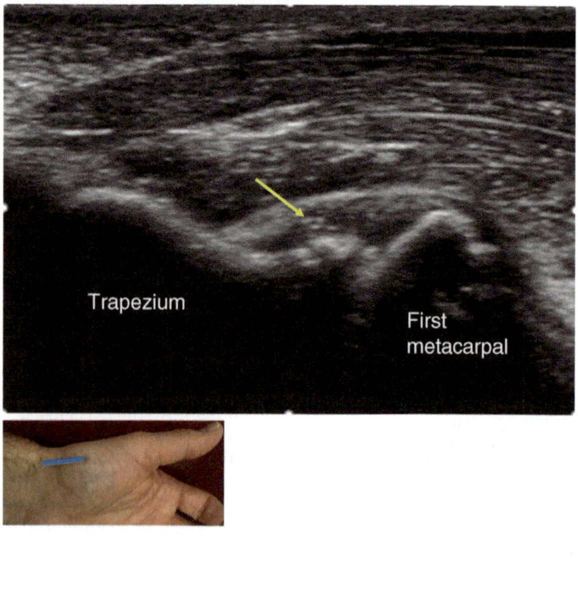

Fig. 13.1 Osteoarthritis. First carpo-metacarpal joint. Palmar long axis view. A cluster of small crystals is seen within the joint cavity (arrow)

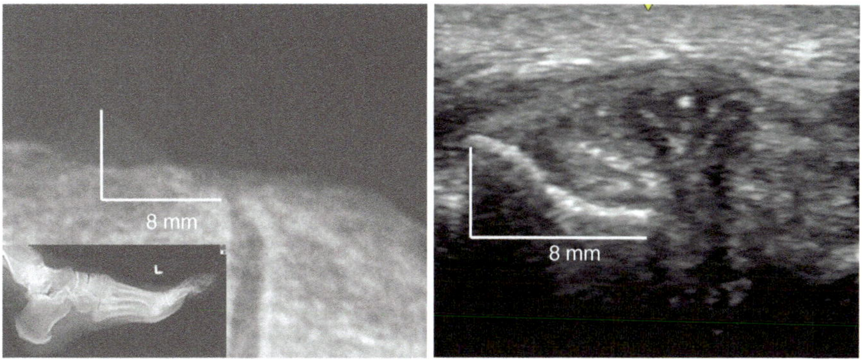

Fig. 13.2 Osteoarthritis. Radiograph of foot, left. Ultrasound of midfoot, right. Dorsal long axis view of same area, right. Hyperechoic material is noted

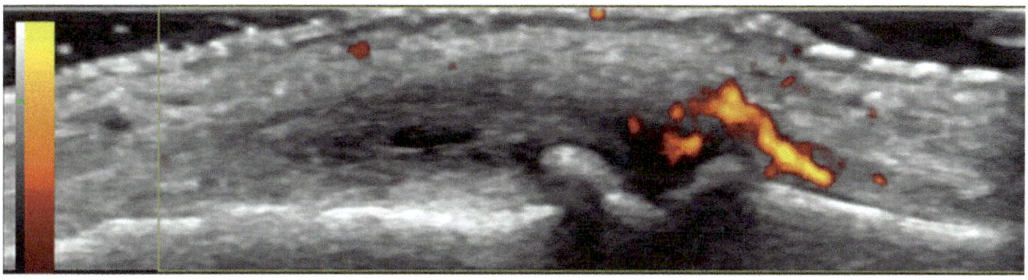

Fig. 13.3 Osteoarthritis. Dorsal long axis view of PIP joint. Bone spur formation is noted. There is hypoechoic thickening of the synovial lining seen, and mildly increased power Doppler signal

can be visualized by ultrasound include the basal joint of the thumb, best seen from a palmar aspect; PIP or DIP joints; or foot joints. Besides OA involving MTP 1, chronic recurrent midfoot pain can be caused by BCP or CPPD crystals, and they can be seen sonographically (Fig. 13.2). The presence of osteophytes or BCP crystals can rarely be associated with synovial thickening. Synovial proliferation in OA is typically less pronounced than in the classic inflammatory arthropathies. If synovial thickening is seen, assessment with power or color Doppler ultrasonography can help identify chronic subclinical inflammation (Fig. 13.3). BCP crystal aggregates in OA are very small, and high-frequency transducers of 18 MHZ and higher are needed to detect them (Fig. 13.4).

Calcific tendinitis is very common, with a prevalence of 2–22% of the population. It affects persons in their productive years, commonly 30- to 60-year-olds, persons with a sedentary job more often than manual laborers, women more commonly than men. In contrast to the appearance in other crystal arthropathies, the calcific deposits in rotator cuff tendinopathy consist of amorphous and poorly crystalline carbonated hydroxyapatite [15, 16]. Sonographically, these crystalline masses can form large, ovoid-shaped deposits in tendons, with a relatively homogeneous echotexture. Ultrasound-guided needle tenotomy, also known as barbotage, can be used therapeutically, with lavage (repeated saline injection) and re-aspiration to extract calcium from the tendon (Fig. 13.5). This is followed by targeted physical therapy [17].

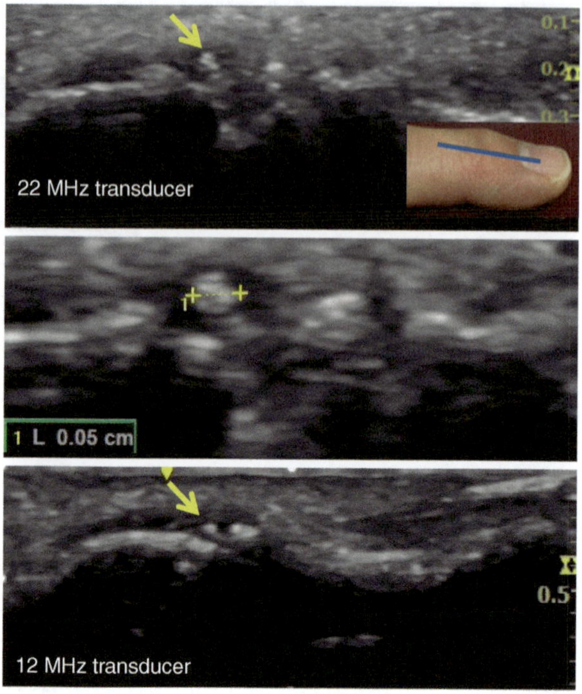

Fig. 13.4 Basic calcium phosphate disease: early osteoarthritis of DIP joint. Size of BCP crystal complex: 0.5 mm 22 MHz transducer, zoom. 12 vs. 22 MHz transducer: small crystal deposits are best seen with high frequency transducers

Calcium Pyrophosphate Dihydrate

Calcium pyrophosphate dihydrate (CPPD) deposition can lead to chondrocalcinosis – deposition in hyaline cartilage or fibrocartilage – and can be associated with arthritis [18]. Hemochromatosis and other secondary metabolic conditions can be associated with CPPD disease. Radiographically and sonographically, "hook osteophytes" can be seen at the radial aspect of metacarpal heads. Sonographically, CPPD deposits are characteristically found within the center of hyaline cartilage, where they can form a layer of hyperechoic material, often formed by aggregation of punctate deposits. Similarly, hyperechoic material can be seen in the center of fibrocartilage. Typical locations would be the triangular fibrocartilage complex of the wrist or the menisci of the knee (Fig. 13.6). The reason for this characteristic sonographic location is the locus of formation. The formation of CPP crystals occurs in the articular cartilage pericellular matrix and is facilitated by extracellular vesicles known as articular cartilage vesicles. Pyrophosphate is generated from extracellular ATP and forms complexes with calcium to create CPP crystals [19]. CPP crystals can break free from the confines of cartilage and distribute in the synovial space. This can occasionally lead to attacks of pseudogout. More commonly, these crystals will then deposit on available surfaces and may create a layer of hyperechoic material on the surface of cartilage. This can rarely create the

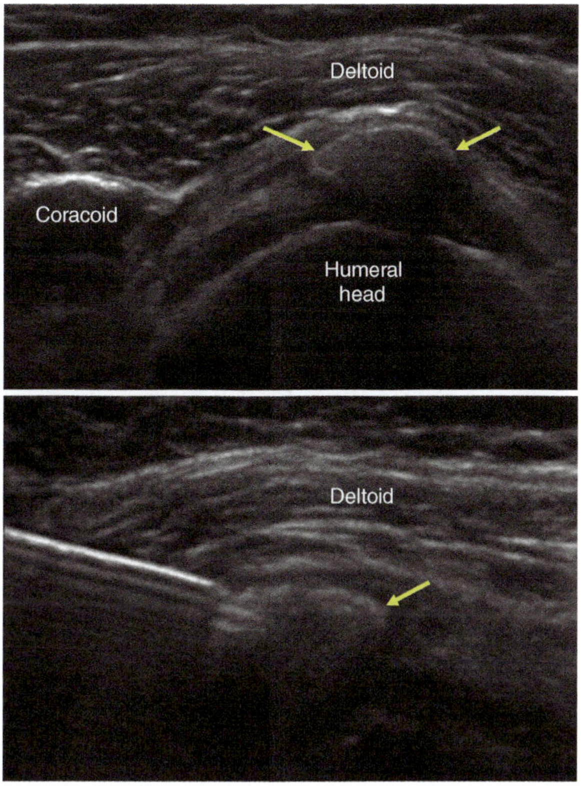

Fig. 13.5 Carbonate apatite disease: calcific tendinitis. Top: short axis view of supraspinatus tendon. Modified Crass position. An ovoid calcification is seen dissecting the tendon, between arrows. Bottom: needle approaching same calcification (arrow)

appearance of a sonographic "double contour sign" and needs to be distinguished from gout. In a study of 414 cases with monosodium urate (MSU)-positive gout and 98 CPPD-positive controls, Ogdie et al. found a double contour sign in 60% of gout patients but only 7% of CPPD controls [20]. If this is seen in CPPD disease, additional hyperechoic material may be seen in the center of cartilage, and radiographs may show calcific material or hook osteophytes (Fig. 13.7) OMERACT (Outcome Measures in Rheumatology) has published ultrasound criteria for CPPD (Table 13.1) [21].

GOUT

Gout

Gout is the most common inflammatory arthropathy, and sonography of gout is one of the main indications for the use of ultrasound in rheumatology. Ultrasound findings of gout have become part of the ACR/EULAR classification criteria [22, 23]. Visualization of gout crystals by ultrasound is informed by the pathogenesis of gout and

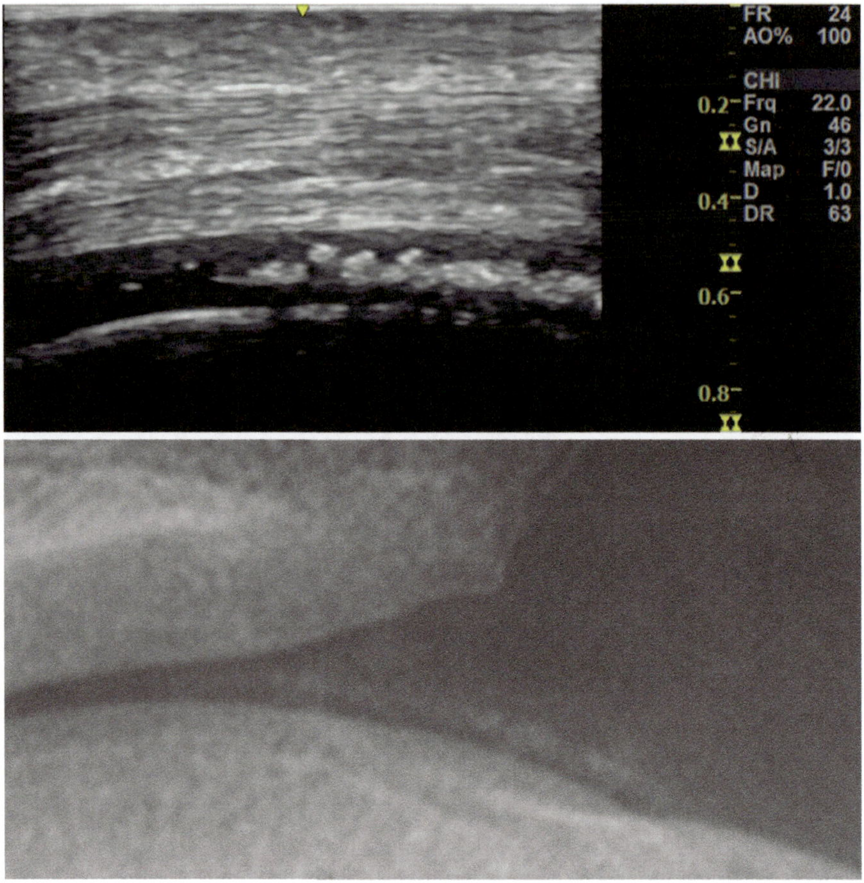

Fig. 13.6 CPPD disease. Top: hyperechoic material is seen in the center of hyaline cartilage over the femoral condyle of knee. Bottom: same location in knee on conventional radiograph. Calcific deposits are seen here as well

monosodium tophi. If serum or tissue urate concentrations exceed the solubility at 6.8 mg/dL, crystal precipitation can occur. Precipitation is facilitated in body areas with slightly lower temperatures, such as fingers and toes, anterior knee, and posterior elbow (and occasionally ears), and in tissues that undergo dynamic stress, such as the insertion of quadriceps tendon, patellar ligament or Achilles tendon, and repetitive pressure, such as olecranon and prepatellar bursae, and medial aspect of first metatarsal head [24, 25]. These represent high-yield areas for the ultrasound assessment of gout.

Within joints, MSU crystals can deposit over hyaline cartilage (double contour sign), within synovial tissue (aggregates), or form larger tophus complexes. Rarely, crystals can be seen floating within synovial fluid (snowstorm appearance). Outside of the joint cavity, tophi can be seen sonographically as ovoid structures, often embedded in fibrovascular granulation tissue. Erosions due to gout have a

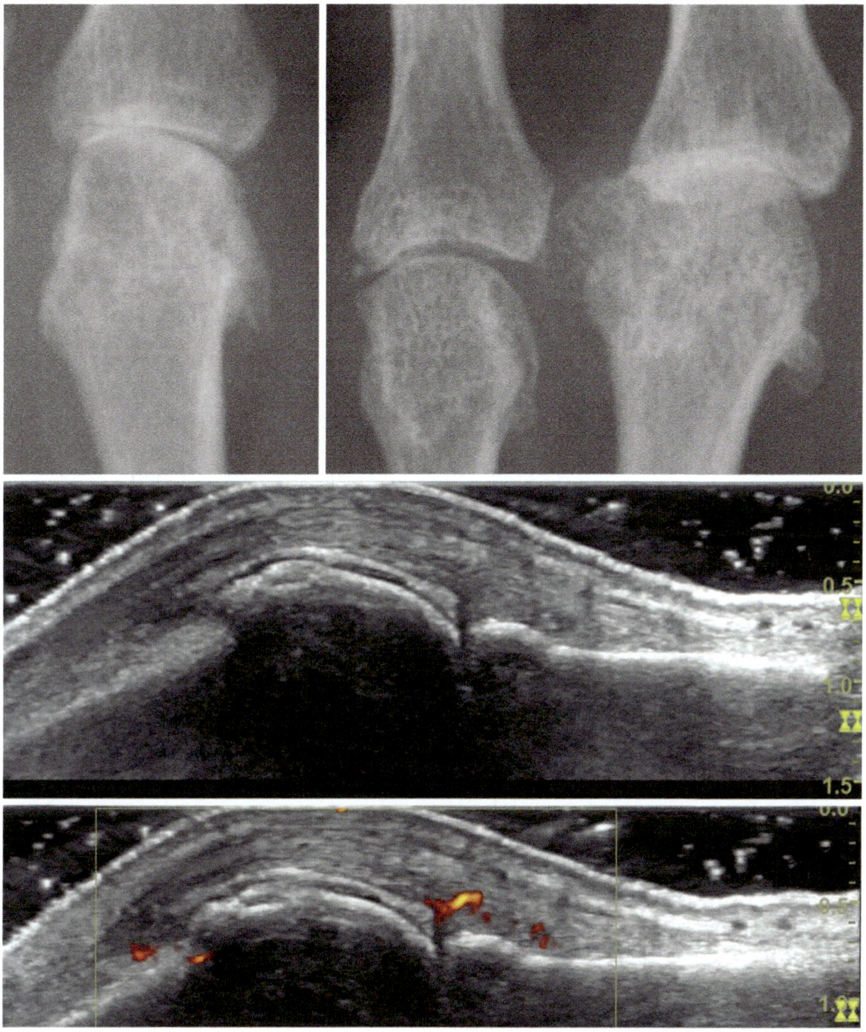

Fig. 13.7 Top: radiographs showing hook osteophytes and small radiodense, calcific deposits. Calcium-dense material is seen over metacarpal head on right, similar to ultrasound findings. Middle: a "pseudo double contour sign" is created by deposits of calcific material. A thin hyperechoic line is seen within the cartilage as well. Bottom image shows mild associated hyperemia

characteristic "punched out" appearance, with relatively smooth walls and typical thin, "eggshell" marginal overhangs [26]. OMERACT has published definitions for ultrasound lesions in gout (Table 13.2) [27].

Double Contour Sign

Identification of a sonographic double contour sign, a characteristic of gout, has become part of the ACR/EULAR classification criteria of gout in 2014. MSU

Table 13.1 OMERACT definitions of ultrasound findings in CPPD disease [21]

Structure	Shape	Echogenicity	Localization	Behavior at dynamic scanning
Fibrocartilage	Deposits of variable shape	Hyperechoic (similar to echogenicity of bony cortex)	Localized within the fibrocartilage structure	Remain fixed and move together with the fibrocartilage during dynamic assessment (i.e., joint movement and probe compression)
Hyaline cartilage	Deposits varying in size and shape	Hyperechoic (similar to echogenicity of bony cortex) that does not create posterior shadowing	Localized within the hyaline cartilage	The deposits remain fixed and move together with the hyaline cartilage (i.e., joint movement and probe compression).
Tendon	Multiple linear (parallel to the tendon fibrillar structure and not in continuity with the bone profile) deposits	Hyperechoic (in relation to the tendon echogenicity) that generally does not create posterior shadowing. The deposits maintain their high degree of echogenicity even at very low levels of gain and are not affected by anisotropy as the surrounding tendon.	Localized within the tendon	Remain fixed and move together with the tendon during movement and probe compression
Synovial fluid	Deposits of variable size (from punctate to large)	Hyperechoic (similar to echogenicity of bony cortex) that generally does not create posterior shadowing	Localized within the synovial fluid	Are mobile according to joint movement and probe pressure

Table 13.2 OMERACT definitions of elemental lesions of gout [27]

Elemental lesion	Definition
Double contour sign	Abnormal hyperechoic band over the superficial margin of the articular hyaline cartilage, independent of the angle of insonation and which may be either irregular or regular, continuous or intermittent, and can be distinguished from the cartilage interface sign
Tophus	Independent of location (e.g., extra-articular/intra-articular/intra-tendinous): A circumscribed, inhomogeneous, hyperechoic and/or hypoechoic aggregation (which may or may not generate posterior acoustic shadow), which may be surrounded by a small anechoic rim
Aggregates	Independent of location (intra-articular/intra-tendinous): Heterogeneous hyperechoic foci that maintain their high degree of reflectivity even when the gain setting is minimized or the insonation angle is changed and which occasionally may generate posterior acoustic shadow
Erosion	An intra- and/or extra-articular discontinuity of the bone surface (visible in two perpendicular planes)

crystals can deposit on the luminal surface of hyaline cartilage within the joint cavity. The cortex of the subchondral bone is echogenic independent of transducer angle (the angle of insonation) and appears as a bright curved outline on the ultrasound screen. The overlying hyaline cartilage has high water content and reflects little of the incident sound waves. It appears as an anechoic, dark band overlying the bright-appearing cortex. If a layer of MSU crystals is present over the cartilage, it reflects sound waves strongly and appears as a bright band, in parallel to the underlying bony cortex. The densely packed crystals reflect sound waves in all directions. The appearance of a double contour sign is therefore independent from the angle of insonation. The double contour sign may occasionally be discontinuous and may not cover the entire cartilaginous surface. The luminal surface often has a rough, granular appearance (Fig. 13.8). This granular surface appearance may be attenuated by ultrasound software that decreases pixelation and smooths the ultrasound images *(also known as speckle noise smoothing)* (Fig. 13.9).

The sonographic double contour sign needs to be distinguished from an interface artifact. A bright appearing line will appear at the interface of anechoic "black" hyaline cartilage and anechoic "black" overlying synovial fluid (an analogy may be oil over water in a glass tube, where both are translucent, but an interface is seen where they meet). At this interface, the greatest reflection occurs at the angle of perpendicular incidence, the apparent "apex" of the cartilage on the ultrasound

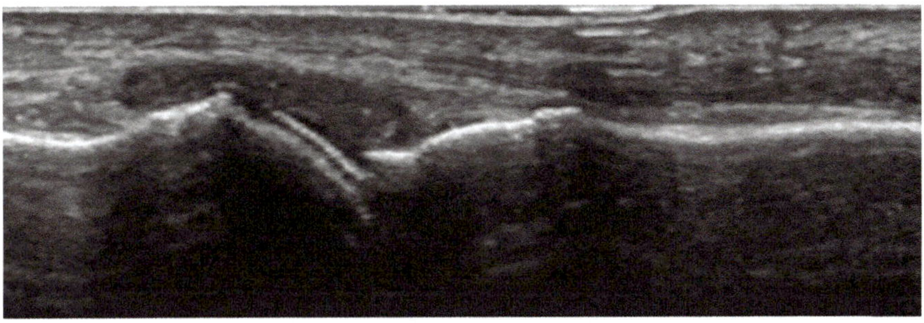

Fig. 13.8 Gout. Double contour sign over metatarsal head. Dorsal long axis view. A hyperechoic granular layer of crystals is seen over the anechoic hyaline cartilage

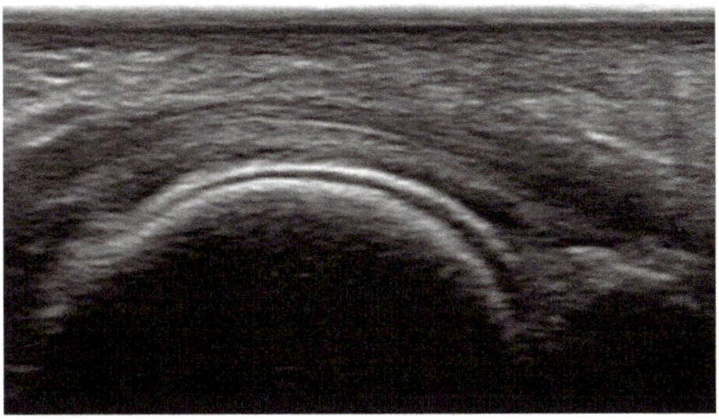

Fig. 13.9 Gout. Double contour sign over metatarsal head. Plantar long axis view. Less grainy appearance due to software modification

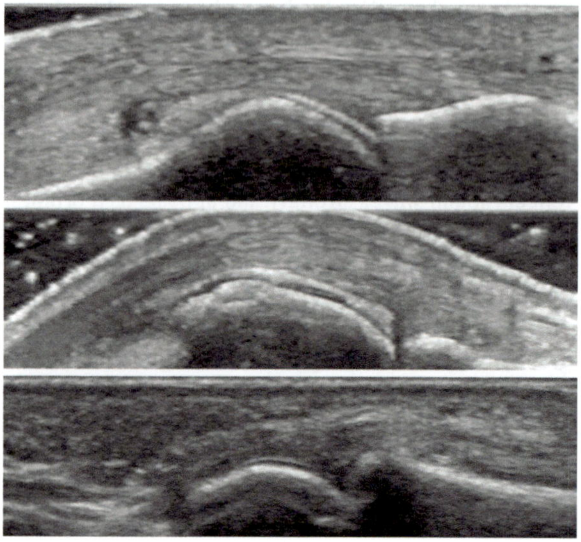

Fig. 13.10 Gout (top image). CPPD disease (middle image). Cartilage interface (bottom image)

image, where the sound waves meet the cartilage straight on and are being reflected back to the transducer directly. Where the cartilage curves away from the transducer, less sound energy is reflected straight back to the transducer, and the interface artifact appears less pronounced further away from the angle of perpendicular incidence (Fig. 13.10). This artifact will change apparent location with transducer movement.

Tophus

Gouty tophi have been described as an organized chronic giant cell granulomatous structure consisting of MSU crystals, innate and adaptive immune cells, and fibrovascular tissue [28]. Components of the tophus complex that can be observed sonographically include (1) a crystalline center is an acellular ("necrotic") collection of MSU crystals; (2) the crystalline center is surrounded by a corona zone consisting of multinucleated giant cells of the foreign body type, histiocytes, fibroblasts, lymphocytes, and plasma cells [29]; and (3) the corona zone is surrounded by a fibrovascular zone that is sparsely infiltrated with mononucleated cells. Calcification is observed in some tophi [30].

This corresponds to the ultrasound appearance of the tophus complex of an often ovoid, mostly hyperechoic structure with a granular "wet clumps of sugar" appearance that is typically surrounded by a small anechoic rim and embedded in fibrovascular matrix tissue that may show vascularity on power Doppler studies even in the absence of clinical symptoms [31] (Fig. 13.11). Pro-inflammatory cytokines, such as IL-1β and TNF, and the anti-inflammatory cytokine TGFβ1 are expressed in the

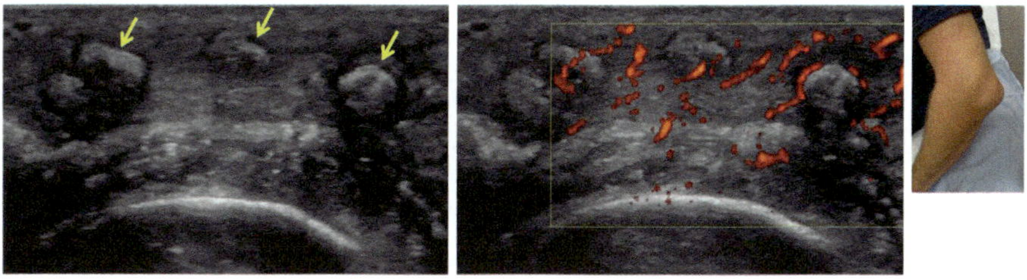

Fig. 13.11 Asymptomatic gout, fullness in olecranon bursa (photo). Short axis view over olecranon shows monosodium urate tophi (arrows). Addition of power Doppler ultrasound: hyperemia of matrix tissue

tophus, suggesting that there is a cycle of chronic inflammation, attempted resolution, and tissue remodeling [29, 32].

In the musculoskeletal system, MSU tophi localize often in areas of dynamic stress, particularly near tendon or ligament entheses such as distal triceps tendon, proximal and distal patellar ligament, and Achilles tendon.

First Metatarsophalangeal Joint (MTP 1)

A high-yield area for finding tophaceous material sonographically is the medial aspect of the first metatarsophalangeal joint, where precipitation of MSU crystals is fostered by the impact of joint capsule, collateral ligament, and tendon insertion of abductor hallucis against the first metatarsal head. This is further compounded by overlying footwear. The medial plantar artery and first dorsal metatarsal artery anastomose medial to MTP 1 [33], and engorgement of these physiologic vessels can be seen if adjacent tophaceous material is present (Fig. 13.12).

Aggregates

Small aggregates of tophaceous material, but not free MSU crystals, can be deposited in the synovial lining of a joint, bursa, or tendon sheath. Chronic synovitis with microtophi and associated foreign body-type giant cells can ensue [34–36]. On light microscopy, small hyperechoic aggregates of MSU crystals can be detected in synovial lining tissues. This aggregate-associated synovial tissue can appear thickened and proliferative, with "pannus-like" tissue comprising vascular granulation tissue or with a focal villous appearance [37–39]. Sonographically, these aggregates appear hyperechoic and can be associated with proliferative synovial tissue (Fig. 13.13).

A *"snowstorm"* appearance of aggregates of MSU crystals has been described. This is defined as aggregates "floating" within synovial fluid, when agitated by pressure with the transducer, or sonopalpation. In the SUGAR cohort, this was found in 30% of patients with microscopically proven gout and 10% of patients with CPPD disease [20, 40, 41].

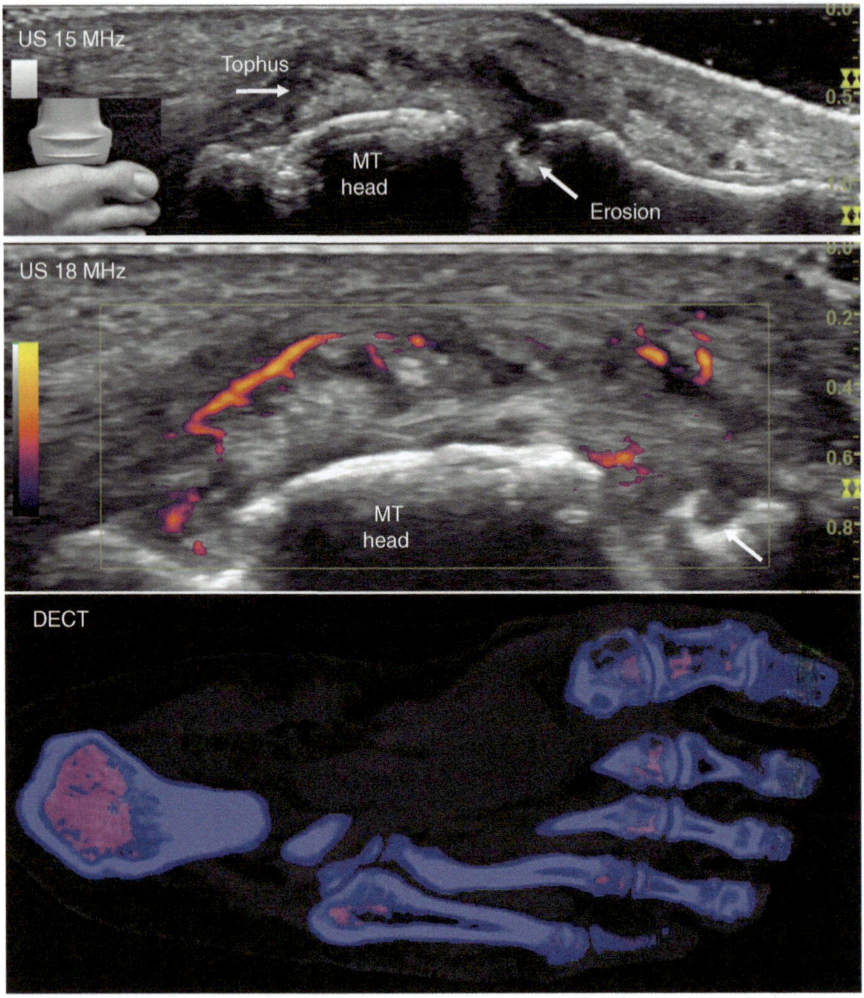

Fig. 13.12 Top: tophaceous gout. Medial long axis view of first metatarsophalangeal joint. Hyperechoic material is seen adjacent to the metatarsal head. A typical "punched out" appearing erosion with a marginal overhang is seen at the base of the proximal phalanx. Middle: hyperemia is seen on Doppler studies. Bottom: dual-energy CT scan of same area. The erosion of the proximal phalanx is seen, but tophaceous material is not seen in this case. Green artifact at the toenail

Erosions

Cortical erosions with a punched-out appearance and a marginal overhang are highly characteristic of gout. These can be seen on conventional radiographs but are detected more readily by ultrasound. In a study of 39 patients and 22 controls, 67% had erosions on ultrasound, and 28% had erosions on conventional radiography [42]. This corresponds to findings in RA, where ultrasound is more sensitive in the detection of erosions [43]. Unlike RA, cortical erosions are not associated with

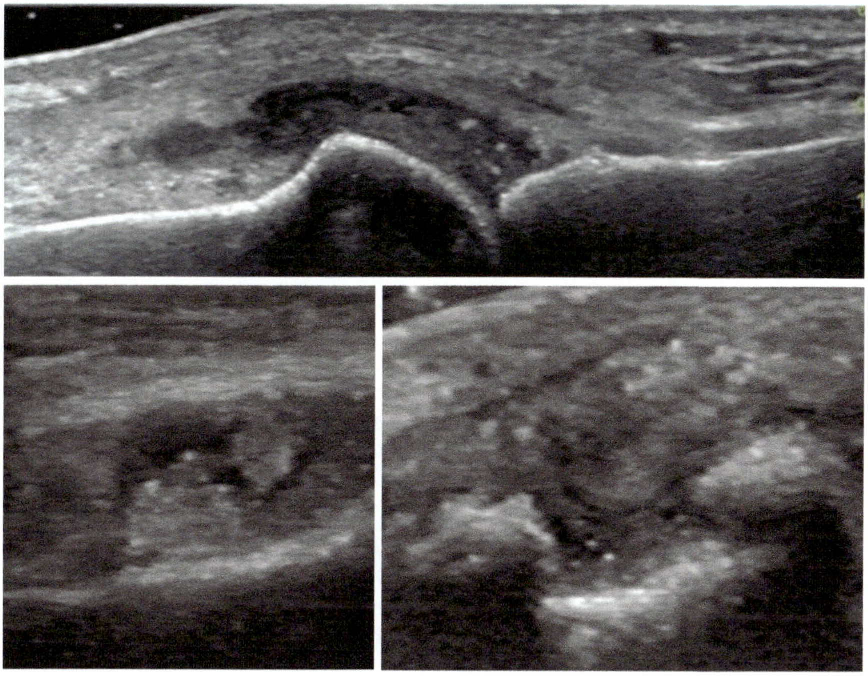

Fig. 13.13 Gout. Three different example images of hyperechoic aggregates

invading pannus tissue but rather with the presence of tophi. Erosions can be found intra- and extra-articularly. At the tophus-bone interface, osteoblasts are decreased, and numerous osteoclast-like cells are found. MSU crystals alter the ratio of RANKL to OPG in stromal cells to favor osteoclastogenesis [44, 45]. Because of the association of tophi with bony erosions, these can typically be found in the same locations (Fig. 13.14).

Comparison of Ultrasonography and Other Imaging Modalities in Gout

Ultrasound, dual-energy CT (DECT) scan, and conventional radiography are well suited to assess gout. MRI is less commonly used due to a relative lack of specific imaging findings. MRI findings were not included in the diagnostic criteria published by the ACR and EULAR [46]. Both dual-energy CT scanning and ultrasound seemed to have good sensitivity and specificity for the detection of gouty tophi in meta-analyses. In one study, ultrasound was found to be more specific, and DECT more sensitive for gout. In a recent study, DECT found more extra-articular tophi in the hand and wrist, but a double contour sign was found

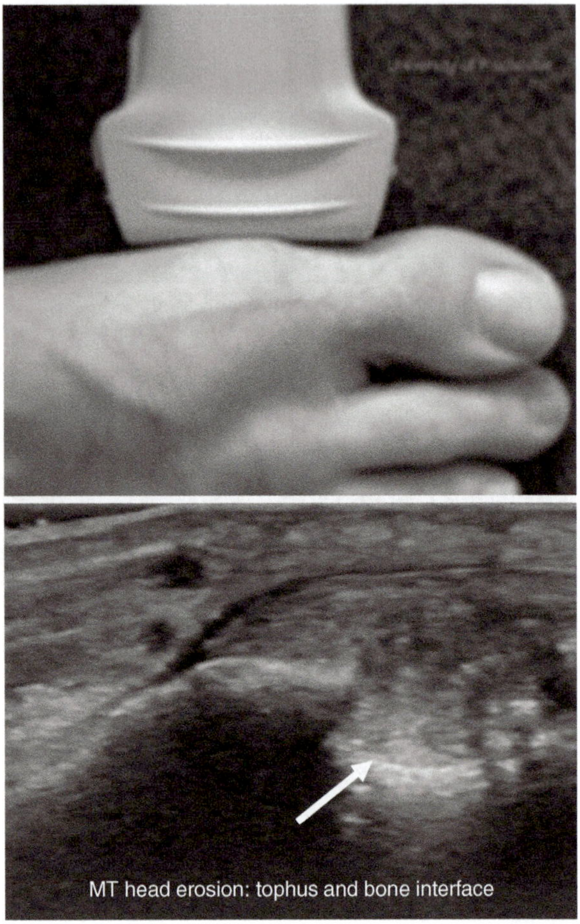

Fig. 13.14 Gout. Medial long axis view of first metatarsal head. A break in the contour of the bony cortex is seen, with hyperechoic material filling the erosion

only sonographically. Small aggregates are typically found more readily by ultrasound than by DECT. Interestingly, the same tophi measure smaller when DECT is used compared to sonographic measurements [47–51] (Fig. 13.15). The tophus-associated fibrovascular matrix tissue can only be appreciated sonographically. Inflammatory changes can be appreciated by Doppler ultrasound or contrast-enhanced MRI, but not by DECT. Ultrasonography depicts tophaceous material in its anatomic environment including bony cortex, cartilage, lumen of joint, joint capsule, tendons, and ligaments, whereas DECT shows tophi only in relation to bone. A distinct advantage of DECT is its visualization of the entire joint area, and 3D reconstructions can be obtained. Ultrasound typically follows a prespecified protocol or focuses on a symptomatic area so that tophi outside of the views of the protocol could potentially be missed (Table 13.3).

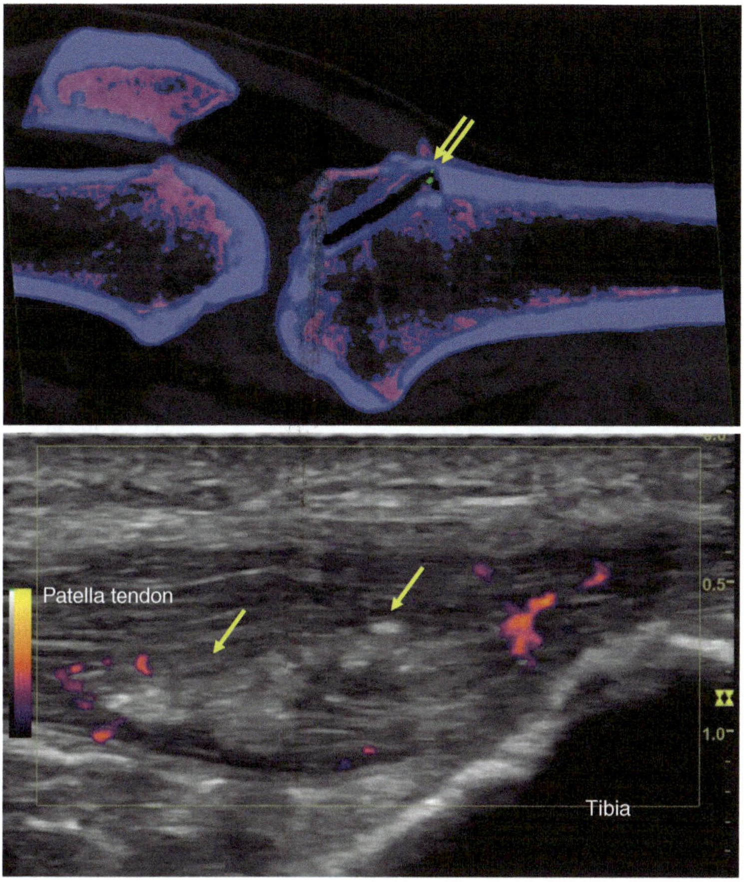

Fig. 13.15 DECT. DECT may underestimate MSU tophus size when compared with US. Ultrasound at 18 MHz

Table 13.3 Comparison of imaging modalities

	Ultrasound	DECT	Conventional radiography
Double contour sign	+		
Aggregates	+		
Fibrovascular matrix	+		
Hyperemia	+		
Tophi	+	+	
Erosions	+	+	+

Assessment of Treatment Response

Ultrasound is sensitive to change in the assessment of gout [52, 53]. If the serum urate level can be lowered consistently below 6 mg/dL, findings of a sonographic

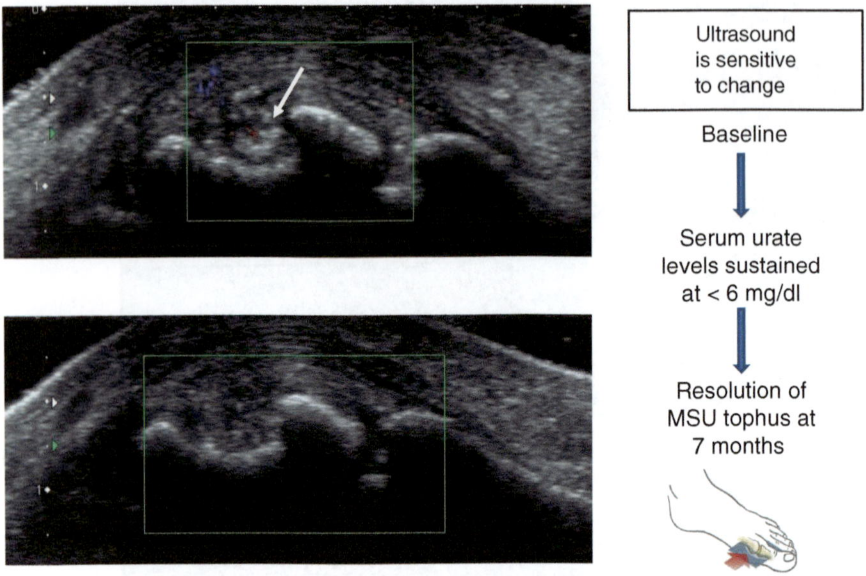

Fig. 13.16 Tophaceous gout, serial imaging. Top: medial long axis view of first metatarsophalangeal joint. A cortical erosion is seen, filled with hyperechoic material and adjacent power Doppler signal. Bottom: follow-up study after 7 months of same area. Serum urate levels had been sustained below 6 mg/dL. The previously seen hyperechoic material has disappeared, and matrix tissue remains. No hyperemia is seen on follow-up study

double contour sign can lessen in extent and thickness or can disappear altogether. A low serum urate level needs to be sustained for at least 6 months. Formed tophi can also decrease in size or dissolve altogether. The matrix tissue in which the MSU tophi were embedded may remain. Typically, the vascularity of this tissue decreases considerably or is not detected on follow-up studies anymore (Fig. 13.16).

Conclusion

Ultrasound is a valuable tool for evaluation of crystalline deposition and is particularly more sensitive and specific than plain x-ray in detecting crystals. Characteristic sonographic appearance and location of crystals of gout vs. calcium-related arthritis can differ, allowing for differentiation of disease processes. Additionally, synovitis and hyperemia associated with crystalline disease, as can be seen in other inflammatory arthritides, can also be visualized and may differentiate a "seronegative arthritis" from disease actually related to crystal deposition disease. Similar to RA, ultrasound findings in gout are sensitive to change and thus can be useful for monitoring treatment response.

Review Questions

1. Which of the following descriptions of a sonographic double contour sign is most appropriate?
   (a) A sonographic double contour sign of gout can typically be detected over either hyaline cartilage or fibrocartilage.
   (b) A sonographic double contour sign changes in location with a change of transducer angle of incidence.
   (c) A sonographic double contour sign can have an irregular superficial margin.
   (d) A sonographic double contour sign is seen only in symptomatic joints.
   (e) A sonographic double contour sign is always seen in a joint affected by gout.
2. Which of the following is true for *CPPD disease*?
   (a) Crystal deposits can be seen in hyaline or fibrocartilage.
   (b) Crystal deposits can be seen in either the central layer or on the articular surface of cartilage with similar frequency.
   (c) CPPD crystals are typically formed in synovial fluid or synovial tissue.
   (d) CPPD crystals can always be distinguished from monosodium urate deposits sonographically.
   (e) The appearance of crystal deposits changes significantly with change of transducer angle.
3. Which of the following is true?
   (a) A "marginal overhang" in gouty arthritis can typically be seen on plain radiographs but not with ultrasound.
   (b) Hyperemia seen as an increased power Doppler signal adjacent to tophaceous material is uncommon in asymptomatic joints.
   (c) An "anechoic rim" is a typical sonographic finding adjacent to tophaceous material.
   (d) Tophaceous material is not typically seen associated with cortical erosions of gout.
   (e) Small aggregates of monosodium urate crystals can be seen in synovial fluid but not the synovial lining.
4. Which of the statements on monosodium urate (MSU), calcium pyrophosphate dihydrate (CPPD), and basic calcium phosphate (BCP) crystals is true?
   (a) MSU, CPPD, and BCP crystals can all be seen with ultrasound, conventional radiography, or polarizing microscopy.
   (b) MSU and CPPD crystals can be seen with ultrasound and polarizing microscopy, and BCP cannot be seen with ultrasound but with polarizing microscopy and conventional radiography.
   (c) MSU crystals are not seen well on conventional radiography but can be seen with ultrasound and polarizing microscopy.
   (d) BCP crystals can be seen with polarizing microscopy but are poorly identified on conventional radiographs.
   (e) CPPD crystals are seen on ultrasound and polarizing microscopy but not with conventional radiography.

5. Which of the following is most appropriate for describing a cartilage interface artifact?
   (a) It appears most pronounced with perpendicular incidence of sound waves on hyaline cartilage.
   (b) It appears weaker when fluid is overlying cartilage.
   (c) It can appear over hyaline or fibrocartilage with similar frequency.
   (d) It is more commonly seen in joints affected by gout.
   (e) It is enhanced by synovial tissue overlying hyaline cartilage.
6. Which of the following crystal arthropathy has the highest prevalence in the United States?
   (a) Gout
   (b) CPPD disease
   (c) Basic calcium phosphate crystal disease (BCP)-associated arthritis
   (d) Gout and basic calcium phosphate crystal disease have similar prevalence.
   (e) Gout and CPPD disease have similar prevalence.
7. Which of the following statements is true?
   (a) Monosodium urate crystals reflect ultrasound waves strongly, and CPPD and basic calcium phosphate crystals are weak reflectors of ultrasound waves.
   (b) Monosodium urate crystals and basic calcium phosphate crystals both reflect ultrasound waves strongly, and CPPD crystals are weak reflectors of ultrasound waves.
   (c) Monosodium urate crystals and CPPD crystals both reflect ultrasound waves strongly, and basic calcium phosphate crystals are weak reflectors of ultrasound waves.
   (d) Monosodium urate crystals are weak reflectors of ultrasound waves, and CPPD and basic calcium phosphate crystals reflect ultrasound waves strongly.
   (e) Monosodium urate crystals, CPPD crystals, and basic calcium phosphate crystals all reflect ultrasound waves strongly.
8. A "tophus complex" with a crystalline center surrounded by a cellular corona zone, embedded in fibrovascular matrix tissue, has characteristically been described for which of the following conditions?
   (a) Gout
   (b) CPPD disease
   (c) Basic calcium phosphate (BCP)-associated arthritis
   (d) Both gout and CPPD disease
   (e) Gout, CPPD disease, and basic calcium phosphate (BCP)-associated arthritis
9. An imaging finding of a "punched-out cortical lesion with a marginal overhang" is characteristically seen in which of the following conditions?
   (a) In gout by conventional radiography but not typically by ultrasound
   (b) In both gout and rheumatoid arthritis by conventional radiography or ultrasound
   (c) In both gout and CPPD disease

   (d) In gout, CPPD disease, or basic calcium phosphate (BCP)-associated arthritis
   (e) In gout by conventional radiography or ultrasound
10. Which of the following is true about CPPD crystals?
   (a) CPPD crystals are typically formed within hyaline cartilage or fibrocartilage.
   (b) CPPD crystals are typically formed within synovial tissue.
   (c) CPPD crystals are typically formed within synovial fluid.
   (d) CPPD crystals are typically formed within cortical bone.
   (e) CPPD crystals are typically formed within the periosteum.

Answers

1. (c) A sonographic double contour sign can have an irregular superficial margin.
2. (a) Crystal deposits can be seen in hyaline or fibrocartilage.
3. (c) An "anechoic rim" is a typical sonographic finding adjacent to tophaceous material.
4. (c) MSU crystals are not seen well on conventional radiography but can be seen with ultrasound and polarizing microscopy.
5. (a) It appears most pronounced with perpendicular incidence of sound waves on hyaline cartilage.
6. (c) Basic calcium phosphate crystal disease (BCP)-associated arthritis
7. (e) Monosodium urate crystals, CPPD crystals, and basic calcium phosphate crystals all reflect ultrasound waves strongly.
8. (a) Gout
9. (e) In gout by conventional radiography or ultrasound
10. (a) CPPD crystals are typically formed within hyaline cartilage or fibrocartilage.

References

1. Schlegel JU, Diggdon P, Cuellar J. The use of ultrasound for localizing renal calculi. J Urol. 1961;86:367–9.
2. Raskind R. Diagnostic ultrasonography. J Am Geriatr Soc. 1965;13(10):887–92.
3. Helmick CG, Felson DT, Lawrence RC, Gabriel S, Hirsch R, Kwoh CK, et al. Estimates of the prevalence of arthritis and other rheumatic conditions in the United States. Part I. Arthritis Rheum. 2008;58(1):15–25.
4. Kotlarz H, Gunnarsson CL, Fang H, Rizzo JA. Insurer and out-of-pocket costs of osteoarthritis in the US: evidence from national survey data. Arthritis Rheum. 2009;60(12):3546–53.
5. Chen-Xu M, Yokose C, Rai SK, Pillinger MH, Choi HK. Contemporary prevalence of gout and hyperuricemia in the United States and decadal trends: the national health and nutrition examination survey, 2007–2016. Arthritis Rheumatol. 2019;71(6):991–9.
6. Lim SY, Lu N, Oza A, Fisher M, Rai SK, Menendez ME, et al. Trends in gout and rheumatoid arthritis hospitalizations in the United States, 1993–2011. JAMA. 2016;315(21):2345–7.
7. Khosla S, Thiele R, Baumhauer JF. Ultrasound guidance for intra-articular injections of the foot and ankle. Foot Ankle Int. 2009;30(9):886–90.

8. Schumacher HR Jr, Sieck MS, Rothfuss S, Clayburne GM, Baumgarten DF, Mochan BS, et al. Reproducibility of synovial fluid analyses. A study among four laboratories. Arthritis Rheum. 1986;29(6):770–4.
9. Hasselbacher P. Variation in synovial fluid analysis by hospital laboratories. Arthritis Rheum. 1987;30(6):637–42.
10. McGill NW, York HF. Reproducibility of synovial fluid examination for crystals. Aust NZ J Med. 1991;21(5):710–3.
11. Gordon C, Swan A, Dieppe P. Detection of crystals in synovial fluids by light microscopy: sensitivity and reliability. Ann Rheum Dis. 1989;48(9):737–42.
12. Stack J, McCarthy G. Basic calcium phosphate crystals and osteoarthritis pathogenesis: novel pathways and potential targets. Curr Opin Rheumatol. 2016;28(2):122–6.
13. Nalbant S, Martinez JA, Kitumnuaypong T, Clayburne G, Sieck M, Schumacher HR Jr. Synovial fluid features and their relations to osteoarthritis severity: new findings from sequential studies. Osteoarthr Cartil. 2003;11(1):50–4.
14. Fuerst M, Bertrand J, Lammers L, Dreier R, Echtermeyer F, Nitschke Y, et al. Calcification of articular cartilage in human osteoarthritis. Arthritis Rheum. 2009;60(9):2694–703.
15. Grases F, Muntaner-Gimbernat L, Vilchez-Mira M, Costa-Bauza A, Tur F, Prieto RM, et al. Characterization of deposits in patients with calcific tendinopathy of the supraspinatus. Role of phytate and osteopontin. J Orthop Res. 2015;33(4):475–82.
16. Hamada J, Ono W, Tamai K, Saotome K, Hoshino T. Analysis of calcium deposits in calcific periarthritis. J Rheumatol. 2001;28(4):809–13.
17. Gatt DL, Charalambous CP. Ultrasound-guided barbotage for calcific tendonitis of the shoulder: a systematic review including 908 patients. Arthroscopy. 2014;30(9):1166–72.
18. Conway R, McCarthy GM. Calcium-containing crystals and osteoarthritis: an unhealthy alliance. Curr Rheumatol Rep. 2018;20(3):13.
19. Rosenthal AK, Ryan LM. Calcium pyrophosphate deposition disease. N Engl J Med. 2016;374(26):2575–84.
20. Ogdie A, Taylor WJ, Neogi T, Fransen J, Jansen TL, Schumacher HR, et al. Performance of ultrasound in the diagnosis of gout in a multicenter study: comparison with monosodium urate monohydrate crystal analysis as the gold standard. Arthritis Rheumatol. 2017;69(2):429–38.
21. Filippou G, Scire CA, Damjanov N, Adinolfi A, Carrara G, Picerno V, et al. Definition and reliability assessment of elementary ultrasonographic findings in calcium pyrophosphate deposition disease: a study by the OMERACT calcium pyrophosphate deposition disease ultrasound subtask force. J Rheumatol. 2017;44(11):1744–9.
22. Zaka R, Williams CJ. New developments in the epidemiology and genetics of gout. Curr Rheumatol Rep. 2006;8(3):215–23.
23. Neogi T, Jansen TL, Dalbeth N, Fransen J, Schumacher HR, Berendsen D, et al. 2015 Gout classification criteria: an American College of Rheumatology/European League Against Rheumatism collaborative initiative. Ann Rheum Dis. 2015;74(10):1789–98.
24. Loeb JN. The influence of temperature on the solubility of monosodium urate. Arthritis Rheum. 1972;15(2):189–92.
25. Thiele RG, Schlesinger N. Diagnosis of gout by ultrasound. Rheumatology (Oxford). 2007;46(7):1116–21.
26. Martel W. The overhanging margin of bone: a roentgenologic manifestation of gout. Radiology. 1968;91(4):755–6.
27. Gutierrez M, Schmidt WA, Thiele RG, Keen HI, Kaeley GS, Naredo E, et al. International Consensus for ultrasound lesions in gout: results of Delphi process and web-reliability exercise. Rheumatology (Oxford). 2015;54(10):1797–805.
28. Towiwat P, Chhana A, Dalbeth N. The anatomical pathology of gout: a systematic literature review. BMC Musculoskelet Disord. 2019;20(1):140.
29. Dalbeth N, Pool B, Gamble GD, Smith T, Callon KE, McQueen FM, et al. Cellular characterization of the gouty tophus: a quantitative analysis. Arthritis Rheum. 2010;62(5):1549–56.
30. Traut EF, Knight AA, Szanto PB, Passerelli EW. Specific vascular changes in gout. J Am Med Assoc. 1954;156(6):591–3.

31. Araujo EG, Manger B, Perez-Ruiz F, Thiele RG. Imaging of gout: new tools and biomarkers? Best Pract Res Clin Rheumatol. 2016;30(4):638–52.
32. Schweyer S, Hemmerlein B, Radzun HJ, Fayyazi A. Continuous recruitment, co-expression of tumour necrosis factor-alpha and matrix metalloproteinases, and apoptosis of macrophages in gout tophi. Virchows Arch. 2000;437(5):534–9.
33. Standring S. Gray's anatomy. 41Elsevier Health Sciences 2016. 1418–1451.e2.
34. Agudelo CA, Schumacher HR. The synovitis of acute gouty arthritis. A light and electron microscopic study. Hum Pathol. 1973;4(2):265–79.
35. Schumacher HR. Pathology of the synovial membrane in gout. Light and electron microscopic studies. Interpretation of crystals in electron micrographs. Arthritis Rheum. 1975;18(6 Suppl):771–82.
36. Rodnan GP, Yunis EJ, Totten RS. Experience with punch biopsy of synovium in the study of joint disease. Ann Intern Med. 1960;53:319–31.
37. Sherman MS. Pathologic changes in gouty arthritis. Arch Pathol (Chic). 1946;42(6):557–63.
38. Martin DJ, Merenda G, McDonald DJ, Sundaram M. Recurrent hemarthrosis associated with gout. Clin Orthop Relat Res. 1992;277:262–5.
39. Hawkins CF, Ellis HA, Rawson A. Malignant gout with tophaceous small intestine and megaloblastic anaemia. Ann Rheum Dis. 1965;24:224–33.
40. Grassi W, Meenagh G, Pascual E, Filippucci E. "Crystal clear"-sonographic assessment of gout and calcium pyrophosphate deposition disease. Semin Arthritis Rheum. 2006;36(3):197–202.
41. Lamers-Karnebeek FB, Van Riel PL, Jansen TL. Additive value for ultrasonographic signal in a screening algorithm for patients presenting with acute mono-/oligoarthritis in whom gout is suspected. Clin Rheumatol. 2014;33(4):555–9.
42. Wright SA, Filippucci E, McVeigh C, Grey A, McCarron M, Grassi W, et al. High-resolution ultrasonography of the first metatarsal phalangeal joint in gout: a controlled study. Ann Rheum Dis. 2007;66(7):859–64.
43. Szkudlarek M, Terslev L, Wakefield RJ, Backhaus M, Balint PV, Bruyn GA, et al. Summary findings of a systematic literature review of the ultrasound assessment of bone erosions in rheumatoid arthritis. J Rheumatol. 2016;43(1):12–21.
44. Dalbeth N, Smith T, Nicolson B, Clark B, Callon K, Naot D, et al. Enhanced osteoclastogenesis in patients with tophaceous gout: urate crystals promote osteoclast development through interactions with stromal cells. Arthritis Rheum. 2008;58(6):1854–65.
45. Chhana A, Callon KE, Pool B, Naot D, Watson M, Gamble GD, et al. Monosodium urate monohydrate crystals inhibit osteoblast viability and function: implications for development of bone erosion in gout. Ann Rheum Dis. 2011;70(9):1684–91.
46. Davies J, Riede P, van Langevelde K, Teh J. Recent developments in advanced imaging in gout. Ther Adv Musculoskelet Dis. 2019;11 https://doi.org/10.1177/1759720X19844429.
47. Huppertz A, Hermann KG, Diekhoff T, Wagner M, Hamm B, Schmidt WA. Systemic staging for urate crystal deposits with dual-energy CT and ultrasound in patients with suspected gout. Rheumatol Int. 2014;34(6):763–71.
48. Dalbeth N, Schauer C, Macdonald P, Perez-Ruiz F, Schumacher HR, Hamburger S, et al. Methods of tophus assessment in clinical trials of chronic gout: a systematic literature review and pictorial reference guide. Ann Rheum Dis. 2011;70(4):597–604.
49. Klauser AS, Halpern EJ, Strobl S, Abd Ellah MMH, Gruber J, Bellmann-Weiler R, et al. Gout of hand and wrist: the value of US as compared with DECT. Eur Radiol. 2018;28(10):4174–81.
50. Lee YH, Song GG. Diagnostic accuracy of ultrasound in patients with gout: a meta-analysis. Semin Arthritis Rheum. 2018;47(5):703–9.
51. Lee YH, Song GG. Diagnostic accuracy of dual-energy computed tomography in patients with gout: a meta-analysis. Semin Arthritis Rheum. 2017;47(1):95–101.
52. Thiele RG, Schlesinger N. Ultrasonography shows disappearance of monosodium urate crystal deposition on hyaline cartilage after sustained normouricemia is achieved. Rheumatol Int. 2010;30(4):495–503.
53. Peiteado D, Villalba A, Martin-Mola E, Balsa A, De Miguel E. Ultrasound sensitivity to changes in gout: a longitudinal study after two years of treatment. Clin Exp Rheumatol. 2017;35(5):746–51.

Ultrasound in Osteoarthritis

14

Amanda E. Nelson

Key Points

- Osteoarthritis, the most common form of arthritis, is on the rise along with increasing age and body weight in the population.
- Ultrasound is more sensitive than conventional radiography, and more cost-effective and accessible than MRI, for assessing many of the key features of osteoarthritis in a variety of joint sites for clinical and research purposes.
- By utilizing standardized protocols for obtaining ultrasound images and applying standardized atlas-based scoring systems, ultrasound can be a reliable tool for research assessment in osteoarthritis.

Introduction

Osteoarthritis (OA) is by far the most common form of arthritis, with even the most recent figure of 50 million Americans with OA likely underestimating the true burden of this common and often debilitating disease [1, 2]. Although for many years OA was thought of as a "degenerative" or "wear and tear" condition mostly affecting cartilage, it has become evident recently that OA is much more complex. The OA Research Society International (OARSI) has proposed the following definition to capture this complexity:

A. E. Nelson (✉)
Thurston Arthritis Research Center and Division of Rheumatology, Allergy, and Immunology, University of North Carolina at Chapel Hill, Chapel Hill, NC, USA
e-mail: amanda_nelson@med.unc.edu

M. J. Kohler (ed.), *Musculoskeletal Ultrasound in Rheumatology Review*,
https://doi.org/10.1007/978-3-030-73555-5_14

> Osteoarthritis is a disorder involving movable joints characterized by cell stress and extracellular matrix degradation initiated by micro- and macro-injury that activates maladaptive repair responses including pro-inflammatory pathways of innate immunity. The disease manifests first as a molecular derangement (abnormal joint tissue metabolism) followed by anatomic, and/or physiologic derangements (characterized by cartilage degradation, bone remodeling, osteophyte formation, joint inflammation and loss of normal joint function), that can culminate in illness. (https://www.oarsi.org/research/standardization-osteoarthritis-definitions)

Additionally, the OARSI published a white paper in 2016 detailing the high burden of OA on affected individuals and on society, making it clear that OA is a serious disease [3]. While OA is primarily a clinical diagnosis [4–6], radiographic criteria [such as a Kellgren-Lawrence grade (KLG) [7] of 2 or more, osteophytes, and joint space narrowing] are most often used for clinical trial enrollment and assessment of structural progression. However, as noted in the above definition, the features driving OA are cartilage degradation, bone remodeling, osteophyte formation, and joint inflammation, which can be better visualized using other modalities. Advanced imaging [to date, primarily magnetic resonance imaging (MRI)] has played a key role in our understanding of the pathophysiology of this disease, identifying the features most associated with pain, and in the ongoing development of criteria for pre-radiographic, early disease which might be more amenable to treatment [8–10]. Importantly, ultrasound (US) imaging can also capture many of these key features and in a much more cost-effective, accessible, and acceptable manner than MRI for patients and study participants. This chapter will cover what has been done using diagnostic US in OA by joint site, compare benefits and drawbacks of various imaging modalities in OA, and provide an overview of the author's ongoing work in this area, including development of an ultrasound atlas for knee OA.

Ultrasound Findings in Osteoarthritis

The Outcome Measures in Rheumatology (OMERACT) group recently released updated definitions of US-detected pathologies [11]; those most relevant to OA are listed below.

Synovitis "Presence of a hypoechoic synovial hypertrophy regardless of the presence of effusion or any grade of Doppler signal." The synovium may be involved in OA although generally not to the extent of more inflammatory arthritides such as rheumatoid arthritis; such synovitis has been associated with pain in OA (Fig. 14.1) [12–15].

Enthesitis "Hypoechoic and/or thickened insertion of the tendon close to the bone (within 2 mm from the bony cortex) which exhibits Doppler signal if active and that may show erosions, enthesophytes/calcifications as a sign of structural damage." Although enthesophytes can be seen in OA [16, 17], they are more characteristic of psoriatic arthritis and other seronegative spondyloarthropathies, which are often in the differential particularly for distal interphalangeal joint-predominant OA. The location of bone spurs can be useful as osteophytes in hand OA are typically palmar or dorsal, while the proliferative changes of psoriatic arthritis are more often on the radial side of the joint and associated with entheses [18].

Erosion "Intra- and/or extra-articular discontinuity of bone surface (visible in two perpendicular planes)." Erosions can be seen particularly in erosive OA in the hands (and likely the same entity in the feet although this has not yet been studied), further detailed below.

Evaluation of a number of other joint pathologies is possible using US, with a recent summary available from Okano et al. [19], although some are not detailed by OMERACT.

Cartilage degradation is a main feature of OA. Normal cartilage is visible on US as a homogeneous anechoic layer lining the bony cortex with clear, hyperechoic margins; loss of these characteristics indicates pathologic change (Fig. 14.2) [19]. Articular cartilage at the knee has a normal thickness of

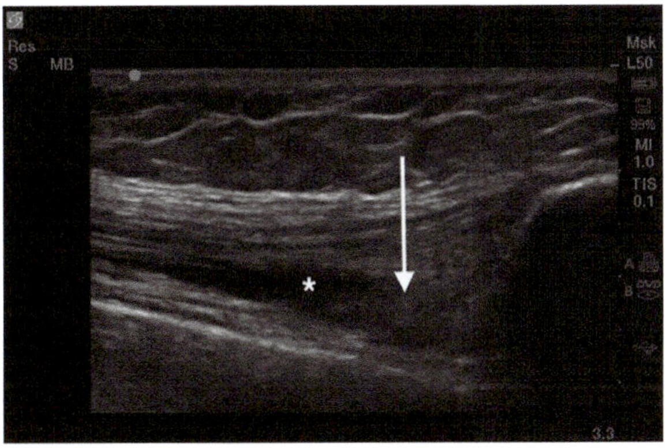

Fig. 14.1 Suprapatellar longitudinal view showing mild synovitis (arrow) and a small effusion (*), courtesy of the Sonography of OA by Rheumatologists (SOAR) project

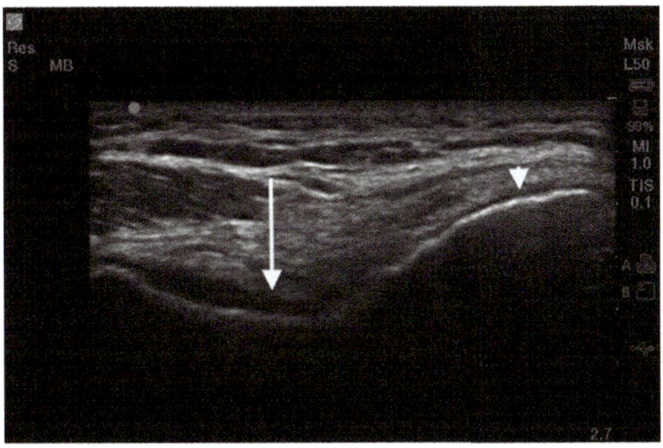

Fig. 14.2 Suprapatellar transverse in maximal flexion showing moderate medial (arrow, grade = 2) and severe lateral (arrowhead, grade = 3) cartilage damage, courtesy of the SOAR project

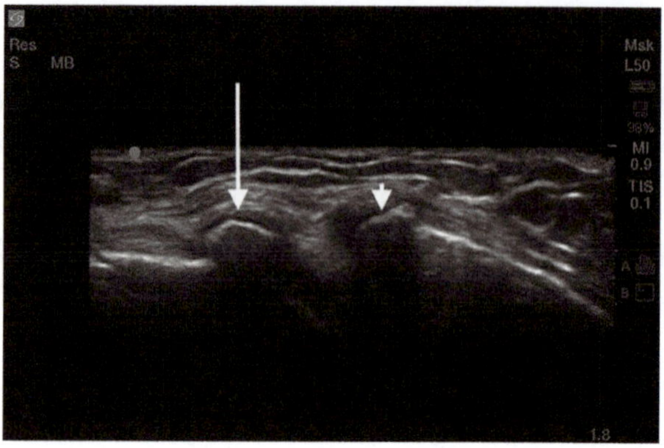

Fig. 14.3 Medial longitudinal image showing large, bulky osteophytes on the femoral (arrow) and tibial (arrowhead) side of the joint, courtesy of the SOAR project

approximately 3 mm [20]. In OA, the cartilage is asymmetrically thinned and can become less sharply defined. In a series of cadaveric knees, measurement of the articular cartilage in maximum flexion was reproducible within and between readers (ICC > 0.70) and was accurate when compared to direct anatomic measurements in knees with minimal to moderate damage. US measurements were less accurate in more severely damaged knees [21]. US measurement was also comparable in accuracy to arthroscopic measurements, particularly at the medial condyle [22].

Osteophytes involve a step-up rather than the usual step-down discontinuity seen in bony erosion, often at the margin of the joint (Fig. 14.3), and US has excellent sensitivity for their detection [19].

Reliability of Ultrasound in Osteoarthritis

Ultrasound is commonly criticized as being operator dependent and of questionable reliability. It is essential to recognize that other imaging assessments are not exempt from operator/reader dependency although this limitation is not often acknowledged. For example, a large study of reliability of radiographic KLG and semiquantitative joint space narrowing in knee OA reported kappa values ranging from 0.56 to 0.72 [23], while in a systematic review of semiquantitative MRI grading, inter-reader correlation coefficients (ICCs) ranged from 0.77 (meniscus) to 0.94 (cartilage quality); in 2 studies ($n = 317$) assessing synovium, the kappa was 0.52 [24]. A recent review of the characteristics of US for OA [25] included a review of reliability, finding that pooled estimates of inter-rater reliability at the knee ranged from good to excellent and were higher for popliteal cysts and osteophytes and lower for effusion/synovitis.

For studies of hand OA, agreement ranged from slight for cartilage thickness to excellent for synovitis, effusion, and osteophyte. Only two studies assessed reliability at the hip, which varied from fair to excellent.

At the knee, an OMERACT study demonstrated good reliability for assessment of synovitis, cartilage damage, medial meniscal extrusion, and osteophytes (kappa statistics: 0.67, 0.55, 0.75, 0.73, respectively); this group provided consensus definitions and standard images for each [26]. For hand OA, reliability of assessments of osteophytes, synovitis, and synovial hypertrophy has been substantial to excellent [25]. In 2016, OMERACT published a reliability study for cartilage and osteophytes in finger joints [27], finding better agreement for osteophytes than for cartilage, the latter of which could only be assessed at the metacarpophalangeal joints given challenges with positioning. A recent OMERACT study showed generally moderate agreement for sonographic assessment of OA features in the foot [28].

Ultrasound Features by Joint in Osteoarthritis

General

Several recent reviews have highlighted the status of US for OA, from both a clinical and a research perspective. Drs. Iagnocco and Naredo updated their review series with an overview of US for OA in 2017 [29]. They highlighted the capability of US to evaluate most of the structures involved in OA, including "articular cartilage, bony cortex, synovial recesses, tendons, ligaments, bursae, and peripheral aspect of the menisci." Also of importance is the ability to do limited scans of multiple joint sites at a given visit due to the propensity of OA to affect multiple joint sites [30]. The limitations of US are also noted and are widely recognized, including the limited ability to assess cartilage and bone in some joints, inability to assess subchondral bone, and limitations of Doppler in large or deep joints. US is very useful for injection guidance in OA joints which are often narrowed and affected by bony overgrowth; US for injection guidance is discussed in Chap. 9.

Hand/Wrist

The risk of developing symptomatic hand OA by the age of 85 years is approximately 40% [31]. Radiographic hand OA is common but not always associated with symptoms. The Newcastle Thousand Families birth cohort was the first study to assess the prevalence of US features of OA in a community-based sample [32]. Individuals in this study ($n = 311$) were 61–63 years of age with a mean body mass index (BMI) of 27 kg/m^2, and about half were women. For the dominant hand index finger, osteophytes were seen in 70% of DIP and 41% of thumb base joints, and both were more frequent in women [32]. US in hand OA has demonstrated associations between symptoms and inflammatory features, particularly in erosive OA [29], again in small studies. A study of 93 patients with OA of the thumb base identified synovitis in 56% and power Doppler in 14%; those with Doppler signal compared to those without had more pain but similar function [33]. Ultrasound findings at the thumb base may be more useful than radiography in classifying severity of OA at this joint (Fig. 14.4) [34].

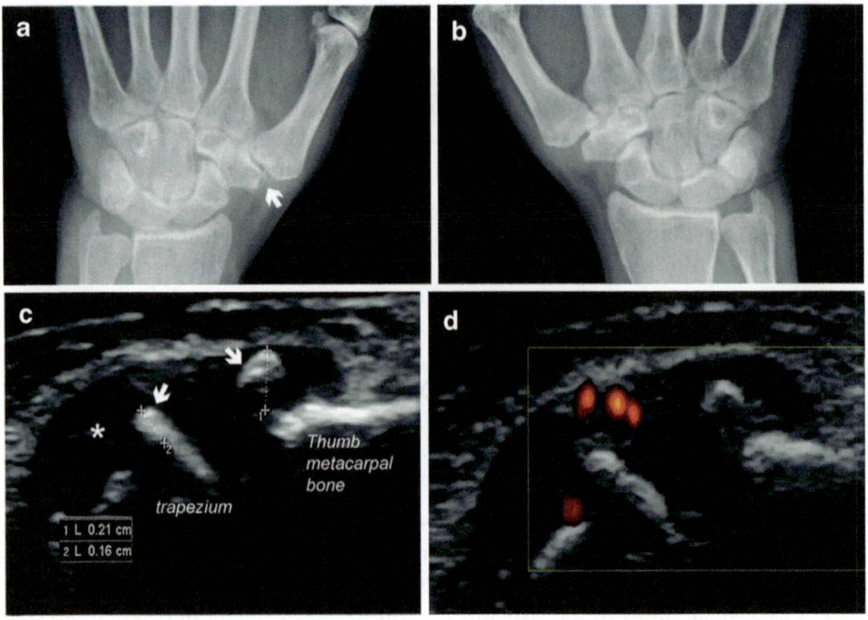

Fig. 14.4 In this patient with right thumb base pain, joint space narrowing and mild sclerosis of the CMC were seen on radiography ((**a**); the left hand was unremarkable (**b**)). Longitudinal ultrasound of the volar aspect of the CMC (**c**) revealed moderate osteophytes (arrows), moderate effusion (asterisk), and a mild power Doppler signal (**d**). (Used with permission from John Wiley and Sons, originally published in: Checa and Panahi [34])

Elbow

Very little has been studied about elbow OA in general as it is not a frequent site of primary OA involvement, and when affected by OA, it is typically secondary to other causes (e.g., occupational or sport exposures) [35]. Even less is available specific to US features of OA in this site although findings similar to other joints would be expected. A review of US for the hand, wrist, and elbow from a physiatrist's perspective is available [36].

Shoulder

While glenohumeral OA is relatively uncommon and often post-traumatic in nature, acromioclavicular (AC) joint OA is clinically very common [37]. Again, most studies of US for OA at the shoulder have focused on guidance of therapeutic injections [29]. In one small study, among 30 consecutive patients with anterior shoulder pain, US frequently identified capsular distention and bony irregularity of the AC joint; less commonly, calcifications, cysts, and subluxation were seen [38].

Hip

The Newcastle study found hip OA (defined as the presence of either osteophytes or femoral head abnormality) in 40% of unselected participants, more commonly in men [32]. However, most studies of US for hip OA to date have focused on injection guidance. Diagnostically, effusion is the most commonly assessed feature at the hip given technical limitations for assessing bony or cartilaginous structures at this joint although synovial hypertrophy and osteophytes can be seen [29]. Importantly, US is able to assess the surrounding soft tissue structures including the greater trochanteric region (for bursitis and tendinopathy) which often coexist or mimic OA in this joint site [39].

Knee

In the Newcastle Thousand Families study, again an unselected sample, 30% of participants had knee osteophytes, and 20–24% had knee effusions; the majority were found to have some evidence of OA [32]. In several small studies, features of inflammation at the knee have been associated with clinical features of OA as well as increased symptoms and more advanced radiographic disease [29]. Findings of effusion and synovitis on US imaging are also associated with knee pain and poorer function [40, 41] and are more common among individuals with knee OA than those with knee pain alone [42].

Meniscal extrusion and popliteal cysts are OA features specifically affecting the knee that are amenable to evaluation with US. Meniscal extrusion can be appreciated on medial and lateral longitudinal joint line views at the knee as meniscal tissue extending beyond the joint borders (Fig. 14.5). In a Japanese study of 270 individuals with knee OA, medial meniscal extrusion at baseline was independently associated with radiographic medial joint space narrowing and osteophyte formation at 3-year follow-up [43]. US is particularly well suited to evaluation of popliteal cysts

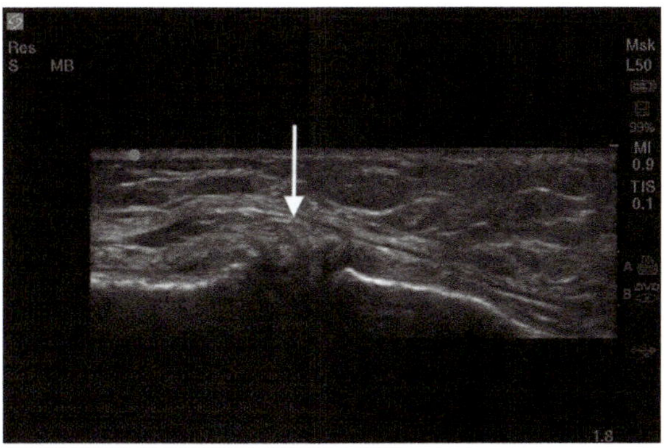

Fig. 14.5 Medial longitudinal image of the right knee showing meniscal extrusion (arrow), courtesy of the SOAR project

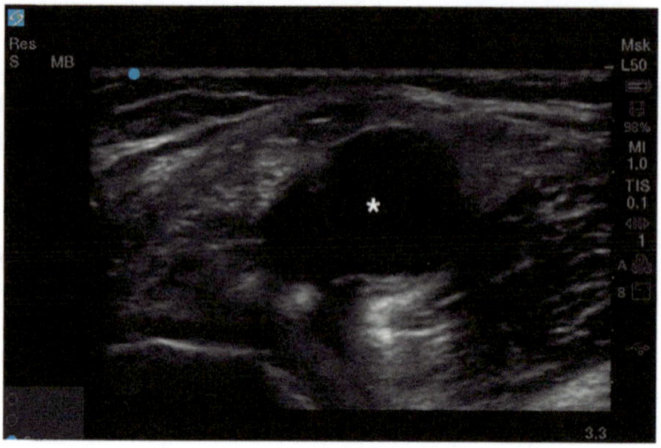

Fig. 14.6 Posterior transverse image of a right knee demonstrating a large popliteal cyst (*), courtesy of the SOAR project

(Fig. 14.6), where it is more sensitive than clinical assessment and can demonstrate response to local injection [29]. A study of 125 individuals with symptomatic knee OA followed over 2 years identified a significant association between US-detected popliteal cysts at baseline and both radiographic and clinical progression (OR 2.8–3.1); synovitis was also associated with progression but did not reach statistical significance (OR 2.1) [44]. Color power Doppler is a specific finding in knee OA [45] and is reflective of treatment response [46].

US is predictive of pain and joint replacement in knee OA. Baseline radiographic grade (hazard ratio [HR] 4.1 [95% CI 2.3–7.1]), ultrasonographic knee effusion (HR 2.6 [95% CI 1.7–4.1]), knee pain intensity (HR 1.8 [95% CI 1.2–2.8]), and disease duration (HR 1.6 [95% CI 1.1–2.5]) were independent predictors of knee joint replacement over 3 years in 531 adult patients with symptomatic knee OA [47]. In a study of 56 OA patients with equal radiographic grades of OA in both knees, three US features were found to be more frequent in symptomatic knees compared with those that were asymptomatic: suprapatellar synovitis, suprapatellar effusion, and medial compartment synovitis. Frequencies of marginal osteophytosis, medial meniscal protrusion, and lateral compartment synovitis did not differ. Medial compartment synovitis was associated with pain by visual analog scale with movement and at rest, and with pain by the WOMAC, more so with increasing severity of synovitis [48].

US is also highly sensitive and specific for calcium crystal deposition [49–51], which is associated with greater inflammation and comorbidities in OA [52–54]. US can also be useful to assess whether crystal-induced arthropathies may be present, either mimicking OA or concomitant with it, as is often the case with calcium pyrophosphate deposition disease (CPPD) (see Chap. 13).

Foot/Ankle

While foot pain and foot OA are highly prevalent [55, 56], the foot has received little attention in OA research; this holds true for studies of ultrasound despite the

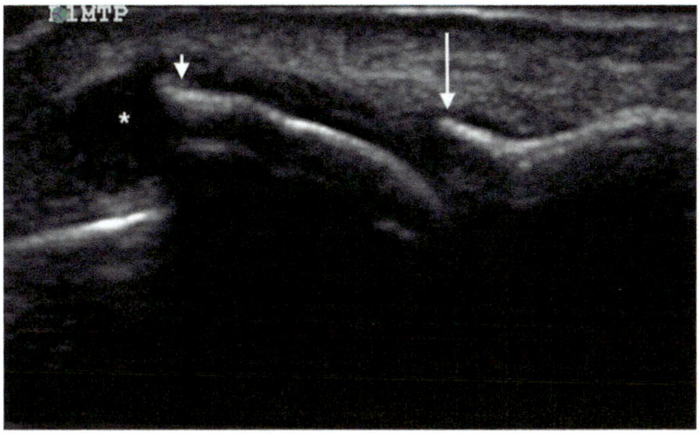

Fig. 14.7 Dorsal longitudinal image of the right first metatarsophalangeal joint showing a bulky osteophyte of the metatarsal (arrowhead), a smaller osteophyte at the base of the proximal phalanx (arrow), and surrounding mild effusion (*), courtesy of the author

obvious applicability of this imaging modality for the small peripheral foot joints, which are similar to those in the hand (Fig. 14.7). An early study of first metatarsophalangeal (MTP) joints in individuals with MTP pain compared to those without MTP pain showed that osteophytes were more frequent in symptomatic MTPs (73% vs. 35% in controls), and power Doppler signal was only present in painful MTPs (21% vs. 0 in controls); both US features were associated with poorer patient-reported function [57]. In a cohort of 100 individuals with clinical and radiographic signs of foot OA, a detailed ultrasonographic evaluation was undertaken including the midfoot and forefoot [58]. In the midfoot, the most commonly involved sites were the subtalar, talonavicular, and navicular-cuneiform joints; the most common pathologies were effusion and osteophytes. In the forefoot, the first MTP was most commonly affected, with effusion and osteophytes again most common, although synovial hypertrophy was also seen; US was more sensitive than clinical exam for detection of abnormalities [58]. No studies focused on ultrasonography for ankle OA were identified.

Image Modality Comparison

Overview

Oo et al. reviewed studies assessing the validity of US against radiography, MRI, histology, or arthroscopy at knee, hand, and hip [25]. Between US and radiography at the knee, there were strong correlations for osteophytes, moderate for effusion and meniscal extrusion, but weak correlations for cartilage thickness. US and MRI at the knee demonstrated strong correlations, while agreement between histology and US was moderate in two studies, and between US and arthroscopy was strong for osteophytes and moderate with cartilage grading. Fewer studies have considered validity of hand US, finding weak to moderate correlations with other imaging modalities. Joint sites other than hand, hip, and knee have been minimally studied, if at all.

Knee

As noted in the introduction, US is more sensitive for early OA changes such as osteophytes and joint space narrowing compared with conventional radiography [59] at the knee. Knee US has high specificity and sensitivity for effusion when compared to MRI [60] and moderate correlations overall for synovitis, effusion, synovial hypertrophy, cartilage thickness, and popliteal cysts [25]. US of the knee is responsive to changes in synovial thickness, effusion size, and popliteal cyst size [61]. A small study compared US, MRI, and histopathology among 15 rheumatoid arthritis (RA) and five OA patients undergoing joint replacement, finding that US features were significantly correlated with inflammatory infiltrates and vascularity on histology and that color power Doppler was more sensitive for vascularity (100% vs. 75%) compared with contrast-enhanced MRI and was more specific for all features (Doppler specificity range 69–88% vs. 8–13% for CE-MRI) [62]. Another group compared osteophyte assessments by US and radiography and compared these to arthroscopic cartilage damage, finding moderate agreement between readers and significant correlations between US and radiographs for osteophytes [63]. Although the correlation between US and radiographs was highest in the medial compartment, only US osteophyte grade was associated with medial arthroscopic cartilage grade ($r = 0.75$ for US, $r = 0.29$ for radiographs) [63]. Okano et al. compared osteophytes and medial femoral cartilage grades from US to radiographic grades in 84 patients with primary knee OA, finding a correlation of 0.71 between radiographic medial joint space narrowing and US medial cartilage grade, 0.75 for medial osteophytes, and 0.69 for lateral osteophytes by US and radiography [64].

Hip

Steer et al. considered the presence of effusion synovitis by either US or MR at the hip joint, finding that among 97 patients with hip OA referred for IA corticosteroid injection, US and MR assessments of bone-capsular distance at week 0 (pre-IASI) and week 8 (post IASI) were significantly correlated, particularly at the femoral neck, but were not associated with post-IASI outcomes [65].

Hand

Among 127 patients with hand OA, US was more sensitive for detecting joints with osteophytes compared with radiography or clinical exam (53%, 30%, and 37%, respectively); US also detected osteophytes in more joints (median number of joints with osteophytes by US, exam, or radiography was 16, 11, and 8, respectively) [66]. In a longitudinal study of 78 participants with hand OA, grayscale synovitis (odds ratio [OR] 3.3, 95% confidence interval [CI] 2.4–4.6) and power Doppler (OR 5.0, 95% CI 2.6–9.4) detected on ultrasound were associated with overall radiographic progression over 5 years (Fig. 14.8); these features also predicted erosive development, joint space narrowing, and osteophyte progression [67]. The same group

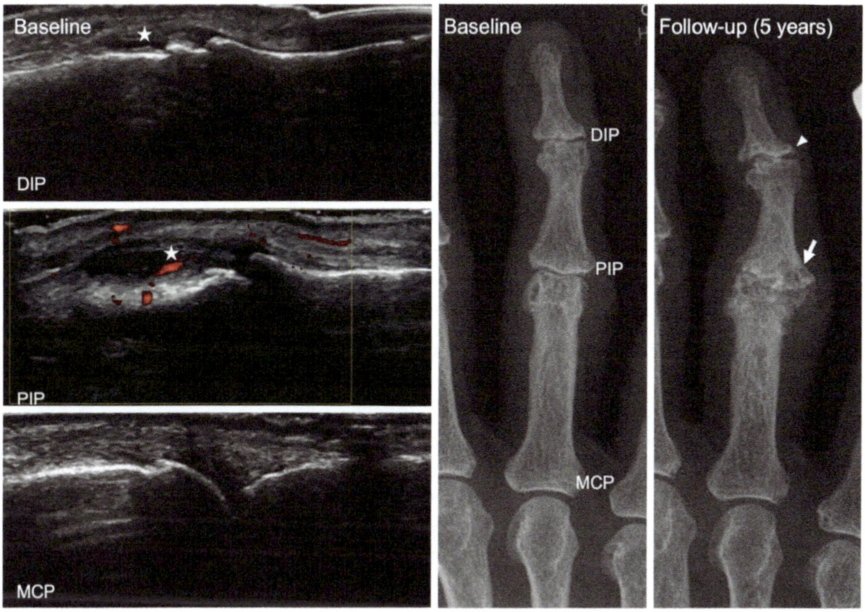

Fig. 14.8 Baseline ultrasound with corresponding baseline and 5-year follow-up radiographs in a patient with hand OA. The baseline ultrasound shows grayscale synovitis of the DIP and PIP joint, with mild power Doppler signal in the PIP and a normal MCP. Radiography of the same digit demonstrates moderate progression at the DIP and severe progression at the PIP at follow-up. DIP distal interphalangeal, PIP proximal interphalangeal, MCP metacarpophalangeal. (Used with permission from Elsevier, originally published in: Best Pract Res Clin Rheumatol. 2016;30(4):653–669, Fig. 14.3, p. 661, https://doi.org/10.1016/j.berh.2016.09.007)

demonstrated that osteophytes detected by ultrasound were predictive of development of radiographic and clinical hand OA over 5 years [68]. Similarly, among 62 patients with hand pain and no obvious clinical diagnosis, US identified nearly twice as many osteophytes compared with radiographs, and osteophytes on US were more strongly correlated with joint tenderness than those found on radiographs [69]. Ultrasound has been of particular interest for the subgroup of individuals with erosive hand OA; two small studies demonstrated high sensitivity, specificity, and agreement for US compared with MRI (including contrast-enhanced MRI) [70, 71].

Sonography of Osteoarthritis for Rheumatologists (SOAR)

The lack of standardized protocols and atlases developed or available for the application of US in OA (in contrast to several available in inflammatory arthritis) led to a funded Rheumatology Research Foundation grant, Sonography of OsteoArthritis by Rheumatologists (SOAR, PI: Nelson, collaborators included Drs. M Kohler, C Bakewell, J Samuels, and J Lin). This funding allowed development of a standardized protocol and scoring atlas for use in a large community-based cohort, the Johnston County Osteoarthritis Project (previously described in detail) [72–74].

The initial work involved the training of local staff to perform standardized imaging, for which we developed a standardized protocol for use in all patients. This protocol describes probe placement, patient positioning, image labeling, and expected landmarks. It includes an image of the probe in place and a representative US image including the expected features. Once the infrastructure was in place, the training complete, and acceptable images being routinely obtained, we convened a series of Web conferences to determine scoring criteria and discuss discordant scores, views, etc. The final set of views, features, scoring range, and definitions is shown in Table 14.1. An initial training set of 50 images was read by all four

Table 14.1 Ultrasound features including views, scoring range, and definitions of scoring levels in SOAR

US feature	Range	Scoring description
View: Suprapatellar longitudinal and transverse in 30 degree flexion		
Effusion/synovitis	0–3	0: None 1: JCD parallel to bone or a small anechoic or hypoechoic line beneath the capsule 2: JCD horizontal or elevated parallel to the joint line 3: Convex/bulging JCD
Synovitis	0–3	0: None 1: Minimal JCD by abnormal internal hypoechoic or anechoic material 2: JCD elevated parallel/flat superficial limit 3: JCD with convex/bulging superficial limit
Effusion	0–1	0: None 1: Abnormal anechoic or hypoechoic IA material
Color power Doppler	0–3	0: None 1: Trace to 10% of IA area with color signal 2: 10–50% of IA area with color signal 3: >50% of IA area with color signal
View: Suprapatellar transverse in maximal flexion (medial and lateral scored separately)		
Cartilage damage (medial/lateral)	0–3	0: Normal 1: Minimal thinning 2: Mild or local thinning 3: Complete loss of cartilage
View: Longitudinal at the medial or lateral femorotibial joint in 30 degrees flexion		
Osteophytes (medial/lateral)	0–3	0: None 1: Small but distinct 2: Medium/intermediate 3: Large, bulky, and prominent
Meniscal extrusion (medial/lateral)	0–1	0: None 1: Definitely partially or completely extruded
View: Posterior medial transverse		
Popliteal cyst	0–2	0: Absent 1: Small/possible 2: Definite
View: Assessed in all views		
Calcium crystal deposition	0–1	0: Absent 1: Hyperechoic deposits in cartilage, meniscus, or synovial fluid in each view

JCD joint capsular distention, *IA* intra-articular

Table 14.2 Reliability assessments for 4 readers in 6 pairs and 30 knees (15 participants)

US feature	Kappa[a]		Kendall	Percentage
	Minimum	*Maximum*	coefficient[b]	agreement[c]
Effusion/synovitis	0.23	0.59	0.71	50
Synovitis	0.21	0.49	0.62	49
Effusion	0.10	0.72	na	74
Color power Doppler	0.36	0.67	0.69	69
Osteophytes				
Medial	0.52	0.79	0.81	69
Lateral	0.57	0.82	0.88	73
Meniscal extrusion				
Medial	0.09	0.47	na	72
Lateral	0.29	0.44	na	64
Cartilage damage				
Medial	0.42	0.67	0.84	57
Lateral	0.26	0.58	0.75	54
Popliteal cyst	0.19	0.57	0.66	58

[a]Weighted kappa for multiple levels, simple kappa for binary, assessed for each reader pair and presented as a range (minimum-maximum) across these pairs

[b]Kendall concordance coefficient, 0–1, appropriate when multiple levels of scoring (but not for binary scores, n/a)

[c]Percentage (%) agreement, for all possible 2 × 2 combinations (6 2 × 2 comparisons and 30 instances = 180 total instances)

rheumatology readers followed by a Web conference discussion to further hone the definitions. This was followed by a final reliability exercise in 15 participants with a range of pathology work which was presented at the annual OARSI meeting in 2019 (Table 14.2) [75]. This project demonstrated feasibility of this training, of obtaining standardized images (10-minute acquisition, 3–5 minutes for reading), and reliability of US in this setting.

The second part of the project assessed correlations between US and XR features, in work presented at the American College of Rheumatology 2019 meeting [76]. Data were from 203 consecutive individuals participating in the fourth follow-up of the Johnston County OA Project (2016–18) who had bilateral knee US according to our standardized protocol and read using the atlas developed specifically for this project. There were statistically significant correlations between nearly all US features below (Table 14.1) and radiographic KLG, with the exception of medial calcium deposition and lateral cartilage damage. The strongest correlations were between US medial and lateral osteophytes and KLG (Spearman correlation $r = 0.62$ and 0.54, respectively) and between US medial and lateral osteophytes and radiographic osteophytes ($r = 0.58$ and 0.57 for medial and lateral, respectively). US medial meniscal extrusion was significantly associated with both radiographic KLG and with medial joint space narrowing ($r = 0.42$ and 0.36, respectively), while US medial meniscal damage was weakly correlated with KLG but not medial joint space narrowing ($r = 0.15$ and 0.10, respectively). Additionally, stronger correlations were seen between medial osteophytes by US and pain as assessed by the KOOS (Knee Injury and Osteoarthritis Outcome Score, $r = 0.34$) compared with radiographic osteophytes ($r = 0.16$). US medial and lateral osteophytes, medial meniscal extrusion, medial cartilage damage, and popliteal cysts were all significantly associated with the presence of radiographic symptomatic knee OA ($r = 0.15–0.43$). A manuscript related to this work, including the protocol and scoring atlas, is available [77].

Summary

The main features of osteoarthritis are readily imaged by ultrasonography. This widely available and cost-effective modality is particularly applicable to this disease state as it is (1) able to image multiple joint sites in one visit, and OA often affects multiple joints; (2) noninvasive and lacks ionizing radiation, allowing for repeated examinations in this chronic slowly progressive disease; (3) universally applicable, able to image any patient, regardless of body size, joint size, implants, pregnancy status, claustrophobia, or other factors that can limit use of MRI; (4) more sensitive to early disease features and change over time than conventional radiography; (5) able to image all joint tissues simultaneously, given the understanding that OA is a disease of the whole joint. The continued development of standardized protocols and scoring systems should increase the applicability of this promising modality for both clinical and research use.

Review Questions

1. All of these features relevant to osteoarthritis are readily evaluated using ultrasound EXCEPT:
   (a) Osteophytes
   (b) Effusion/synovitis
   (c) Bone marrow lesions
   (d) Cartilage damage
2. The reliability of ultrasound in knee OA is:
   (a) Comparable to that of other imaging modalities
   (b) Best for cartilage damage
   (c) Well characterized in numerous large studies
   (d) Worse than that of other imaging modalities
3. Osteoarthritis is best characterized as a:
   (a) Wear and tear process
   (b) Consequence of normal aging
   (c) Disease of cartilage breakdown
   (d) Complex disease of all joint tissues
4. Benefits of radiographs compared with ultrasonography for OA assessment include which of the following?
   (a) Enhanced sensitivity to early changes
   (b) Enhanced sensitivity to change
   (c) Widely accepted standardized scoring
   (d) Better ability to assess soft tissues

5. Ultrasound assessment in OA has been best characterized at which joints?
   (a) Hand and knee
   (b) Hip and SI
   (c) Foot and ankle
   (d) Shoulder and elbow
6. Progression of knee OA (either radiographically or to joint replacement) has been associated with what US features at baseline?
   (a) Medial meniscal extrusion
   (b) Popliteal cysts
   (c) Effusion
   (d) All of the above
7. Radiographic or clinical progression of hand OA is associated with all of the listed US features at baseline EXCEPT:
   (a) Grayscale synovitis
   (b) Power Doppler signal
   (c) Osteophytes
   (d) Cartilage damage
8. Cartilage thickness is best assessed with the joint of interest in what position?
   (a) Full extension
   (b) Thirty degrees flexion
   (c) Maximal flexion
   (d) Neutral
9. Ultrasound is useful in the differential diagnosis of OA and can often identify features of which of the following?
   (a) Rheumatoid arthritis
   (b) Psoriatic arthritis
   (c) Crystalline arthritis
   (d) All of the above
10. Which of the four shoulder joints is most frequently affected by osteoarthritis?
   (a) Acromioclavicular
   (b) Sternoclavicular
   (c) Glenohumeral
   (d) Scapulothoracic

Answers

1. (c) Bone marrow lesions (sound waves cannot penetrate cortex)
2. (a) Comparable to that of other imaging modalities
3. (d) Complex disease of all joint tissues
4. (c) Widely accepted standardized scoring (e.g., KLG, osteophyte and joint space narrowing scores)
5. (a) Hand and knee
6. (d) All of the above
7. (d) Cartilage damage (difficult to assess and not significant in multiple studies)
8. (c) Maximal flexion (part of the reason it is hard to assess in finger joints)

9. (d) All of the above (RA-synovitis/erosions, PsA-enthesitis, crystalline-crystal deposition, erosions)
10. (a) Acromioclavicular

References

1. Hootman JM, Helmick CG, Barbour KE, Theis KA, Boring MA. Updated projected prevalence of self-reported doctor-diagnosed arthritis and arthritis-attributable activity limitation among US adults, 2015–2040. Arthritis Rheumatol. 2016;68(7):1582–7. https://doi.org/10.1002/art.39692.
2. Jafarzadeh SR, Felson DT. Corrected estimates for the prevalence of self-reported doctor-diagnosed arthritis among US adults: comment on the article by Hootman et al. Arthritis Rheumatol. 2017;69(8):1701–2. https://doi.org/10.1002/art.40144.
3. Osteoarthritis Research Society International. Osteoarthritis: a serious disease. 2016:1–103. Available from: https://www.oarsi.org/sites/default/files/docs/2016/oarsi_white_paper_oa_serious_disease_121416_1.pdf
4. Altman R, Alarcon G, Appelrouth D, Bloch D, Borenstein D, Brandt K, et al. The American College of Rheumatology criteria for the classification and reporting of osteoarthritis of the hip. Arthritis Rheum. 1991;34(5):505–14.
5. Altman R, Alarcon G, Appelrouth D, Bloch D, Borenstein D, Brandt K, et al. The American College of Rheumatology criteria for the classification and reporting of osteoarthritis of the hand. Arthritis Rheum. 1990;33(11):1601–10.
6. Altman R, Asch E, Bloch D, Bole G, Borenstein D, Brandt K, et al. Development of criteria for the classification and reporting of osteoarthritis. Classification of osteoarthritis of the knee. Diagnostic and Therapeutic Criteria Committee of the American Rheumatism Association. Arthritis Rheum. 1986;29(8):1039–49.
7. Kellgren JH, Lawrence JS. Radiological assessment of osteo-arthrosis. Ann Rheum Dis. 1957;16(4):494–502. https://doi.org/10.1136/ard.16.4.494.
8. van Oudenaarde K, Jobke B, Oostveen AC, Marijnissen AC, Wolterbeek R, Wesseling J, et al. Predictive value of MRI features for development of radiographic osteoarthritis in a cohort of participants with pre-radiographic knee osteoarthritis-the CHECK study. Rheumatology (Oxford). 2017;56(1):113–20. https://doi.org/10.1093/rheumatology/kew368.
9. Emery CA, Whittaker JL, Mahmoudian A, Lohmander LS, Roos EM, Bennell KL, et al. Establishing outcome measures in early knee osteoarthritis. Nat Rev Rheumatol. 2019;15(7):438–48. https://doi.org/10.1038/s41584-019-0237-3.
10. Hunter DJ, Arden N, Conaghan PG, Eckstein F, Gold G, Grainger A, et al. Definition of osteoarthritis on MRI: results of a Delphi exercise. Osteoarthr Cartil. 2011;19(8):963–9. https://doi.org/10.1016/j.joca.2011.04.017.
11. Bruyn GA, Iagnocco A, Naredo E, Balint PV, Gutierrez M, Hammer HB, et al. OMERACT definitions for ultrasonographic pathologies and elementary lesions of rheumatic disorders 15 years on. J Rheumatol. 2019;46(10):1388–93. https://doi.org/10.3899/jrheum.181095.
12. Bastick AN, Runhaar J, Belo JN, Bierma-Zeinstra SM. Prognostic factors for progression of clinical osteoarthritis of the knee: a systematic review of observational studies. Arthritis Res Ther. 2015;17:152. https://doi.org/10.1186/s13075-015-0670-x.
13. Hill CL, Hunter DJ, Niu J, Clancy M, Guermazi A, Genant H, et al. Synovitis detected on magnetic resonance imaging and its relation to pain and cartilage loss in knee osteoarthritis. Ann Rheum Dis. 2007;66(12):1599–603. https://doi.org/10.1136/ard.2006.067470.
14. Torres L, Dunlop DD, Peterfy C, Guermazi A, Prasad P, Hayes KW, et al. The relationship between specific tissue lesions and pain severity in persons with knee osteoarthritis. Osteoarthr Cartil. 2006;14(10):1033–40. https://doi.org/10.1016/j.joca.2006.03.015.

15. Neogi T, Guermazi A, Roemer F, Nevitt MC, Scholz J, Arendt-Nielsen L, et al. Association of joint inflammation with pain sensitization in knee osteoarthritis: the multicenter osteoarthritis study. Arthritis Rheumatol. 2016;68(3):654–61. https://doi.org/10.1002/art.39488.
16. Gibson N, Guermazi A, Clancy M, Niu J, Grayson P, Aliabadi P, et al. Relation of hand enthesophytes with knee enthesopathy: is osteoarthritis related to a systemic enthesopathy? J Rheumatol. 2012;39(2):359–64. https://doi.org/10.3899/jrheum.110718.
17. Rogers J, Shepstone L, Dieppe P. Is osteoarthritis a systemic disorder of bone? Arthritis Rheum. 2004;50(2):452–7. https://doi.org/10.1002/art.20136.
18. Finzel S, Sahinbegovic E, Kocijan R, Engelke K, Englbrecht M, Schett G. Inflammatory bone spur formation in psoriatic arthritis is different from bone spur formation in hand osteoarthritis. Arthritis Rheumatol. 2014;66(11):2968–75. https://doi.org/10.1002/art.38794.
19. Okano T, Mamoto K, Di Carlo M, Salaffi F. Clinical utility and potential of ultrasound in osteoarthritis. Radiol Med. 2019;124(11):1101–11. https://doi.org/10.1007/s11547-019-01013-z.
20. Schmidt WA, Schmidt H, Schicke B, Gromnica-Ihle E. Standard reference values for musculoskeletal ultrasonography. Ann Rheum Dis. 2004;63(8):988–94. https://doi.org/10.1136/ard.2003.015081.
21. Naredo E, Acebes C, Moller I, Canillas F, de Agustin JJ, de Miguel E, et al. Ultrasound validity in the measurement of knee cartilage thickness. Ann Rheum Dis. 2009;68(8):1322–7. https://doi.org/10.1136/ard.2008.090738.
22. Saarakkala S, Waris P, Waris V, Tarkiainen I, Karvanen E, Aarnio J, et al. Diagnostic performance of knee ultrasonography for detecting degenerative changes of articular cartilage. Osteoarthr Cartil. 2012;20(5):376–81. https://doi.org/10.1016/j.joca.2012.01.016.
23. Gossec L, Jordan JM, Mazzuca SA, Lam MA, Suarez-Almazor ME, Renner JB, et al. Comparative evaluation of three semi-quantitative radiographic grading techniques for knee osteoarthritis in terms of validity and reproducibility in 1759 X-rays: report of the OARSI-OMERACT task force. Osteoarthr Cartil. 2008;16(7):742–8. https://doi.org/10.1016/j.joca.2008.02.021.
24. Hunter DJ, Zhang W, Conaghan PG, Hirko K, Menashe L, Reichmann WM, et al. Responsiveness and reliability of MRI in knee osteoarthritis: a meta-analysis of published evidence. Osteoarthr Cartil. 2011;19(5):589–605. https://doi.org/10.1016/j.joca.2010.10.030.
25. Oo WM, Linklater JM, Daniel M, Saarakkala S, Samuels J, Conaghan PG, et al. Clinimetrics of ultrasound pathologies in osteoarthritis: systematic literature review and meta-analysis. Osteoarthr Cartil. 2018;26(5):601–11. https://doi.org/10.1016/j.joca.2018.01.021.
26. Bruyn GA, Naredo E, Damjanov N, Bachta A, Baudoin P, Hammer HB, et al. An OMERACT reliability exercise of inflammatory and structural abnormalities in patients with knee osteoarthritis using ultrasound assessment. Ann Rheum Dis. 2016;75(5):842–6. https://doi.org/10.1136/annrheumdis-2014-206774.
27. Hammer HB, Iagnocco A, Mathiessen A, Filippucci E, Gandjbakhch F, Kortekaas MC, et al. Global ultrasound assessment of structural lesions in osteoarthritis: a reliability study by the OMERACT ultrasonography group on scoring cartilage and osteophytes in finger joints. Ann Rheum Dis. 2016;75(2):402–7. https://doi.org/10.1136/annrheumdis-2014-206289.
28. Zabotti A, Filippou G, Canzoni M, Adinolfi A, Picerno V, Carrara G, et al. OMERACT agreement and reliability study of ultrasonographic elementary lesions in osteoarthritis of the foot. RMD Open. 2019;5(1):e000795. https://doi.org/10.1136/rmdopen-2018-000795.
29. Iagnocco A, Naredo E. Ultrasound of the osteoarthritic joint. Clin Exp Rheumatol. 2017;35(3):527–34.
30. Gullo TR, Golightly YM, Cleveland RJ, Renner JB, Callahan LF, Jordan JM, et al. Defining multiple joint osteoarthritis, its frequency and impact in a community-based cohort. Semin Arthritis Rheum. 2019;48(6):950–7. https://doi.org/10.1016/j.semarthrit.2018.10.001.
31. Qin J, Barbour KE, Murphy LB, Nelson AE, Schwartz TA, Helmick CG, et al. Lifetime risk of symptomatic hand osteoarthritis: the Johnston County Osteoarthritis Project. Arthritis Rheumatol. 2017;69(6):1204–12. https://doi.org/10.1002/art.40097.

32. Abraham AM, Pearce MS, Mann KD, Francis RM, Birrell F. Population prevalence of ultrasound features of osteoarthritis in the hand, knee and hip at age 63 years: the Newcastle thousand families birth cohort. BMC Musculoskelet Disord. 2014;15:162. https://doi.org/10.1186/1471-2474-15-162.
33. Oo WM, Deveza LA, Duong V, Fu K, Linklater JM, Riordan EA, et al. Musculoskeletal ultrasound in symptomatic thumb-base osteoarthritis: clinical, functional, radiological and muscle strength associations. BMC Musculoskelet Disord. 2019;20(1):220. https://doi.org/10.1186/s12891-019-2610-4.
34. Checa A, Panahi E. Clinical images: is ultrasonography better than radiography for determining the need for surgical treatment in patients with carpometacarpal osteoarthritis? Arthritis Rheumatol. 2014;66(7):1954. https://doi.org/10.1002/art.38619.
35. Spahn G, Lipfert JU, Maurer C, Hartmann B, Schiele R, Klemm HT, et al. Risk factors for cartilage damage and osteoarthritis of the elbow joint: case-control study and systematic literature review. Arch Orthop Trauma Surg. 2017;137(4):557–66. https://doi.org/10.1007/s00402-017-2654-6.
36. Bodor M, Fullerton B. Ultrasonography of the hand, wrist, and elbow. Phys Med Rehabil Clin N Am. 2010;21(3):509–31. https://doi.org/10.1016/j.pmr.2010.04.003.
37. Menge TJ, Boykin RE, Bushnell BD, Byram IR. Acromioclavicular osteoarthritis: a common cause of shoulder pain. South Med J. 2014;107(5):324–9. https://doi.org/10.1097/SMJ.0000000000000101.
38. Blankstein A, Ganel A, Givon U, Dudkiewicz I, Perry M, Diamant L, et al. Ultrasonography as a diagnostic modality in acromioclavicular joint pathologies. Isr Med Assoc J. 2005;7(1):28–30.
39. Iagnocco A, Filippucci E, Riente L, Meenagh G, Delle Sedie A, Sakellariu G, et al. Ultrasound imaging for the rheumatologist XLI. Sonographic assessment of the hip in OA patients. Clin Exp Rheumatol. 2012;30(5):652–7.
40. Malas FU, Kara M, Kaymak B, Akinci A, Ozcakar L. Ultrasonographic evaluation in symptomatic knee osteoarthritis: clinical and radiological correlation. Int J Rheum Dis. 2014;17(5):536–40. https://doi.org/10.1111/1756-185X.12190.
41. Abbasi B, Pezeshki-Rad M, Akhavan R, Sahebari M. Association between clinical and sonographic synovitis in patients with painful knee osteoarthritis. Int J Rheum Dis. 2017;20(5):561–6. https://doi.org/10.1111/1756-185X.12834.
42. Sarmanova A, Hall M, Moses J, Doherty M, Zhang W. Synovial changes detected by ultrasound in people with knee osteoarthritis – a meta-analysis of observational studies. Osteoarthr Cartil. 2016;24(8):1376–83. https://doi.org/10.1016/j.joca.2016.03.004.
43. Chiba D, Tsuda E, Maeda S, Sasaki E, Takahashi I, Nakaji S, et al. Evaluation of a quantitative measurement of suprapatellar effusion by ultrasonography and its association with symptoms of radiographic knee osteoarthritis: a cross-sectional observational study. Arthritis Res Ther. 2016;18:181. https://doi.org/10.1186/s13075-016-1078-y.
44. Bevers K, Vriezekolk JE, Bijlsma JW, van den Ende CH, den Broeder AA. Ultrasonographic predictors for clinical and radiological progression in knee osteoarthritis after 2 years of follow-up. Rheumatology (Oxford). 2015;54(11):2000–3. https://doi.org/10.1093/rheumatology/kev224.
45. Sarmanova A, Hall M, Fernandes GS, Valdes AM, Walsh DA, Doherty M, et al. Thresholds of ultrasound synovial abnormalities for knee osteoarthritis - a cross sectional study in the general population. Osteoarthr Cartil. 2019;27(3):435–43. https://doi.org/10.1016/j.joca.2018.09.018.
46. Keen HI, Hensor EM, Wakefield RJ, Mease PJ, Bingham CO 3rd, Conaghan PG. Ultrasound assessment of response to intra-articular therapy in osteoarthritis of the knee. Rheumatology (Oxford). 2015;54(8):1385–91. https://doi.org/10.1093/rheumatology/keu529.
47. Conaghan PG, D'Agostino MA, Le Bars M, Baron G, Schmidely N, Wakefield R, et al. Clinical and ultrasonographic predictors of joint replacement for knee osteoarthritis: results from a large, 3-year, prospective EULAR study. Ann Rheum Dis. 2010;69(4):644–7. https://doi.org/10.1136/ard.2008.099564.

48. Wu PT, Shao CJ, Wu KC, Wu TT, Chern TC, Kuo LC, et al. Pain in patients with equal radiographic grades of osteoarthritis in both knees: the value of gray scale ultrasound. Osteoarthr Cartil. 2012;20(12):1507–13. https://doi.org/10.1016/j.joca.2012.08.021.
49. Gutierrez M, Di Geso L, Salaffi F, Carotti M, Girolimetti R, De Angelis R, et al. Ultrasound detection of cartilage calcification at knee level in calcium pyrophosphate deposition disease. Arthritis Care Res (Hoboken). 2014;66(1):69–73. https://doi.org/10.1002/acr.22190.
50. Filippou G, Adinolfi A, Iagnocco A, Filippucci E, Cimmino MA, Bertoldi I, et al. Ultrasound in the diagnosis of calcium pyrophosphate dihydrate deposition disease. A systematic literature review and a meta-analysis. Osteoarthr Cartil. 2016;24(6):973–81. https://doi.org/10.1016/j.joca.2016.01.136.
51. Lee KA, Lee SH, Kim HR. Diagnostic value of ultrasound in calcium pyrophosphate deposition disease of the knee joint. Osteoarthr Cartil. 2019;27(5):781–7. https://doi.org/10.1016/j.joca.2018.11.013.
52. Zhang W, Doherty M, Bardin T, Barskova V, Guerne PA, Jansen TL, et al. European league against rheumatism recommendations for calcium pyrophosphate deposition. Part I: terminology and diagnosis. Ann Rheum Dis. 2011;70(4):563–70. https://doi.org/10.1136/ard.2010.139105.
53. Han BK, Kim W, Niu J, Basnyat S, Barshay V, Gaughan JP, et al. Association of chondrocalcinosis in knee joints with pain and synovitis: data from the osteoarthritis initiative. Arthritis Care Res (Hoboken). 2017;69(11):1651–8. https://doi.org/10.1002/acr.23208.
54. Karimzadeh H, Sirous M, Sadati SN, Bashshash M, Mottaghi P, Ommani B, et al. Prevalence of chondrocalcinosis in patients above 50 years and the relationship with osteoarthritis. Adv Biomed Res. 2017;6:98. https://doi.org/10.4103/2277-9175.211835.
55. Roddy E, Thomas MJ, Marshall M, Rathod T, Myers H, Menz HB, et al. The population prevalence of symptomatic radiographic foot osteoarthritis in community-dwelling older adults: cross-sectional findings from the clinical assessment study of the foot. Ann Rheum Dis. 2015;74(1):156–63. https://doi.org/10.1136/annrheumdis-2013-203804.
56. Gates LS, Arden NK, Hannan MT, Roddy E, Gill TK, Hill CL, et al. Prevalence of foot pain across an international consortium of population-based cohorts. Arthritis Care Res (Hoboken). 2019;71(5):661–70. https://doi.org/10.1002/acr.23829.
57. Keen HI, Redmond A, Wakefield RJ, Freeston J, Grainger AJ, Hensor EM, et al. An ultrasonographic study of metatarsophalangeal joint pain: synovitis, structural pathology and their relationship to symptoms and function. Ann Rheum Dis. 2011;70(12):2140–3. https://doi.org/10.1136/annrheumdis-2011-200349.
58. Iagnocco A, Filippucci E, Riente L, Meenagh G, Delle Sedie A, Sakellariou G, et al. Ultrasound imaging for the rheumatologist XXXV. Sonographic assessment of the foot in patients with osteoarthritis. Clin Exp Rheumatol. 2011;29(5):757–62.
59. Keen HI, Wakefield RJ, Grainger AJ, Hensor EM, Emery P, Conaghan PG. Can ultrasonography improve on radiographic assessment in osteoarthritis of the hands? A comparison between radiographic and ultrasonographic detected pathology. Ann Rheum Dis. 2008;67(8):1116–20. https://doi.org/10.1136/ard.2007.079483.
60. Draghi F, Urciuoli L, Alessandrino F, Corti R, Scudeller L, Grassi R. Joint effusion of the knee: potentialities and limitations of ultrasonography. J Ultrasound. 2015;18(4):361–71. https://doi.org/10.1007/s40477-015-0180-3.
61. Keen HI, Mease PJ, Bingham CO 3rd, Giles JT, Kaeley G, Conaghan PG. Systematic review of MRI, ultrasound, and scintigraphy as outcome measures for structural pathology in interventional therapeutic studies of knee arthritis: focus on responsiveness. J Rheumatol. 2011;38(1):142–54. https://doi.org/10.3899/jrheum.100377.
62. Takase K, Ohno S, Takeno M, Hama M, Kirino Y, Ihata A, et al. Simultaneous evaluation of long-lasting knee synovitis in patients undergoing arthroplasty by power Doppler ultrasonography and contrast-enhanced MRI in comparison with histopathology. Clin Exp Rheumatol. 2012;30(1):85–92.

63. Koski JM, Kamel A, Waris P, Waris V, Tarkiainen I, Karvanen E, et al. Atlas-based knee osteophyte assessment with ultrasonography and radiography: relationship to arthroscopic degeneration of articular cartilage. Scand J Rheumatol. 2016;45(2):158–64. https://doi.org/10.3109/03009742.2015.1055797.
64. Okano T, Filippucci E, Di Carlo M, Draghessi A, Carotti M, Salaffi F, et al. Ultrasonographic evaluation of joint damage in knee osteoarthritis: feature-specific comparisons with conventional radiography. Rheumatology (Oxford). 2016;55(11):2040–9. https://doi.org/10.1093/rheumatology/kew304.
65. Steer KJD, Bostick GP, Woodhouse LJ, Nguyen TT, Schankath A, Lambert RGW, et al. Can effusion-synovitis measured on ultrasound or MRI predict response to intra-articular steroid injection in hip osteoarthritis? Skelet Radiol. 2019;48(2):227–37. https://doi.org/10.1007/s00256-018-3010-9.
66. Mathiessen A, Haugen IK, Slatkowsky-Christensen B, Boyesen P, Kvien TK, Hammer HB. Ultrasonographic assessment of osteophytes in 127 patients with hand osteoarthritis: exploring reliability and associations with MRI, radiographs and clinical joint findings. Ann Rheum Dis. 2013;72(1):51–6. https://doi.org/10.1136/annrheumdis-2011-201195.
67. Mathiessen A, Slatkowsky-Christensen B, Kvien TK, Hammer HB, Haugen IK. Ultrasound-detected inflammation predicts radiographic progression in hand osteoarthritis after 5 years. Ann Rheum Dis. 2016;75(5):825–30. https://doi.org/10.1136/annrheumdis-2015-207241.
68. Mathiessen A, Slatkowsky-Christensen B, Kvien TK, Haugen IK, Berner HH. Ultrasound-detected osteophytes predict the development of radiographic and clinical features of hand osteoarthritis in the same finger joints 5 years later. RMD Open. 2017;3(2):e000505. https://doi.org/10.1136/rmdopen-2017-000505.
69. Sivakumaran P, Hussain S, Ciurtin C. Comparison between several ultrasound hand joint scores and conventional radiography in diagnosing hand osteoarthritis. Ultrasound Med Biol. 2018;44(3):544–50. https://doi.org/10.1016/j.ultrasmedbio.2017.11.009.
70. Vlychou M, Koutroumpas A, Alexiou I, Fezoulidis I, Sakkas LI. High-resolution ultrasonography and 3.0 T magnetic resonance imaging in erosive and nodal hand osteoarthritis: high frequency of erosions in nodal osteoarthritis. Clin Rheumatol. 2013;32(6):755–62. https://doi.org/10.1007/s10067-013-2166-x.
71. Wittoek R, Jans L, Lambrecht V, Carron P, Verstraete K, Verbruggen G. Reliability and construct validity of ultrasonography of soft tissue and destructive changes in erosive osteoarthritis of the interphalangeal finger joints: a comparison with MRI. Ann Rheum Dis. 2011;70(2):278–83. https://doi.org/10.1136/ard.2010.134932.
72. Jordan JM, Helmick CG, Renner JB, Luta G, Dragomir AD, Woodard J, et al. Prevalence of knee symptoms and radiographic and symptomatic knee osteoarthritis in African Americans and Caucasians: the Johnston County Osteoarthritis Project. J Rheumatol. 2007;34(1):172–80.
73. Jordan JM, Helmick CG, Renner JB, Luta G, Dragomir AD, Woodard J, et al. Prevalence of hip symptoms and radiographic and symptomatic hip osteoarthritis in African Americans and Caucasians: the Johnston County Osteoarthritis Project. J Rheumatol. 2009;36(4):809–15. https://doi.org/10.3899/jrheum.080677.
74. Jordan JM, Linder GF, Renner JB, Fryer JG. The impact of arthritis in rural populations. Arthritis Care Res. 1995;8(4):242–50. https://doi.org/10.1002/art.1790080407.
75. Alvarez C, Schwartz TA, Savage-Guin S, Bakewell CJ, Kohler MJ, Lin J, et al. Reliability of knee ultrasound in a community based cohort. Osteoarthr Cartil. 2019;27(S1):S335–S6. https://doi.org/10.1016/j.joca.2019.02.741.
76. Yerich NV, Alvarez C, Schwartz TA, Savage-Guin S, Bakewell CJ, Kohler MJ, et al. Frequency of ultrasound features of knee osteoarthritis and their association with radiographic features and symptoms in a community-based cohort. Arthritis Rheum. 2019;71:443–4.
77. Yerich NV, Alvarez C, Schwartz TA, Savage-Guin S, Renner JB, Bakewell CJ, et al. A standardized, pragmatic approach to knee ultrasound for clinical research in osteoarthritis: the Johnston County Osteoarthritis Project. ACR Open Rheumatol. 2020;2(7):438–48.

Ultrasound in Systemic Sclerosis and Systemic Lupus Erythematosus

15

Robert M. Fairchild and Diane Mar

Key Points

- Ultrasound is useful across a broad range of systemic sclerosis disease manifestations including articular and periarticular disease, calcinosis, skin involvement, peripheral vasculopathy and neuropathy, and interstitial lung disease.
- Ultrasound is useful to identify joint and tendon involvement in systemic lupus erythematosus; while erosions are more likely in the overlap syndrome of rheumatoid arthritis and lupus, also known as "rhupus", they may be seen across the entire spectrum of articular disease in systemic lupus erythematosus.
- Ultrasound has revealed that synovitis, erosions, tendinopathy and tenosynovitis, and enthesopathy are all more common than previously thought in systemic lupus erythematosus.

Ultrasound in Systemic Sclerosis

Introduction

Systemic sclerosis (SSc, also known as scleroderma) is a chronic connective tissue disease with a broad range of manifestations resulting from characteristic vascular and fibrotic changes. As the disease progresses, involvement of the skin, joints, soft tissue, vasculature, and other organs can lead to progressive functional decline and significantly impacts activities of daily living and quality of life [1, 2]. Patterns of organ, vascular, and soft tissue involvement help to determine disease subtype,

R. M. Fairchild (✉) · D. Mar
Division of Immunology and Rheumatology, Stanford University School of Medicine, Palo Alto, CA, USA
e-mail: rfairchi@stanford.edu

M. J. Kohler (ed.), *Musculoskeletal Ultrasound in Rheumatology Review*,
https://doi.org/10.1007/978-3-030-73555-5_15

severity, and prognosis. Early and accurate detection of SSc-related pathology is critical to improve outcomes relating to the life-threatening complications of SSc, including interstitial lung disease (ILD), pulmonary arterial hypertension, renal crisis, and digital ischemia.

Peripheral disease in SSc may reveal any combination of skin thickening, pitting and digital ulceration, nail fold capillary changes, decreased peripheral perfusion and Raynaud's phenomena, calcinosis, joint contractures, synovitis, paresthesia, and telangiectasias [3]. Often skin tightening, "puffy" edematous fingers, and contractures, which are common in SSc, obscure underlying peripheral pathology sought on physical exam, and alternative methods for identifying and grading disease in the periphery are important [4]. Organ involvement is evaluated by a combination of laboratory, imaging, functional measurements, and invasive procedures, but these techniques can be costly, time-consuming, and expose patients to significant radiation.

The dramatic vascular and fibrotic changes associated with SSc are particularly amenable to evaluation by ultrasound (US), which has the benefits of being a low cost, nonionizing, point-of-care imaging modality. Continuing advances in US processing algorithms and the recent availability of higher-frequency US probes affords greater imaging detail and resolution. In parallel with this progression, the applications of US in SSc are increasingly diversified, expanding beyond typical joint and soft tissue evaluation to include uses in SSc-associated skin, vascular, and pulmonary disease. In this section, we will explore the role of US in SSc, review evidence for its use, and discuss how it may be incorporated into everyday clinical practice.

Joint and Tendon Disease in Systemic Sclerosis

Arthralgias are a typical finding in SSc encountered in 24–97% of patients during the course of their disease [5]. However, their exact cause is poorly understood due to the multiplicity of peripheral joint and soft tissue manifestations [6, 7]. US is particularly useful in SSc to identify articular disease, including synovitis, erosions, and osteophytes, as well as periarticular disease such as tendinopathy and calcinosis.

Articular Disease in Systemic Sclerosis

Clinically, inflammatory arthritis in SSc has been reported with a low incidence. Multiple ultrasound studies in SSc have found higher than expected frequencies of synovitis although the range varies between 19% and 58% in the general SSc population [8–12]. Articular US findings of synovitis were compared between SSc and rheumatoid arthritis (RA) cohorts in three studies (synovitis defined here as any degree of synovial hypertrophy on B-mode ultrasound) [8, 10, 11]. These US studies found the prevalence of SSc synovitis (22–46%) to be roughly half the prevalence seen in RA, with power Doppler noted in 20–57% of SSc patients. Studies by Cuomo et al. and Gohar et al. found synovitis primarily in the MCP and PIP joints, while Elhai et al. noted an even distribution among the joints of the fingers and the wrists [8, 10, 11].

Abdel-Magied et al. and Chitale et al. compared US to magnetic resonance imaging (MRI) in a subset of SSc patients reporting ongoing arthralgias, evaluating for synovitis defined as having both synovial hypertrophy on B-mode and power Doppler activity [6, 7]. In the former study, 16 patients were evaluated with synovitis on US seen in 4 (25%) patients at baseline and 5 (31%) at 6-month follow-up, at which time MRI was also obtained revealing 14 (88%) with synovitis [7]. In the latter study, 17 SSc patients were evaluated with synovitis on US seen in 1 (6%) and 3 (23%) at baseline and 6-month follow-up, respectively. Of eight unselected patients who underwent MRI at 6 months, all eight (100%) demonstrated articular synovitis [6].

There are several complicating factors to consider when interpreting the results of these studies and when considering sonography to evaluate for synovitis in SSc in clinical practice. Firstly, several definitions for US synovitis are used between studies with some authors defined synovitis as synovial hypertrophy on B-mode ultrasound alone, while others also required the presence of power Doppler activity, which may be responsible for the wide range of frequencies of synovitis reported. Secondly, it is important to remember that synovitis is a pathologic feature and not a disease. While synovitis is the hallmark of inflammatory arthritis in rheumatoid arthritis, its significance in SSc is less clear, particularly in light of the multiplicity of articular and periarticular manifestations encountered in this disease. Along these lines, the severity of synovial hypertrophy on B-mode ultrasound may be a distinguishing feature among the various causes of articular pathology in SSc, but severity was not assessed in the majority of these studies. Our group attempted to address this issue by evaluating the joints and tendons of 43 SSc patients by US with semi-quantitative grayscale scoring (grade 0–3) based on OMERACT definitions (Outcome Measures in Rheumatology) developed for RA [13]. We found that 86% of SSc patients had some degree of synovial hypertrophy, of which, 49% were scored as grade 1 (mild), a finding that is often encountered in even normal individuals. In our SSc cohort only 19% were found to have power Doppler activity suggesting active inflammation (Fig. 15.1) [9].

The presence of erosions and osteophytes may provide additional insights into the underlying drivers of synovial change in SSc. Across the studies outlined above, US-detected erosions were seen in 0–19% of SSc patients, a relatively infrequent finding. Cuomo et al. encountered osteophytes on US in 59% of SSc patients [11], while our group noted osteophytosis in 49% [9]. In the latter study, osteophytes

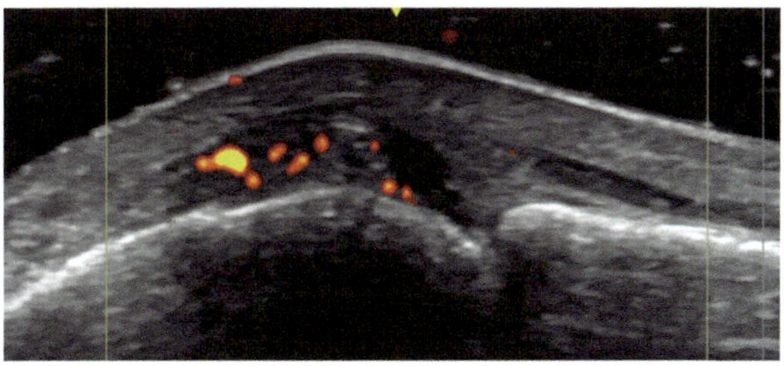

Fig. 15.1 Ultrasound of the dorsal metacarpophalangeal (MCP) joint in an SSc patient with synovitis demonstrated by hypoechoic synovium with associated hyperemia indicated by power Doppler activity

were seen in 54% of SSc patients who demonstrated synovial hypertrophy on B-mode, and 74% of patients with tender joints, suggesting osteophytes, may have a role in synovial hypertrophy findings on ultrasound and joint pain in SSc. Interestingly, many SSc patients appear to have findings similar to those encountered in inflammatory/erosive osteoarthritis including severe osteophytosis, synovial hypertrophy, and associated hyperemia (Fig. 15.2).

Acro-osteolysis (resorption of the distal phalanges) is often encountered in SSc on physical examination and radiography; on ultrasound acro-osteolysis is identified by loss or abrupt end of the normally straight or slightly concave dorsal cortical architecture of the distal phalanx (Fig. 15.3) [14].

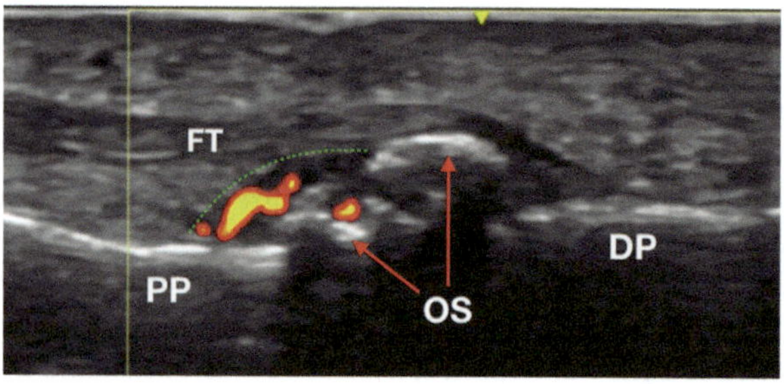

Fig. 15.2 Volar view of a distal interphalangeal (DIP) joint on ultrasound in an SSc patient with an inflammatory osteoarthritis appearance with features of severe osteophytosis and synovitis. FT, flexor tendon, OS, osteophytes, PP, proximal phalanx, DP, distal phalanx, green line, synovial border

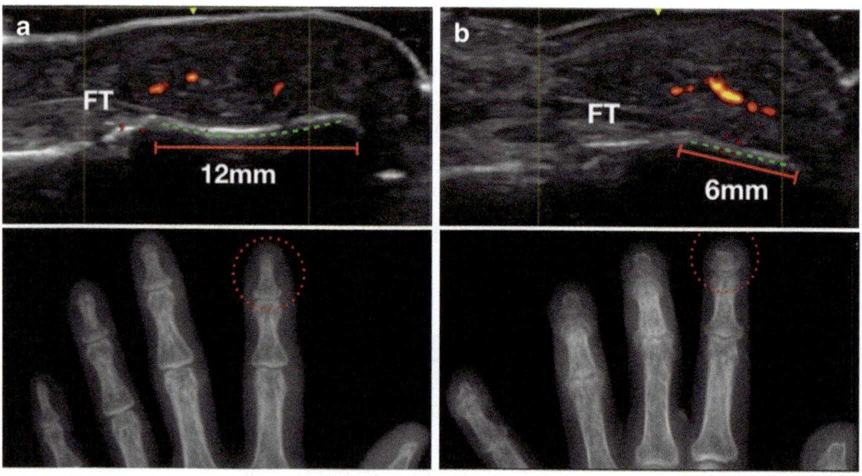

Fig. 15.3 X-ray and ultrasound (volar view) of the distal finger. (**a**) Normal individual, (**b**) acro-osteolysis in an individual with SSc. Notice the normal curvature of the distal phalanx in (**a**) is lost in (**b**) (dotted green line). Measurement from the flexor tendon insertion on the distal phalanx to its tip shows severe shortening of the distal digit in acro-osteolysis. FT, flexor tendon

Taken altogether, these SSc US studies provide valuable insight into joint disease in SSc, suggesting (1) a higher burden of synovitis than is seen on clinical examination alone, (2) less frequent synovitis and erosions compared to rheumatoid arthritis, and (3) a high frequency of osteophytosis in SSc joints. Further work is needed to validate sonographic definitions of synovitis and to expand our understanding of articular pathology in SSc. Clinical US assessment may be helpful in SSc patients with arthralgias to identify synovitis, erosions, inflammation, and osteophytes in everyday practice, which can provide additional information to help guide therapeutic decisions.

Tendinopathy in Systemic Sclerosis

US can identify both inflammatory and sclerotic changes in the tendons of patients with SSc and have been reported in ranges of 23–88% and 40–43%, respectively [3, 6–10]. Typical pathological inflammatory findings include hypoechoic tendons with loss of fibrillar pattern, surrounding edema and in areas where tendon sheaths are present, hypoechoic to anechoic surrounding tissue with or without associated hyperemia (Fig. 15.4).

Sclerotic tendons appear to be a unique feature in SSc but are poorly defined in the literature. In our experience sclerotic tendons are easy to identify by their hyperechoic thickened outline located on the superficial or deep aspects of the tendon, located in areas with or without tendon sheaths, and may be found independently or associated with tenosynovitis or tendonitis (Fig. 15.5). Tendon friction rubs are thought to be due to fibrin deposition [15], and it is tempting to speculate there may be a connection between ultrasound identified tendon sclerosis and clinically identified friction rubs. Cuomo et al. found that SSc patients with friction rubs had an increased retinacular thickness by US compared to those without, but studies focused on US-identified tendon sclerosis are lacking [16].

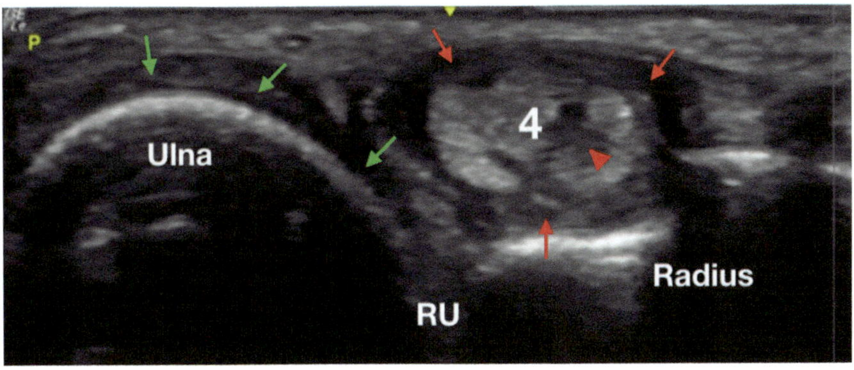

Fig. 15.4 Ultrasound of the proximal transverse view of the wrist in an individual with SSc showing both articular synovitis (green arrows) and tenosynovitis (red arrows). 4, fourth compartment extensor tendons of the wrist; red arrowhead, synovial proliferation invading into the inter-tendon space of the fourth compartment tendons; RU, radioulnar joint

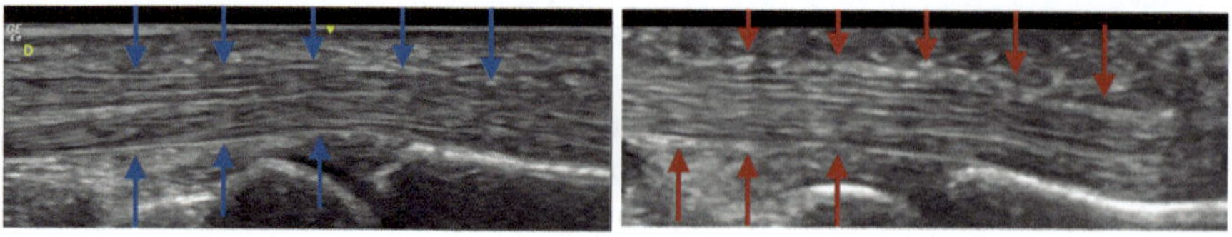

Fig. 15.5 Ultrasound of the volar flexor tendon at the level of the metacarpophalangeal joint (MCP). Left: normal tendon. Right: SSc patient with a sclerotic tendon indicated by a hyperechoic and thickened tendon sheath

Vascular Disease and Associated Pathology in Systemic Sclerosis

Vascular pathology is responsible for many disease manifestations seen in SSc. In the periphery, destructive and obliterative vasculopathy leads to capillary loss, narrowing, and occlusion of palmar and ulnar arteries leading to Raynaud's phenomena, digital ischemia, ulceration, and gangrene and may be contributing factors to the development of calcinosis and acro-osteolysis [17–19]. Nail fold capillary evaluation by capillaroscopy or using a low magnification device is a simple method to evaluate vascular disease. More recently, US has proven utility in assessing both micro- and macrovascular involvement [17]. Conveniently, US allows tissue imaging capabilities for vasculopathy-related disease manifestations and has been used to evaluate digital ulcers, calcinosis, and acro-osteolysis, making it a central tool for both research and clinical SSc evaluation and management.

Raynaud's Phenomena

Studies on Raynaud's phenomena (RP) demonstrated an ability of ultrasound to discriminate between healthy, primary RP, and secondary RP. Keberle et al. showed nail bed and fingertip color Doppler measurements at baseline were similar between healthy controls and those with primary RP but were statistically less dense in patient with SLE and SSc. Furthermore, after cold challenge, both primary and secondary RP showed greater loss of Doppler compared to healthy individuals [20]. A similar study using power Doppler underscored ultrasound's ability to correctly classify healthy patients, primary RP, and secondary RP and demonstrated strong correlation with nail fold capillaroscopy ($\kappa = 0.658$) to differentiate between primary and secondary RP [21]. On a macrovascular level, studies evaluating the radial, ulnar, and palmar arteries by US showed pathologic vessel changes and response to cold stimuli to be distinguishing features of secondary RP compared to primary RP, in particular, severe disease characterized by narrowing and chronic occlusion of the proper digital arteries appeared to be a characteristic feature of SSc-associated RP [22, 23]. In addition to RP, Luders et al. found digital artery involvement on US to be associated with digital ulcers [24].

Ulnar Artery Occlusion and Finger Pulp Blood Flow

Outside of the hands, SSc seems to preferentially target the ulnar arteries [25], and occlusion of this vessel is associated with a variety of disease manifestations

(Fig. 15.6). Association between ulnar artery occlusion on ultrasound in SSc and new or recurrent digital ulcers has been shown in several studies [26–28].

Lescoat et al. also used US to show concordance between ulnar artery occlusion, finger pulp blood flow, and microvascular disease on capillaroscopy and that these measures of vessel disease associate with digital pits, ulcers, acro-osteolysis, and calcinosis. Ulnar artery occlusion on US also associated with markers of disease severity including higher modified Rodnan skin score (MRSS), lower diffusion capacity for carbon monoxide (DL_{CO}), and anti-centromere positivity [18, 28]. Fairchild et al. also noted an association between US-identified ulnar artery occlusion and calcinosis in SSc patients (OR 8.08, 95% CI 2.45–26.60, $p < 0.001$) [29]. Collectively, these studies provide powerful evidence linking vasculopathy to many SSc-related peripheral manifestations and disease severity and may inform future treatment approaches (Fig. 15.7).

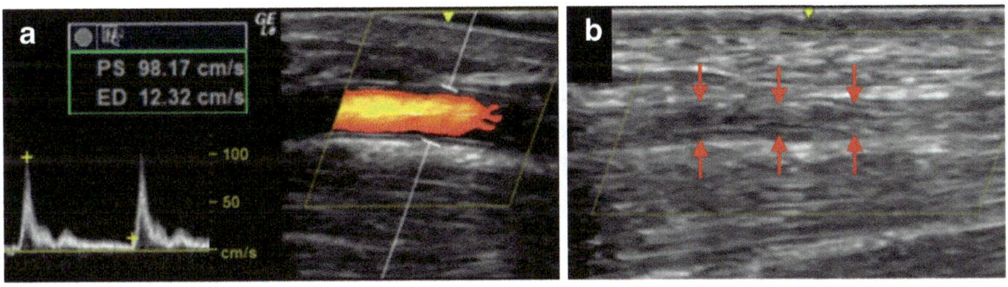

Fig. 15.6 (**a**) Normal ulnar artery architecture and flow parameters on pulsed wave Doppler ultrasound, (**b**) pathologic occlusion of the ulnar artery in SSc showing a thickened fibrotic wall and lack of blood flow on power Doppler ultrasound, confirmed on transverse view (not shown)

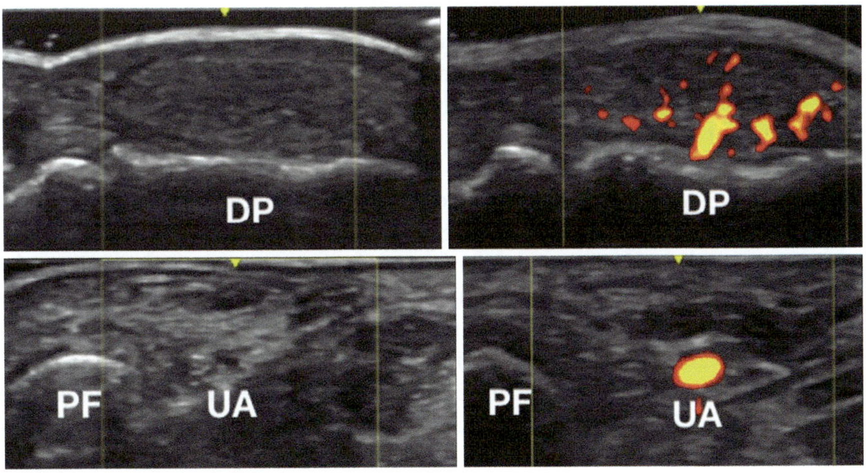

Fig. 15.7 Top right: finger pulp with normal perfusion on power Doppler ultrasound Top left: finger pulp with lack of flow. Bottom left: volar transverse wrist showing ulnar artery occlusion. Bottom right: normal ulnar artery flow. DP= distal phalanx; PF= pisiform; UA= ulnar artery

Digital Ulcers

In SSc, digital ulcers are painful and can cause significant disability, herald worsening digital ischemia, and may result in gangrene and sepsis [30]. Digital ulcers are also an important outcome measure in SSc-related research. Two recent studies have applied US to identify and characterize digital ulcers in SSc. The feasibility of high-frequency (35 MHz) ultrasound evaluation of digital ulcers was assessed by Hughes et al. showing 13 of 15 ulcers evaluated were amenable to both width and depth measurements for classification and was well tolerated by patients [31]. Further work by Suliman et al. defined ultrasonographic features of digital ulcers as focal epidermal loss with or without partial dermal loss or similar findings with the addition of epidermal replacement by irregular hyperechoic tissues below the level of the normal epidermis [32]. Using a more readily available 5–16 MHz linear probe for evaluation, they found significantly increased lesional depth and power Doppler activity in ulcers versus non-ulcer lesions. The authors suggest increased power Doppler, and discontinuity in the epidermis and dermis on ultrasound might discriminate between infected and uninfected ulcers. Although intriguing, further work is needed to evaluate this hypothesis. In our experience, US evaluation of the skin takes little time to perform, and identification and characterization of the epidermis, dermis, and subdermis can be achieved on middle- to high-frequency linear probes which are readily available on most newer ultrasound equipment (see *Skin Thickening in Systemic Sclerosis*). Ulcer evaluation is more challenging if the lesions are small or if ulcers are directly adjacent to or underneath the nail bed. If validated in future studies, ultrasound evaluation of digital ulcers may prove useful as an outcome measure and for clinical decision-making.

Calcinosis

Calcinosis occurs in 22–25% of patients with SSc, commonly occurring in the hands and fingers with associated pain and functional impairment [33]. Researchers have yet to identify a clear pathophysiologic mechanism behind the development of calcinosis, but chronic inflammation and hypoxia are thought to have a role (see *Ulnar Artery Occlusion and Finger Pulp Blood Flow*). On ultrasound, calcinosis appears as hyperechoic punctate to confluent lesions with or without associated shadowing, depending on the size and density of the lesions (Fig. 15.8). Ultrasound has identified calcinosis in the hands and wrists in multiple SSc ultrasound studies. Friere et al. identified calcinosis by ultrasound with a sensitivity of 89% versus X-rays per patient [14]. Fairchild et al. utilized a novel screening technique to identify lesions by 22 zones previously outlined in a validated novel X-ray scoring system for calcinosis [34]. To perform the exam, each hand was examined by ultrasound while submerged in water to provide easy interrogation of all surfaces, and calcinosis was recorded by each zone. The sensitivity and specificity for ultrasound detection of calcinosis versus X-ray was 61% and 95% by zone, 78% and 98% by hand, and 76% and 100% by patient, respectively [29].

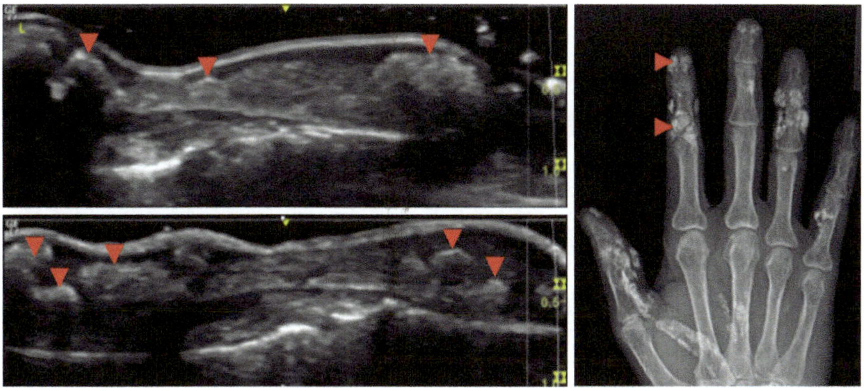

Fig. 15.8 Left top: ultrasound of the palmar distal finger over the distal interphalangeal (DIP) joint showing calcinosis (red arrowheads) with dense shadowing lesions. Left bottom: similar findings with through transmission seen in calcinosis lesions in the distal fingertip. Right: X-ray showing extensive calcinosis

In our experience, US provides a detailed image of calcinosis lesions, particularly in the fingers, and has the potential to be used as an outcome measure in therapeutic trials. Measuring inflammation associated with calcinosis via color or power Doppler is obscured by twinkling artifact, a phenomenon resulting from phase shifting from multiple reflections occurring within calcifications [35]. Whether this artifactual finding could be exploited in the detection of calcinosis has yet to be explored [36].

Peripheral Neuropathy in SSc

Involvement of the peripheral nervous system in SSc is well documented, the majority of which are sensory disturbances [37, 38]. In the upper extremities, carpal tunnel- and cubital tunnel-like syndromes are seen, and there continues to be debate whether these phenotypes are entirely due to compressive neuropathy or perhaps a result of nerve ischemia resulting from the dysangiogenesis and vascular disease seen in SSc [39, 40]. One study from Thailand surveyed 75 SSc patients and found 44% with mild to severe median neuropathy on nerve conduction studies of which only 12% were symptomatic [41]. Several studies have attempted to explore peripheral neuropathy in SSc using ultrasonography. Tagliagico et al. found no statistical difference in sonographic cross-sectional area measurements of the median and ulnar nerves between all-comer SSc patients and controls. Of five patients with carpal tunnel symptoms, two median nerves showed pathologically enlarged cross-sectional areas by ultrasonography, and the remaining three patients were normal by US and electrophysiologic studies. Five patients had cubital tunnel symptoms; of these patients, US showed three ulnar nerves were enlarged, while the other two nerves were obscured by calcifications, and entrapment was instead confirmed by

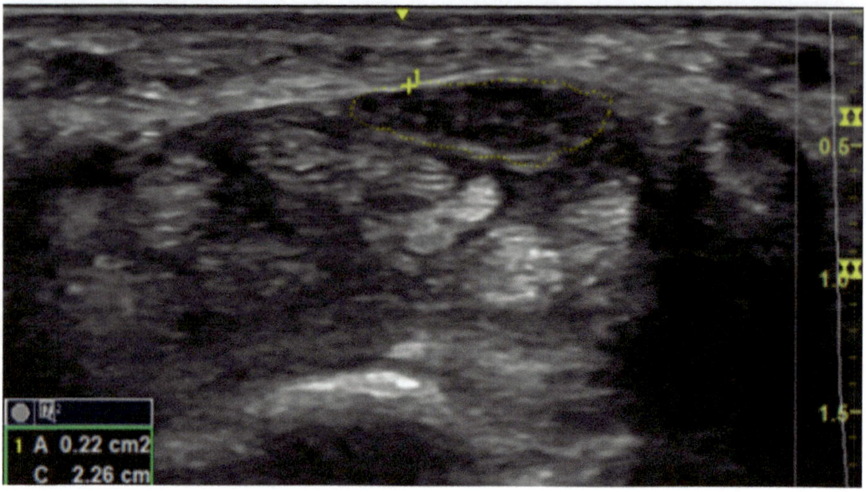

Fig. 15.9 Volar transverse view of the wrist demonstrating median neuropathy in a patient with SSc characterized by an enlarged, hypoechoic, and fusiform (longitudinal view not shown) appearance. Yellow dotted circle: median nerve, 22 mm^2 in cross-sectional area consistent with ultrasound diagnosis of median neuropathy

pathologic changes on MRI [39]. Bignotti et al. used US with computer-aided quantification to show decreased median nerve density in SSc patients vs. controls at the level of the elbow [42]. Bandenelli et al. evaluated 64 SSc patients by US who had no sensory complaints and found a significant enlargement in the median nerve at the level of the carpal tunnel as compared to healthy controls, independent of disease duration and phase of skin involvement [43]. Taken together, these studies suggest support for both a vasculopathic and compressive dependent neuropathy in SSc patients (Fig. 15.9).

In day-to-day practice, SSc patients with peripheral sensory complaints US can be used to evaluate for compressive neuropathy using methods outlined earlier in this book. Space-occupying calcific lesions, common in SSc, may also lead to a compressive picture. Further research is needed to know whether SSc patients with negative US findings for compressive neuropathy, but with suggestive clinical features, may benefit from therapies to improve tissue oxygenation.

Skin Thickening in Systemic Sclerosis

Skin evaluation in SSc patients is important for disease classification, monitoring, and prognostication [44]. Although clinical examination is commonly used for this purpose, the semiquantitative modified Rodnan skin score (mRSS) suffers from observer variability and low sensitivity to change and does not differentiate skin thickness from tightness [45–47]. Additionally, skin palpation is known to overlook areas of skin fibrosis confirmed on biopsy and durometry [48, 49].

Around the time the Rodnan skin score was developed in 1979, US evaluation of the skin was beginning to be explored [50]. With technological advances in US equipment and higher-frequency probes becoming more readily available, high-resolution imaging of the skin is possible (Fig. 15.10). Sonographic skin evaluation in SSc has become an area of research interest [51–55]. By measuring epidermal-dermal thickness, US is capable of reliably detecting SSc with good sensitivity and specificity, with low intra-observer and interobserver variability. In several studies, US detected statistically significant skin thickening in clinically uninvolved areas in both diffuse and limited SSc [56–59].

More nuanced US studies by Akesson [47] and Hesselstrand [60] showed that skin thickening regresses over time in SSc, while echogenicity increases, likely reflecting transition from the early edematous phase of SSc to the late indurated phase (Fig. 15.11). Although mRSS correlates with US skin thickness and inversely correlates with echogenicity, it does not distinguish between these two sonographic findings, highlighting its limitations in discriminating pathophysiologic skin

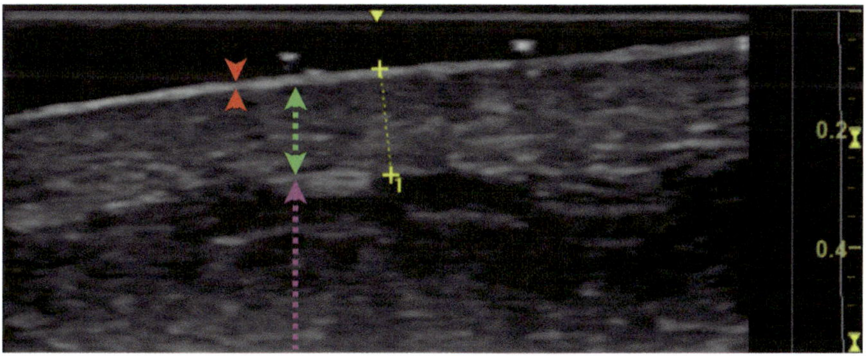

Fig. 15.10 High-frequency B-mode ultrasound evaluation of normal skin. Red, epidermis; green, dermis; pink, subdermis; yellow line, epidermal-dermal thickness measurement taken orthogonal to the skin surface

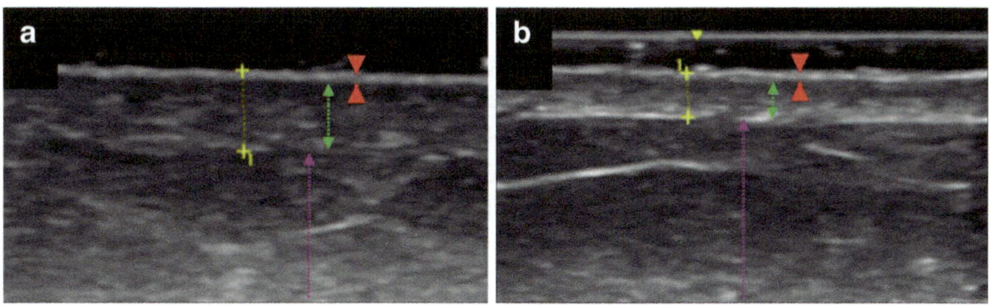

Fig. 15.11 High-frequency B-mode ultrasound evaluation of the skin of the dorsal hand in diffuse SSc at 8 months (**a**) and 89 months (**b**). In early disease (**a**), the dermis is hypoechoic and thicker (17 mm). In late disease (**b**), the dermis is thinner (9 mm), more dense/hyperechoic. Red, epidermis; green, dermis; pink, subdermis; yellow, thickness measurements

changes in SSc over time [60, 61]. More recently, Hesselstrand et al. showed that in early SSc, US skin thickness correlates with serum cartilage oligomeric matrix protein, mRSS, and hand functional measures [46].

Limited studies on US elastography in SSc skin disease showed distinct changes on imaging associated with reduced dermal elasticity [62, 63]. Exploiting these findings, elastography was used to highlight the dermis-hypodermis interface, improving SSc skin thickness measurements on B-mode [64]. See Chap. 19 for further information on the possibilities of US elastography.

These studies highlight distinct ultrasonographic features of SSc skin disease not easily assessed by other modalities which may be useful as outcome measures in therapeutic trials or in the clinical diagnosis, monitoring, and prognosis in SSc. Further studies defining the role of SSc skin US in these domains are needed.

Practically, skin measurements on US are relatively simple to perform. Although higher-frequency probes improve measurement accuracy, the epidermis, dermis, and hypodermis can be identified and measured with linear probes as low as 10 MHz in our experience. Skin thickness is measured from the skin surface to the dermis-hypodermis interface, taking care that the probe and the digital measurement are both orthogonal to the skin surface (Fig. 15.10). In some areas this interface is obvious, in other areas (e.g., the fingers) the dermis-hypodermis interface may be difficult to identify. One trick is to translate the probe a short distance over the skin and identify arterioles or venules which run parallel to the skin surface and highlight the most superficial aspect of the hypodermis. Another technique is to fan the probe which accentuates anisotropic differences between the dermal and subdermal layers making their interface more conspicuous. With some practice, US skin measurements in SSc can be taken quickly and reliably.

Lung Ultrasound in Systemic Sclerosis

Interstitial lung disease (ILD) is a major cause of morbidity and mortality in SSc and is seen in roughly half of SSc patients [65–67]. Currently high-resolution computed tomography (HRCT) is the gold standard for SSc-ILD diagnosis and is performed when patients have suggestive symptoms or signs, imaging, or pulmonary function tests [68]. Dependence on HRCT for screening, characterization, and monitoring for progression and recurrence exposes SSc patients to significant cumulative radiation, financial burden, and treatment delays stemming from time lost between dates of suspected disease to HRCT acquisition [69].

Lung ultrasonography (LUS), described more broadly in Chap. 18, is a potential alternative imaging modality for SSc-ILD. Nonspecific interstitial pneumonia (NSIP) and usual interstitial pneumonia (UIP) make up the vast majority of SSc-ILD patterns of ILD and are well suited to ultrasonography due to their peripheral and basilar lung distribution [70]. LUS findings of B-lines, pleural irregularity, and pleural thickening are all known to be associated with the presence of underlying

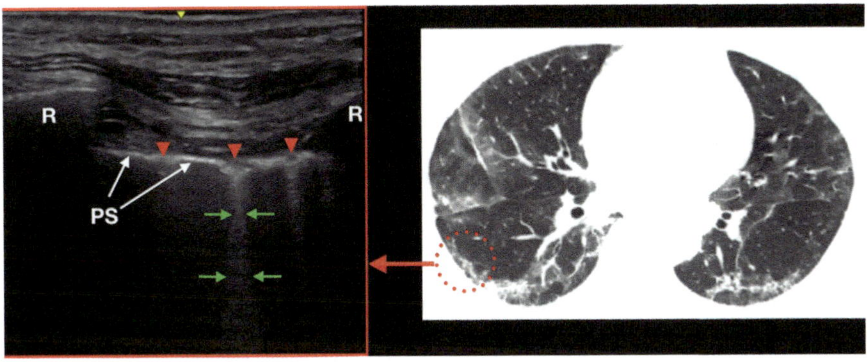

Fig. 15.12 Ultrasound and high-resolution computed tomography (HRCT) of in SSc-associated interstitial lung disease. Right: HRCT shows typical findings of subpleural ground glass opacities and mild reticulation in a patient with nonspecific interstitial pneumonia (NSIP). Left: corresponding US demonstrates pleural irregularity (red arrowheads), B-lines (green arrows), and mild pleural thickening to the right of the image. R, ribs; PS, pleural surface

ILD in SSc and can predict progression (Fig. 15.12) [71–76]. Studies have shown a high diagnostic accuracy for SSc-ILD detection compared to HRCT [71–75, 77, 78]. B-line quantification has traditionally been the focus of the majority of studies on SSc-ILD; however, with the continuing technologic advances in sonographic imaging, pleural thickening and pleural irregularity may be visualized and provide better specificity for SSc-ILD [79].

While significant variability exists in LUS acquisition technique, typically, LUS can be performed by examining the anterior intercostal spaces with the patient supine and the posterior spaces in a seated position [73, 78, 80]. Although exhaustive lung surface evaluation is possible, we perform our LUS examinations using a simplified examination of 14 lung intercostal spaces outlined by Gutierrez et al. [73] (second parasternal, fourth mid-clavicular, anterior axillary, and mid-axillary, and the eighth paravertebral, subscapular, and posterior axillary intercostal spaces, bilaterally), which typically takes 10–15 min to complete. B-lines are an US artifact whose presence and quantity varies by machine settings and reader; B-lines are also not specific to ILD [81, 82]. Due to these drawbacks, we prefer to identify SSc-ILD by examining for US pleural irregularity (hypoechoic pleural defects and cavitations) and pleural thickening (hyperechoic thickening and granularity of the pleura) [79]. When performing the examination, the probe can be oriented either parallel to the ribs or orthogonal (spanning the ribs). Although the former provides a larger unobstructed field of view, we prefer the latter technique as lesions can be tracked with respiration as they slide along the axis of the probe. Regardless of technique used, lung US studies report consistently high sensitivities and specificities for detection of SSc-ILD versus HRCT [71–75, 77–79]. Although this technique shows great promise in SSc-ILD, it suffers from a lack of well-defined and validated US interpretation criteria, and additional studies are needed to determine whether LUS can differentiate ILD subtype, severity, activity, and monitor response to therapy.

Ultrasound in Systemic Lupus Erythematosus

Introduction

Systemic lupus erythematosus (SLE) is a heterogeneous multisystem autoimmune disease in which musculoskeletal complaints are seen in 70–95% of patients during their disease course [83–88]. In this section, we will focus on the role of ultrasonography in SLE-associated joint and tendon disease. Similar to other areas of research in SLE, US studies are complicated by heterogeneity intrinsic to the disease, with significant variation in clinical presentation and severity, treatment, and demographics. SLE US studies differ greatly in scope and focus, varying by pathology examined, US measures employed, and regions studied. These factors, combined with the intrinsic inter-machine and inter-user variability of US, make comparison among SLE US studies challenging.

Arthropathy in Systemic Lupus Erythematosus

Distinct patterns of SLE arthropathy observed on physical examination and radiography have long been recognized. In 1998, Vugt et al. attempted to formalize these findings under a system based on the presence or absence of deformities and erosions [89]. Under this system, nondeforming nonerosive arthritis (NDNE) makes up the vast majority of patients with SLE-associated arthritis, whereas approximately 5–15% develop deforming arthritis [83, 87, 89, 90]. Deforming arthritis is further subdivided into either erosive or nonerosive disease. The former is typically considered an overlap with RA or "Rhupus," while the nonerosive Jaccoud's arthropathy is believed to result from disease involvement of the ligaments and tendons [83, 87, 89–91]. With advances in more sensitive imaging modalities including MRI and US, the distinctions between these groups are less clear with a higher degree of

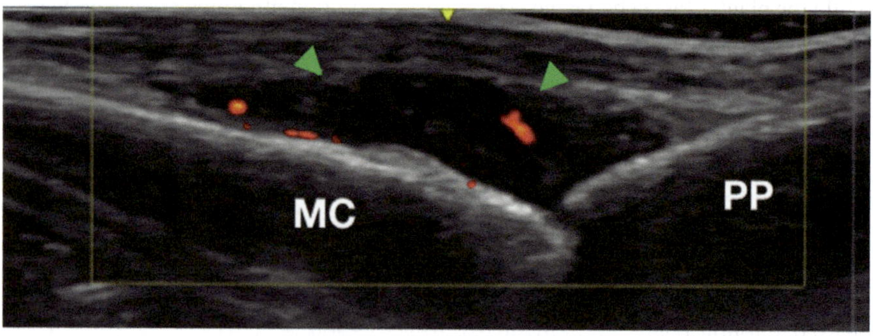

Fig. 15.13 Ultrasound of the dorsal metacarpophalangeal joint in SLE with Jaccoud's arthropathy and inflammatory arthritis. Ultrasound reveals joint hyperextension characteristic of a Boutonnieres deformity and synovitis with a hypoechoic semi-compressible synovium extended from the joint (green arrowheads) with included sparse Doppler activity. MC, metacarpal; PP, proximal phalanx

erosions, synovitis, and various other articular and periarticular pathologies identified across each of these SLE arthropathy subtypes (Fig. 15.13) [85, 91].

In symptomatic SLE patients, US-detected articular synovitis (by B-mode and/or power Doppler) is encountered at a higher-frequency compared to asymptomatic patients, ranging widely across multiple studies from roughly 20% to 80% [90, 92–101]. Synovitis is commonly reported in the MCPs, wrists, MTPs, and tibiotalar joints [98, 102–104] although this distribution may be confounded by selection and omission biases. Involvement of the knees is reported in some studies, but this finding has not been extensively studied [105, 106].

When SLE patients experience musculoskeletal symptoms, pathologic findings of US synovitis and power Doppler activity reduce after therapeutic intervention [107]. Global SLE outcome measures such as the SLEDAI (Systemic Lupus Erythematosus Disease Activity Index), BILAG (British Isles Lupus Assessment Group Index), and SRI-4 (SLE responders index-4) variably correlate with US abnormalities, which is not surprising given the small articular component of each of these measures [92, 98, 102, 105, 108]. In contrast, joint-specific measures including the DAS28-CRP (Disease Activity Score), SDAI (Simple Disease Activity Index), and CDAI (Clinical Disease Activity Index) show positive correlation with US findings [109]. In this respect, clinical monitoring and clinical trials utilizing SLE specific outcome measures may lack sensitivity for musculoskeletal changes and argue for the inclusion of US and joint specific outcome measures [107].

Correlation between US findings in SLE and inflammatory markers has shown mixed results. Mosca et al. found both US synovial hypertrophy on B-mode and power Doppler activity to be associated with CRP [100]. In support of this finding, Ball et al. noted a correlation between US inflammatory joint and tendon findings and IL-6, but not TNF-alpha or BLys levels [110]. In contrast, studies by Iagnocco et al. found no association between US joint pathology and ESR (erythrocyte sedimentation rate) or CRP (C-reactive protein) [94, 102]. These findings could suggest that CRP is more sensitive than ESR to underlying US inflammatory pathology, but this question has yet to be addressed. DsDNA and hypocomplementemia do not appear to correlate with US findings in SLE, while RF (rheumatoid factor) and ACPA (anti-citrullinated protein antibody) were associated with US findings of inflammation (see section "Rhupus and Erosive Arthropathy" below) [100, 102].

Asymptomatic Arthropathy

In SLE patients without signs or symptoms of musculoskeletal disease, US and MRI studies reveal a higher prevalence of subclinical joint involvement than previously recognized [92, 104, 111, 112]. Accurate determination of subclinical synovitis by US highlights the importance of semiquantitative severity assessments, particularly when measuring synovial hypertrophy. In a study by Ruano et al. using OMERACT RA definitions for semiquantitative scoring, 50% of controls demonstrated grayscale synovial hypertrophy grade 1 or higher compared to 77% of asymptomatic SLE patients and 100% of symptomatic SLE patients (Fig. 15.14). Grade 2 or higher synovial hypertrophy was seen in 0% of controls and 13% and 83% of asymptomatic and symptomatic SLE patients, respectively, highlighting a lack of specificity of low-grade synovial

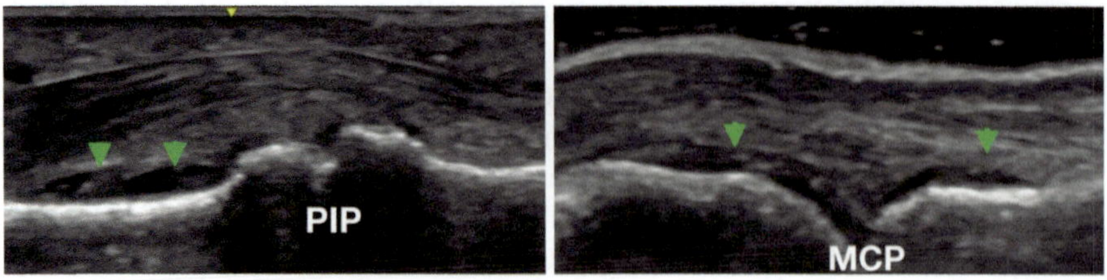

Fig. 15.14 Ultrasound of the volar proximal interphalangeal joint (PIP, left) and dorsal metacarpophalangeal joint (MCP, right) in two patients with SLE. Semiquantitative scoring systems can be helpful to identify and compare severity among patients with mild to moderate synovial changes. Left PIP joint demonstrates grade 2 synovial hypertrophy suggesting articular pathology, while on the right, the MCP joint reveals a grayscale score of 1, which may be pathologic, but is also frequently encountered in normal individuals

hypertrophy for true joint pathology [112]. Similar conclusions can be made from work by Han and Yoon's groups [104, 111]. With respect to power Doppler activity in asymptomatic patients, articular power Doppler findings ranged from 0% to 20% across three studies; all observed power Doppler signal was found to be grade 1 with the exception of one patient [97, 111, 112]. When healthy controls were included in SLE studies, they did not demonstrate articular power Doppler signal [101, 112].

In SLE-subclinical disease, Han et al. showed correlations between synovial hypertrophy and ESR but not CRP, complements C3 and C4, ANA (antinuclear antibodies), extractable nuclear antibodies, RF (rheumatoid factor), ACPA (anti-citrullinated protein antibodies), or antiphospholipid antibodies [104]. However, Yoon et al. found that power Doppler and ultrasound synovitis correlated positively with both anti-dsDNA antibodies and ESR [111]. These findings are distinct from the SLE all-comer or symptomatic patients described earlier and could suggest a different pathologic process in SLE patients with subclinical ultrasound pathology. In contrast to this, Ruano et al. found no correlation between ultrasound power Doppler and RF, ACPA, anti-dsDNA antibodies, C3, C4, and ESR in subclinical SLE patients [112]. Further work is needed on the prognostic and therapeutic implications of subclinical joint disease seen on ultrasound in SLE.

Nondeforming, Nonerosive (NDNE) Arthropathy and Jaccoud's Arthropathy

The majority of SLE patients who present with symptoms of arthritis are assumed to have NDNE arthropathy, traditionally described as clinical arthritis in SLE lacking severe deformity or erosions [89]. NDNE is thought to be a potential precursor to Jaccoud's arthropathy, which is seen in roughly 5% of SLE patients and is characterized by reducible joint deformities, including ulnar deviation, Boutonniere's, and swan neck deformities, to name a few [90, 101, 113].

US of SLE patients with NDNE reveals fewer inflammatory changes compared to rhupus or Jaccoud's arthropathy patients [90]. When NDNE patients are followed longitudinally, Piga et al. showed roughly 1 in 20 progresses to Jaccoud's arthropathy at 5 years. Baseline US findings do not appear to predict this progression; however, baseline synovial power Doppler severity in NDNE patients was associated with musculoskeletal flare within 2 years [117].

There are limited studies on SLE-associated Jaccoud's arthropathy, but findings of synovitis, tenosynovitis, and capsular enlargement are common [113–115] and appear to be increased compared to non-Jaccoud's arthropathy patients [116]. Synovitis and tenosynovitis seen on US in SLE-associated Jaccoud's arthropathy correlate with clinical swollen and tender joints but not SLEDAI, further demonstrating a lack of sensitivity of SLEDAI for underlying musculoskeletal disease in SLE [115, 116].

Rhupus and Erosive Arthropathy

Similar to non-SLE studies, US is more sensitive than radiography but less sensitive than CT or MRI in the detection of erosions (Fig. 15.15) [100, 108, 117]. When present, erosions are often seen in the MCPs, wrists, and MTPs of SLE patients [90, 92–95, 98, 100]. Historically, erosive disease in SLE was typically attributed to an overlap between SLE and RA, also known as "rhupus." Advances in imaging technology have challenged this paradigm, revealing erosive disease in Jaccoud's arthropathy and even NDNE arthropathy. Gabba et al. compared the hands and wrists of SLE patients with NDNE, rhupus, and Jaccoud's by ultrasonography noting erosions in 21%, 88%, and 17% of patients, respectively [90]. Other investigators noted a wide range of US-detected erosions in SLE patients with Jaccoud's arthropathy with a prevalence as high as 58.8%, similar to MRI work done by Ostendorf et al. and Sa Ribeiro et al. [113–118]. In a prospective study monitoring the progression of SLE patients from NDNE to Jaccoud's arthropathy over 5 years, the burden of US erosions slightly increased over time, but erosions were not predictive of deformities or accrued erosive damage [117]. Compared to Jaccoud's arthropathy and NDNE arthropathy, rhupus patients display a greater degree of inflammatory disease, with increased synovial proliferation and larger and more prevalent erosions seen on US [90, 117, 119, 120]. These findings appear to be associated with higher titers of RF, CCP, and anti-carbamylated protein antibodies [90, 119–121].

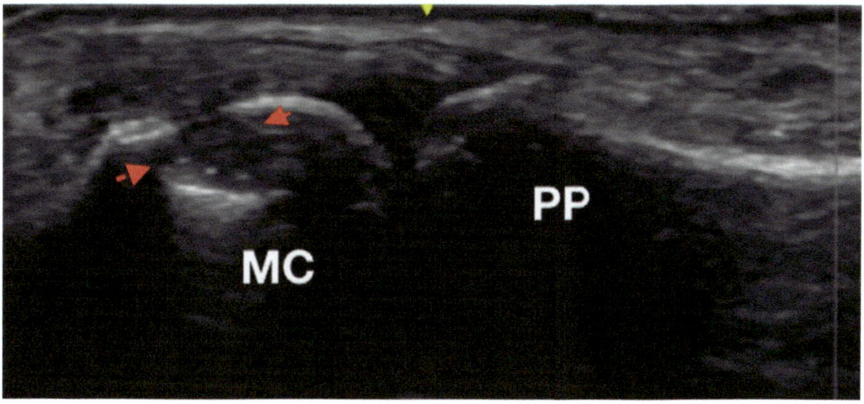

Fig. 15.15 Ultrasound of the lateral aspect of the metacarpophalangeal joint (MCP) revealing a large erosion on the metacarpal head in a patient with SLE and "rhupus." MC, metacarpal bone; PP, proximal phalanx

Reviews of these studies suggest that although erosive disease is more severe in rhupus, erosions alone are not specific for rhupus and can be found across the entire spectrum of SLE clinical arthropathy. Sonographic evaluation, regardless of SLE arthropathy subtype, may help identify patients with potentially destructive disease. Further studies on erosive disease in SLE and its longitudinal consequence are needed.

Tendinopathy in Systemic Lupus Erythematosus

Tendon pathology in SLE is diverse including tendinosis, tendonitis, tenosynovitis, as well as tendon dislocations, ruptures, thinning, and entheseal disease [87]. Inflammatory tendon involvement in SLE seen on US is reported in a wide range and as high as 93% of SLE patients, with tenosynovitis being more common than previously thought (Fig. 15.16) [88, 90, 92–97, 104, 115, 122, 123].

Compared to RA, SLE patients may have a greater burden of tendinopathy which may be a significant source of clinical symptoms [122]. Tenosynovitis is common in Jaccoud's arthropathy [90, 115, 116]. Interestingly, in treatment naive SLE patients compared to RA patients, tendon involvement was less likely to be concordant with joint involvement, suggesting an independent development of tendon from joint inflammation; this finding may explain why deforming Jaccoud's arthropathy in SLE is less associated with joint erosions [122]. Tendon involvement is observed in both the flexor and extensor tendons of the hands and wrists and in the lower extremities in the tibialis tendons of the ankles, although a broader distribution of tendinopathy is likely given the limited examinations prescribed in most studies (Fig. 15.17) [90, 92, 93, 96–98, 104, 116, 122].

US studies have shown enthesopathy to be more common in SLE than was previously recognized. Di Matteo et al. reported entheseal pathology in 20–68% SLE

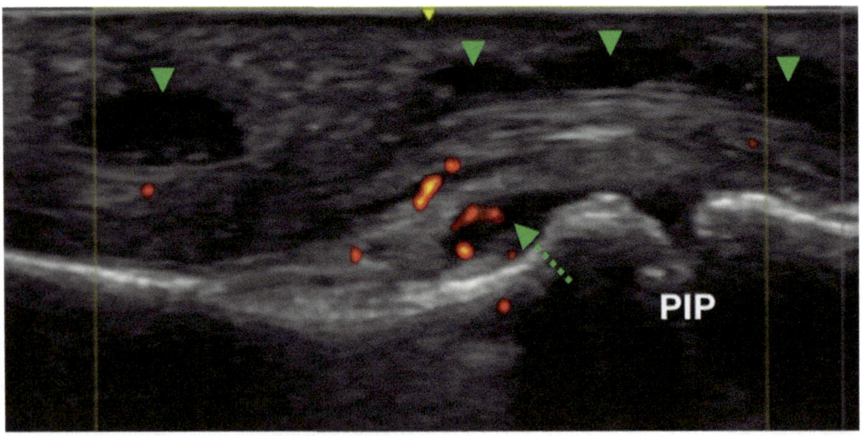

Fig. 15.16 Ultrasound showing flexor tenosynovitis and articular synovitis in a patient with SLE. Green arrowheads, tenosynovial proliferation with small effusions; green arrow, proximal interphalangeal joint synovitis (PIP) with synovial proliferation and hyperemia

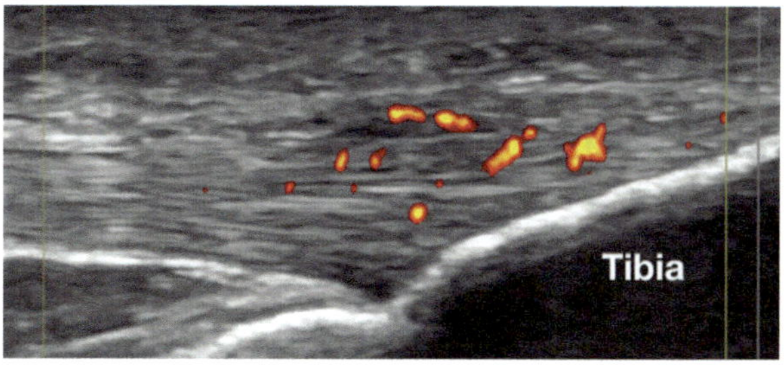

Fig. 15.17 Ultrasound in an SLE patient with infrapatellar ligament tendonitis indicated by pre-insertional tendon thickening, hypoechogenicity, and power Doppler signal, but without clear evidence of entheseal involvement

patients, described by entheseal hypoechogenicity, pre-insertional tendon thickening, erosions and enthesophytes, and power Doppler signal. SLE-associated enthesitis is most commonly noted at the distal patellar tendon insertion but is also seen in the insertions/origins of the quadriceps tendon, proximal patellar tendon, Achilles tendon, and plantar fascia [124, 125]. Morales-Lozano et al. found plantar fascia insertional enthesopathy and associated calcaneal enthesophytes in 10% and 5% of SLE patients, respectively, compared to 0% of controls [98].

Conclusion

US has great potential to be applied to a broad array of practical applications in both clinical and research settings for both SSc and SLE. In SSc, US has helped to reveal associations between vascular disease and many of the peripheral disease manifestations of SSc; and lung US shows promise as a potential tool for screening and monitoring of SSc-associated interstitial lung disease. US may also be a useful outcome measure in studies on SSc-associated skin disease, calcinosis, and lung disease. In SLE, US may be useful for identifying synovitis, tendinopathy, and erosive disease, complementing the clinical exam and diagnostic workup to aid diagnosis and therapeutic decision-making. Further research studies to validate ultrasound findings and develop reproducible scoring systems to be incorporated into clinical trials are needed to further advance the use of US in these rheumatic diseases.

Review Questions

1. Which of the following may play a role in joint pain *and* articular synovial hypertrophy in systemic sclerosis patients?
   (a) Calcinosis
   (b) Osteophytosis
   (c) Tendinopathy
   (d) Acro-osteolysis
   (e) Erosions

2. Acro-osteolysis on ultrasound is identified by which of the following?
   (a) Synovial hypertrophy on B-mode ultrasound and power Doppler activity
   (b) Severe osteophytosis, synovial hypertrophy on B-mode ultrasound, and hyperemia
   (c) Focal epidermal loss with or without partial dermal loss

   (d) Loss or abrupt end of normally straight or concave dorsal cortical architecture of the distal phalanx
   (e) Hyperechoic punctate to fluent lesions with or without associated shadowing
3. Which of the following ultrasound findings are commonly seen in systemic sclerosis but are atypical for other connective tissue diseases?
   (a) Hypoechoic tendons with loss of fibrillarity, surrounding edema
   (b) Hyperechoic thickened tendon borders
   (c) Loss of finger pulp blood flow
   (d) Hypoechoic and enlarged median nerves
   (e) Severe osteophytosis and associated synovial hypertrophy
4. Which of the following are ultrasound findings that can be seen in systemic sclerosis associated Raynaud's phenomenon?
   (a) Less dense nail bed and fingertip color Doppler measurements
   (b) Focal epidermal loss with or without partial dermal loss
   (c) Hyperechoic punctate to confluent lesions
   (d) Narrowing and chronic occlusion of the proper digital arteries
   (e) Both (a) and (d)
5. Ulnar artery occlusion is associated with which of the following in systemic sclerosis?
   (a) Scl-70 negativity
   (b) Digital ulcers and calcinosis
   (c) Higher DLCO
   (d) Lower Rodnan skin score
   (e) Synovitis
6. Which of the following ultrasound artifacts can be seen on power Doppler in calcinosis?
   (a) Mirror image artifact
   (b) Anisotropy
   (c) Reverberation artifact
   (d) "Interface" sign
   (e) Twinkling artifact
7. In systemic sclerosis patients, peripheral sensory complaints of numbness and tingling may be associated with which of the following?
   (a) Compressive neuropathy and vasculopathy
   (b) Severe osteophytosis and compressive neuropathy
   (c) Vasculopathy and epidermal replacement by irregular hyperechoic tissues below the level of the normal epidermis
   (d) Severe osteophytosis and discontinuity in the epidermis and dermis
   (e) Hypoechoic tendons with loss of fibrillarity and compressive neuropathy
8. Compared to normal individuals, in early systemic sclerosis, on ultrasound the dermis is more ________ and in later disease it becomes relatively more ________?
   (a) Hypoechoic and thin; hyperechoic and thick
   (b) Hyperechoic and thin; hypoechoic and thick
   (c) Hypoechoic and thin; hyperechoic and thin

(d) Hypoechoic and thick; hyperechoic and thin
(e) Hyperechoic and thick; hyperechoic and thick

9. Which of the following is *not* associated with interstitial lung disease (ILD) in systemic sclerosis on ultrasound?
   (a) A-lines
   (b) B-lines
   (c) Pleural irregularities
   (d) Pleural thickening
10. Which of the following subtypes of SLE-associated arthropathy display the greatest degree of inflammatory changes on ultrasound?
   (a) Subclinical
   (b) Non deforming, nonerosive arthropathy
   (c) "Rhupus"
   (d) Jaccoud's
   (e) Both (b) and (d)
11. Compared to rheumatoid arthritis patients, SLE patients may show a greater burden of which of the following?
   (a) Tendinopathy
   (b) Erosions
   (c) Osteophytes
   (d) Synovitis
   (e) Power Doppler signal
12. Erosions on ultrasound *may* be found in which of the following types of arthropathy in SLE?
   (a) Jaccoud's
   (b) NDNE arthropathy
   (c) Rhupus
   (d) All of the above
   (e) None of the above
13. What ultrasound feature of enthesopathy is unique to SLE?
   (a) Power Doppler signal.
   (b) Enthesophytes.
   (c) Pre-insertional tendon thickening and hypoechogenicity.
   (d) Erosions.
   (e) There are no ultrasound features of enthesopathy that are unique to SLE.

Answers

1. (b) Osteophytosis
2. (d) Loss or abrupt end of normally straight or slightly concave dorsal cortical architecture of the distal phalanx
3. (b) Hyperechoic thickened tendon borders
4. (e) Both (a) and (d)
5. (b) Digital ulcers and calcinosis
6. (e) Twinkling artifact

7. (a) Compressive neuropathy and vasculopathy
8. (d) hypoechoic and thick; hyperechoic and thin
9. (a) A lines
10. (c) Rhupus
11. (a) Tendinopathy
12. (d) All of the above
13. (e) There are no ultrasound features of enthesopathy that are unique to SLE.

References

1. Randone SB, Guiducci S, Cerinic MM. Musculoskeletal involvement in systemic sclerosis. Best Pract Res Clin Rheumatol. 2008;22:339–50.
2. El Sawy N, Suliman I, Nouh M, Naguib A. Hand function in systemic sclerosis: a clinical and ultrasonographic study. Egypt Rheumatologist. Egyptian Society for Joint Diseases and Arthritis. 2012;34:167–78.
3. Avouac J, Walker U, Tyndall A, Kahan A, Matucci-Cerinic M, Allanore Y, et al. Characteristics of joint involvement and relationships with systemic inflammation in systemic sclerosis: results from the EULAR Scleroderma Trial and Research Group (EUSTAR) database. J Rheumatol. 2010;37:1488–501.
4. Tagliafico A, Panico N, Serafini G, Ghio M, Martinoli C. The thickness of the A1 pulleys reflects the disability of hand mobility in scleroderma. A pilot study using high-frequency ultrasound. Eur J Radiol. Elsevier Ireland Ltd. 2011;77:254–7.
5. Baron M, Lee P, Keystone EC. The articular manifestations of progressive systemic sclerosis (scleroderma). Ann Rheum Dis. 9th ed. BMJ Publishing Group Ltd. 1982;41:147–52.
6. Chitale S, Ciapetti A, Hodgson R, Grainger A, O'Connor P, Goodson NJ, et al. Magnetic resonance imaging and musculoskeletal ultrasonography detect and characterize covert inflammatory arthropathy in systemic sclerosis patients with arthralgia. Rheumatology. 2010;49:2357–61.
7. Abdel-Magied RA, Lotfi A, AbdelGawad EA. Magnetic resonance imaging versus musculoskeletal ultrasonography in detecting inflammatory arthropathy in systemic sclerosis patients with hand arthralgia. Rheumatol Int. 8th ed. 2013;33:1961–6.
8. Elhai M, Guerini H, Bazeli R, Avouac J, Freire V, Drapé J-L, et al. Ultrasonographic hand features in systemic sclerosis and correlates with clinical, biological and radiographic findings. Arthritis Care Res. 2012;63:1244–9.
9. Fairchild R, Horomanski A, Sharpless L, Chung M, Li S, Hong J, et al. Ultrasound Evaluation of the Hands and Wrists in Patients with Systemic Sclerosis: Osteophytosis is a Major Contributor to Tender Joints. Semin Arthritis Rheum. 2021 May. Epub ahead of print.
10. Gohar N, Ezzat Y, Naeem N, El Shazly R. A comparative study between ultrasonographic hand features in systemic sclerosis and rheumatoid arthritis patients: relation to disease activity, clinical and radiological findings. Egypt Rheumatologist. Egyptian Society for Joint Diseases and Arthritis. 2015;37:177–84.
11. Cuomo G, Zappia M, Abignano G, Iudici M, Rotondo A, Valentini G. Ultrasonographic features of the hand and wrist in systemic sclerosis. Rheumatology. 2009;48:1414–7.
12. Iagnocco A, Vavala C, Vasile M, Stefanantoni K, Valesini G, Riccieri V. Power Doppler ultrasound of the hand and wrist joints in systemic sclerosis. Clin Exp Rheumatol. 2013;31:89–95.
13. D'Agostino M-A, Terslev L, Aegerter P, Backhaus M, Balint P, Bruyn GA, et al. Scoring ultrasound synovitis in rheumatoid arthritis: a EULAR-OMERACT ultrasound taskforce—Part 1: definition and development of a standardised, consensus-based scoring system. RMD Open. BMJ Specialist Journals. 2017;3:e000428–9.

14. Freire V, Bazeli R, Elhai M, Campagna R, Pessis É, Avouac J, et al. Hand and wrist involvement in systemic sclerosis: US features. Radiology. 2013;269:824–30.
15. Steen VD, Medsger TA. The palpable tendon friction rub: an important physical examination finding in patients with systemic sclerosis. Arthritis Rheum. 1997;40:1146–51.
16. Cuomo G, Zappia M, Iudici M, Abignano G, Rotondo A, Valentini G. The origin of tendon friction rubs in patients with systemic sclerosis: a sonographic explanation. Arthritis Rheum. 2012;64:1291–3.
17. McMahan ZH, Wigley FM. Raynaud's phenomenon and digital ischemia: a practical approach to risk stratification, diagnosis and management. Int J Clin Rheumtol. 2010;5:355–70.
18. Lescoat A, Coiffier G, de Carlan M, Droitcourt C, Ballerie A, Cazalets C, et al. Combination of capillaroscopic and ultrasonographic evaluations in systemic sclerosis: results of a cross-sectional study. Arthritis Care Res. 2018;70:938–43.
19. Baron M, Pope J, Robinson D, Jones N, Khalidi N, Docherty P, et al. Calcinosis is associated with digital ischaemia in systemic sclerosis—a longitudinal study. Rheumatology. 2016;55:2148–55.
20. Keberle M, Tony HP, Jahns R, Hau M, Haerten R, Jenett M. Assessment of microvascular changes in Raynaud's phenomenon and connective tissue disease using colour Doppler ultrasound. Rheumatology. 2000;39:1206–13.
21. Lee SI, Lee SY, Yoo WH. The usefulness of power Doppler ultrasonography in differentiating primary and secondary Raynaud's phenomenon. Clin Rheumatol. 2nd ed. 2006;25:814–8.
22. Schmidt WA, Krause A, Schicke B, Wernicke D. Color Doppler ultrasonography of hand and finger arteries to differentiate primary from secondary forms of Raynaud's phenomenon. J Rheumatol. 2008;35:1591–8.
23. Toprak U, Hayretci M, Erhuner Z, Tascilar K, Ates A, Karaaslan Y, et al. Dynamic Doppler evaluation of the hand arteries to distinguish between primary and secondary Raynaud phenomenon. Am J Roentgenol. 2011;197:W175–80.
24. Lüders S, Friedrich S, Ohrndorf S, Glimm A-M, Burmester G-R, Riemekasten G, et al. Detection of severe digital vasculopathy in systemic sclerosis by colour Doppler sonography is associated with digital ulcers. Rheumatology. 2017;56:1865–73.
25. Stafford L, Englert H, Gover J, Bertouch J. Distribution of macrovascular disease in scleroderma. Ann Rheum Dis. 1998;57:476–9.
26. Frerix M, Stegbauer J, Dragun D, Kreuter A, Weiner SM. Ulnar artery occlusion is predictive of digital ulcers in SSc: a duplex sonography study. Rheumatology. 2012;51:735–42.
27. Lescoat A, Coiffier G, Rouil A, Droitcourt C, Cazalets C, de Carlan M, et al. Vascular evaluation of the hand by power Doppler ultrasonography and new predictive markers of ischemic digital ulcers in systemic sclerosis: results of a prospective pilot study. Arthritis Care Res. 2017;69:543–51.
28. Lescoat A, Yelnik CM, Coiffier G, Wargny M, Lamotte C, Cazalets C, et al. Ulnar artery occlusion and severity markers of vasculopathy in systemic sclerosis: a multicenter cross-sectional study. Arthritis Rheumatol. 2019;71:983–90.
29. Fairchild R, Chung M, Sharpless L, Li S, Chung L. Ultrasound detection of calcinosis and association with ulnar artery occlusion in patients with systemic sclerosis. Arthritis Care Res. 2020; https://doi.org/10.1002/acr.24327. Epub ahead of print.
30. Li W, Frech TM. The critical need for accurately defining digital ulcers in scleroderma. J Scleroderma Relat Disord. 2018;2:69–71.
31. Hughes M, Moore T, Manning J, Dinsdale G, Herrick AL, Murray A. A pilot study using high-frequency ultrasound to measure digital ulcers: a possible outcome measure in systemic sclerosis clinical trials? Clin Exp Rheumatol. 2017;35(Suppl 106):218–9.
32. Suliman YA, Kafaja S, Fitzgerald J, Wortsman X, Grotts J, Matucci-Cerrinic M, et al. Ultrasound characterization of cutaneous ulcers in systemic sclerosis. Clin Rheumatol. 2018;37:1555–61.
33. Valenzuela A, Chung L. Calcinosis. Curr Opin Rheumatol. 2015;27:542–8.

34. Chung L, Valenzuela A, Fiorentino D, Stevens K, Li S, Harris J, et al. Validation of a novel radiographic scoring system for calcinosis affecting the hands of patients with systemic sclerosis. Arthritis Care Res. 2015;67:425–30.
35. Kamaya A, Tuthill T, Rubin JM. Twinkling artifact on color Doppler sonography: dependence on machine parameters and underlying cause. Am J Roentgenol. 2003;180:215–22.
36. Pracoń G, Płaza M, Walentowska-Janowicz M, Sudoł-Szopińska I. Wartość badania ultrasonograficznego w diagnostyce twardziny ograniczonej – opis przypadku klinicznego. J Ultrason. 2015;15:326–31.
37. Frech TM, Smith G, Reily M, Chamberlain J, Murtaugh MA, Penrod J, et al. Peripheral neuropathy: a complication of systemic sclerosis. Clin Rheumatol. 2013;32:885–8.
38. Amaral TN, Peres FA, Lapa AT, Marques-Neto JF, Appenzeller S. Neurologic involvement in scleroderma: a systematic review. Semin Arthritis Rheum. 2013;43:335–47.
39. Tagliafico A, Panico N, Resmini E, Derchi LE, Ghio M, Martinoli C. The role of ultrasound imaging in the evaluation of peripheral nerve in systemic sclerosis (scleroderma). Eur J Radiol. Elsevier Ireland Ltd. 2011;77:377–82.
40. Poncelet AN, Connolly MK. Peripheral neuropathy in scleroderma. Muscle Nerve. John Wiley & Sons, Ltd. 2003;28:330–5.
41. Nimitbancha T, Sirasaporn P, Wattanapan P, Foocharoen C. The prevalence of median neuropathy at wrist in systemic sclerosis patients at Srinagarind Hospital. J Sci Soc. 2015;42:180–5.
42. Bignotti B, Ghio M, Panico N, Tagliafico G, Martinoli C, Tagliafico A. High-resolution ultrasound of peripheral nerves in systemic sclerosis: a pilot study of computer-aided quantitative assessment of nerve density. Skelet Radiol. 2015;44:1761–7.
43. Bandinelli F, Kaloudi O, Candelieri A, Conforti ML, Casale R, Cammarata S, et al. Early detection of median nerve syndrome at the carpal tunnel with high-resolution 18 MHz ultrasonography in systemic sclerosis patients. Clin Exp Rheumatol. 2010;28:S15–8.
44. Clements PJ, Lachenbruch PA, Ng SC, Simmons M, Sterz M, Furst DE. Skin score. A semi-quantitative measure of cutaneous involvement that improves prediction of prognosis in systemic sclerosis. Arthritis Rheum. 1990;33:1256–63.
45. Clements P, Lachenbruch P, Siebold J, White B, Weiner S, Martin R, et al. Inter and intraobserver variability of total skin thickness score (modified Rodnan TSS) in systemic sclerosis. J Rheumatol. 1995;22:1281–5.
46. Hesselstrand R, Carlestam J, Wildt M, Sandqvist G, Andréasson K. High frequency ultrasound of skin involvement in systemic sclerosis – a follow-up study. Arthritis Res Ther. 2015;17:329.
47. Akesson A. Longitudinal development of skin involvement and reliability of high frequency ultrasound in systemic sclerosis. Ann Rheum Dis. 2004;63:791–6.
48. Claman HN, Giorno RC, Seibold JR. Endothelial and fibroblastic activation in scleroderma. The myth of the "uninvolved skin". Arthritis Rheum. 1991;34:1495–501.
49. Kissin EY, Schiller AM, Gelbard RB, Anderson JJ, Falanga V, Simms RW, et al. Durometry for the assessment of skin disease in systemic sclerosis. Arthritis Rheum. 2006;55:603–9.
50. Alexander H, Miller DL. Determining skin thickness with pulsed ultra sound. J Invest Dermatol. 1979;72:17–9.
51. Myers SL, Cohen JS, Sheets PW, Bies JR. B-mode ultrasound evaluation of skin thickness in progressive systemic sclerosis. J Rheumatol. 1986;13:577–80.
52. Serup J. Quantification of acrosclerosis: measurement of skin thickness and skin-phalanx distance in females with 15 MHz pulsed ultrasound. Acta Derm Venereol. 1984;64:35–40.
53. Akesson A, Forsberg L, Hederström E, Wollheim F. Ultrasound examination of skin thickness in patients with progressive systemic sclerosis (scleroderma). Acta Radiol Diagn (Stockh). 1986;27:91–4.
54. Seidenari S, Belletti B, Conti A. A quantitative description of echographic images of sclerotic skin in patients with systemic sclerosis, as assessed by computerized image analysis on 20 MHz B-scan recordings. Acta Derm Venereol. 1996;76:361–4.
55. Brocks K, Stender I, Karlsmark T, Ullman S, Halberg P, Jacobsen S. Ultrasonic measurement of skin thickness in patients with systemic sclerosis. Acta Derm Venereol. 2000;80:59–60.

56. Moore TL. Seventeen-point dermal ultrasound scoring system--a reliable measure of skin thickness in patients with systemic sclerosis. Rheumatology. 2003;42:1559–63.
57. Kaloudi O, Bandinelli F, Filippucci E, Conforti ML, Miniati I, Guiducci S, et al. High frequency ultrasound measurement of digital dermal thickness in systemic sclerosis. Ann Rheum Dis. 2010;69:1140–3.
58. Ihn H, Shimozuma M, Fujimoto M, Sato S, Kikuchi K, Igarashi A, et al. Ultrasound measurement of skin thickness in systemic sclerosis. Br J Rheumatol. 1995;34:535–8.
59. Sulli A, Ruaro B, Smith V, Paolino S, Pizzorni C, Pesce G, et al. Subclinical dermal involvement is detectable by high frequency ultrasound even in patients with limited cutaneous systemic sclerosis. Arthritis Res Ther. 2017;19:61.
60. Hesselstrand R, Scheja A, Wildt M, Akesson A. High-frequency ultrasound of skin involvement in systemic sclerosis reflects oedema, extension and severity in early disease. Rheumatology. 2008;47:84–7.
61. Sedky MM, Fawzy SM, El Baki NA, El Eishi NH, El Bohy AEMM. Systemic sclerosis: an ultrasonographic study of skin and subcutaneous tissue in relation to clinical findings. Skin Res Technol. 2nd ed. 2012;19:e78–84.
62. Iagnocco A, Kaloudi O, Perella C, Bandinelli F, Riccieri V, Vasile M, et al. Ultrasound elastography assessment of skin involvement in systemic sclerosis: lights and shadows. J Rheumatol. 2010;37:1688–91.
63. Wang L, Yan F, Yang Y, Xiang X, Qiu L. Quantitative assessment of skin stiffness in localized scleroderma using ultrasound shear-wave elastography. Ultrasound Med Biol. Elsevier Inc. 2017;43:1339–47.
64. Di Geso L, Filippucci E, Girolimetti R, Tardella M, Gutierrez M, De Angelis R, et al. Reliability of ultrasound measurements of dermal thickness at digits in systemic sclerosis: role of elastosonography. Clin Exp Rheumatol. 2011;29:926–32.
65. Walker UA, Tyndall A, Czirjak L, Denton C, Farge-Bancel D, Kowal-Bielecka O, et al. Clinical risk assessment of organ manifestations in systemic sclerosis: a report from the EULAR Scleroderma Trials and Research group database. Ann Rheum Dis. BMJ Publishing Group Ltd. 2007;66:754–63.
66. Walker UA, Tyndall A, Czirjak L, Denton CP, Farge-Bancel D, Kowal-Bielecka O, et al. Geographical variation of disease manifestations in systemic sclerosis: a report from the EULAR Scleroderma Trials and Research (EUSTAR) group database. Ann Rheum Dis. 2009;68:856–62.
67. Hoffmann-Vold A-M, Fretheim H, Halse A-K, Seip M, Bitter H, Wallenius M, et al. Tracking impact of interstitial lung disease in systemic sclerosis in a complete nationwide cohort. Am J Respir Crit Care Med. 2019;200(10):1258–66.
68. Meyer KC. Diagnosis and management of interstitial lung disease. Transl Respir Med. 2nd ed. SpringerOpen. 2014;2:4.
69. Bradley B, Branley HM, Egan JJ, Greaves MS, Hansell DM, Harrison NK, et al. Interstitial lung disease guideline: the British Thoracic Society in collaboration with the Thoracic Society of Australia and New Zealand and the Irish Thoracic Society. Thorax. 2008;63(Suppl 5):v1–58.
70. Gutsche M, Rosen GD, Swigris JJ. Connective tissue disease-associated interstitial lung disease: a review. Curr Respir Care Rep. Current Science Inc. 2012;1:224–32.
71. Wang Y, Gargani L, Barskova T, Furst DE, Cerinic MM. Usefulness of lung ultrasound B-lines in connective tissue disease-associated interstitial lung disease: a literature review. Arthritis Res Ther. 2017;19:206.
72. Pinal-Fernandez I, Pallisa-Nuñez E, Selva-O'Callaghan A, Castella-Fierro E, Simeon-Aznar CP, Fonollosa-Pla V, et al. Pleural irregularity, a new ultrasound sign for the study of interstitial lung disease in systemic sclerosis and antisynthetase syndrome. Clin Exp Rheumatol. 2015;33:S136–41.
73. Gutierrez M, Salaffi F, Carotti M, Tardella M, Pineda C, Bertolazzi C, et al. Utility of a simplified ultrasound assessment to assess interstitial pulmonary fibrosis in connective tissue disorders – preliminary results. Arthritis Res Ther. BioMed Central Ltd. 2011;13:R134.

74. Gutierrez M, Soto-Fajardo C, Pineda C, Alfaro-Rodriguez A, Terslev L, Bruyn G, et al. Ultrasound in the assessment of interstitial lung disease in systemic sclerosis. A systematic literature review by the OMERACT Ultrasound Group. J Rheumatol. 2020;47(7):991–1000.
75. Song GG, Bae S-C, Lee YH. Diagnostic accuracy of lung ultrasound for interstitial lung disease in patients with connective tissue diseases: a meta-analysis. Clin Exp Rheumatol. 2016;34:11–6.
76. Gasperini ML, Gigante A, Iacolare A, Pellicano C, Lucci S, Rosato E. The predictive role of lung ultrasound in progression of scleroderma interstitial lung disease. Clin Rheumatol. 2020;39:119–23.
77. Tardella M, Di Carlo M, Carotti M, Filippucci E, Grassi W, Salaffi F. Ultrasound B-lines in the evaluation of interstitial lung disease in patients with systemic sclerosis. Medicine. 2018;97:e0566–7.
78. Barskova T, Gargani L, Guiducci S, Randone SB, Bruni C, Carnesecchi G, et al. Lung ultrasound for the screening of interstitial lung disease in very early systemic sclerosis. Ann Rheum Dis. 2013;72:390–5.
79. Fairchild R, Chung M, Yang D, Sharpless L, Li S, Chung L. Development and assessment of a novel lung ultrasound interpretation criteria for the detection of interstitial lung disease in systemic sclerosis. Arthritis Care Res. 2020; https://doi.org/10.1002/acr.24338. Epub ahead of print.
80. Gargani L, Doveri M, D'Errico L, Frassi F, Bazzichi ML, Sedie AD, et al. Ultrasound lung comets in systemic sclerosis: a chest sonography hallmark of pulmonary interstitial fibrosis. Rheumatology. 2009;48:1382–7.
81. Sperandeo M, De Cata A, Molinaro F, Trovato FM, Catalano D, Simeone A, et al. Ultrasound signs of pulmonary fibrosis in systemic sclerosis as timely indicators for chest computed tomography. Scand J Rheumatol. Informa UK Ltd. 2015;44:1–30.
82. Dietrich CF, Mathis G, Blaivas M, Volpicelli G, Seibel A, Wastl D, et al. Lung B-line artefacts and their use. J Thorac Dis. 2016;8:1356–65.
83. Mahmoud K, Zayat A, Vital EM. Musculoskeletal manifestations of systemic lupus erythematosus. Curr Opin Rheumatol. 2017;29:486–92.
84. Zoma A. Musculoskeletal involvement in systemic lupus erythematosus. Lupus. 2004;13:851–3.
85. Murphy G, Isenberg DA. Connective tissue diseases: SLE-associated arthropathy: truly a benign entity? Nat Rev Rheumatol. Nature Publishing Group. 2012;8(12):695–6.
86. Torrente-Segarra V, Monte TCS, Corominas H. Musculoskeletal involvement and ultrasonography update in systemic lupus erythematosus: new insights and review. Eur J Rheumatol. 2018;5:127–30.
87. Di Matteo A, Isidori M, Corradini D, Cipolletta E, McShane A, De Angelis R, et al. Ultrasound in the assessment of musculoskeletal involvement in systemic lupus erythematosus: state of the art and perspectives. Lupus. 2019;28:583–90.
88. Wong PC, Lee G, Sedie AD, Hanova P, Inanc N, Jousse-Joulin S, et al. Musculoskeletal ultrasound in systemic lupus erythematosus: systematic literature review by the Lupus Task Force of the OMERACT Ultrasound Working Group. J Rheumatol. 2019;46(10):1379–87.
89. van Vugt RM, Derksen RH, Kater L, Bijlsma JW. Deforming arthropathy or lupus and rhupus hands in systemic lupus erythematosus. Ann Rheum Dis. BMJ Publishing Group Ltd. 1998;57:540–4.
90. Gabba A, Piga M, Vacca A, Porru G, Garau P, Cauli A, et al. Joint and tendon involvement in systemic lupus erythematosus: an ultrasound study of hands and wrists in 108 patients. Rheumatology (Oxford). 2012;51:2278–85.
91. Zayat AS, Md Yusof MY, Wakefield RJ, Conaghan PG, Emery P, Vital EM. The role of ultrasound in assessing musculoskeletal symptoms of systemic lupus erythematosus: a systematic literature review. Rheumatology. 2016;55(3):485–94.
92. Salliot C, Denis A, Dernis E, Andre V, Perdriger A, Albert J-D, et al. Ultrasonography and detection of subclinical joints and tendons involvements in systemic lupus erythematosus (SLE) patients: a cross-sectional multicenter study. Joint Bone Spine. Elsevier Masson SAS. 2018;85:741–5.

93. Wright S, Filippucci E, Grassi W, Grey A, Bell A. Hand arthritis in systemic lupus erythematosus: an ultrasound pictorial essay. Lupus. 2016;15:501–6.
94. Iagnocco A, Ossandon A, Coari G, Conti F, Priori R, Alessandri C, et al. Wrist joint involvement in systemic lupus erythematosus. An ultrasonographic study. Clin Exp Rheumatol. 2004;22:621–4.
95. Delle Sedie A, Riente L, Scirè CA, Iagnocco A, Filippucci E, Meenagh G, et al. Ultrasound imaging for the rheumatologist. XXIV. Sonographic evaluation of wrist and hand joint and tendon involvement in systemic lupus erythematosus. Clin Exp Rheumatol. 2009;27:897–901.
96. Dreyer L, Jacobsen S, Juul L, Terslev L. Ultrasonographic abnormalities and inter-reader reliability in Danish patients with systemic lupus erythematosus – a comparison with clinical examination of wrist and metacarpophalangeal joints. Lupus. 6th ed. 2014;24:712–9.
97. Torrente-Segarra V, Lisbona MP, Rotés-Sala D, Muñoz-Ortego J, Padró-Blanch I, Maymó-Guarch J, et al. Hand and wrist arthralgia in systemic lupus erythematosus is associated to ultrasonographic abnormalities. Joint Bone Spine. Elsevier Masson SAS. 2013;80:402–6.
98. Morales-Lozano R, Martínez-Barrio J, González-Fernández ML, López-Longo FJ, Ovalles-Bonilla JG, Valor L, et al. The feet in systemic lupus erythematosus; are we underestimating their involvement and functional impact? Clin Exp Rheumatol. 2016;34:609–17.
99. Di Matteo A, De Angelis R, Cipolletta E, Filippucci E, Grassi W. Systemic lupus erythematosus arthropathy: the sonographic perspective. Lupus. 2017;27:794–801.
100. Mosca M, Tani C, Carli L, Vagnani S, Possemato N, Delle Sedie A, et al. The role of imaging in the evaluation of joint involvement in 102 consecutive patients with systemic lupus erythematosus. Autoimmun Rev. 2015;14:10–5.
101. Piga M, Saba L, Gabba A, Congia M, Balestrieri A, Mathieu A, et al. Ultrasonographic assessment of bone erosions in the different subtypes of systemic lupus erythematosus arthritis: comparison with computed tomography. Arthritis Res Ther. 2016;18:222.
102. Iagnocco A, Ceccarelli F, Rizzo C, Truglia S, Massaro L, Spinelli FR, et al. Ultrasound evaluation of hand, wrist and foot joint synovitis in systemic lupus erythematosus. Rheumatology. 2014;53:465–72.
103. Mukherjee S, Cherry L, Zarroug J, Culliford D, Bowen C, Arden N, et al. A pilot investigation of the prevalence of US-detectable forefoot joint pathology and reported foot-related disability in participants with systemic lupus erythematosus. J Foot Ankle Res. 2016;9:27.
104. Han N, Tian X. Detection of subclinical synovial hypertrophy by musculoskeletal gray-scale/power Doppler ultrasonography in systemic lupus erythematosus patients: a cross-sectional study. Int J Rheum Dis. 2019;22:1058–69.
105. Ossandon A, Iagnocco A, Alessandri C, Priori R, Conti F, Valesini G. Ultrasonographic depiction of knee joint alterations in systemic lupus erythematosus. Clin Exp Rheumatol. 2009;27:329–32.
106. Demirkaya E, Özçakar L, Türker T, Haghari S, Ayaz NA, Bakkaloğlu A, et al. Musculoskeletal sonography in juvenile systemic lupus erythematosus. Arthritis Care Res. 2008;61:58–60.
107. Mahmoud K, Zayat AS, Yusof Y, Hensor E, Conaghan PG, Emery P, et al. Responsiveness of clinical and ultrasound outcome measures in musculoskeletal systemic lupus erythematosus. Rheumatology. 2019;62:222–8.
108. Lei L, Morgan S, Ntatsaki E, Ciurtin C. Comparative assessment of hand joint ultrasound findings in symptomatic patients with systemic lupus erythematosus and Sjögren's syndrome: a pilot study. Ultrasound Med Biol. Elsevier Inc. 2019;45:452–60.
109. Ceccarelli F, Perricone C, Cipriano E, Massaro L, Natalucci F, Spinelli FR, et al. Usefulness of composite indices in the assessment of joint involvement in systemic lupus erythematosus patients: correlation with ultrasonographic score. Lupus. 2019;28:383–8.
110. Ball E, Gibson DS, Bell AL, Rooney MR. Plasma IL-6 levels correlate with clinical and ultrasound measures of arthritis in patients with systemic lupus erythematosus. Lupus. 2013;23:46–56.
111. Yoon H-S, Kim K-J, Baek I-W, Park Y-J, Kim W-U, Yoon C-H, et al. Ultrasonography is useful to detect subclinical synovitis in SLE patients without musculoskeletal involvement before symptoms appear. Clin Rheumatol. Springer London. 2014;33:341–8.

112. Ruano CA, Malheiro R, Oliveira JF, Pinheiro S, Vieira LS, Moraes-Fontes MF. Ultrasound detects subclinical joint inflammation in the hands and wrists of patients with systemic lupus erythematosus without musculoskeletal symptoms. Lupus Sci Med. 2017;4:e000184–8.
113. Sá Ribeiro D, Galvão V, Luiz Fernandes J, de Araújo Neto C, D'Almeida F, Santiago M. Magnetic resonance imaging of Jaccoud's arthropathy in systemic lupus erythematosus. Joint Bone Spine. Elsevier Masson. 2010;77:241–5.
114. Ostendorf B, Scherer A, Specker C, Mödder U, Schneider M. Jaccoud's arthropathy in systemic lupus erythematosus: differentiation of deforming and erosive patterns by magnetic resonance imaging. Arthritis Rheum. John Wiley & Sons, Ltd. 2003;48:157–65.
115. Lins CF, de Sá Ribeiro DL, Santos WGD, Rosa G, Machicado V, Pedreira AL, et al. Sonographic findings of hands and wrists in systemic lupus erythematosus patients with Jaccoud arthropathy. J Clin Rheumatol. 2018;24:70–4.
116. Ribeiro DS, Lins CF, Galvão V, Santos WGD, Rosa G, Machicado V, et al. Association of CXCL13 serum level and ultrasonographic findings of joints in patients with systemic lupus erythematosus and Jaccoud's arthropathy. Lupus. 2018;27:939–46.
117. Piga M, Gabba A, Congia M, Figus F, Cauli A, Mathieu A. Predictors of musculoskeletal flares and Jaccoud's arthropathy in patients with systemic lupus erythematosus: a 5-year prospective study. Semin Arthritis Rheum. Elsevier. 2016;46:217–24.
118. Ceccarelli F, Massaro L, Perricone C, Pendolino M, Cipriano E, Truglia S, et al. Jaccoud's arthropathy in systemic lupus erythematosus: clinical, laboratory and ultrasonographic features. Clin Exp Rheumatol. 2017;35:674–7.
119. Ziegelasch M, van Delft MAM, Wallin P, Skogh T, Magro-Checa C, Steup-Beekman GM, et al. Antibodies against carbamylated proteins and cyclic citrullinated peptides in systemic lupus erythematosus: results from two well-defined European cohorts. Arthritis Res Ther. 2016;18:289.
120. Tani C, D'Aniello D, Sedie AD, Carli L, Cagnoni M, Possemato N, et al. Rhupus syndrome: assessment of its prevalence and its clinical and instrumental characteristics in a prospective cohort of 103 SLE patients. Autoimmun Rev. Elsevier B.V. 2013;12:537–41.
121. Ceccarelli F, Perricone C, Colasanti T, Massaro L, Cipriano E, Pendolino M, et al. Anti-carbamylated protein antibodies as a new biomarker of erosive joint damage in systemic lupus erythematosus. Arthritis Res Ther. 2018;20:126.
122. Ogura T, Hirata A, Hayashi N, Takenaka S, Ito H, Mizushina K, et al. Comparison of ultrasonographic joint and tendon findings in hands between early, treatment-naïve patients with systemic lupus erythematosus and rheumatoid arthritis. Lupus. 2016;26:707–14.
123. Lins CF, de Sá Ribeiro DL, Santos WGD, Rosa G, Machicado V, Pedreira AL, et al. Ultrasound findings on hands and wrists of patients with systemic lupus erythematosus: relationship with physical examination. Ultrasound Med Biol. Elsevier Inc. 2017;43:1764–8.
124. Di Matteo A, Filippucci E, Cipolletta E, Satulu I, Hurnakova J, Lato V, et al. Entheseal involvement in patients with systemic lupus erythematosus: an ultrasound study. Rheumatology. 6th ed. 2018;57:1822–9.
125. Di Matteo A, Satulu I, Di Carlo M, Lato V, Filippucci E, Grassi W. Entheseal involvement in systemic lupus erythematosus: are we missing something? Lupus. 2016;26:320–8.

Part II

Beyond Musculoskeletal Ultrasound

Ultrasound in Vasculitis

16

Andreas P. Diamantopoulos

Key Points

- Ultrasound has a high sensitivity and specificity in the diagnosis of giant cell arteritis in experienced sonographers.
- The "halo" sign represents inflamed, thickened intimal wall of the artery as visualized by ultrasound.
- Appropriate training of the ultrasonographer and adjustments of ultrasound equipment settings are essential for accurate diagnostics.

Introduction

General Considerations

The systemic vasculitides are a group of autoimmune diseases affecting the blood vessel wall. Systemic vasculitides can cause stenosis, occlusions, and thrombosis with subsequent ischemia or destructive changes causing aneurysms and blood vessel rupture [1]. According to Chapel Hill consensus in 2012, the vasculitides are classified with regard to blood vessel size, affecting large, medium, small, and variable-sized vessels [1].

Large-vessel vasculitis (LVV) affects the large and medium-sized vessels [1]. The main systemic vasculitides affecting the large vessels are giant cell arteritis (GCA), Takayasu's arteritis (TA), and idiopathic aortitis. GCA can present as

A. P. Diamantopoulos (✉)
Department of Rheumatology, Martina Hansens Hospital, Bærum, Norway

Department of Rheumatology, Akershus University Hospital, Lørenskog, Norway

M. J. Kohler (ed.), *Musculoskeletal Ultrasound in Rheumatology Review*,
https://doi.org/10.1007/978-3-030-73555-5_16

cranial arteritis (CA), large-vessel vasculitis, or as a combination of cranial and large-vessel vasculitis. Single-organ or isolated aortitis is also a variant of large-vessel vasculitis affecting the aorta; however, whether or not this form of aortitis is a limited variant of TA or GCA is unknown [1]. Epidemiologic data on isolated aortitis is currently lacking.

A different arterial distribution has been observed between GCA and TA, with GCA affecting mainly the temporal artery, thoracic aorta, subclavian, and axillary arteries and TA affecting the aorta, abdominal vessels, carotid, and subclavian arteries [1, 2]. In approximately 55% of GCA patients, there is ultrasonographic evidence of vasculitis in the infra-aortic arteries; however, it seems that vasculitis of the large vessels of the lower extremities is always accompanied by inflammation of the cranial and/or supraaortic vessels [3].

Evidence-Based Background for the Use of Ultrasound in Vasculitis

Ultrasound has been widely used in inflammatory joint diseases for diagnosis and monitoring of treatment response [4]. Nonetheless, the use of ultrasound in the diagnosis of GCA has been controversial; imaging of the temporal arteries, in particular, reports sensitivities ranging from excellent to not better than a thorough clinical evaluation [5].

Ultrasound has been used as early as the 1980s as a diagnostic modality in cranial GCA, initially in the form of Doppler flow [6]. However, the first prospective study of color duplex ultrasonography was performed by WA Schmidt in 1997 and reported the use of ultrasound as an imaging modality with high sensitivity and specificity in the diagnostics of GCA [7]. In the following years, a plethora of studies were performed showing great variation in the sensitivity and specificity of ultrasound in GCA. Three meta-analyses have shown a relatively high sensitivity and specificity of the ultrasound versus the American College of Rheumatology (ACR) GCA classification criteria (Table 16.1).

The reasons for wide variation of previously published diagnostic ultrasound results could be attributed to the low-quality resolution of equipment used, erroneous technique, and erroneous adjustments of the ultrasound equipment settings in an inexperienced ultrasonographer [8, 9]; however, with advances in technology

Table 16.1 Summary of the meta-analyses examining ultrasound in GCA

	Karassa FB, Ann Int Med 2005 [11][a]	Arida A, BMC Musculoskelet Disord, 2010 [10][b]	Ball EL, Br J Surg, 2010 [12][a]	Duftner C, RMD Open, 2018[a,b] [31]
# of studies evaluated	3	8	7	8
Sensitivity	87%	68%	78%	77%
Specificity	96%	91%	88%	96%

number
[a]Halo, occlusion or stenosis vs ACR GCA classification criteria
[b]Halo vs ACR GCA classification criteria

and availability of higher frequency probes, better image processing and possibilities of artificial intelligence and machine learning, as well as educational teaching for appropriate techniques and image optimization, the use of diagnostic ultrasound for vasculitis has great potential for diagnostic and even potentially monitoring purposes. In a survey of diverse articles regarding ultrasonography in GCA performed by the author, fundamental errors in both technique and adjustments of ultrasound equipment settings were found and obvious in the accompanied published images.

Ultrasound appears to be more sensitive than the biopsy of the temporal artery in the diagnostics of cranial GCA [10–12]. Ultrasound can image the whole length of the temporal and occipital arteries and the distal part of the facial arteries [13, 14], which is an advantage over biopsy that often cannot exceed 1 cm of vascular tissue [8]. However, Germano et al. evaluated ultrasound-guided temporal artery biopsies vs standard temporal artery biopsies in the diagnosis of GCA and found no difference in the rate of positive biopsies between the two groups [15]. Limitations of this study included small sample size, varying lengths of time on corticosteroids prior to biopsy, different surgeons performing the biopsies, and the possibility for false negative biopsies despite marking, due to the segmental nature of temporal artery inflammation.

Numerous studies have shown the usefulness of ultrasound in the imaging of inflammatory changes of the large vessels (in up to 54% of GCA patients) [3, 8, 16–21]. The axillary artery is by far the most affected artery in LVV GCA (98%) [22]. Ultrasound examination of the carotid artery in addition to temporal and axillary artery raises the sensitivity on the diagnostics of GCA up to 100% [8]. Implementation of ultrasound in the "fast-track" outpatient GCA clinics seems to reduce the rate of blindness among GCA patients [23]. In TA, ultrasound can visualize changes in the supraaortic vessels and abdominal aorta, nonetheless, wall abnormalities of the abdominal blood vessels and descending aorta can be difficult to visualize [24].

Compared to other imaging modalities, ultrasound appears to have a number of advantages. Ultrasound has a comparable sensitivity to MRA (1.5 T and up) in cranial arteritis [25] and to PET-CT scan in LVV-GCA [17, 18]. Ultrasound also has better contrast resolution than CTA, MRA, and PET-CT scan (a transducer of 18 MHz gives a resolution of 0.15 mm) [26]. From a safety perspective, no ionized radiation or contrast admission is required with ultrasonography, unlike CTA, MRA (contrast), and PET-CT [27]. Use of potentially nephrotoxic contrast agents are contraindicated in patients with kidney failure and may limit use of these more expensive imaging modalities [28]. Ultrasound examination can be useful in patients who cannot undergo MR due to claustrophobia, in patients with a pacemaker, metallic parts in the body, or in pregnant women [28]. Furthermore, CTA and MRA cannot estimate precisely to what extent arteries like the axillary are affected [29, 30], whereas ultrasound has higher spatial resolution than other imaging modalities. Ultrasound is by far the most economical imaging modality in the diagnostics of GCA [26].

A recent meta-analysis confirmed the high sensitivity and specificity of ultrasound in cranial GCA [31] and has been used as the main source of evidence for the development of the European League Against Rheumatism's (EULAR) guidelines on the use of imaging modalities in LVV. These guidelines strongly advise the use of ultrasound of the temporal and axillary arteries as a first-line examination for diagnosing cranial GCA [32]. The British Society for Rheumatology also recently published guidelines on the diagnosis and treatment of GCA, with a strong recommendation that patients with suspected GCA should obtain a confirmatory diagnostic test. This could be either a temporal artery biopsy at least 1 cm in length or an ultrasound of the temporal and axillary arteries or both [33].

Medium-Sized and Small Vessel Vasculitides

Polyarteritis nodosa (PAN) and Kawasaki's disease predominantly assault the medium-sized vessels [1]. Ultrasound can depict the extension of cardiac vessel affection in Kawasaki by transthoracic echocardiography or carotid artery ultrasonography [34, 35]. Affection of renal, hepatic, and mesenteric arteries is seen frequently in PAN. Nonetheless, the quality of images is moderate and varies according to patient's habitus. Other modalities, like conventional angiography and/or cross-sectional imaging with CT or MR, are better suited for accurate imaging of affected medium-sized vessels. In some cases with Raynaud signs, ultrasound can reveal vasculitis of the medium-sized vessels as the digital arteries [22]. However, in the small vessel vasculitides (ANCA-associated, etc.), ultrasound is not sensitive and should not be used for diagnostic or follow-up purposes.

Caution should be given to the involvement of the temporal artery by other than GCA vasculitides (PAN, AVV) [8], and ultrasound findings should always be interpreted in conjunction with the appropriately related clinical context.

Polymyalgia Rheumatica

Polymyalgia rheumatica (PMR) is an inflammatory disorder that affects older individuals and is often linked with GCA. As noted in Chaps. 5 and 6 (ultrasound of the shoulder and hip, respectively), the 2012 EULAR/ACR classification criteria includes ultrasound findings of shoulder and hip periarthritis in the criteria [36]. Preliminary prospective studies have also looked at the incidence of temporal arteritis diagnosed by ultrasound in patients with PMR [37]. Of 102 patients with "pure" PMR, 8% had ultrasonographic findings consistent with concomitant temporal arteritis. Of the controls, none had a halo sign and four had stenoses. In a case-control study of 176 consecutive patients with newly diagnosed GCA, ultrasound of the temporal, subclavian, axillary, and proximal brachial arteries was performed in all patients with suspected temporal arteritis, PMR, arm claudication, unclear inflammation, or fever of unknown origin. Interestingly, performing axillary artery ultrasound in these patients was found to increase the diagnostic yield for LVV-GCA [38]. These studies suggest that ultrasound has a potential role in diagnosing GCA-LVV in patients presenting initially with symptoms of PMR.

Ultrasound Adjustments for Vasculitis: Proper Equipment and Settings

Proper Equipment, B-Mode, and Color Doppler Adjustments

The intima media thickness (IMT) is the part of the artery that can be evaluated by ultrasound. IMT is "the area of tissue starting at the luminal edge of the artery and ending at the boundary between the media and the adventitia" [39]. The measurement of IMT is performed from the internal hypoechoic line to the external hyperechoic line (Fig. 16.1). In vasculitis, due to inflammatory changes, the IMT appears thickened and hypoechoic, while in atherosclerosis it appears hyperechoic.

Color Doppler use is highly advised, and one can acquire information on flow characteristics (aliasing, persisting diastolic phase, or retrograde flow) that can assist in the diagnosis of ambivalent cases [40]. Duplex ultrasonography (the combination of grayscale, color Doppler and flow patterns) can also be used to indirectly obtain information on stenotic areas proximal or distal to the studied arterial segment. Ultrasound can also be useful in patients with retrograde flow (e.g., subclavian steel syndrome).

To examine the thoracic aorta, a low-frequency transducer is required, preferably a curvilinear (abdominal) or a phased array (cardiac) probe. The aortic valve and the ascending aorta can be examined with low resolution. The major part of the descending aorta remains inaccessible by ultrasound, although the use of an invasive transesophageal probe could potentially provide some visualization. The abdominal aorta also requires a low-frequency probe (6 MHz-curved array); it can sometimes be difficult to obtain images of satisfactory quality in patients with large body habitus or after a meal. Therefore, examination of the abdominal aorta in a fasting individual is highly advised.

The infra-aortic vessels (iliac, femoral, popliteal artery) can be easily visualized by ultrasound and are often affected in GCA patients [3]. Nevertheless, due to the common occurrence of atherosclerotic changes in older individuals observed in these arteries and limited time for ultrasound scanning, we advise the examination of the infra-aortic vessels only in patients presenting with claudication symptoms of the lower extremities.

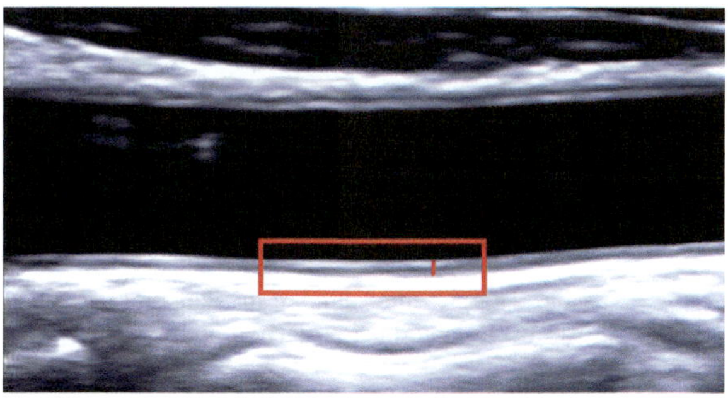

Fig. 16.1 The intima media complex thickness (red vertical line) of the carotid artery in a healthy young individual

Atherosclerosis is considered the main diagnostic challenge in ultrasonography for vasculitis. Even so, atherosclerosis is present in the majority of patients appearing nonhomogeneous and hyperechoic (due to calcifications). In addition, atherosclerosis rarely affects the temporal and axillary arteries. A hypoechoic, thickened IMC, localized in the bifurcation in elderly individuals, should always raise the suspicion of atherosclerosis (soft plaque) and should be distinguished from vasculitis. *See* Fig. 16.2.

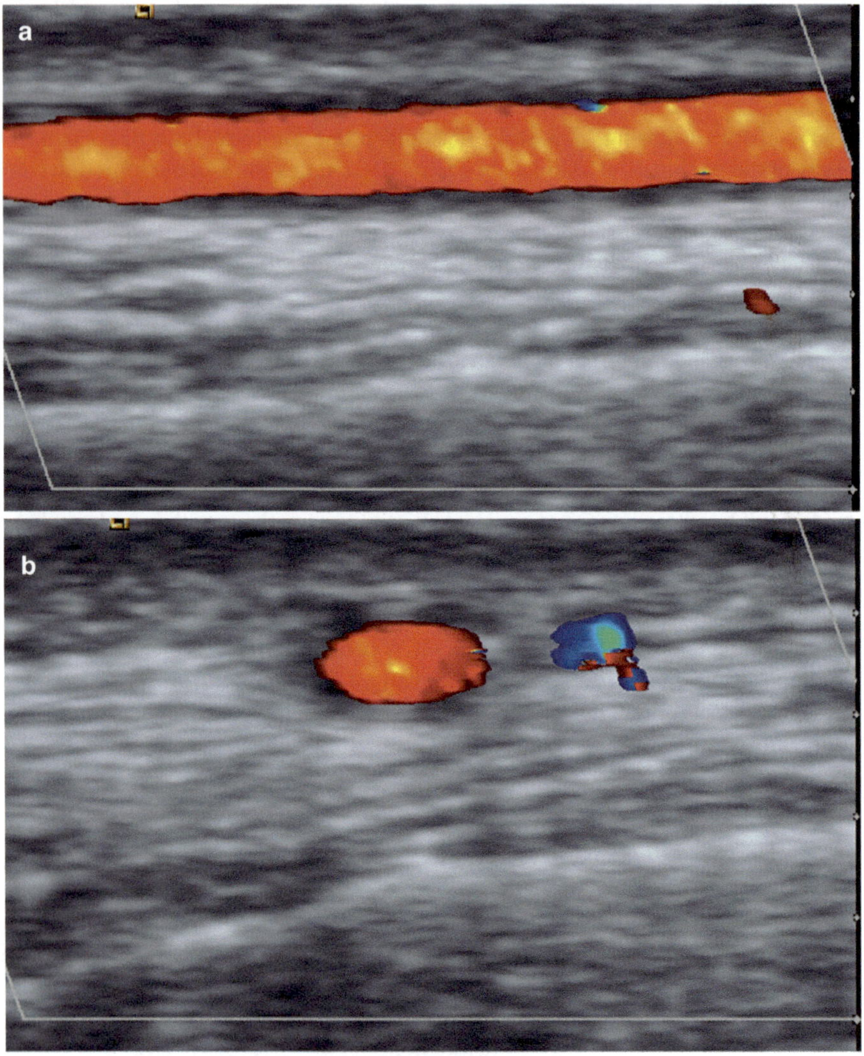

Fig. 16.2 Color Doppler ultrasound of the temporal parietal artery of a patient with generalized atherosclerosis. (**a**) Longitudinal view (**b**) transverse view

B-Mode Adjustments

The examination should start with proper adjustment of the ultrasound equipment. To perform vascular ultrasonography, use of high-end equipment is required. The temporal artery has a diameter from 1.7 mm for the main branch to 0.7–0.8 mm for the facial and parietal branches [7]. Consecutively, a transducer with an axial resolution theoretically less than 0.7 and practically less than 0.4 mm should be used. This necessitates a transducer with a frequency of at least 10 MHz. The newer ultrasound machines are equipped with 18 MHz transducers, which warrant a spatial resolution of approximately 0.15 mm. The distal part of the facial artery and the proximal part of the occipital artery are also easy accessible due to their superficial position [13, 14]. The diameter of the facial and occipital arteries is approximately the same as that of the common branch of the temporal artery.

It is important for the examination of the cranial arteries to keep the axial resolution as high as possible; thus the highest available frequency should be chosen. The depth of the examination should be kept at 1.5 cm or less for the temporal artery and facial artery and at 2–2.5 cm for the occipital artery. The B-mode gain should permit the identification of the hypoechoic IMC thickness seen in vasculitis, and, therefore, very low gain (too dark images) or very high gain (too bright images) should be avoided. To improve the contrast, a reduction of dynamic range should be considered.

For the large vessels and especially the deeper ones, a lower frequency should be used. This allows better penetration and imaging of the deeper structures but at the cost of lower resolution. In patients with large body habitus, a curvilinear transducer can be useful for the examination of the brachiocephalic trunk and subclavian arteries. For the carotid, subclavian, and brachiocephalic trunk in patients with normal habitus, a multifrequency linear transducer is usually enough. Some ultrasound equipment vendors offer transducers especially for vascular examination; however, such equipment is usually not required (Table 16.2).

Table 16.2 B and color Doppler adjustments for the examination of the cranial and large vessels

Artery	Frequency of the B-mode	Frequency of the color Doppler	Pulse repetition frequency (PRF)	Comments
Temporal, facial	Higher possible	7–10 MHz	2 KHz	
Occipital	Higher possible	~ 6 MHz	1.5 KHz or lower	
Carotid	10–15 MHz	6 MHz	3.5 KHz	
Subclavian	10–15 MHz or lower (obese patients)	6 MHz or lower	3.5 KHz	In obese patients, consider the use of curvilinear transducer
Axillary	Higher possible	6–10 MHz	3.5 KHz	
Abdominal aorta	3–6 MHz	3–6 MHz	1–1.5 KHz	Curvilinear transducer

Color Doppler Adjustments

It is important to remember that color Doppler is different from power Doppler. With power Doppler, one is getting information on energy from the movement of the blood cells; in color Doppler, also known as color flow Doppler, it is the direction of the movement that will be measured. This is directly a consequence of the Doppler shift equation, and one needs to keep in mind that an angle of 90 degrees gives a zero Doppler shift and thus no color inside the blood vessel. An angle of insonation between 30 and 60 degrees is preferred (Fig. 16.3).

Pitfalls

Vascular ultrasonography requires appropriate training and correct adjustment of ultrasound equipment settings. Otherwise, the risk of overcalling inflammatory changes in the vessel wall or to overdiagnose GCA is high. Below we present the most common pitfalls and ways to avoid them.

Not Steering the Color Box

Solution Steer the color box appropriately in order for the sound waves to meet the blood flow in an angle between 30 and 60 degrees (Fig. 16.1).

Pseudohalo

This could be due to low color gain or high PRF and in deep vessels because of high Doppler frequency (Fig. 16.3).

Solution Adjust the color gain correctly in healthy individuals before examining patients suspected to have GCA. Adjust the PRF appropriately. Lower the color Doppler frequency when examining deep vessels. Try to keep the color box as small as possible. Use the compression maneuver (Table 16.1; Fig. 16.4).

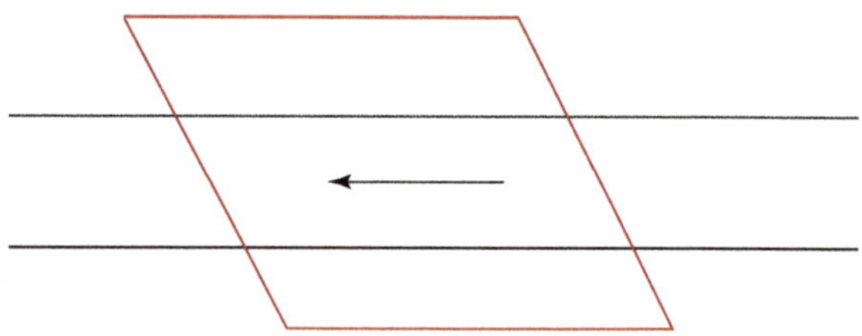

Fig. 16.3 The correct adjustment of the color box is between 30 and 60 degrees

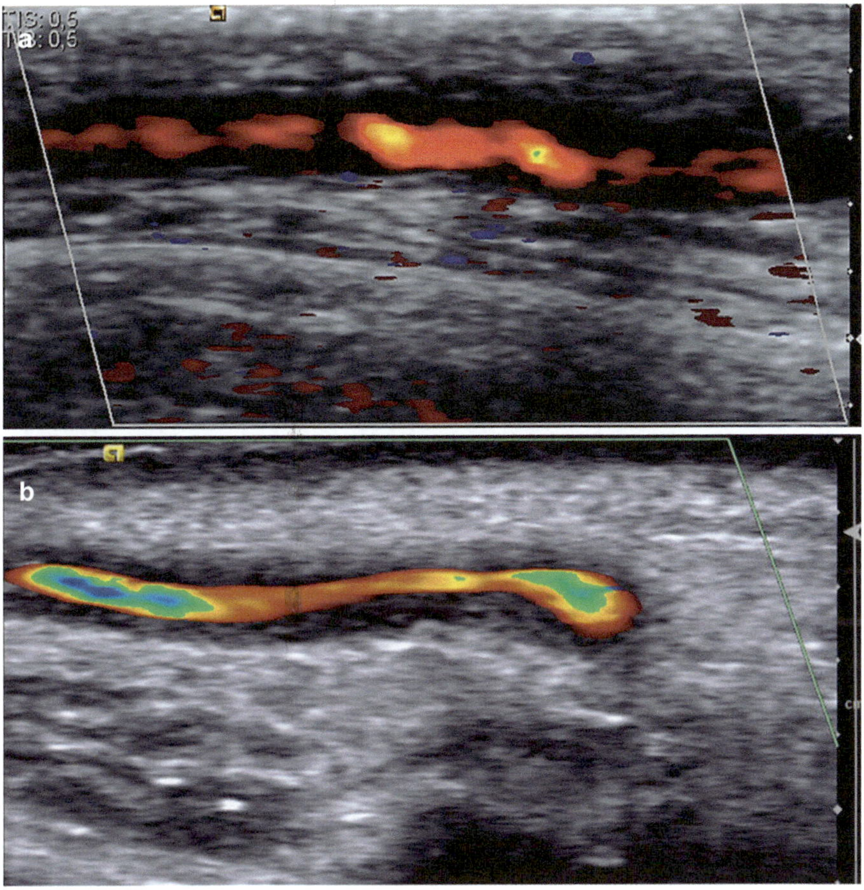

Fig. 16.4 False halo in the temporal artery due to low color gain. The "thickness" of the vessel wall appears anechoic (**a**) and no hypoechoic as it should be expected in a patient with vasculitis (**b**)

Blooming

The color that exceeds beyond the artery walls. In such a case, the color gain is too high or PRF is too low (Fig. 16.5).

Solution Adjust the color gain and PRF accordingly.

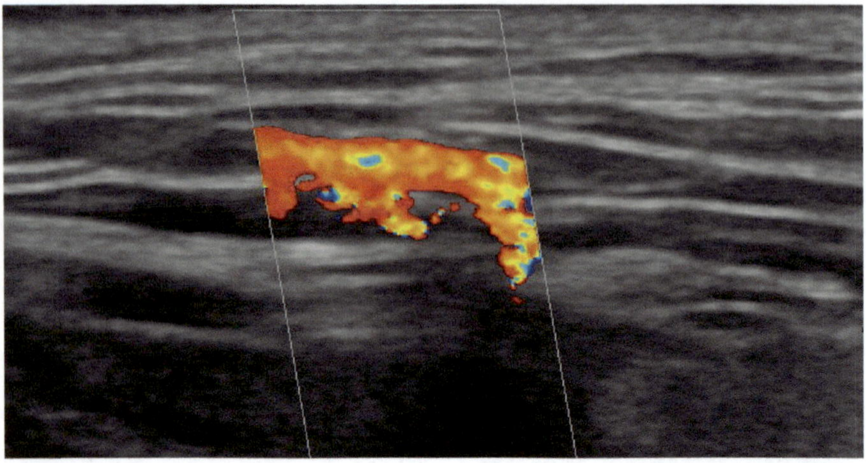

Fig. 16.5 Blooming in the temporal artery due to high color gain. The color extends beyond the vessel wall

Hair

Solution Raise the B-gain, use copious amounts of gel, and gently press the transducer toward cranium.

Use of Power and Not Color Doppler

The margins of power Doppler are often unclear, and a black rim around the color is often present. In addition, no information on aliasing (mixing of colors due to stenosis) can be seen.

Solution Use color Doppler.

Atherosclerosis

Atherosclerosis is seen in the majority of the patients as hyperechoic, nonhomogeneous, and localized plaques (Fig. 16.2).

Solution Examine 30 control patients in their cranial and supraaortic vessels before advancing to the examination of GCA patients.

The IMC Thickness Disappears with Treatment

Solution Patients suspected to have GCA should be evaluated as soon as possible after the initiation of corticosteroids, optimally before the treatment is started.

Inflammatory Changes Due to Other Diseases (Infection, Other Systemic Vasculitides, Amyloidosis, etc.)

Solution Obtain appropriate clinical and laboratory evaluation of every patient suspected to have GCA.

Normal Vascular Ultrasound Anatomy and Examination Techniques

Temporal Artery

1. Start the examination in the front of the ear longitudinally (Fig. 16.6).
2. Proceed to the parietal branch until the top of the head and then turn transversely (Fig. 16.7).
3. Continue transversely to bifurcation and identify the frontal artery longitudinally (Fig. 16.8).
4. Follow the frontal branch up to frontal area and then transversely backward to bifurcation.
5. Terminate with the examination in transverse view of the common branch (Fig. 16.6).

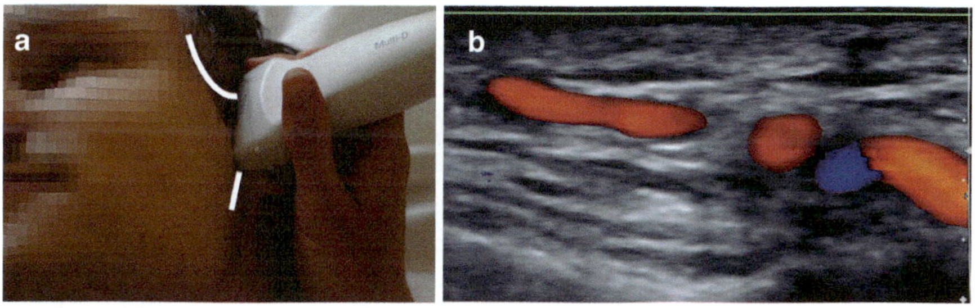

Fig. 16.6 Examination of the common temporal branch (**a**, **b**)

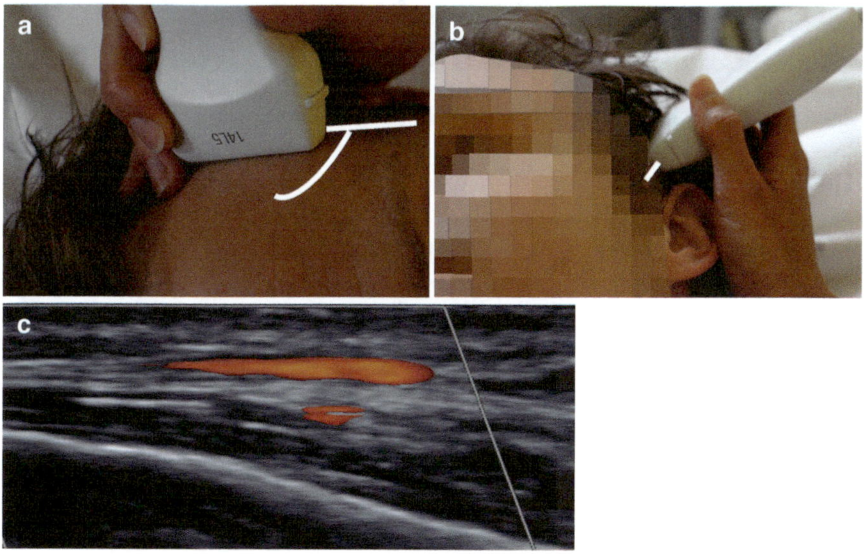

Fig. 16.7 Examination of the temporal parietal branch (**a**–**c**)

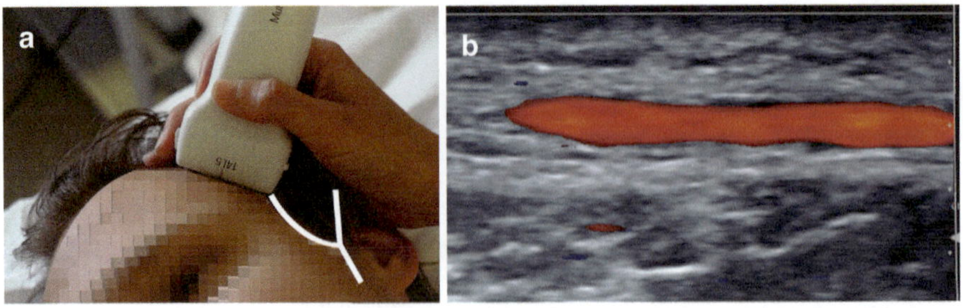

Fig. 16.8 Examination of the temporal frontal branch (**a**, **b**)

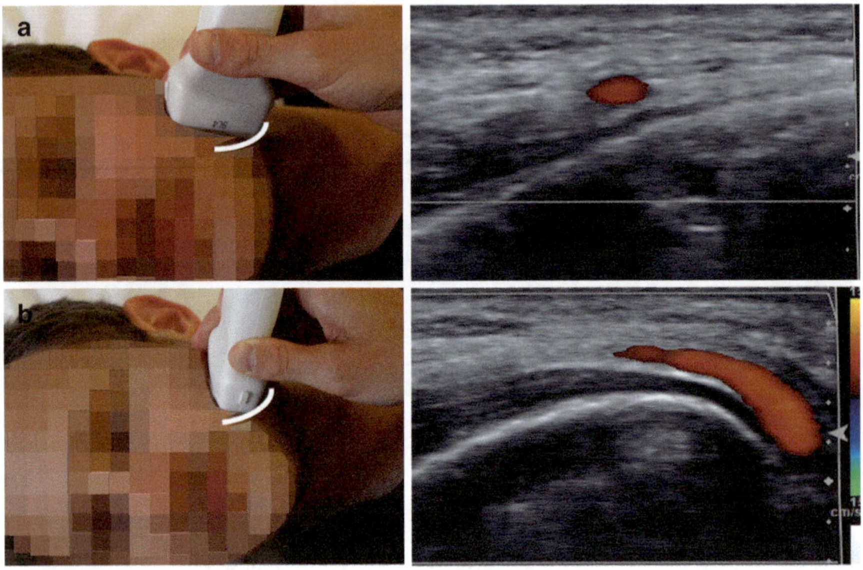

Fig. 16.9 Examination of the facial artery: (**a**) longitudinal and (**b**) transverse views

Distal Facial Artery

1. The examination starts with the identification of the facial artery in transverse view in the middle of the jaw.
2. A longitudinal view is obtained by switching the probe parallel to mandible (Fig. 16.9).

Carotid Artery

1. Start the examination at the middle of neck just above the clavicle in transverse view.
2. The artery should be followed in the whole length proximally to the clavicle and distally to skull base. Internal and external arteries should be identified.

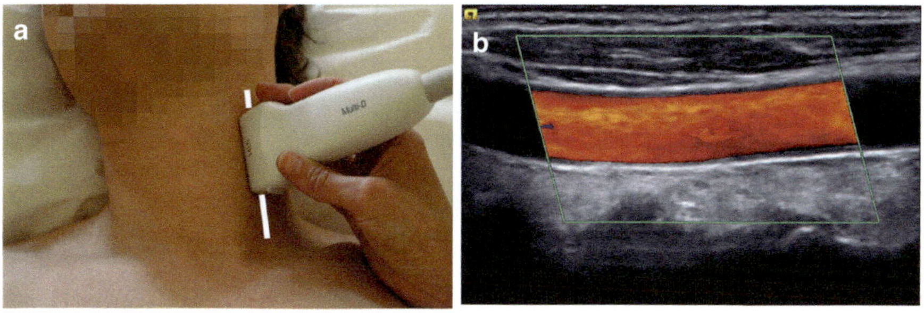

Fig. 16.10 Examination of the carotid artery: (**a**) longitudinal and (**b**) transverse view

3. Thereafter an evaluation in longitudinal plane should be performed, and the IMC thickness is measured at the thickest point both in longitudinal and transverse planes (Fig. 16.10).

Subclavian Artery

1. Identify the carotid artery in transverse plan: then follow the artery proximal; the probe should now be in contact with the clavicle, and the subclavian artery arises longitudinally at the left side of the screen.
2. Follow the subclavian artery distally to the beginning of clavicle.
3. Rotate the probe to get transverse views.
4. The vertebral artery lies just distally to carotid. Identify the beginning for stenosis occlusions (Fig. 16.11).

Axillary Artery

1. The transducer is placed in the infraclavicular fossa (transversal plan), and the artery is identified and followed along its course to the axilla distally.
2. The proximal and distal parts of the artery are identified both transversely and longitudinally.
3. The examination should be continued distally until the brachial artery is visible in the upper arm from a medial position.
4. In occlusion, the artery in B-mode can mistakenly been taken as normal (hypoechogenicity of the artery wall inflammation).
5. Use color Doppler to confirm the existence of normal blood flow (Fig. 16.12).

Abdominal Aorta

1. Use a curved transducer with a low frequency (3.5–5 MHz).
2. Identify the aorta just below the diaphragm transversely.
3. The vessel is followed in transverse orientation down to the separation into the iliac arteries (aortic bifurcation).
4. Continue with an evaluation in the longitudinal plane (Fig. 16.13).

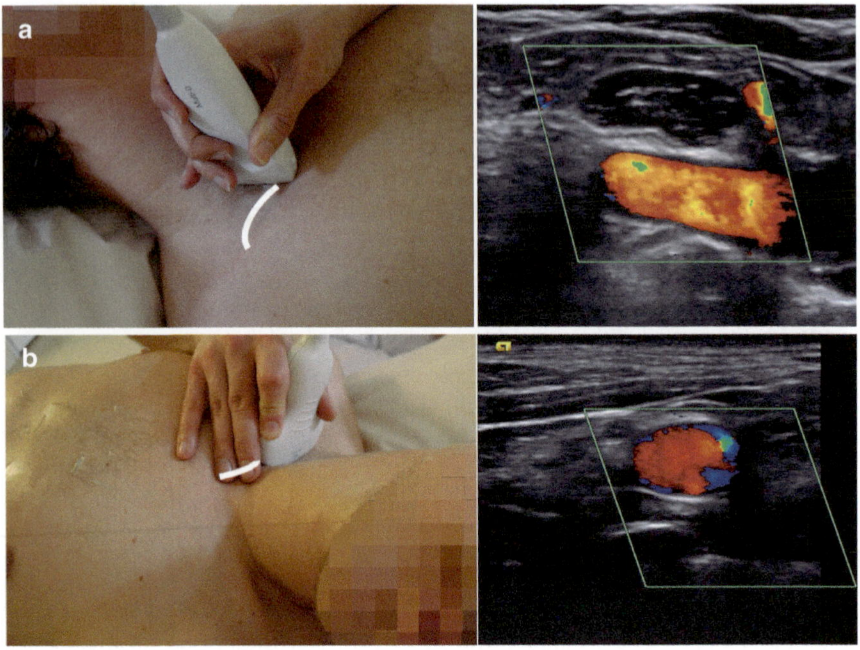

Fig. 16.11 Examination of the subclavian artery: (**a**) longitudinal and (**b**) transverse view

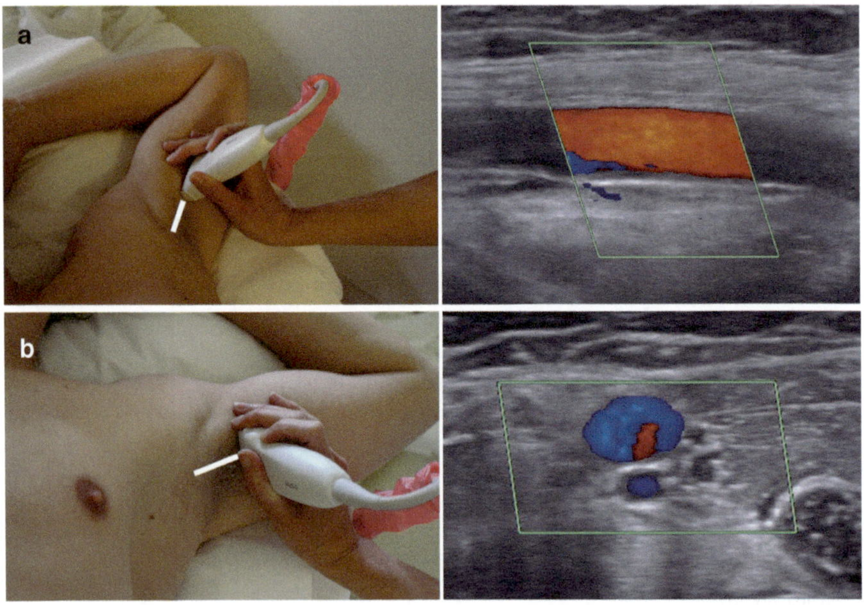

Fig. 16.12 Examination of the axillary artery: (**a**) longitudinal and (**b**) transverse view

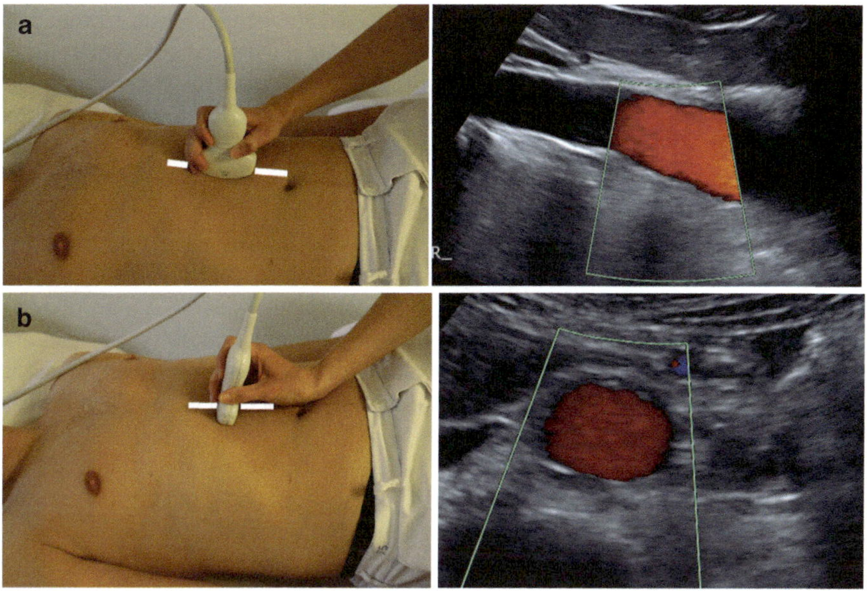

Fig. 16.13 Examination of the abdominal aorta: (**a**) longitudinal and (**b**) transverse view

Sonopathology in Large-Vessel Vasculitis

The inflammation of the vessel wall is visualized by ultrasound by the *halo sign* defined as a homogenous, hypoechoic wall thickening, well delineated toward the luminal side, visible both in longitudinal and transverse planes, most commonly concentric in transverse scans [7, 8, 41]. It has also been described to look similar to a ring (circumferential) or a half moon (eccentric) [7, 8]. In some cases, due to long-standing disease (especially in Takayasu's arteritis patients), the appearance of the edematous wall can be mid-echoic. The vertebral artery lies laterally to carotid artery, and while is not often involved in GCA or TA should be examined in older patients with vertebrobasilar stroke of unknown etiology or when stenosis or occlusion of the proximal part of the left subclavian or innominate artery is suspected (retrograde flow). In addition, with use of color Doppler, important information on blood flow characteristics can be collected. With duplex ultrasonography, information on velocity and pulsatility of the blood flow can be obtained. However, these techniques are more advanced and out of the scope of this book.

Vasculitis (increased IMC thickness) should be visualized in both transverse and longitudinal planes. If it is possible, video clips of the examination should be obtained and kept with the patient's stored images.

In the presence of a suspected halo, the *compression sign*, where one sonopalpates the probe to compress the artery walls together, can also be performed and measured [7, 41]. A compression sign is considered positive when the thickened arterial wall remains visible upon compression; the hypoechogenic vasculitic vessel wall thickening contrasts with the mid-echogenic to hyperechogenic surrounding tissue. Excellent reliability of the definitions for normal temporal and axillary arteries, "halo" sign, and "compression" sign has been shown with inter-rater agreements of 91–99% on web-based assessments and K inter/intra-rater reliabilities 0.83–0.98 [41]. The "halo" and "compression" signs are regarded as the most important ultrasound abnormalities for GCA.

Recently, an ultrasonographic halo score was developed to quantify the extent of vascular inflammation and investigate its diagnostic accuracy and association with clinical factors in GCA [42]. This prospective study included 89 patients suspected of having GCA of whom 58 had a confirmed clinical diagnosis of GCA after 6-month follow-up. Bilateral ultrasound examination of the three temporal artery segments and axillary arteries were completed, prior to temporal artery biopsy. The extent of vascular inflammation was quantified by (1) counting the number of temporal and axillary artery segments with a halo and (2) calculating a composite halo score that also incorporated the thickness of each halo. Halo counts and halo scores were found to have moderate diagnostic accuracy for a clinical diagnosis of GCA and correlated positively with systemic inflammation. When compared with the halo count, the halo score correlated better with CRP levels and allowed to firmly establish the diagnosis of GCA in more patients. Higher halo counts and halo scores were associated with a higher risk of ocular ischemia [42]. The halo score is also being investigated, not only for diagnostic purposes but also as a prognostic and disease monitoring tool [43].

Cranial Arteritis

Temporal Arteritis

Figure 16.14 shows a longitudinal and transverse view.

Facial Arteritis

Figure 16.15 shows a longitudinal and transverse view.

Supraaortic Arteritis

Carotid Arteritis

Figure 16.16 shows a longitudinal and transverse view.

Subclavian Arteritis

Figure 16.17 shows a longitudinal and transverse view.

Axillary Arteritis

Figure 16.18 shows a longitudinal and transverse view.

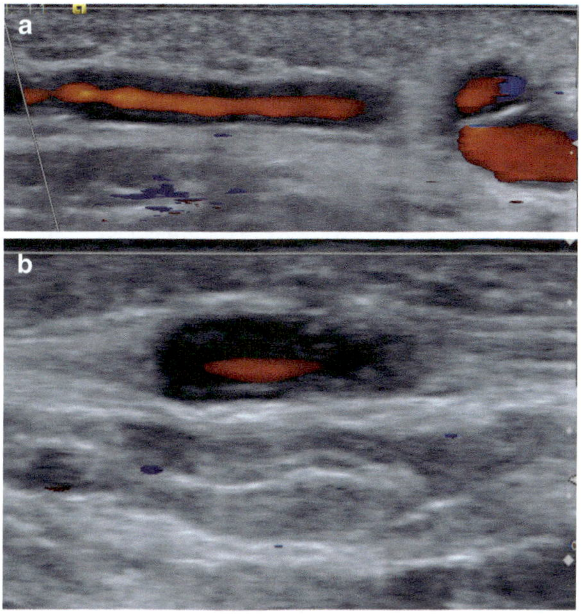

Fig. 16.14 Temporal arteritis (**a**) longitudinal and (**b**) transverse view

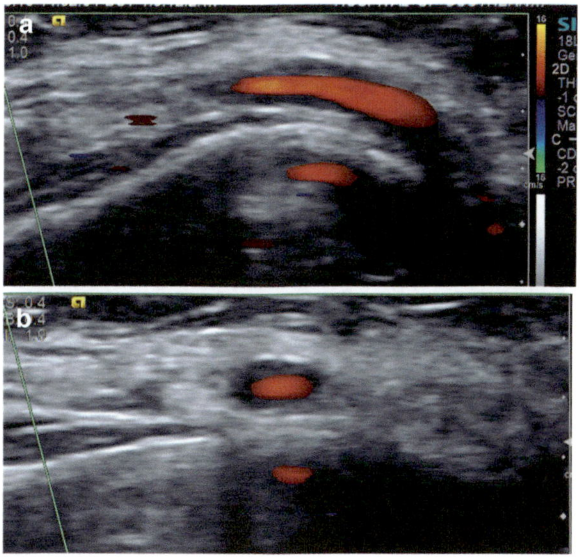

Fig. 16.15 Facial arteritis (**a**) longitudinal and (**b**) transverse view

Abdominal Aortitis

Figure 16.19 shows a longitudinal and transverse view.

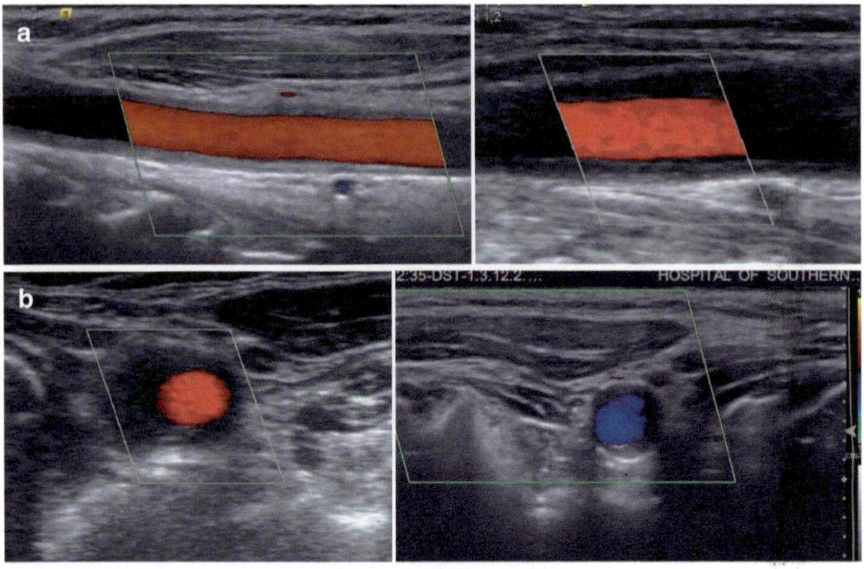

Fig. 16.16 Carotid arteritis (**a**) longitudinal and (**b**) transverse view

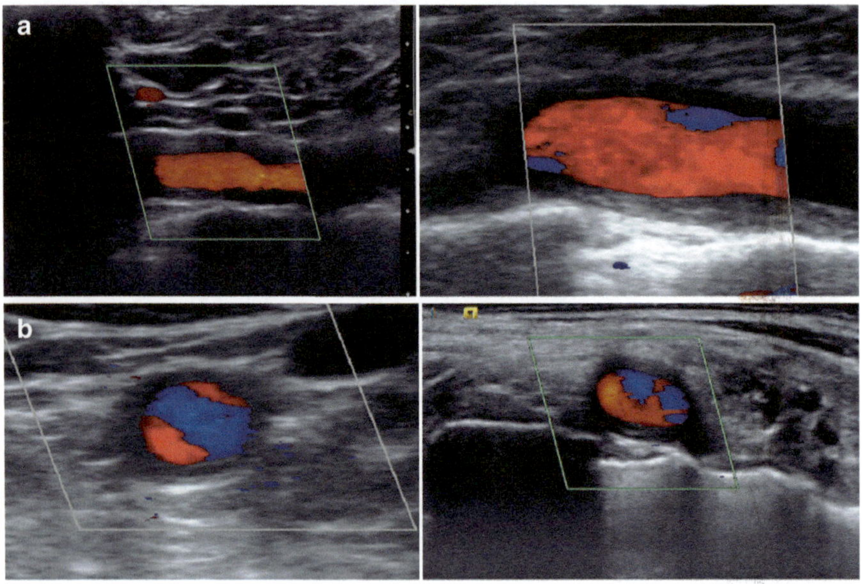

Fig. 16.17 Subclavian arteritis (**a**) longitudinal and (**b**) transverse view

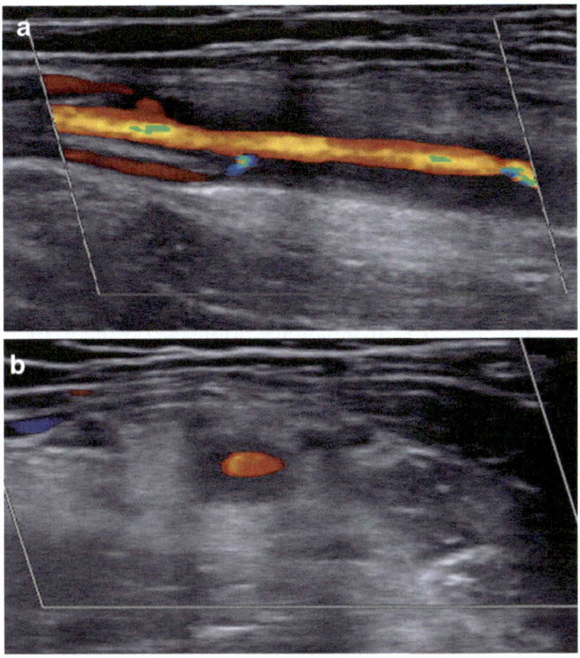

Fig. 16.18 Axillary arteritis (**a**) longitudinal and (**b**) transverse view

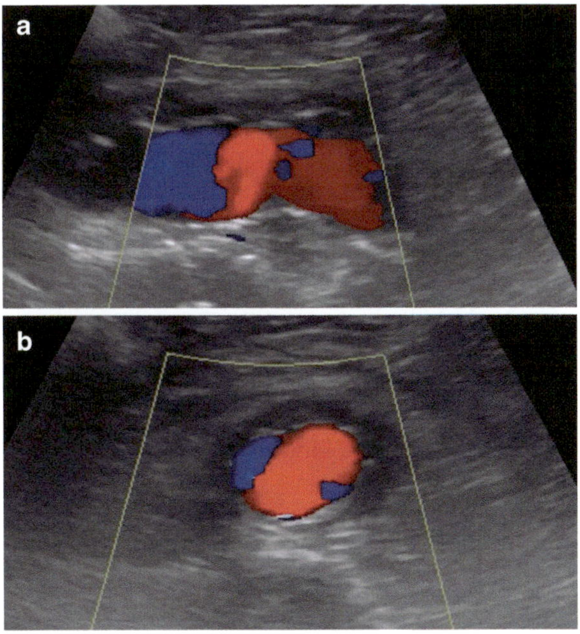

Fig. 16.19 Abdominal aortitis (**a**) longitudinal and (**b**) transverse view

Review Questions

1. What is the intima media complex (IMC) thickness?
   (a) The distance between the upper and lower borders of the color flow
   (b) The distance between the outer and the inner hyperechoic lines on the vessel wall
   (c) The distance between the outer anechoic and inner hyperechoic lines on the vessel wall
   (d) None of the above
2. Why should one steer the window in color Doppler ultrasound examination?
   (a) To get more stable images while moving the transducer
   (b) To get sufficient color filling according to the Doppler swift acquisition
   (c) To visualize the whole length of the artery
   (d) No need to steer the window
3. Which diseases can present with halo sign in the temporal arteries?
   (a) GCA
   (b) Other medium vessel vasculitides
   (c) Infections
   (d) All the above
4. How do you avoid a false halo in a patient with thick hair?
   (a) Apply hard pressure with the transducer
   (b) Shave the hair
   (c) Use copious amounts of gel
   (d) Apply gently pressure with the transducer
   (e) c and d
5. Which is the appropriate frequency and PRF adjustment of the color Doppler in order to examine the cranial arteries?
   (a) 10 MHz and 2.0 MHz
   (b) 3.5 MHz for the frequency and 2 MHz for the PRF
   (c) As low as possible for the frequency and PRF
   (d) 13 MHz and 5 MHz
6. Why is it important to use high-end ultrasound equipment to visualize the temporal artery?
   (a) Because you are able to visualize the whole temporal artery with excellent resolution and not miss inflammation
   (b) Because it is easier to perform ultrasound with high-end equipment
   (c) Because the power Doppler is performing excellent in high-end equipment
   (d) a and b
7. How often are the blood vessels in under extremities affected in GCA (ultrasound evaluation)?
   (a) Never
   (b) 20%
   (c) 50%
   (d) 90%

8. Which are the supraaortic arteries that are routinely evaluated in GCA patients?
   (a) None, we do not need to perform ultrasound of large vessels in GCA, the disease affects only the cranial arteries
   (b) Carotid, axillary, subclavian arteries
   (c) Vertebral artery, cervicocephalic trunk, mastic artery
   (d) Carotid arteries
9. Which is the difference between color and power Doppler?
   (a) Only the color
   (b) No difference – we can use both equally in the examination of blood vessels
   (c) Color Doppler is measuring the velocity while power Doppler the energy
   (d) Power Doppler is more sensitive than color Doppler in visualizing intimal wall inflammation
10. What is the sensitivity of color Doppler of temporal artery and large vessels in GCA diagnostics according to recent studies?
   (a) 20%
   (b) 55%
   (c) 80%
   (d) 100%

Answers

1. (b) The distance between the outer and the inner hyperechoic lines on the vessel wall
2. (b) To get sufficient color filling according to the Doppler swift acquisition
3. (d) All the above
4. (e) c and d
5. (a) 10 MHz and 2.0 MHz
6. (d) a and b
7. (c) 50%
8. (b) Carotid, axillary, subclavian arteries
9. (c) Color Doppler is measuring the velocity while power Doppler the energy
10. (c) 80%

References

1. Jennette JC, Falk RJ, Bacon PA, Basu N, Cid MC, Ferrario F, et al. 2012 revised international Chapel Hill consensus conference nomenclature of Vasculitides. Arthritis Rheum. 2013;65(1):1–11.
2. Grayson PC, Maksimowicz-McKinnon K, Clark TM, Tomasson G, Cuthbertson D, Carette S, et al. Distribution of arterial lesions in Takayasu's arteritis and giant cell arteritis. Ann Rheum Dis. 2012;71(8):1329–34.
3. Aschwanden M, Kesten F, Stern M, Thalhammer C, Walker UA, Tyndall A, et al. Vascular involvement in patients with giant cell arteritis determined by duplex sonography of 2x11 arterial regions. Ann Rheum Dis. 2010;69(7):1356–9.
4. Kang T, Lanni S, Nam J, Emery P, Wakefield RJ. The evolution of ultrasound in rheumatology. Ther Adv Musculoskelet Dis. 2012;4(6):399–411.

5. Salvarani C, Silingardi M, Ghirarduzzi A, Lo Scocco G, Macchioni P, Bajocchi G, et al. Is duplex ultrasonography useful for the diagnosis of giant-cell arteritis? Ann Intern Med. 2002;137(4):232–8.
6. Menkes CJ, Branche I, Feldmann JL, Chauveau M, Delbarre F. Application of the Doppler effect to the detection of Horton's temporal arteritis. La Nouvelle Presse Medicale. 1981;10(28):2371.
7. Schmidt WA, Kraft HE, Vorpahl K, Volker L, Gromnica-Ihle EJ. Color duplex ultrasonography in the diagnosis of temporal arteritis. N Engl J Med. 1997;337(19):1336–42.
8. Diamantopoulos AP, Haugeberg G, Hetland H, Soldal DM, Bie R, Myklebust G. The diagnostic value of color Doppler ultrasonography of temporal arteries and large vessels in giant cell arteritis: a consecutive case series. Arthritis Care Res. 2013;66(1):113–9.
9. Jennifer Piper ASS, Ponte C, Singh S, Dasgupta B, Schmidt WA, McNally E, Diamantopoulos A, Hutchings A, Luqmani R. A diagnostic protocol for giant cell arteritis using ultrasound assessment. Rheumatology (Oxford). 2015;54(suppl 1):i33-i.
10. Arida A, Kyprianou M, Kanakis M, Sfikakis PP. The diagnostic value of ultrasonography-derived edema of the temporal artery wall in giant cell arteritis: a second meta-analysis. BMC Musculoskelet Disord. 2010;11:44.
11. Karassa FB, Matsagas MI, Schmidt WA, Ioannidis JP. Meta-analysis: test performance of ultrasonography for giant-cell arteritis. Ann Intern Med. 2005;142(5):359–69.
12. Ball EL, Walsh SR, Tang TY, Gohil R, Clarke JM. Role of ultrasonography in the diagnosis of temporal arteritis. Br J Surg. 2010;97(12):1765–71.
13. Schmidt WA, Natusch A, Moller DE, Vorpahl K, Gromnica-Ihle E. Involvement of peripheral arteries in giant cell arteritis: a color Doppler sonography study. Clin Exp Rheumatol. 2002;20(3):309–18.
14. Pfadenhauer K, Weber H. Giant cell arteritis of the occipital arteries–a prospective color coded duplex sonography study in 78 patients. J Neurol. 2003;250(7):844–9.
15. Germano G, Muratore F, Cimino L, Lo Gullo A, Possemato N, Macchioni P, et al. Is colour duplex sonography-guided temporal artery biopsy useful in the diagnosis of giant cell arteritis? A randomized study. Rheumatology (Oxford). 2014;54(3):400–4.
16. Ghinoi A, Pipitone N, Nicolini A, Boiardi L, Silingardi M, Germano G, et al. Large-vessel involvement in recent-onset giant cell arteritis: a case-control colour-Doppler sonography study. Rheumatology (Oxford). 2011;51(4):730–4.
17. Czihal M, Tato F, Forster S, Rademacher A, Schulze-Koops H, Hoffmann U. Fever of unknown origin as initial manifestation of large vessel giant cell arteritis: diagnosis by colour-coded sonography and 18-FDG-PET. Clin Exp Rheumatol. 2010;28(4):549–52.
18. Forster S, Tato F, Weiss M, Czihal M, Rominger A, Bartenstein P, et al. Patterns of extracranial involvement in newly diagnosed giant cell arteritis assessed by physical examination, colour coded duplex sonography and FDG-PET. Vasa. 2011;40(3):219–27.
19. Czihal M, Tato F, Rademacher A, Kuhlencordt P, Schulze-Koops H, Hoffmann U. Involvement of the femoropopliteal arteries in giant cell arteritis: clinical and color duplex sonography. J Rheumatol. 2012;39(2):314–21.
20. Czihal M, Zanker S, Rademacher A, Tato F, Kuhlencordt PJ, Schulze-Koops H, et al. Sonographic and clinical pattern of extracranial and cranial giant cell arteritis. Scand J Rheumatol. 2012;41(3):231–6.
21. Blockmans D, Bley T, Schmidt W. Imaging for large-vessel vasculitis. Curr Opin Rheumatol. 2009;21(1):19–28.
22. Schmidt WA, Krause A, Schicke B, Wernicke D. Color Doppler ultrasonography of hand and finger arteries to differentiate primary from secondary forms of Raynaud's phenomenon. J Rheumatol. 2008;35(8):1591–8.
23. Diamantopoulos AP, Haugeberg G, Hetland H, Soldal DM, Myklebust G. "Fast track" giant cell arteritis outpatient clinic: A useful tool to reduce the morbidity of the disease?. EULAR Madrid 2013.
24. Schmidt WA. Role of ultrasound in the understanding and management of vasculitis. Ther Adv Musculoskelet Dis. 2014;6(2):39–47.

25. Bley TA, Reinhard M, Hauenstein C, Markl M, Warnatz K, Hetzel A, et al. Comparison of duplex sonography and high-resolution magnetic resonance imaging in the diagnosis of giant cell (temporal) arteritis. Arthritis Rheum. 2008;58(8):2574–8.
26. Schmidt WA. Imaging in vasculitis. Best Pract Res Clin Rheumatol. 2013;27(1):107–18.
27. Pipitone N, Versari A, Salvarani C. Role of imaging studies in the diagnosis and follow-up of large-vessel vasculitis: an update. Rheumatology (Oxford). 2008;47(4):403–8.
28. HelseNorge. MR-undersøkelse (magnetisk resonans). Available from: https://helsenorge.no/Sykdomogbehandling/Sider/MR-undersokelse.aspx.
29. Prieto-Gonzalez S, Arguis P, Garcia-Martinez A, Espigol-Frigole G, Tavera-Bahillo I, Butjosa M, et al. Large vessel involvement in biopsy-proven giant cell arteritis: prospective study in 40 newly diagnosed patients using CT angiography. Ann Rheum Dis. 2012;71(7):1170–6.
30. Kissin EY, Merkel PA. Diagnostic imaging in Takayasu arteritis. Curr Opin Rheumatol. 2004;16(1):31–7.
31. Duftner C, Dejaco C, Sepriano A, Falzon L, Schmidt WA, Ramiro S. Imaging in diagnosis, outcome prediction and monitoring of large vessel vasculitis: a systematic literature review and meta-analysis informing the EULAR recommendations. RMD Open. 2018;4(1):e000612.
32. Dejaco C, Ramiro S, Duftner C, Besson FL, Bley TA, Blockmans D, et al. EULAR recommendations for the use of imaging in large vessel vasculitis in clinical practice. Ann Rheum Dis. 2018;77(5):636–43.
33. Mackie SL, Dejaco C, Appenzeller S, et al. British Society for Rheumatology guideline on diagnosis and treatment of giant cell arteritis: executive summary. Rheumatology (Oxford). 2020;59(3):487–94.
34. Wu TH, Kuo HC, Tain YL, Lin KM, Kuo HC, Chien SJ. Common carotid artery intima-media thickness is useful for diagnosis of the acute stage of Kawasaki disease. BMC Pediatr. 2014;14:98.
35. Baer AZ, Rubin LG, Shapiro CA, Sood SK, Rajan S, Shapir Y, et al. Prevalence of coronary artery lesions on the initial echocardiogram in Kawasaki syndrome. Arch Pediatr Adolesc Med. 2006;160(7):686–90.
36. Dasgupta B, Cimmino MA, Kremers HM, Schmidt WA, Schirmer M, Salvarani C, et al. 2012 provisional classification criteria for polymyalgia rheumatica: a European League Against Rheumatism/American College of Rheumatology collaborative initiative. Arthritis Rheum. 2012;64(4):943–54.
37. Schmidt WA, Gromnica-Ihle E. Incidence of temporal arteritis in patients with polymyalgia rheumatica: a prospective study using colour Doppler ultrasonography of the temporal arteries. Rheumatology (Oxford). 2002;41(1):46–52.
38. Schmidt WA, Seifert A, Gromnica-Ihle E, Krause A, Natusch A. Ultrasound of proximal upper extremity arteries to increase the diagnostic yield in large-vessel giant cell arteritis. Rheumatology (Oxford). 2008;47(1):96–101.
39. Touboul PJ, Hennerici MG, Meairs S, Adams H, Amarenco P, Bornstein N, et al. Mannheim carotid intima-media thickness and plaque consensus (2004-2006-2011). An update on behalf of the advisory board of the 3rd, 4th and 5th watching the risk symposia, at the 13th, 15th and 20th European Stroke Conferences, Mannheim, Germany, 2004, Brussels, Belgium, 2006, and Hamburg, Germany, 2011. Cerebrovasc Dis. 2012;34(4):290–6.
40. Schmidt WA. Ultrasound in vasculitis. Clin Exp Rheumatol. 2014;32(1 Suppl 80):S71–7.
41. Chrysidis S, Duftner C, Dejaco C, et al. Definitions and reliability assessment of elementary ultrasound lesions in giant cell arteritis: a study from the OMERACT Large Vessel Vasculitis Ultrasound Working Group. RMD Open. 2018;4(1):e000598.
42. van der Geest KSM, Borg F, Kayani A, et al. Novel ultrasonographic halo score for giant cell arteritis: assessment of diagnostic accuracy and association with ocular ischaemia. Ann Rheum Dis. 2020;79(3):393–9.
43. Sebastian A, van der Geest KSM, Coath F, et al. Halo score (temporal artery, its branches and axillary artery) as a diagnostic, prognostic and disease monitoring tool for Giant Cell Arteritis (GCA). BMC Rheumatol. 2020;4:35. Published 2020 Aug 18. https://doi.org/10.1186/s41927-020-00136-5.

17 Salivary Gland Ultrasound for Sjögren's Syndrome

Eugene Y. Kissin and Veronika Sharp

Key Points
- Ultrasound is a noninvasive technique that can be used to scan the entire parotid and submandibular glands in orthogonal planes.
- Salivary gland ultrasonography improves the diagnostic performance of the 2012 American College of Rheumatology classification criteria for Sjögren's syndrome.
- Increased parenchymal inhomogeneity correlates with poorer prognostic features.
- Differential diagnoses of Sjögren's syndrome based on ultrasound features should be considered, including sarcoidosis and IgG4-related disease.

Introduction

Sjögren's syndrome is a systemic autoimmune disease that targets the salivary and lacrimal glands resulting in decreased saliva and tear production and dryness. There are established clinical, laboratory, radiological, and pathological criteria that are used in suspected cases to diagnose the disease, but these are not highly specific,

E. Y. Kissin
Division of Rheumatology, Department of Medicine, Boston University Medical Center, Boston, MA, USA
e-mail: eukissin@bu.edu

V. Sharp (✉)
Division of Rheumatology, Department of Medicine, Santa Clara Valley Medical Center, San Jose, CA, USA
e-mail: Veronika.Sharp@hhs.sccgov.org

M. J. Kohler (ed.), *Musculoskeletal Ultrasound in Rheumatology Review*,
https://doi.org/10.1007/978-3-030-73555-5_17

and some tests are invasive. Ultrasound (US) is a noninvasive technique which can be used at the point-of-care and provides valuable information to assist in the diagnosis of Sjögren's syndrome [1].

Salivary Gland Anatomy

For sonographic evaluation for Sjögren's syndrome, the two largest pairs of salivary glands, the parotid and the submandibular glands, are examined.

The parotid gland is the largest of the major salivary glands. It is located in the retromandibular fossa. It is irregular and wedge shaped (Fig. 17.1) [1]. The gland contains a large superficial lobe (80% of the gland) and a smaller deep lobe (20% of the gland). The superficial lobe extends anteriorly over the masseter muscle (overlying the ramus and angle of the mandible). Posteriorly, it is bordered by to the external auditory canal. Proximally, the distal superficial lobe extends from the level of the external auditory canal to the angle of the mandible. The deep, or retromandibular lobe, extends deep into the stylomandibular tunnel posterior to the ramus of the mandible and anterior to the styloid process and the sternocleidomastoid muscle. The superficial and deep lobes do not appear as separate structures on ultrasound. The retromandibular vein and the external carotid artery are located at the border of the two lobes. The retromandibular vein marks the location of the facial nerve which lies just lateral to the vein but is not routinely seen on US [2–4].

The submandibular gland is about half the size of the parotid gland. It is located in the posterior aspect of the submandibular triangle bordered by the body of the mandible laterally, the anterior belly of the digastric muscle medially, and the posterior belly of the digastric muscle posteriorly. It is triangular shaped. The mylohyoid muscle partially indents the gland anteriorly. The facial artery crosses the gland in a tortuous course. The facial vein is located lateral to the gland adjacent to the body of the mandible [2].

The parotid gland contains lymph nodes. The most commonly seen lymph nodes are one visible in the superior pole and one in the inferior pole. There are several regional lymph nodes groups surrounding the submandibular gland, but the submandibular gland itself does not contain lymph nodes. This difference is explained by the embryological development. The parotid gland is encapsulated later, after the formation of lymph nodes, while the submandibular gland is encapsulated early, prior to lymph node formation [2].

The intraglandular ducts within the parotid and submandibular glands are collapsed and not visible or appear as thin linear hyperechoic stripes in a non-stimulated gland [2].

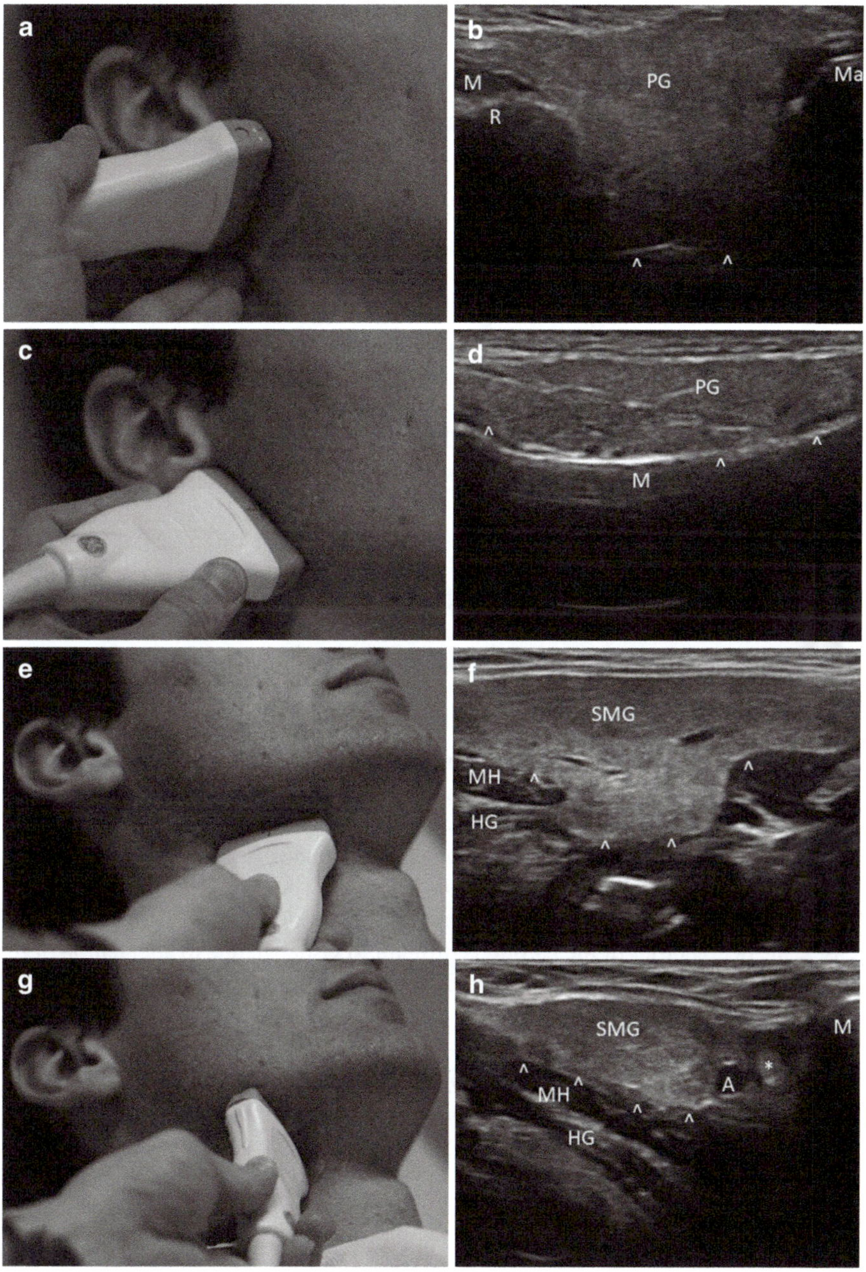

Fig. 17.1 Normal salivary glands. Photographic depiction of the transducer position to obtain the views of the salivary glands: (**a**) transverse/axial view of the parotid gland, (**c**) longitudinal/coronal view of the parotid gland, (**e**) longitudinal/sagittal view of the submandibular gland, and (**g**) transverse/coronal view of the submandibular gland. The corresponding US images are shown: (**b**) transverse parotid gland, (**d**) longitudinal parotid gland, (**f**) longitudinal submandibular gland, and (**h**) transverse submandibular gland. Masseter muscle (M), ramus of the mandible (R), mastoid process (Ma), parotid gland (PG), submandibular gland (SMG), mylohyoid muscle (MH), hyoglossus muscle (HG), facial artery (A), lymph node (*). The arrows (^) show the posterior (deep) border of the glands

Scanning Technique

To scan the parotid and submandibular glands, a linear high-frequency probe is used (preferably 12 MHz or higher frequency). Due to the marked attenuation of the sonographic waves in the parotid gland in some individuals, a lower-frequency probe may be needed to visualize the deep portion of the gland.

To scan either the parotid or submandibular gland, the patient is positioned in a recumbent or semi-recumbent position with the neck slightly extended and rotated to the opposite side of the gland examined. The entire gland is examined in transverse and in longitudinal planes (Fig. 17.1) [2].

The echotexture and homogeneity of the parotid and submandibular glands are compared to the thyroid gland. For this reason, an image of the thyroid gland should also be taken. This is most easily obtained by placing the probe over the trachea in a transverse (axial) plane (Fig. 17.3c) [2].

Power Doppler US of both glands is done for evaluation of hypervascularity of the parenchyma [1].

Ultrasonographic Features of the Normal Salivary Glands

Both the parotid and the submandibular glands are similar to the thyroid in echogenicity and homogeneity. The parotid gland has higher fat content, and therefore, it is hyperechoic compared to the surrounding muscles. The submandibular gland has slightly less fat content than the parotid, but it is still hyperechoic compared to the surrounding muscles. The submandibular gland is lightly more homogeneous in appearance compared to the parotid gland [1]. Lymph nodes may be found in the parotid gland but not within the submandibular gland. Normal lymph nodes are elongated and may contain a hyperechoic hilum with central vessels which may be Doppler positive [2]. The borders of each gland should be well defined. In some cases, the deep border of the parotid is difficult to visualize due to attenuation of the US waves, and lower frequency may be required for examination [4].

Ultrasonographic Features in Sjögren's Syndrome

US is a validated imaging tool for evaluation of Sjögren's syndrome [5]. The disease tends to affect the parotid gland earlier than the submandibular gland [3]. The most characteristic (and most important) change described in Sjögren's syndrome is the development of multiple small, round or oval hypoechoic areas scattered throughout the gland resulting in an inhomogeneous appearance [4]. While these areas resemble cysts, unlike cysts, these do not create posterior acoustic enhancement and are in fact dilated ducts (sialectasis) and destroyed parenchyma filled with lymphocytic infiltrate. The size of these globular collections enlarges with progression of disease as demonstrated with MR sialogram [6]. Increased parenchymal blood flow can be present at times of flare [4].

Scoring and Diagnosis of Sjögren's Syndrome

There are over 30 scoring systems developed for the evaluation of Sjögren's syndrome, but most include evaluation of gland tissue echogenicity, homogeneity, hypoechoic areas, hyperechoic areas, and border clarity. Intra- and interobserver reliability is best for homogeneity [7]. The most extensive scoring system is the Hocevar system which has been reported to show a specificity of 99% and sensitivity of 59% for Sjögren's syndrome when the American-European Consensus group classification criteria served as the gold standard [8]. A scoring system proposed by DeVita et al. on a 0–4 scale was found in a recent meta-analysis to have similar sensitivity and specificity to the Hocevar system but had less heterogeneity of results between studies and is faster to use (Table 17.1) [9, 10]. This scoring system evaluating hypoechoic areas, calcification, and hyperechoic bands was added to the ACR 2012 Sjögren's criteria and showed increased sensitivity and essentially unchanged specificity [11, 12]. Addition of this scoring system to the ACR/EULAR 2016 Sjögren's criteria showed increased accuracy [13]. Unilateral scan of one parotid and one submandibular gland has also been evaluated and showed good predictability of the ACR/EULAR 2016 criteria for Sjögren's syndrome [14]. Recently, a semiquantitative scoring system of salivary gland scan video clips was shown to have good intra-reader and excellent inter-reader reliability [15]. This offers the potential to be used for prognostic and therapeutic studies in the future. Sjögren's disease is characterized by episodic increase in parenchymal blood flow; however, this feature has not been incorporated into scoring systems reliably [1].

Table 17.1 Sjögren's syndrome scoring: the Hocevar and the modified DeVita scoring systems

Author/year Score performance	Characteristics	Score range
Hocevar 2005 Sensitivity 75% Specificity 95%	Parenchymal echogenicity	0–1 (decreased = 1)
	Homogeneity	0–3 (gross inhomogeneous = 3)
	Hypoechoic areas	0–3 (numerous areas = 3)
	Hyperechoic reflections	0–3 parotid (numerous = 3) 0–1 submandibular (present = 1)
	Clearness of gland border	0–3 (border not visible = 3)
		Score range 0–48
DeVita 1992 Sensitivity 75% Specificity 93%	Parenchymal inhomogeneity	0 = normal 1 = few confluent hypoechoic lesions 2 = numerous hypoechoic areas <2 mm 3 = moderate large hypoechoic areas 2–6 mm 4 = severe large hypoechoic areas >6 mm
		Score range 0–4

Differential Diagnoses

While the scattered hypoechoic oval areas with hyperechoic septal lines within the glands are characteristic for Sjögren's syndrome, these are not pathognomonic. Similar changes are found in other diseases resulting in chronic sialadenitis such as sarcoid and other granulomatous diseases, disseminated lymphoma (NHL), HIV-associated salivary gland disease, amyloidosis, and IgG4-related disease (Figs. 17.2 and 17.3) [4]. Other causes of bilateral salivary gland enlargement include diabetes mellitus, alcoholism, liver cirrhosis, and bulimia.

Noninflammatory/Nonmalignant Causes

In a study that recruited 50 consecutive patients with parotid swelling, 35 were found to have sialosis – noninflammatory/nonmalignant causes [16]. Seventeen of these thirty-five (49%) had diabetes mellitus, while nine (26%) had alcoholism, seven (20%) had liver disease, and one had bulimia. Thus, 74% of patients with noninflammatory parotid gland enlargement were accounted for by these four diagnoses. On US, sialosis has been described as enlarged, hyperechoic glandular tissue with a poorly visible deep border but without heterogeneity, hypoechoic lesions, or hyperechoic septae [17]. In diabetes mellitus, these alterations are thought to be due to increased fat content within the glands [18].

IgG4-Related Disease

A recently discovered mimic of Sjögren's syndrome, IgG4-related disease can also cause bilateral salivary gland enlargement, and salivary glands are affected in 27–53% of cases [19]. In a cross-sectional study of 39 patients with IgG4-related disease, 90% showed sonographic signs of disease in the salivary glands with 90% having submandibular gland infiltration compared to 35% in the parotid gland (Tables 17.2, 17.3, and Fig. 17.3) [20, 21]. The most common pattern of infiltration resulted in a superficial hypoechoic pattern (60%), while the multiple hypoechoic, reticulated pattern more typical for Sjögren's was detected in 23% of lesions. A more recent study of nine patient found bilateral, nodular, hyperemic submandibular involvement in 8/9 patients, but none in the parotid glands [22]. See Fig. 17.4 for an example of submandibular disease in IgG4-related disease.

HIV-Associated Disease

Oval, hypoechoic lesions diffusely distributed though glandular parenchyma can be seen in Sjögren's as well as HIV-associated salivary gland disease, granulomatous disease, acute inflammation, lymphoma, and hematogenous metastases [23]. In

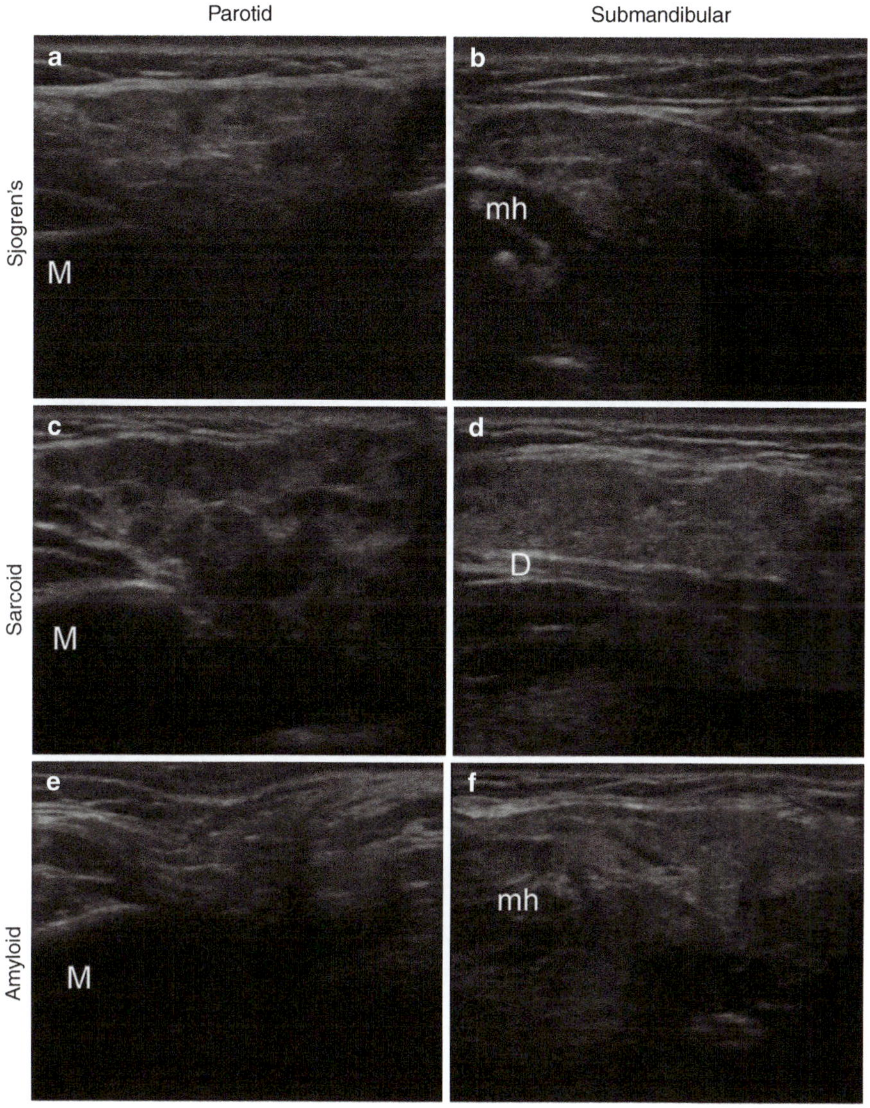

Fig. 17.2 Chronic sialadenitis. US image of (**a**) the parotid gland and the (**b**) submandibular gland in Sjögren's syndrome. US image of the (**c**) parotid gland and the (**d**) submandibular gland in sarcoidosis. US image of the (**e**) parotid and (**f**) submandibular gland in amyloidosis. Note the multiple intraglandular "cyst"-like changes in all three conditions as well as gland tissues hypoechogenicity relative to the thyroid gland tissue. Mandible (M), mylohyoid muscle (mh), anterior belly of the digastric muscle (D)

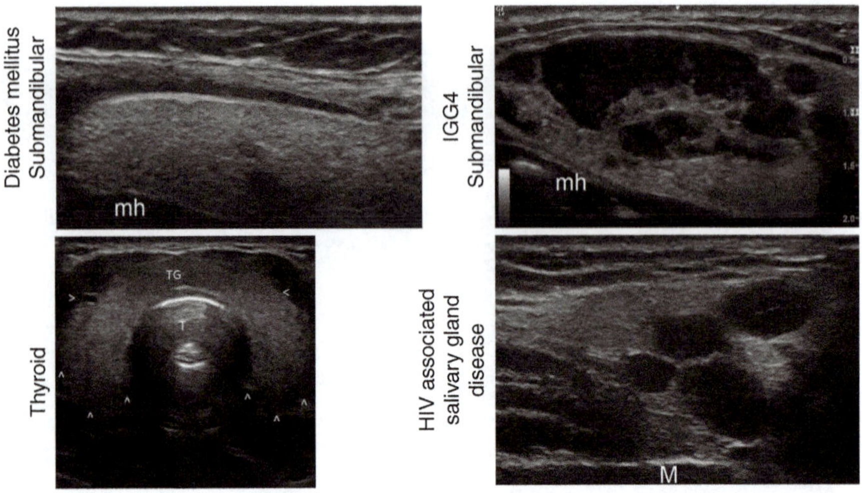

Fig. 17.3 Chronic sialadenitis. US image of the (**a**) submandibular gland in diabetes mellitus, (**b**) submandibular gland in IgG4-related disease, (**c**) normal thyroid, (**d**) parotid gland in HIV-associated salivary gland disease. Note the hyperechoic gland in diabetes and the large size of the cysts in HIV

Table 17.2 Ultrasound features of conditions with bilateral salivary gland enlargement

Disease	Parotid/ submandibular	Doppler	Diffuse/ focal	Echogenicity
Sjögren's	Both	+/−	Diffuse	Hypo
Sarcoid	Both	+/−	Diffuse or focal	Hypo
Amyloid	Both	+/−	Diffuse	Hypo
IgG4	Submandibular	+	Focal	Hypo
Diabetes mellitus	Both	−	Diffuse	Hyper
Diffuse Infiltrative Lymphocytosis syndrome (DILS)	Parotid	+/−	Focal	Iso

diffuse infiltrative lymphocytosis syndrome (DILS), the nodules are particularly large and represent multiple lymphoepithelial cysts. In distinction, benign lymphoepithelial lesions in HIV have been described to produce ultrasound findings from simple cysts to mixed masses with solid components. Benign lymphoepithelial lesions in HIV differ from Sjögren's in that they are usually larger, fewer, more focal, and without change in echogenicity of the surrounding gland tissue and spare the submandibular glands (Fig. 17.3) [24].

Table 17.3 Comparison of US features of conditions which can cause bilateral salivary gland enlargement

Condition	Echogenicity	Infiltrate heterogeneity	Gland distribution
Sjögren's	Hypo	Multiple hypoechoic "cysts"	Parotid = submandibular
Sarcoidosis	Hypo	Multiple hypoechoic "cysts"	Parotid = submandibular
Amyloidosis	Hypo	Multiple hypoechoic "cysts"	Parotid = submandibular
IgG4	Hypo	Infiltrated hypoechoic masses > hypoechoic "cysts"	Submandibular > parotid
Benign lymphoepithelial lesions in HIV	Iso	Large, few "cysts"	Parotid > submandibular
Diabetes mellitus	Hyper	None	Parotid = submandibular

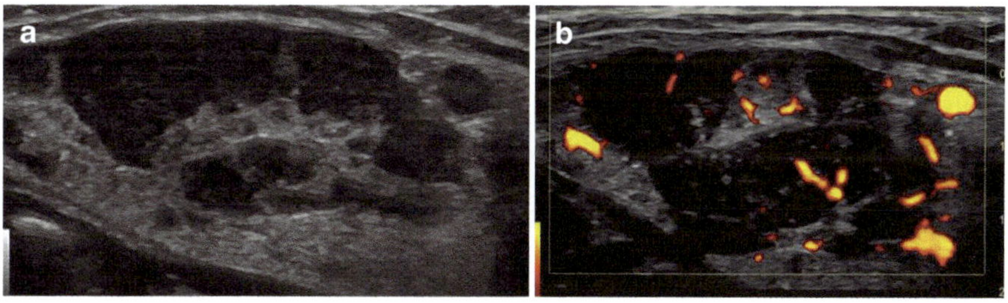

Fig. 17.4 Ultrasound image example of IgG4-related submandibular disease in gray scale and with power Doppler activity. (Image courtesy of Minna Kohler, MD, RhMSUS)

Sarcoidosis, Amyloidosis

Sarcoidosis involvement of the salivary glands has not been extensively studied by ultrasonography. A case series of six patients describes two with rounded hypoechoic nodules of various sizes throughout the parenchyma similar to what is described in Sjögren's, while two others had echogenic septa without the hypoechoic nodules [25]. Our own experience with 27 patients with sarcoidosis is that US-detectable lesions are seen in about a third of the patients, involving both parotid and submandibular glands, and appear similar to Sjögren's (Fig. 17.2).

We could find only one published article reporting US imaging of AA amyloidosis of the salivary gland. This article noted "ill-defined hypoechoic nodules" of the parotid glands [26]. Their description matches our own experience with 22 patients with AL amyloidosis where lesions were again similar to what is seen in Sjögren's syndrome and involve both parotid and submandibular glands (Fig. 17.2).

Ultrasound in Prognostication and Therapeutic Response

Sjögren's syndrome is a slowly progressive disease. US features were evaluated in early disease at baseline and nearly 2 years later, and no significant change was found in the sonographic features of the glands [27]. Therapeutic response was evaluated in two randomized controlled trials using rituximab. In the TRACTISS study, definition of the deep (posterior) border of the glands improved with therapy [28]. In the TEARS study, improvement in parotid and submandibular gland echotexture was observed after rituximab therapy [29]. Higher baseline gland involvement correlated with poorer therapeutic response to rituximab [30]. Increased parenchymal inhomogeneity does correlate with poorer prognostic features [5]. Further US research is needed to better define damage, improve reader reliability, and define the role of US in disease surveillance.

Conclusion

Salivary gland US is a noninvasive technique that can be easily used in the office to visualize parotid and submandibular glands in orthogonal planes. Scoring systems have been developed to better characterize sonographic features that can differentiate a normal gland from a disease-affected gland. Salivary gland US has been shown to improve the diagnostic performance of the 2012 American College of Rheumatology classification criteria for Sjögren's syndrome. There is great potential for future work to further develop the role of US in prognostication and disease surveillance in Sjögren's syndrome, as well as other diseases affecting the salivary gland. Studies are ongoing to evaluate novel techniques such as sonoelastography and use of artificial intelligence in image interpretation to enhance the role of US in these disease processes [31].

Review Questions

1. Which ultrasound feature of the parotid and submandibular glands has the best reliability for detection of Sjögren's syndrome?
   (a) Presence of hyperechoic bands
   (b) Presence of parenchymal calcifications
   (c) Presence of scattered round or oval anechoic areas
   (d) Indistinct appearance of the deep glandular borders
2. Sonographic appearance of the normal submandibular gland is:
   (a) Hyperechoic compared to the surrounding muscles
   (b) Less echogenic than the thyroid gland
   (c) Less homogeneous than the parotid gland
   (d) More echogenic than the parotid gland
3. Simplified scoring that was added to the ACR 2012 and the ACR/EULAR 2016 criteria for Sjögren's syndrome to improve diagnostic accuracy includes all except:
   (a) Presence of hypoechoic areas

   (b) Presence of Doppler signal
   (c) Presence of echogenic bands
   (d) Presence of calcifications
4. Which of the following causes of chronic sialadenitis is much more likely to affect the submandibular gland than the parotid gland?
   (a) Sjögren's syndrome
   (b) Sarcoidosis
   (c) IgG4-related disease
   (d) Benign lymphoepithelial lesions in HIV
5. What is the optimal ultrasound probe and choice of frequency for examination of the parotid glands?
   (a) Phased array probe
   (b) Curved probe with low frequency
   (c) Linear probe with high frequency
   (d) Linear probe with low frequency
6. Which salivary glands are routinely examined with ultrasound for evaluation for Sjögren's syndrome?
   (a) The parotid and the sublingual glands
   (b) The parotid and the submandibular glands
   (c) The submandibular and the sublingual glands
   (d) The parotid, submandibular, and sublingual glands
7. Can lymph nodes be detected in normal salivary glands with ultrasound?
   (a) No, there are no lymph nodes in normal salivary glands.
   (b) Yes, lymph nodes can be found in normal submandibular glands but not in the parotid glands.
   (c) Yes, lymph nodes can be found in the normal parotid glands but not in the normal submandibular glands.
   (d) Yes, lymph nodes can be found in both the normal parotid and submandibular salivary glands.
8. What is the appearance of the salivary glands in noninflammatory diseases that cause salivary gland enlargement such as diabetes mellitus, alcoholism, liver disease, or bulimia?
   (a) Heterogeneous, hyperechoic parenchyma with well-defined posterior border
   (b) Homogeneous, hyperechoic parenchyma with poorly visible posterior border
   (c) Heterogeneous parenchyma with hypoechoic oval lesions and hyperechoic septae
   (d) Homogeneous hypoechoic parenchyma with well-defined posterior border
9. What are the characteristic ultrasound findings of the major salivary glands that differ between benign lymphoepithelial lesions in HIV and Sjögren's syndrome?
   (a) Benign lymphoepithelial lesions are larger, fewer, and more focal.
   (b) Benign lymphoepithelial lesions in HIV are larger, fewer, but present more diffusely.

   (c) Benign lymphoepithelial lesions in HIV are larger, more abundant, and present more diffusely.
   (d) Benign lymphoepithelial lesions in HIV are smaller, more abundant, and present more diffusely.
10. Which of the following causes of chronic sialadenitis usually does not affect the submandibular gland?
   (a) Sarcoidosis
   (b) Amyloidosis
   (c) Sjögren's syndrome
   (d) Benign lymphoepithelial disease of HIV

Answers

1. (c) The most characteristic (and most important) change described in Sjögren's syndrome is the development of multiple small, round or oval hypoechoic areas scattered throughout the gland resulting in inhomogeneous appearance [4]. These are dilated ducts and destructed parenchyma filled with lymphocytic infiltrate. While hyperechoic bands (fibrous tissue), calcifications, and indistinct deep (posterior) border are also features of Sjögren's, these have been found to have lower intra- and inter-reader reliability [7].
2. (a) The submandibular gland has slightly less fat content than the parotid, but it is still hyperechoic compared to the surrounding muscles and has similar echogenicity to the thyroid gland. Both salivary glands are homogeneous similar to the thyroid, but the submandibular gland is slightly more homogeneous in appearance compared to the parotid gland [1].
3. (b) A simplified version of the Hocevar scoring system evaluating for the presence or absence of hypoechoic areas, calcification, and hyperechoic bands was added to the ACR 2012 Sjögren's criteria and showed increased sensitivity and essentially unchanged specificity [11, 12]. Addition of this scoring system to the ACR/EULAR 2016 Sjögren's criteria showed increased accuracy [13].
4. (c) IgG4 disease affects the submandibular gland 90% of the time compared to 35% in the parotid gland [21]. The glands are affected relatively evenly in Sjögren's syndrome and sarcoidosis. The submandibular gland is typically spared in benign lymphoepithelial lesions in HIV [24].
5. (c) In general, linear probe with high frequency (12 MHz or higher frequency) is preferred to examine the parenchyma or the salivary glands. A lower frequency is needed to visualize the posterior border of the gland due to marked attenuation of the ultrasound waves in the parotid gland in a portion of patients [2].
6. (b) For sonographic evaluation for Sjögren's syndrome, the largest salivary glands, the parotid, and the submandibular glands are examined. The parotid glands and the submandibular glands are much larger than the sublingual glands; therefore, it is easier to evaluate the parenchyma of these glands for abnormalities [2].
7. (c) The normal parotid gland contains lymph nodes. Commonly, one lymph node is seen in the superior pole and one in the inferior pole with ultrasound.

The submandibular gland does not contain lymph nodes, but several regional lymph nodes can be found surrounding the gland with ultrasound [2].

8. (b) Noninflammatory diseases affecting the salivary glands that cause glandular enlargement such as diabetes mellitus, alcoholism, liver disease, and bulimia present as homogeneous hyperechoic glandular parenchyma on ultrasound exam. The gland is enlarged and is hyperechoic due to increased fat content. The posterior border is poorly visible due to attenuation of the ultrasound waves in the hyperechoic glandular parenchyma [18].
9. (a) Benign lymphoepithelial lesions differ from Sjögren's in that the lesions are usually larger, fewer, and more focal. Additionally, unlike in Sjögren's syndrome, there is no change of echogenicity of the surrounding glandular tissue, and the submandibular gland is spared [24].
10. (d) Benign lymphoepithelial disease of HIV usually spares the submandibular glands. Sarcoidosis, amyloidosis, and Sjögren's affect both the parotid glands and the submandibular glands [4, 24, 25, 26].

References

1. Jousse-Joulin S. Salivary glands. In: Essential applications of musculoskeletal ultrasound in rheumatology. Philadelphia: Elsevier/Saunders; 2010. p. 199–206.
2. Bhatia KSS, Dai Y-L. Routine and advanced ultrasound of major salivary glands. Neuroimaging Clin N Am. 2018;28(2):273–93.
3. Curtin HD, Som PM, editors. Head and neck imaging. St. Louis: Mosby; 2011.
4. Bialek EJ, Jakubowski W, Zajkowski P, Szopinski KT, Osmolski A. US of the major salivary glands: anatomy and spatial relationships, pathologic conditions, and pitfalls. Radiogr Rev Publ Radiol Soc N Am Inc. 2006;26(3):745–63.
5. Martire MV, Santiago ML, Cazenave T, Gutierrez M. Latest advances in ultrasound assessment of salivary glands in Sjögren syndrome. J Clin Rheumatol Pract Rep Rheum Musculoskelet Dis. 2018;24(4):218–23.
6. Kojima I, et al. Diagnostic performance of MR imaging of three major salivary glands for Sjögren's syndrome. Oral Dis. 2017;23(1):84–90.
7. Jousse-Joulin S, et al. Salivary gland ultrasound abnormalities in primary Sjögren's syndrome: consensual US-SG core items definition and reliability. RMD Open. 2017;3(1):e000364.
8. Hočevar A, Ambrožič A, Rozman B, Kveder T, Tomšič M. Ultrasonographic changes of major salivary glands in primary Sjögren's syndrome. Diagnostic value of a novel scoring system. Rheumatology. 2005;44(6):768–72.
9. Zhou M, et al. Diagnostic accuracy of salivary gland ultrasonography with different scoring systems in Sjögren's syndrome: a systematic review and meta-analysis. Sci Rep. 2018;8(1):17128.
10. De Vita S, Lorenzon G, Rossi G, Sabella M, Fossaluzza V. Salivary gland echography in primary and secondary Sjögren's syndrome. Clin Exp Rheumatol. 1992;10(4):351–6.
11. Cornec D, et al. Salivary gland ultrasonography improves the diagnostic performance of the 2012 American College of Rheumatology classification criteria for Sjögren's syndrome. Rheumatol Oxf Engl. 2014;53(9):1604–7.
12. Cornec D, et al. Contribution of salivary gland ultrasonography to the diagnosis of Sjögren's syndrome: toward new diagnostic criteria? Arthritis Rheum. 2013;65(1):216–25.
13. Takagi Y, et al. Combined classification system based on ACR/EULAR and ultrasonographic scores for improving the diagnosis of Sjögren's syndrome. PLoS One. 2018;13(4):e0195113.

14. Mossel E, et al. Scoring hypoechogenic areas in one parotid and one submandibular gland increases feasibility of ultrasound in primary Sjögren's syndrome. Ann Rheum Dis. 2018;77(4):556–62.
15. Jousse-Joulin S, et al. Video clip assessment of a salivary gland ultrasound scoring system in Sjögren's syndrome using consensual definitions: an OMERACT ultrasound working group reliability exercise. Ann Rheum Dis. 2019;78(7):967–73.
16. Scully C, Bagán JV, Eveson JW, Barnard N, Turner FM. Sialosis: 35 cases of persistent parotid swelling from two countries. Br J Oral Maxillofac Surg. 2008;46(6):468–72.
17. Gritzmann N, Rettenbacher T, Hollerweger A, Macheiner P, Hübner E. Sonography of the salivary glands. Eur Radiol. 2003;13(5):964–75.
18. Lindeberg H, Andersen L. The size and composition of the submandibular glands in late-onset diabetes. Arch Otorhinolaryngol. 1987;244(2):100–3.
19. Puxeddu I, Capecchi R, Carta F, Tavoni AG, Migliorini P, Puxeddu R. Salivary gland pathology in IgG4-related disease: a comprehensive review. J Immunol Res. 2018;2018:6936727.
20. Li W, et al. Ultrasonographic features of immunoglobulin G4-related sialadenitis. Ultrasound Med Biol. 2016;42(1):167–75.
21. Shimizu M, et al. Effectiveness of imaging modalities for screening IgG4-related dacryoadenitis and sialadenitis (Mikulicz's disease) and for differentiating it from Sjögren's syndrome (SS), with an emphasis on sonography. Arthritis Res Ther. 2015;17:223.
22. Shimizu M, et al. Sonographic diagnosis for Mikulicz disease. Oral Surg Oral Med Oral Pathol Oral Radiol Endod. 2009;108(1):105–13.
23. Białek EJ, Jakubowski W. Mistakes in ultrasound examination of salivary glands. J Ultrason. 2016;16(65):191–203.
24. Martinoli C, Pretolesi F, Del Bono V, Derchi LE, Mecca D, Chiaramondia M. Benign lymphoepithelial parotid lesions in HIV-positive patients: spectrum of findings at gray-scale and Doppler sonography. AJR Am J Roentgenol. 1995;165(4):975–9.
25. Teymoortash A, Werner JA. Parotid gland involvement in sarcoidosis: sonographic features. J Clin Ultrasound. 2009;37(9):507–10.
26. Cho CM, et al. Unusual parotid gland lesions: a pictorial review. J Clin Ultrasound. 2013;41(8):501–8.
27. Gazeau P, Cornec D, Jousse-Joulin S, Guellec D, Saraux A, Devauchelle-Pensec V. Time-course of ultrasound abnormalities of major salivary glands in suspected Sjögren's syndrome. Joint Bone Spine Rev Rhum. 2018;85(2):227–32.
28. Fisher BA, et al. Effect of rituximab on a salivary gland ultrasound score in primary Sjögren's syndrome: results of the TRACTISS randomised double-blind multicentre substudy. Ann Rheum Dis. 2018;77(3):412–6.
29. Jousse-Joulin S, et al. Brief report: ultrasonographic assessment of salivary gland response to rituximab in primary Sjögren's syndrome. Arthritis Rheumatol. 2015;67(6):1623–8.
30. Cornec D, et al. High-grade salivary-gland involvement, assessed by histology or ultrasonography, is associated with a poor response to a single rituximab course in primary Sjögren's syndrome: data from the TEARS randomized trial. PLoS One. 2016;11(9):e0162787.
31. Devauchelle-Pensec V, Zabotti A, Carvajal-Alegria G, Filipovic N, Jousse-Joulin S, De Vita S. Salivary gland ultrasonography in primary Sjögren's syndrome: opportunities and challenges. Rheumatology. 2019:kez079. https://doi.org/10.1093/rheumatology/kez079.

Lung Ultrasound for Rheumatic Diseases

18

Karina D. Torralba, Vaneet K. Sandhu, and Anna M. Lafian

Key Points

- Point-of-care lung ultrasound has comparable efficacy to high-resolution computed tomography in detecting interstitial lung disease, even in its early stages.
- Lung ultrasound is a feasible skill for rheumatologists to acquire, based on using knowledge about artifacts to differentiate normal versus pathologic lung.
- Lung ultrasound has been studied in patients with rheumatic disease, particularly systemic sclerosis and rheumatoid arthritis.

Introduction

Ultrasonography entails emission of high-frequency sound through tissue via a transducer. Reflection of the ultrasound beam back to the transducer at tissue interfaces projects a directed image. The attenuating effects of bone (chest wall cage) and air (lungs) have historically limited the use of lung ultrasound [1, 2]. However, a progressive understanding of the sonographic appearance of diseased lung states, where the air-fluid balance is disrupted resulting in an acoustic mismatch between the lung and the surrounding tissues allowing for greater tissue penetration, has led

K. D. Torralba (✉) · V. K. Sandhu · A. M. Lafian
Division of Rheumatology, Department of Medicine, Loma Linda University School of Medicine, Loma Linda, CA, USA
e-mail: ktorralba@llu.edu

M. J. Kohler (ed.), *Musculoskeletal Ultrasound in Rheumatology Review*,
https://doi.org/10.1007/978-3-030-73555-5_18

to the widespread adoption of point-of-care or bedside lung ultrasound (LUS), especially in the critical care or emergency department.

Considered part of "critical care ultrasound," LUS offers advantages over chest X-ray (CXR) and high-resolution computed tomography (HRCT) which collectively involve radiation and transportation to a radiology unit that may not be feasible for critically ill patients. The International Liaison Committee on Lung Ultrasound (ILC-LUS) for the International Consensus Conference on Lung Ultrasound (ICC-LUS) released evidence-based recommendations for point-of-care lung ultrasound in the evaluation of various pulmonary pathologies, highlighting its ease of use and efficacy in detecting pathology over other imaging modalities [3].

With musculoskeletal ultrasound (MSUS) being widely used in rheumatology practice, the translatability of such knowledge and skill sets toward ultrasound evaluation of lung manifestations in connective tissue diseases (CTDs) needs to be considered and has already demonstrated achievability. Gasho et al. demonstrated that a training program (initiated by pulmonology fellows and faculty for their musculoskeletal ultrasound (MSUS)-experienced rheumatology counterparts) comprised of a combination of didactics, hands-on scanning sessions, and case-based scanning enabled sustained competency in LUS skills and knowledge within a 6-month period [4]. In context, cardiologists who took LUS training had a significant learning curve entailing a maximum of ten examinations [5]. It is possible for rheumatologists who have MSUS experience and a basic understanding of artifacts to more easily learn LUS. Point-of-care ultrasound (POCUS) is increasingly being taught in many medical schools and residency programs to teach basic and clinical medicine; trainees entering rheumatology fellowship may have had prior experience with LUS due to early POCUS exposure [6].

The purpose of this chapter is to provide rheumatologists an overview of the role of ultrasound in the evaluation of lung pathologies in CTDs. We also seek to provide a context for rheumatologists, whether with or without experience in MSUS, on the potential role of LUS in the evaluation of pulmonary manifestations of rheumatic diseases. More detailed and in-depth discussions on specific areas may require additional reading, and specific references have been recommended.

Lung Involvement in Rheumatic Diseases

Lung manifestations are common in CTDs [7–18] (Table 18.1).

Most studies of lung disease in CTDs have focused on interstitial lung disease (ILD) and pleural diseases. ILD, also known as interstitial pneumonia (IP), manifests in several major CTDs such as systemic sclerosis (SSc), rheumatoid arthritis (RA), and systemic lupus erythematosus (SLE). Nonspecific interstitial pneumonia (NSIP) and usual interstitial pneumonia (UIP) are the most common types of ILD found in CTDs [19]. It is estimated that 15% of patients presenting with a diagnosis of ILD were diagnosed with a CTD at the time of evaluation. About 25% of ILDs occur in patients with undiagnosed CTD [20]. Interstitial pneumonia with autoimmune features (IPAF) is a term used to describe ILD in patients with features of a CTD but not

Table 18.1 Lung manifestations of major rheumatic diseases

	Interstitial lung disease									
	Frequency (%)	NSIP	UIP	OP	LIP	DAD	Vascular	DAH	Pleural	Comments
SSc	70	+++	+	+	−	+	+++	−	−	Higher mortality in older age, UIP pattern, high score for GGO, and traction bronchiectasis [7–9]
RA	25	++	+++	++	+	+	−	−	++	NSIP more favorable prognosis than UIP. Higher mortality with older age, smoking, seropositive, physiologic impairment [10–12]
PM/DM	20–50	+++	+	+++	−	++	+	−	+/−	Antibodies associated with anti-ARS-ILD in order of predominance: anti-EJ, anti Jo-1, anti-PL-7, anti-PL-12, anti-KS, anti-OJ [13]
SjS	25	++	+	−	++	=	+	−	+	GGO, consolidation, reticular and nodular opacities common. UIP with more progression of disease [14]
MCTD	20–60	++	+	+	−	−	++	−	+	Reticular patterns consistent with fibrosis. Fibrosis uniform in lower parts of lungs [15]

(continued)

Table 18.1 (continued)

	Interstitial lung disease									
	Frequency (%)	NSIP	UIP	OP	LIP	DAD	Vascular	DAH	Pleural	Comments
SLE	2–8	+	+	+	+	++	+	++	+++	Pneumonitis and anti-RNP antibodies and photosensitivity and oral ulcers associated with shorter and longer time, respectively, to occurrence of pulmonary damage [16]
AAV	10–60	+	++	–	–	+	++	+++	+	Central airway disease and nodular disease mostly in PR3-AAV; ILD can predate diagnosis of AAV [17, 18]

Legend: *SSc* systemic sclerosis, *RA* rheumatoid arthritis, *PM* polymyositis, *DM* dermatomyositis, *SjS* Sjogren syndrome, *MCTD* mixed connective tissue disease, *SLE* systemic lupus erythematosus, *AAV* ANCA-associated vasculitis, *NSIP* nonspecific interstitial pneumonia, *UIP* usual interstitial pneumonia, *OP* organizing pneumonia, *LIP* lymphocytic interstitial pneumonia, *DAD* diffuse alveolar damage, *DAH* diffuse alveolar hemorrhage, *GGO* ground-glass opacity, *Anti-ARS* antibodies to aminoacyl tRNA synthetases

necessarily meeting classification criteria for the diagnosis of one [21]. IPAF patients have marginally better survival when compared to those with idiopathic pulmonary fibrosis but overall fare worse than those with ILD associated with discrete CTDs [22]. Improved survival is noted in individuals without UIP and certain rheumatic manifestations including mechanic's hands, digital tip ulceration, palmar telangiectasia, inflammatory arthritis, Raynaud's phenomenon, and Gottron's sign [23].

HRCT is the current preferred lung imaging modality, especially for ILD, with CXR as the initial imaging option. Table 18.2 demonstrates the HRCT features of interstitial pneumonias seen in rheumatic diseases, as described by the American Thoracic Society and the European Respiratory Society [19]. HRCT abnormalities considered for semiquantitative scoring methods look at the presence and grading of ground-glass opacities, irregular pleural margin, septal or subpleural lines, subpleural cyst, and honeycombing [24, 25]. Widespread fibrosis characterized by extensive reticulation and honeycombing predicts high risks of mortality in RA and SSc [9, 10]. NSIP features on HRCT include bilateral predominantly lower lobe ground-glass opacities with traction bronchiectasis and lower lobe volume loss with subpleural sparing. In UIP, there is peribronchovascular ground-glass and reticular opacities with traction bronchiectasis [21].

Table 18.2 HRCT patterns seen in CTD-ILDs: descriptions as per the ATS/ERS Classification of the Idiopathic Interstitial Pneumonia [19]

Usual interstitial pneumonia (UIP)
Key features: Predominantly basal, reticular abnormality with volume loss. Typical findings of honeycombing, traction bronchiectasis/bronchiolectasis, focal ground glass (arrows)
Distribution: Peripheral, subpleural, basal
Most commonly found in RA

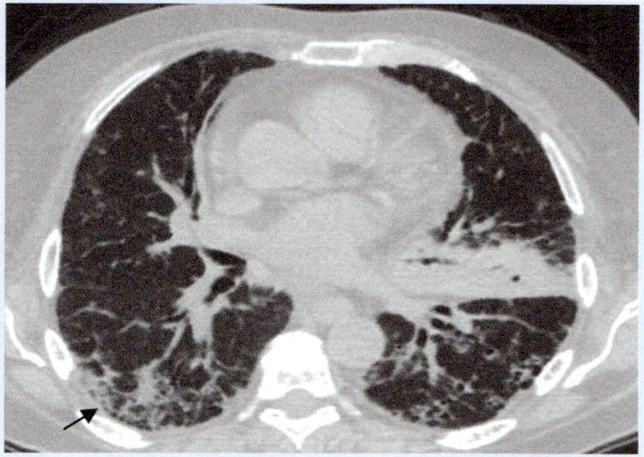

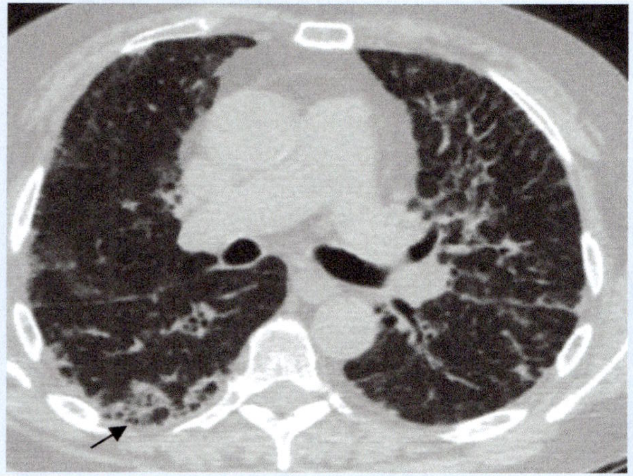

Nonspecific interstitial pneumonia (NSIP)
Key features: Bilateral ground-glass opacities. Irregular reticular opacities, traction bronchiectasis, and bronchiolectasis (in 75% of cases).
Distribution: Subpleural sparing; lower lobe involvement
Most commonly found in scleroderma patients

(continued)

Table 18.2 (continued)

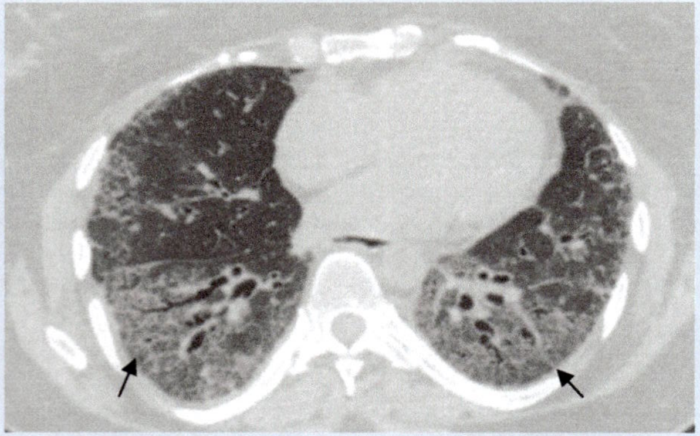

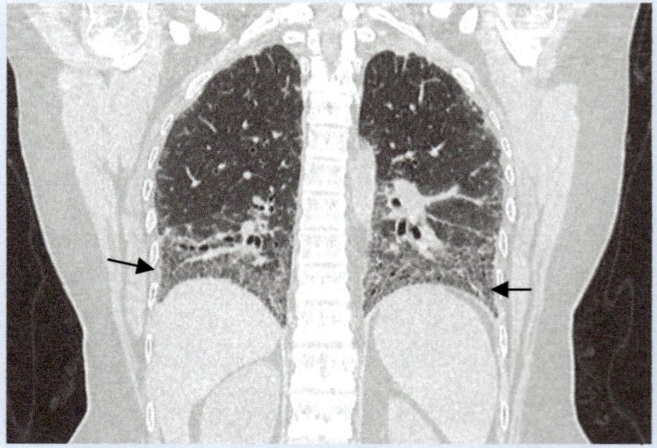

Lymphocytic interstitial pneumonia (LIP)
Key features: Centrilobular nodules, ground-glass attenuation, septal and bronchovascular thickening, thin wall cysts (arrows)
Distribution: Diffuse
Most commonly found in Sjogren's syndrome patients

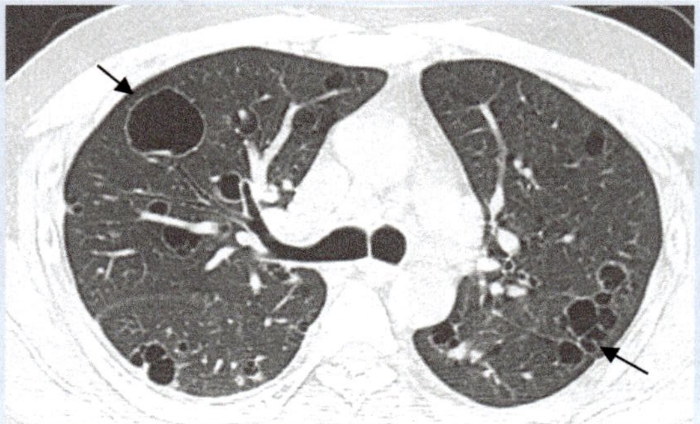

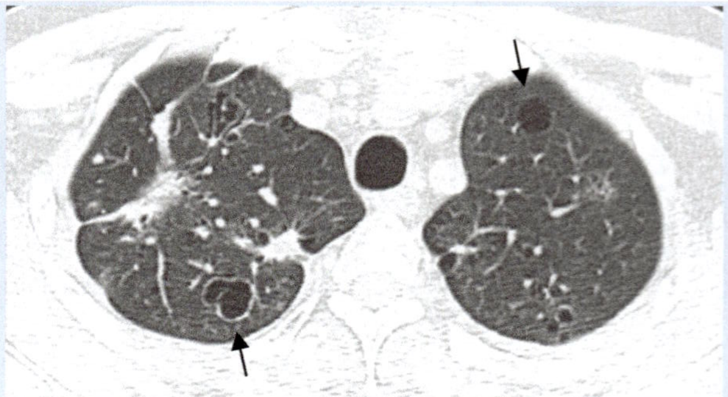

Organizing pneumonia (OP)

Key features: Patchy and migratory consolidations, air bronchograms. Associated with ground-glass opacity (arrows)

Distribution: Subpleural, peribronchial, bronchocentric

Usually present as subacute illness with cough and dyspnea, with duration <3 months

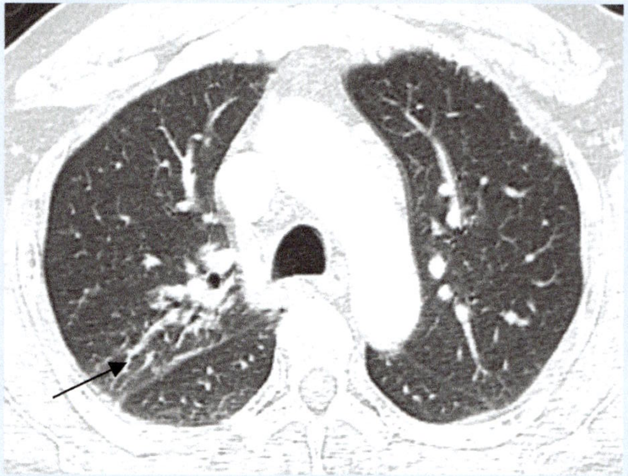

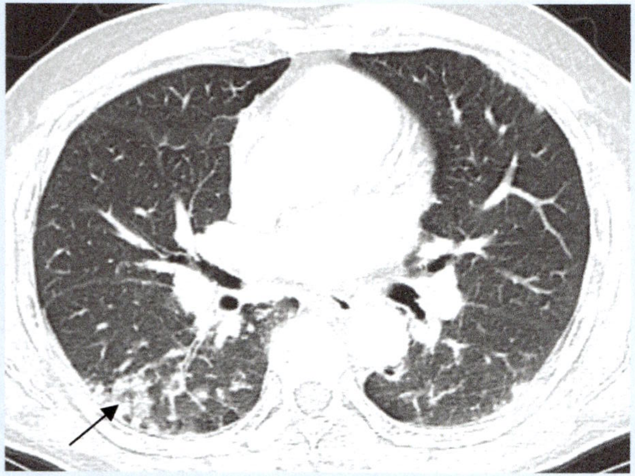

Acute interstitial pneumonia (AIP)/Diffuse Alveolar Damage (DAD)

Key features: Early exudative phase – bilateral patchy ground-glass opacities (arrows) with consolidation; Later organizing stage – traction bronchiectasis

Distribution: Bronchovascular

(continued)

Table 18.2 (continued)

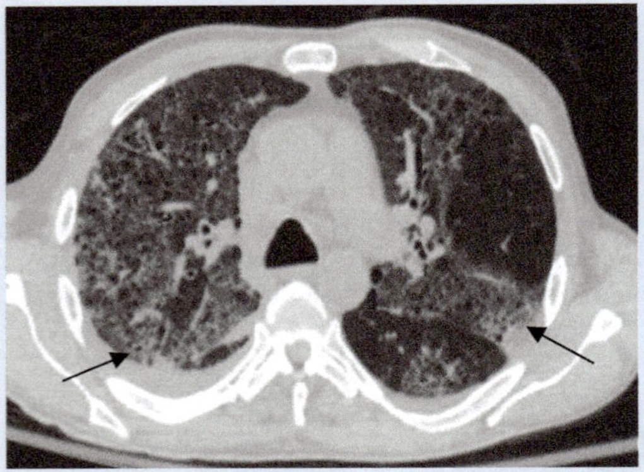

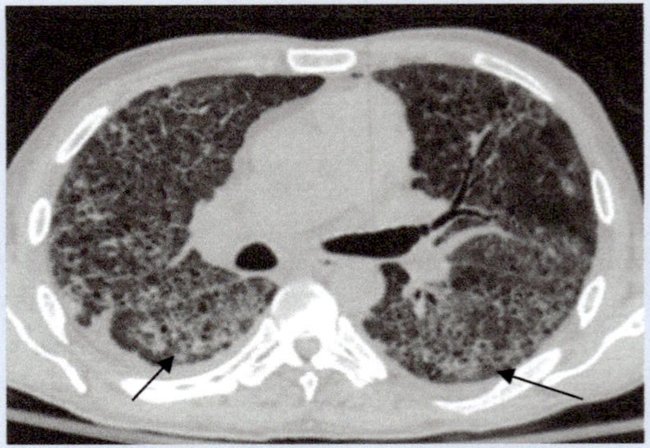

Acknowledgment: Images courtesy of Dr. Niranjan Jeganathan, Assistant Professor of Medicine, Division of Pulmonology and Critical Care Medicine, Loma Linda University School of Medicine

It has been noted that while CXR and LUS are different, they are complementary in nature, and the combined use of these two modalities may reduce the need for HRCT, and thus added radiation, in the evaluation of ILD [26].

The approval by the Food and Drug Administration of nintedanib for ILD in scleroderma and recent studies showing its efficacy for progressive fibrosing lung diseases in general are notable advancements in the management of lung manifestations in CTDs [27–29]. These studies utilized HRCT as the imaging parameter. LUS, in the evaluation of CTDs, has gained attention over the past 20 years with much of the research geared toward comparing its effectiveness to detect disease when compared with CXR and HRCT and looking at the early detection of ILD in SSc.

Normal Lung Imaging

When the probe is placed on the chest wall of a normal lung, the projected image includes the chest wall (skin, subcutaneous fat), the hyperechoic pleural line (or the lung-wall interface), and a mirroring image of the chest wall beneath the pleural line composed of A-lines (Fig. 18.1a–c). The standard window for LUS frames longitudinally between two ribs due to penetration defects of any tissue underlying the ribs [30]. The rib bones generate acoustic shadowing artifacts posterior to it. The pleural line is noted between the two ribs, demonstrating an image that resembles a bat, also known as "bat sign." Turning the probe along the lung intercostal space (LICS) allows for an oblique scan to expand this window for better visualization of potential pathology [1]. A-lines are horizontal linear echogenic lines at regular intervals

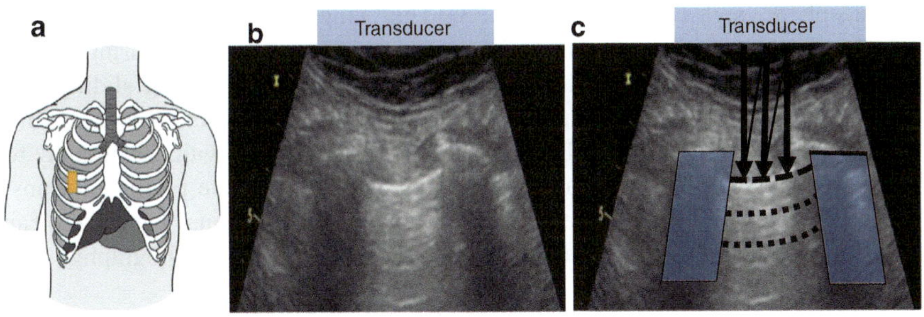

Fig. 18.1 Normal lung ultrasound. (**a**) Diagram of thoracic cage with ultrasound transducer at fourth right intercostal space. (**b**) Normal lung ultrasound – scan of an intercostal space assuming the transducer placed in (**a**) generates this figure. The pleural line, a hyperechoic horizontal line (horizontal arrowheads), is below the rib line (vertical arrowheads). These hyperechoic landmarks are collectively called the bat sign. (**c**) Scan of an intercostal space. Ribs generate acoustic shadowing typified by the signal void (transparent fill) posteriorly. The pleural line indicating apart from parietal pleura in all cases also includes visceral pleura. On dynamic imaging, the pleural line exhibits to-and-fro movement, called lung sliding. A-lines (short dashed lines), generated as horizontal repetitions below the pleural line (long dashed lines), indicate gas. Equidistant A-lines (dashed lines) are reverberation artifacts generated by sound waves reflected back and forth between the pleural line and the transducer

[3]. In addition to A-lines, the phenomenon of lung sliding (sliding motion of the pleural line during respiration) is thought to be due to artifacts caused by a difference in the acoustic impedances of the overlying soft tissue and underlying alveoli. In the M-mode (motion display), the "seashore sign" is seen mimicking a pattern of sand below the pleural line which is created by the dynamics of lung sliding [31]. The parietal pleura appears as a "fine" echogenic line and is far better to visualize than the visceral pleura which has been described as a "delicate" echogenic line [32].

The Abnormal Lung

A multidisciplinary international group of experts in LUS established evidence-based recommendations for point-of-care LUS in the evaluation of pneumothorax, interstitial syndrome, lung consolidation, pleural effusion, monitoring of lung diseases (e.g., acute lung injury or acute respiratory distress syndrome, cardiogenic pulmonary edema, pneumonia), and in neonatal and pediatric conditions (e.g., respiratory distress syndrome, transient tachypnea of the newborn) [3] (Table 18.3). LUS is comparable to, if not more accurate than, CXR for the evaluation of the conditions below [3].

Pneumothorax

Lung sliding and B-lines are absent when air is present between the parietal and visceral pleura. Lack of motion at the pleural line replaces the seashore sign with a linear, laminar pattern superficial and deep to the pleural line and is termed the "stratosphere" sign (Table 18.3) [31, 33]. The "lung point" is a landmark on the chest wall beneath which the lung adheres again to the parietal layer during inspiration and demonstrates lung sliding, while expiration abolishes lung sliding [34]. Lung pulse, which is the movement of the lung on the parietal pleura during cardiac beats, is also absent [35]. The Extended Focused Assessment with Sonography for Trauma (EFAST) protocol is used in cases of trauma to isolate presence of post-traumatic pneumothorax by intensivists and ER physicians and may have significant value in picking up missed pneumothoraces on AP supine chest radiography [36].

Interstitial Syndrome

Interstitial syndrome refers to a variety of conditions affecting the interstitium and causing abnormalities in the alveolar-capillary interface. Interstitial syndromes include pulmonary fibrosis, ILD, IP, acute respiratory distress syndrome, cardiogenic pulmonary edema, and acute lung injury.

Table 18.3 Sonographic signs per the International Liaison Committee on Lung Ultrasound (ILC-LUS) for International Consensus Conference on Lung Ultrasound (ICC-LUS) of pneumothorax, interstitial syndrome, lung consolidation, and pleural effusion [3]

Pneumothorax Presence of "lung point" sign Absence of lung sliding Absence of lung pulse Absence of B-lines "Stratosphere" sign seen in Motion mode (a single pattern of horizontal lines)	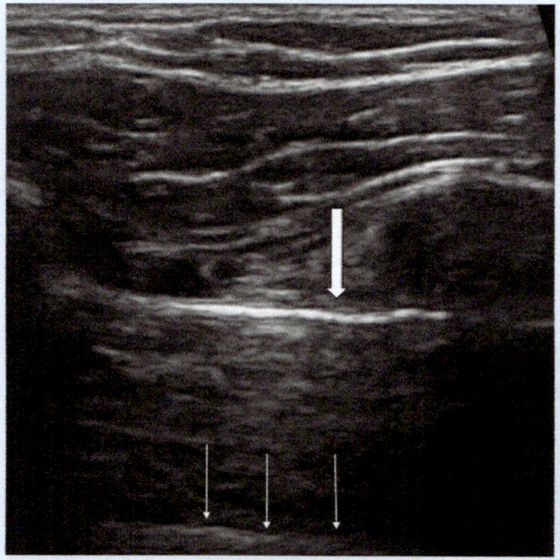 Pneumothorax noted between parietal pleura (thick white arrow) and the visceral pleura (thin white arrows).	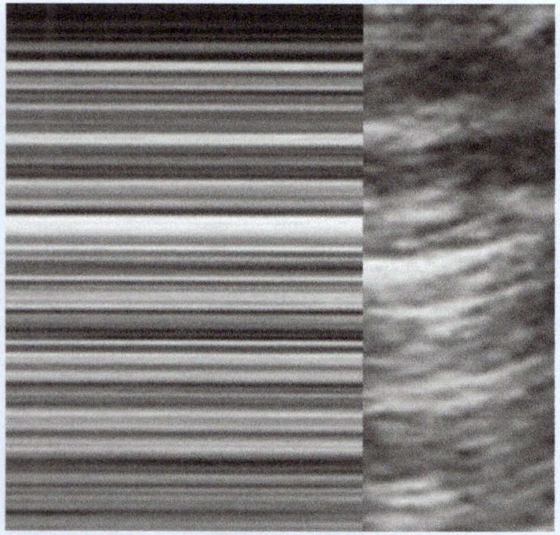 Stratosphere sign (or Barcode sign) – seen in M or Motion mode (on left) showing a single pattern uninterrupted lines indicative of an unaerated lung. B mode on right.

(continued)

Table 18.3 (continued)

Interstitial syndrome Multiple B-lines (more than 2 regions bilaterally with ≥3 B-lines in a longitudinal plane between 2 ribs; if using 28 rib space technique, count B-line number per rib up to 10 and divide by 10)	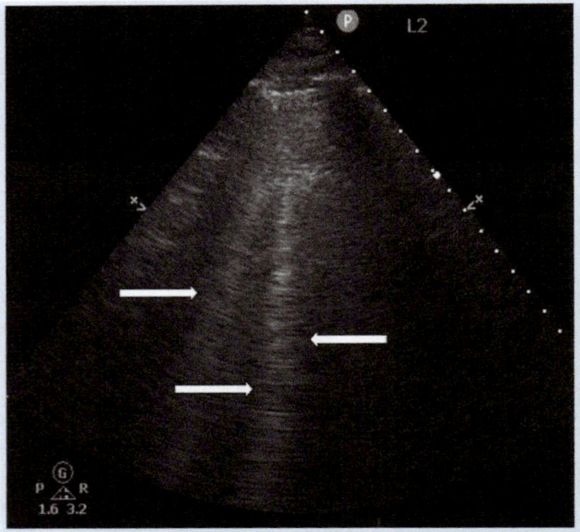 Interstitial syndrome depicted by multiple B-lines (white arrowheads)	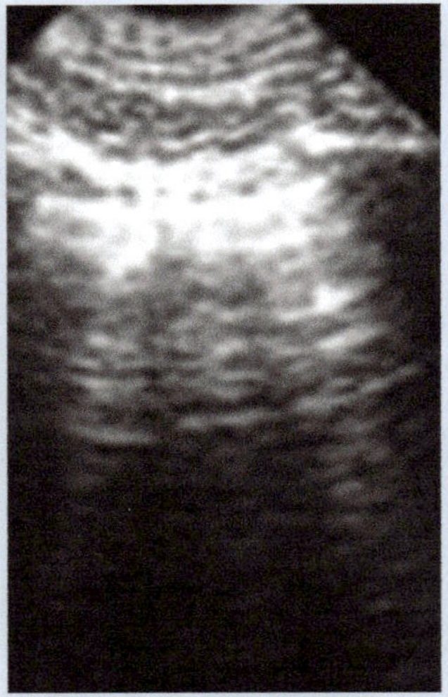 Z-lines – ill-defined hazy lines that do not obliterate the A-lines

Lung consolidation Subpleural echo-poor or tissue-like echogenicity Comet tail reverberation artifacts at the far-field margin Air and/or fluid bronchograms Vascular pattern within the consolidation	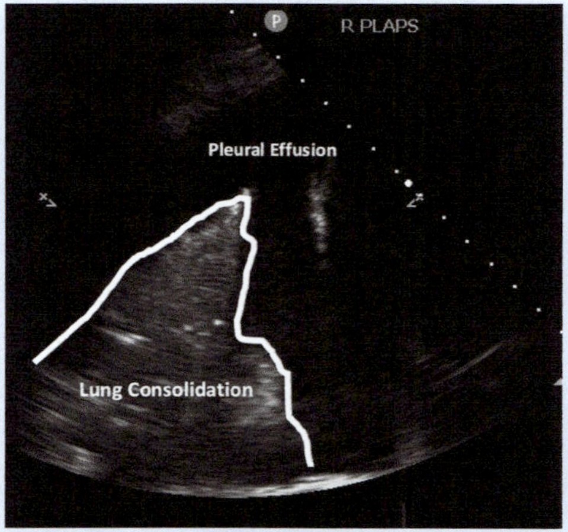 Lung consolidation (outlined) at left lower quadrant with tissue-like echogenicity and vascular pattern. Adjacent to the consolidation is a large anechoic pleural effusion	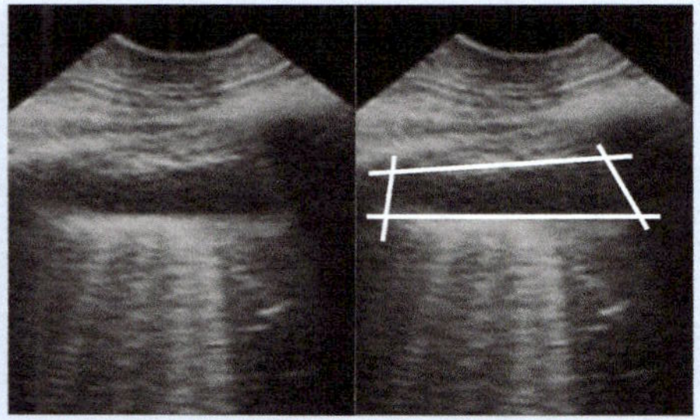 Quad sign: quadrangular image with edges made up by pleural line, visceral line, and shadow of ribs
Pleural effusion Anechoic (dark) space between parietal and visceral pleura depicts fluid, pleural effusion Internal echoes within pleural effusion may suggest exudate or hemorrhage Quad sign Sinusoid sign		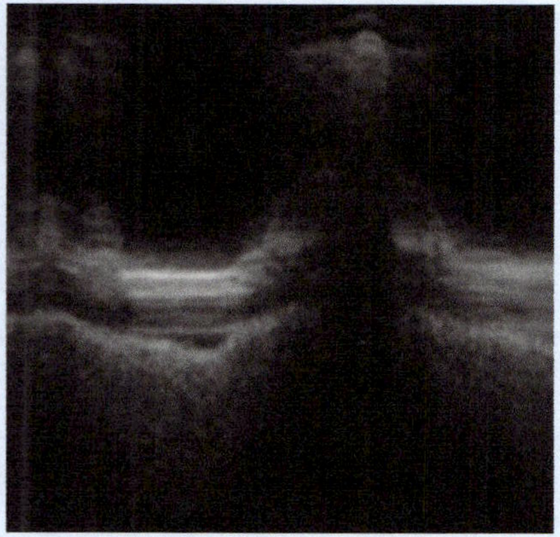 Sinusoid sign: seen in motion mode, cyclic motion of lung parenchyma

Images courtesy of Vi Dinh, MD, Division of Pulmonary and Critical Medicine, Loma Linda University School of Medicine and Karina Torralba, MD, Division of Rheumatology, Loma Linda University School of Medicine

B-Lines

B-lines are defined as "discrete laser-like vertical hyperechoic reverberation artifacts that arise from the pleural line and extend to the bottom of the screen without fading and move synchronously with lung sliding" [3, 37–39]. Previously described as "comet tails," B-lines are common in ILD. In ILD, fluid shifts result in thickening of the lung interstitium and interlobular septa, resulting in B-lines [40, 41]. Multiple B-lines are typical of ILD; increasing B-lines indicates disease progression [41]. When scanning in a longitudinal plane between two ribs, three or more B-lines are considered a positive region [3]. B-lines are not to be mistaken for Z-lines (Table 18.3), which are ill-defined, hazy lines that, unlike B-lines, do not replace A-lines [31]. While the consensus method of imaging utilizes the eight-region technique, critically ill patients may be evaluated by the anterior two-region scan to exclude an interstitial process.

"B-pattern" is used in place of "lung rockets" or "B-PLUS" to describe multiple B-lines as seen in individuals with interstitial lung disease [3]. When differentiating the B-pattern of pulmonary edema from acute respiratory distress syndrome or pulmonary fibrosis, additional sonographic signs are noted. It is still unclear how to distinguish B-lines as a result of early cellular inflammation versus those resulting from chronic fibrotic damage [42]. It is also important to note that B-lines can sometimes be found in normal healthy controls [43].

The source of ring-down artifacts has been theorized to be due to the presence of bubbles or acoustic events stemming from changes in the tissue-fluid relationship in the lung, accounting for the sonographic changes in interstitial lung disease. More studies are needed to determine how B-lines are generated. A more detailed review of the physics involved in LUS and the production of normal and abnormal sonographic lung anatomy, including the physics of B-line generation, is beyond the scope of this chapter but has been elegantly and concisely explained elsewhere [1, 39, 44, 45].

Consolidation

Consolidation is caused by a decrease in air content and a fluid predominance, and is seen in infection, thromboembolic disease, acute lung injury, malignancy, atelectasis, or trauma [30]. The decreased air content opens the lung acoustic window with impedances that are more similar to the surrounding tissues, yielding echo-poor or tissue-like echogenicity [3]. Bronchograms and vascular patterns within consolidation and B-lines can help determine the cause. Dynamic air bronchograms correlate with pneumonia as opposed to atelectasis [35]. Highly vascularized pattern within the consolidation may represent malignancy [32].

Pleural Effusions

Readily detected via LUS, an effusion is depicted by an anechoic or hypoechoic region between the two pleural layers with adjacent lung that is typically consolidated or aerated [30]. Free pleural effusions are evaluated at the posterolateral alveolar and/or pleural syndrome (PLAPS)-point, defined by the intersection of a "horizontal line at the level of the lower BLUE-point and a vertical line at the posterior axillary line" [35]. Two signs depict a pleural effusion: (1) quad sign, a quadrangular image with edges made up by pleural line, visceral line, and rib shadows, and the (2) sinusoid sign, a cyclic motion of the lung line toward the pleural line during inspiration and expiration on M-mode (Table 18.3) [31].

Pleural Disease

It has been observed that B-lines are related to pleural changes [24]. A more detailed discussion of pleural disease is incorporated into the section on LUS in CTDs.

Lung Scanning Protocols

A pragmatic approach to sonography of the lungs has been described by Dietrich et al. [32]. Various scanning protocols have been created to allow the use of ultrasound to diagnose causes of respiratory failure. The BLUE-protocol is a 3-min approach used in dyspneic ICU patients – when it is combined with various signs and associated with a location, seven profiles result. The various profiles (e.g., B, A/B, C profiles) correlate with diagnoses of pulmonary edema, pulmonary embolism, pneumonia, chronic obstructive pulmonary disease, asthma, and pneumothorax. These are beyond the scope of this chapter but are eloquently described by Lichtenstein [31].

Ultrasound Assessment for ILD and Pleural Disease in CTDs

Research on the use of ultrasound for lung disease in CTDs has focused primarily on the evaluation of ILD. However, it is notable that much of the underlying problems in the lung parenchyma and the accompanying pathology noted on ultrasound may emanate from problems in the pleura [2, 24, 46]. The Outcomes Measures in Rheumatoid Arthritis Clinical Trials (OMERACT) ultrasound subcommittee developed definitions for ILD ultrasound pathology for patients with autoimmune diseases (Table 18.4) focusing on the presence of B-lines and pleural irregularities [47].

Table 18.4 OMERACT definitions for interstitial lung disease pathology by lung ultrasound with normal lung ultrasound image for comparison [47]

Key feature	Definition	Representative images	Normal lung ultrasound
B-lines	A vertical hyperechoic reverberation artifact that arise from the pleural line, extend to the bottom of the screen without fading, and move synchronously with lung sliding	Note distinctive B-line (arrowheads). Pleural line also has some irregularity (arrows) 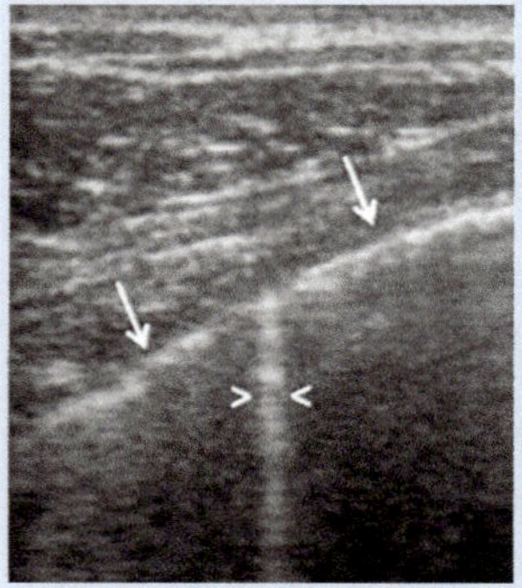	Lack of irregularity of the pleural line (arrows), lack of B-lines, faint A-lines depicted by horizontal equidistant lines parallel to the pleural line 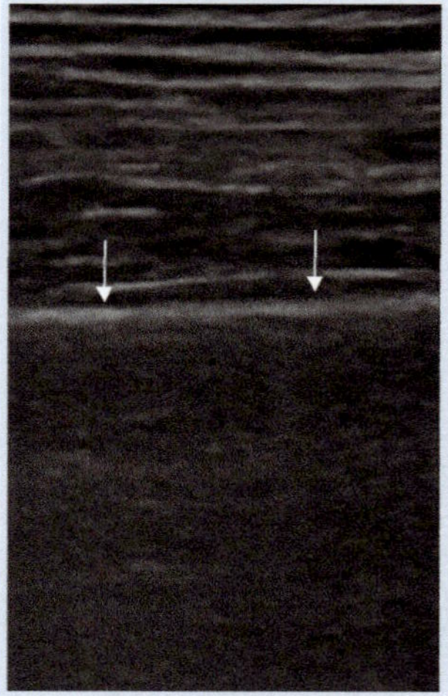
Pleural irregularity	A loss of regularity that may be associated with an increase in thickness, focal, diffuse, or nodular	Note irregularity of pleural line (arrowheads) 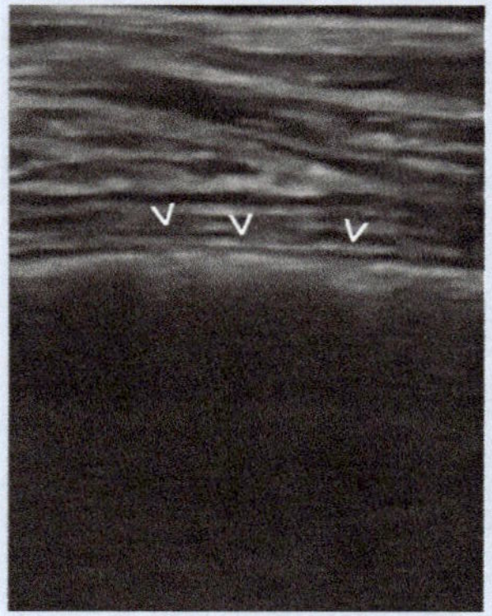	

Image on B-lines from [46]
Legend: *OMERACT* Outcome Measures in Rheumatoid Arthritis Clinical Trials

LUS is comparable to HRCT and pulmonary function test results in the evaluation of CTD-ILD. In a study looking at 1700 LICS ($n = 34$), a significant correlation between the ultrasound score and HRCT score, and DLCO values were noted [48]. A meta-analysis involving five studies ($n = 349$) concluded that LUS has high diagnostic accuracy and correlates well with HRCT findings (sensitivity 91.5%, specificity 81.3%) [49]. Gutierrez et al. have comprehensively looked at studies published over the last 20 years on CTD-related ILD, looking at the reliability rates, sensitivity, specificity, positive and negative predictive values of each study, equipment and settings used, and basic demographics and disease diagnoses information [50].

Pleural abnormalities usually accompany lung fibrosis and ILD. Some early features of lung fibrosis on ultrasound may show pleural line changes (irregularity, raggedness, thickening, blurring, or fragmentation), so-called artifacts that are now considered part of standard lung ultrasound evaluation (single B-lines, numerous B-lines, white lung, Am lines), and consolidation (small 5 or less mm or large >5 mm) [24].

Majority of studies on LUS in rheumatic diseases focus on SSc. However, other conditions such as RA are not uncommonly present with ILD, predominantly of UIP type. RA-ILD is highly associated with seropositivity, smoking history, and higher mortality rates [11, 12]. ILD, while rare in ANCA-associated vasculitis, can predate vasculitis diagnosis and can have a detrimental effect on prognosis [18]. These studies, which involved patients with various CTDs and other non-scleroderma populations, are presented in Table 18.5 [43, 48, 51–59].

Ultrasound in Systemic Sclerosis Lung Disease

Lung disease is quite common in SSc, affecting 70% of the population [7–9]. Most SSc LUS studies focus on ILD. It tends to occur early in the disease course, is more common in diffuse SSc vs. limited SSc or CREST syndrome, and is associated with significant morbidity and mortality [60, 61]. NSIP and UIP are the most common patterns of SSc-ILD, with NSIP being more common and UIP portending a shorter survival [8].

In studies looking at SSc-ILD populations, there is a positive correlation between HRCT and LUS findings (Table 18.6) [62–74]. The number of B-lines was higher in patients with positive SCL-70 autoantibodies [62]. About 51% of SSc patients had >10 B-lines, especially among patients with diffuse SSc vs. those with limited SSc [63]. The sensitivity and specificity of LUS were about 100% and 34%, respectively, and because of this, a low lung ultrasound score (Picano scoring system) obviates the need for HRCT [72]. A minimum of 10 B-lines is highly predictive for ILD on HRCT, contributing to the argument that LUS may be used as an initial tool to improve timing of chest HRCT.

Pleural abnormalities were also significantly more common in SSc patients over healthy normals [65]. In a study looking at both SSc and anti-synthetase syndrome patients, pleural irregularity scores correlated with HRCT Warrick scoring and Wells scoring and DLCO; pleural irregularity appeared to be superior but not

Table 18.5 Interstitial lung disease ultrasound studies in rheumatic diseases, covering studies involving a mix of CTD patients, and non-scleroderma studies published as of September 2019

Author, year published (Ref)	Subjects *N*, gender, mean age in years (SD or range)	CTD types	Equipment	US scoring/scanning protocol	Comments
Sperandeo 2009 [51]	*N* = 84 cases with ILD 51 M, 33 F Age range 46–73 years *N* = 162 controls 78 M, 84 F Age range 18–76 years	18 SSc, 4 RA, 4 MCTD, 4 SjS, 2 PM, 1 PBC	Technos MPX scanner (Esaote, Genova, Italy), 3.5 MHz convex and 8–12 MHz linear transducers	Pleural line – thickening (>3 mm), gliding; reverberations are those horizontal concentric hyperechoic lines representing the pleural-thoracic wall interface Patients were examined in the seated position or lying down (supine, prone or lateral decubitus) position	Lung ultrasound can detect early and late changes. Findings: (1) fragmented, irregular pleural thickening; (2) subpleural cysts (68% cases of moderate-severe disease); (3) reduction or absence of "gliding sign" (39%), increased number of horizontal reverberation artifacts (34%)
Gutierrez 2011 [52]	*N* = 36 4 M, 32 F Mean age 57 (13), range 20–78 years	28 SSc 2 SjS 1 UCTD 2 Anti-SS 2 DM 1 MCTD	MyLab 70 (Esaote), 2–7 MHz convex transducer	Comprehensive (50 LIS) and simplified (14 LIS) semiquantitative scoring: grade 0 (normal) <10 B-lines; grade 1 (mild) 11–20 B-lines; grade 2 (moderate) 21–50 B-lines, and grade 3 (marked) >50 B-lines	Kappa values for the interobserver simplified assessment were in a range from 0.769 to 0.885, whereas the concordance correlation coefficient values for the intra-observer were 0.856–0.955 Time spent on comprehensive (mean 23.3 ± SD 4.5 min) with respect to the simplified assessment (mean 8.6 ± SD 1.4) ($p < 0.00001$). Significant correlation between simplified and comprehensive assessment; between simplified assessment and HRCT

Aghdashi 2013 [53]	$N = 31$ Mean ± SD age was 48.29 (9.7 SD) years, range 30–66 years Mean duration was 68 (23.1 SD) months, range 4–122 months	19 SSc 8 RA 2 Overlap syndrome 1 SjS 1 DM	Siemens Sonoline G-40, 7–10 MHz linear multifrequency transducer	Modified TTUS B-lines assessment of ten LIS bilaterally; >5 B-lines = pulmonary involvement and positive results	Compared to HRCT, the sensitivity, specificity, positive, and negative predictive value of TTUS was 73.58%, 88.23%, 95.12% and 51.72%, respectively
Cogliati 2014 [54]	$N = 39$ 29 F, 10 M Mean age 64.87	39 RA	Envisor (Philips, Andover, MA, USA), 5–12 MHz convex probe	72 segments – 28 anterior, 44 posterior B-lines counted in each segment; score >10 indicated a positive exam	Sensitivity and specificity of standard ultrasound vs. HRCT were 92% and 56%, respectively B-line score significantly correlated with HRCT score ($r = 0.806$) Sensitivity and specificity for pocket-size ultrasound vs. HRCT were 89% and 50%
Hasan 2014 [55]	$N = 61$ 38 M, 23 F Mean age 49.41 (11.69) years	Collagen vascular diseases (8), sarcoidosis (4); other cases: lung fibrosis (30), sarcoidosis (4), hypersensitivity pneumonitis (9), and 10 cases with the following: lymphangitis carcinomatosis, silicosis, radiation pneumonitis, and viral pneumonias	Aloka Prosound (Yokohama, Japan), 3.5-MHz convex probe	Scanned eight regions. Four chest areas per side considered for complete ultrasound examination. Areas 1 and 2 denote the upper anterior and lower anterior areas, respectively. Areas 3 and 4 denote the upper lateral and basal lateral areas, respectively	PFTs and HRCT as comparison Distance between B-lines correlate with findings on HRCT and PFTs B3 (the distance was 3 mm) correlated with ground-glass opacity and B7 (7 mm) correlated with extensive fibrosis and honey combing

(continued)

Table 18.5 (continued)

Author, year published (Ref)	Subjects N, gender, mean age in years (SD or range)	CTD types	Equipment	US scoring/scanning protocol	Comments
Moazedi-Fuerst 2014 [43]	$N = 64$ RA 10 M, 54 F Age 59 (12 SD) years; 6% current smokers; 61 (93%) RF+, 57 (89%) CCP+ $N = 40$ controls 15 M, 25 F 52 (22 SD) years	17 RA with ILD, 46 ILD	GE Logiq 7, 3.5 MHz convex transducer for the parenchyma, linear probe for the pleural changes	B-lines Pleural line, pleural nodules	28% of RA patients showed pleural nodules or B-line phenomena. In these patients, CT scans showed signs of incipient ILD. Ultrasound showed sporadic abnormalities in 7% of the healthy controls
Tardella 2015 [48]	$N = 34$ cases 32 M, 20 F $N = 34$ controls 18 M, 16 F	26 SSc 2 SjS 2 Anti-SS 2 DM 1 MCTD 1 UCTD	MyLab 70 XVG (Esaote Biomedica, Genoa, Italy), 2–7 MHz broadband convex multifrequency transducer.	Semiquantitative scoring: grade 0 (normal) <10 B-lines; grade 1 (mild) 11–20 B-lines; grade 2 (moderate) 21–50 B-lines, and grade 3 (marked) >50 B-lines	Significant linear correlation noted between ultrasound score and HRCT score ($p < 0.001$) Positive correlation between B-line assessment and DLCO values ($p = 0.014$)
Moazedi-Fuerst 2015 [56]	$N = 45$ cases $N = 40$ controls	25 RA 14 SSc 6 SLE	GE Logiq 7, 3.5 MHz convex transducer, linear probe	Chest wall divided into 18 regions; anterior surfaces scanned supine, lateral and posterior surfaces scanned sitting. Scans were performed in a longitudinal or intercostal plane; comet-score of 0, without positive areas; (1) with one to five positive areas; (2) >5 abnormal areas. Pleural "thickening" or pleural line irregularities >3 mm was defined to be pathologic	28% of RA, 64% of SSc, 4/6 SLE had ILD on HRCT Subpleural nodes noted in 100% of RA, 22% SSc, 50% SLE Irregular pleural line >3 mm noted in 100% SSc and SLE with ILD vs. 86% of ILD with RA Pathology more frequent in ILD group than in non-ILD group

Pinal-Fernandez 2015 [57]	$N = 37$ 13 M, 24 F Mean age 51.5 (14.2 SD)	13 probable/definite DM, 6 PM; 2 Anti-SS associated ILD without myositis. 8 limited SSc, 5 diffuse SSc 3 SSc sine scleroderma	MyLabTwice (Esaote, Genoa), 5 MHz 5 cm linear probe (LA 527)	Patients in supine position – anterior and anterolateral points (up to 28), and in sitting position for the posterior and posterolateral ones (up to 44). The 72 points corresponded to the anatomical distribution defined by Gargani	Pleural irregularity is a new ultrasound sign to incorporate in the study of ILD in SSc and anti-SS patients Ultrasound correlates with several HRCT and PFT parameters and performed well as a diagnostic tool for detecting and determining the extent of ILD
Buda 2016 [24]	$N = 52$ with autoimmune disease Mean age 50 (24 SD) 32 M, 20 F $N = 50$ controls Mean age 47 (25 SD) 4 M, 16 F	Not specified	GE Logiq 7, 8–11 MHz linear probe and 2.5–5 MHz convex probe	Each LICS was assessed. Lungs were divided into upper, middle and lower fields Artifacts: single B-lines (≤3 per one scan), numerous B-lines (≥4 per one scan), white lung, Am lines Pleural line changes: irregularity, ragged, fragmentary, thickened, blurred Consolidation: small (≤5 mm) large (>5 mm)	First reported Am lines, pleural line blurring Scale of severity of lung fibrosis Ultrasound-based criteria for lung fibrosis looking at pleural line irregularity, tightening, fragmentary nature, blurring, thickening; B-lines, Am line, subpleural consolidations
Vasco 2017 [58]	$N = 13$ females Mean age 63.62 years (range 39–88)	SjS; 78.5% with primary SjS	GE Logiq 7, 2–5.5 MHz 60-mm wide-band convex array probe (4CRS) or 3.3–10-MHz linear array transducer (9L-RS)	Eight zones of the lungs, using the parasternal, anterior, and posterior axillary lines	Intra-rater reliability k is 1. To detect ILD, ultrasound has a sensitivity of 1 (95% CI 0.398–1.0), specificity 0.89 (95% CI 0.518–0.997), positive probability reason 9.00 (95% CI 7.1–11.3) Ultrasound has excellent correlation with HRCT in Sjs-ILD and might be a useful technique in daily clinical practice for the assessment of lung disease in sicca syndrome

(continued)

Table 18.5 (continued)

Author, year published (Ref)	Subjects *N*, gender, mean age in years (SD or range)	CTD types	Equipment	US scoring/scanning protocol	Comments
Buda 2019 [59]	*N* = 38 18 M, 20 F 18 M, 20 F Mean age 51.7 years (19–80 years)	31 GPA 18 F, 13 M 7 MPA 2 F, 5 M	Machine not specified 2–6 MHz convex and 4–12 MHz linear transducers	LICS over the chest wall (anterior, lateral, and inferior) in the following lines: parasternal, middle clavicular, axillary (anterior, middle, and posterior), scapular, and paraspinal	Fibrosis noted in 11 HRCT and ultrasound images of pulmonary lesions were consistent but highly variable

Legend: CTD connective tissue diseases, *PM* polymyositis, *DM* dermatomyositis, *UCTD* undifferentiated connective tissue disease, *MCTD* mixed connective tissue disease, *SSc* systemic sclerosis, *RA* rheumatoid arthritis, *ILD* interstitial lung disease, *SjS* Sjogren syndrome, *anti-SS* anti-synthetase syndrome, *PBC* primary biliary cirrhosis, *SLE* systemic lupus erythematosus, *GPA* granulomatosis with polyangiitis, *MPA* microscopic polyangiitis, *M* male, *F* female, *MHz* megahertz, *HRCT* high-resolution computed tomography, *PFT* pulmonary function testing, *RF* rheumatoid factor, *CCP* cyclic citrullinated peptide, *LICS* lung intercostal space

Table 18.6 Interstitial lung disease (ILD) ultrasound studies involving systemic sclerosis (SSc) patients only

Author and year published (Ref)	Equipment	Subjects number, gender, mean age in years (SD)	US scoring/scanning protocol (author/year of publication if adopted from another study)	Major findings, other comments
Doveri 2008 [62]	Optigo Philips, 2.5–3.5 MHz probe	*N* = 30 7 M, 23 F Mean age 54 (13)	Jambrik 2004 Picano 2006	Lung comets higher in SCL70+ patients and correlated to HRCT score, not to presence of pulmonary hypertension No intra- or inter-reader variability, less structured score for HRCT
Gargani 2009 [63]	Optigo HP Sonos 7500, and IE33 (Philips Medical Systems); Famiglia Mylab25 (Esaote) 2.5–3.5 MHz cardiac sector transducer	*N* = 33 3 M, 30 F Mean age 54 (13)	Jambrik 2004 Picano – modified lung comets (>10 lung comets)	Lung comets are found in SSc, more in dSSc. Lung comets correlate well with HRCT-diagnosed lung fibrosis. B-lines correlate with HRCT Weak but significant correlation with TLC, VC, DLCO Intra- and interobserver variability between two blinded and independent sonographers
Delle Sedie 2010 [64]	Toshiba PowerVision 6000 linear 6 MHz and Optigo Philips cardiac 2.5–3.5 MHz	*N* = 25 3 M, 22 F Mean age 53 (10)	No midaxillary line scanning to avoid duplicate counting of B-lines	B-lines detectable using linear probe ICC = 0.681 between both probes, better results for anterior than posterior Moderate-good ICC between cardiac or linear prob. and HRCT (0.547 and 0.600, respectively) Pathologic cut offs for B-lines – 5 for cardiac, 11 for linear

(continued)

Table 18.6 (continued)

Author and year published (Ref)	Equipment	Subjects number, gender, mean age in years (SD)	US scoring/scanning protocol (author/year of publication if adopted from another study)	Major findings, other comments
Moazedi-Fuerst 2012 [65]	GE Logiq 7; convex 3.5 MHz transducer for parenchyma, linear probe for pleural changes	*N* = 25 2 M, 23 F; 1 smoker Mean (SD) age 51 (15) Disease duration (mean, range 6.5 (1–20) years) 40 age- and sex-matched healthy controls; 12 smokers	18 regions; anterior pleural surface done in supine position; lateral and posterior surfaces scanned in sitting position; scans done in longitudinal or intercostal plane	ILD patients had higher pleural and comet scores HRCT confirmed US abnormalities (B-lines) in 44% of SSc patients (in accordance with incidence of lung fibrosis in SSc) Underscores the potential for LUS as a screening method for ILD in SSc Limited by small patient number difficulty blinding ultrasound investigators
Barskova 2012 [66]	IE33, Philips Medical Systems; Vivid-I, GE/Vingmed; 2.5–3.5 MHz phased-array sector scan probe, second harmonic technology and coupled with tissue Doppler imaging	*N* = 58 4 M, 54 F Mean (SD) age 51 32 with very early SSc – 29 F Disease duration mean (SD) 1.9 (3.2) years	Picano 2006 Volpicelli 2012 Gargani 2009	ILD is detected by US in very early SSc B-lines by US correlate with HRCT B-lines in patients without ILD on HRCT – not due to cardiogenic pulmonary interstitial syndrome Limited by long time duration between US and HRCT; larger studies are needed with shorter gap between imaging modalities improve sensitivity/specificity; small patient number; need studies correlating LUS with ground-glass changes or honeycombing

Table 18.6 (continued)

Author and year published (Ref)	Equipment	Subjects number, gender, mean age in years (SD)	US scoring/scanning protocol (author/year of publication if adopted from another study)	Major findings, other comments
Mohammadi 2014 [67]	Medison Accuvix V20, 7–10 MHz broadband linear multifrequency transducer	$N = 70$ 9 M, 60 F excluded h/o lung cancer, heart failure, asthma and smoking	10-LICS; semiquantitative scoring: 0 = normal (≤5 B-lines), 1 = mild (6–15 B-lines), 2 = moderate (16–30 B-lines), 3 = severe (>30 B-lines)	Modified comet tails scoring system could be useful in assessment of the pulmonary involvement in patients with SS Positive correlation between HRCT and LUS Sensitivity 73.58%, specificity 88.23% PPV 95.12%, NPV 51.72% Excellent intra-observer *K* value 0.838
Sperandeo 2015 [68]	Esaote Technos Mpx – Esaote My Lab 30 Gold 3.5–5-MHz convex probe (and 8–12.5-MHz linear prob)	$N = 175$ 9 M, 166 F Mean age 46 (15.33)	Pleural line thickness. B-line counts: >3 as positive and 3 as a negative sign	Ultrasound had good concordance with HRCT patterns indicating lung fibrosis severity. Pleural line thickness measurement is able to rule out lung fibrosis. Ultrasound is able to detect some lung abnormalities previously evident only by HRCT and may reveal subpleural abnormalities (pneumonitis, pleural effusion) even when not yet radiographically evident

(continued)

Table 18.6 (continued)

Author and year published (Ref)	Equipment	Subjects number, gender, mean age in years (SD)	US scoring/scanning protocol (author/year of publication if adopted from another study)	Major findings, other comments
Cakir 2016 [69]	SonoSite, Inc., linear probe, L38E/5–10 MHz	$N = 48$ 2 M, 46 F Mean age 50.8 (11.9)	Interstitial involvement – bilateral symmetric areas containing more than three B-lines	Number of B-lines detected on LUS correlated with Warrick score ($r = 0.89$; $p = 0.0001$) and Medsger disease scale ($r = 0.55$; $p = 0.0001$) and negatively correlated with DLCO ($r = -0.56$; $p = 0.0001$) and FVC ($r = -0.46$; $p = 0.001$) Interobserver reliability for the Warrick score was very good in HRCT evaluation ($r = 0.87$; $p = 0.0001$)
Gigante 2016 [70]	Toshiba's ultrasound system convex 2.5- to 3.5-MHz probe	$N = 39$ 6 M, 33 F Mean age 51 (15.2) 24 dSSc, 15 lSSc	Analyzed anterior and lateral hemithoraces, scanning along the parasternal, midclavicular, anterior axillary, and midaxillary lines, to evaluate location and number of B-lines	Positive correlation between B-lines ($r = 0.81$, $p < 0.0001$) and DLCO ($r = 0.63$, $p < 0.0001$) noted B-lines increased with capillaroscopic damage. Statistically significant difference in number of B-lines between patients with and without ulcers noted Intra-observer variability in B-line assessment was 3.8%

Table 18.6 (continued)

Author and year published (Ref)	Equipment	Subjects number, gender, mean age in years (SD)	US scoring/scanning protocol (author/year of publication if adopted from another study)	Major findings, other comments
Tardella 2018 [71]	MyLab Twice, 4–13 MHz broadband linear transducer	$N = 40$ 6 M, 34 F	Gutierrez 2011 14 LICS: for the anterior chest the second LIS along the parasternal lines and the fourth LIS along the midclavicular, anterior axillary and midaxillary lines; for the posterior chest, the eighth LIS along the paravertebral, subscapular, and posterior axillary lines	Detection of 10 B-lines is highly predictive for the HRCT presence of significant SSc-ILD. Strong correlation between total LUS score and the Warrick score ($p < 0.001$) and between ultrasound score and DLCO ($p < 0.001$) noted. Moderate correlation was seen with SF-36 mental component summary scale score, SF-36 physical component summary scale score (respectively $p < 0.001$ and $p < 0.001$), and with FVC ($p = 0.001$)
Hassan 2018 [72]	Philips Envisor HD; convex transducer 3.5 MHz	$N = 67$ 4 M, 63 F	Gargani 2009 72 intercostal spaces scanned	Ultrasound sensitivity 100%, specificity 34%. Receiver operating characteristic curve analysis showed relation between number of B-lines and presence of ILD on HRCT. Low Warrick score can rule out need for HRCT

(continued)

Table 18.6 (continued)

Author and year published (Ref)	Equipment	Subjects number, gender, mean age in years (SD)	US scoring/scanning protocol (author/year of publication if adopted from another study)	Major findings, other comments
Gasperini 2019 [73]	Toshiba Aplio XV; 2.5–3.5 MHz probe	$N = 41$ 6 M, 35 F Mean age 50 (15.1) 27 dSSc; 14 lSSc	Number of B-lines in 50 scanning sites (bilateral anterior, medial and posterior chest) was counted Semiquantitative scoring: grade 0 (normal) <10 B-lines; grade 1 (mild) 11–20 B-lines; grade 2 (moderate) 21–50 B-lines, and grade 3 (marked) >50 B-lines	Positive correlation between number of B-lines and HRCT score ($r = 0.51$, $p < 0.05$), and negative correlation between number of B-lines and DLCO ($r = -0.49$, $p < 0.05$) and FVC ($r = -0.42$, $p < 0.05$) noted At 12 months, a positive correlation exists between number of B-lines and delta of DLCO. Intra-observer variability in B-line assessment was 3.5%
Reyes-Long 2019 [74]	MyLab Seven (Esaote SpA) 5–13 MHz linear transducer	$N = 68$ 7 M, 61 F Mean age 51.2 (10.2) Disease duration 4.09 (2.3) years 39 dSSC, 29 lSSC	Gutierrez 2011 B-lines 0 = normal, <5 lines; 1 = mild, 6–15 lines, 2 = moderate, 16–30 lines; 3 = severe, >30 lines	Ultrasound should be considered for detection of ILD in early scleroderma Positive correlation between HRCT and ultrasound. Sensitivity 91.2%, specificity 88.6%, $K = 0.72$. Anti-centromere antibodies and Rodnan Skin score were associated with ultrasound and HRCT findings

ILD interstitial lung disease, *PPV* positive predictive value, *NPV* negative predictive value, *DLCO* carbon monoxide diffusing capacity, *FVC* forced vital capacity, *TLC* total lung capacity, *VC* vital capacity, *HRCT* high-resolution computed tomography, *SSc* systemic sclerosis, *LICS* lung intercostal spaces, *dSSc* diffuse systemic sclerosis, *lSSc* limited systemic sclerosis statistically significant for detecting ILD over B-lines and allowed for classification of ILD as either limited or extensive using the Goh algorithm [57, 75].

LUS can detect ILD in patients with negative HRCTs [66, 72]. B-lines have also been detected in "very early" and "early" SSc [65, 66, 74]. LUS may correlate with pulmonary function test findings. In populations of patients already scanned via HRCT, LUS scores correlated with DLCO and FVC; in this study, the sensitivity, specificity, positive predictive value, and negative predictive value of LUS were 100%, <84%, 90%, and 100%, respectively [69]. A negative relationship was noted between the numbers of B-lines and DLCO in another study [70]. LUS also has the potential to predict SSc-ILD progression. A positive correlation exists between numbers of B-lines and change in DLCO, progression of digital microvascular damage, and the overall worsening of ILD [73]. Interestingly, in a study combining the use of LUS with the Borg Dyspnea Index, HRCT, and DLCO, the prevalence of subclinical ILD in SSC was 41% vs. 4.8% among healthy controls; a positive correlation between HRCT and B-lines was noted, and anti-centromere and Rodnan skin scores correlated with presence of ILD [74]. Sensitivity and specificity of ultrasound was 91% and 89%, respectively [74].

Scanning Protocols and Scoring Systems for CTD-LUS

A number of protocols have been used for evaluation of CTD-ILD. The discussion here focuses on how many LICS are needed and how to evaluate for severity of lung disease. In general, latest iterations of expert opinion are leaning toward designating <5 B-lines as ruling out ILD [72] and >10 B-lines as abnormal [50].

Jambrik et al. used a protocol that reportedly took less than 3 min by looking at the number of comet tail signs at LICs 2–4 along the parasternal, midclavicular, anterior axillary, and midaxillary lines over both hemithoraces, with LIC 5 being done only along the right side [76]. Parasternal regions were done with the patient lying lateral decubitus position over the ipsilateral side of the lung being scanned, while anterior axillary scans were done in the supine position. This protocol was supplemented by adding bilateral posterior LICS along the posterior axillary, linea scapularis, and paravertebral lines as part of a study looking at SSc patients [63]. A 14 bilateral LICS protocol was comparable to a 50-LICS protocol and correlated with HRCT findings [52]. Kappa values for interobserver simplified assessment kappa values ranged between 0.769 and 0.885. A 10-LICS scoring system was comparable a HRCT scoring system [67]. Comprehensive scoring systems can take up to 23 ± 4.5 min vs. simplified (8.6 ± 1.4 min) vs. modified systems (5.4 ± 1.8) [67].

A meta-analysis of 11 studies involving 487 CTD-ILD patients noted that a protocol involving scanning of 14 LICS had 98% sensitivity and 88% specificity. Six methods to evaluate LICS were noted with a pooled sensitivity and specificity of 86% and 84%, respectively [77].

One of the more widely used systems for CTD-ILD evaluation was based on a schema developed by Picano et al. [5] where a mild score describes the presence of 6–15 B-lines and either moderate or severe scores (≥16 B-lines). Ultrasound Fibrosis

Index has been proposed describing the severity of pulmonary fibrosis (mild, moderate, severe disease) by utilizing a mix of pleural changes and parenchymal changes [24]. An extensive scoring system was proposed looking at B-lines in 50 LICS: grade 0 (normal) = <0 B-lines, grade 1 (mild) 11–20 B-lines, grade 2 (moderate) = 21 = 50 B-lines, grade 3 (marked) = >50 B-lines [48]. However, in an effort to achieve a realistically feasible method, a much more simplified system looking at 14 LICS and number of B-lines has been proposed with the grading of B-lines designated as follows: grade 0 = normal based on <5 B-lines, grade 1 was mild (6–15 B-lines), grade 2 = moderate (16–30 B-lines), and grade 3 = marked (>30 B-lines) [52].

Lung ultrasound interpretation criteria for SSc-ILD detection have been proposed and validated in a small cohort of 20 patients. In line with observations by other experts that pleural abnormalities yield more information over B-lines, Fairchild et al. noted that lung zones were considered positive for ILD if two sets of criteria are met: (1) the first set requires discontinuation or cavitations in the linear pleural surface or a hyperechoic, granular appearance; (2) the second set requires identification of at least two distinct lesion >2 mm in width or as confluent lesions involving the entire pleural surface, pseudothickening, and tracks with lung movement [78]. Validation using a much larger cohort of SSc and PM/DM patients is forthcoming.

Equipment Issues

Many LUS studies done to study patients with rheumatic diseases have been done using a 2.5–3.5 MHz cardiac sector probe, but 6–12 MHz linear probes typically used for MSUS may also be used. Sector transducers are useful for optimum depth penetration, for evaluation of lungs from the intercostal, subcostal, or parasternal approach, and for evaluation of pleural and peripheral pulmonary lesions [32]. Wide-range (1–16 cm) microconvex probes are helpful for "whole body critical ultrasound" where time is of the essence and there is a need to scan other organs (such as the abdomen, veins) apart from the lung [35]. Linear probes utilized by rheumatologists for musculoskeletal ultrasound can also be used. Others prefer linear array 5–17 MHz transducers. A linear probe, usually used for MSUS, was useful for LUS by comparing scans using a 2.5–3.5 MHz cardiac sector probe vs. a 6–12 MHz linear probe [64]. The one caveat of the linear probe is that is that midaxillary scanning becomes challenging because the 6 cm linear width of the linear probe footprint risks having ultrasound lung comets being numbered twice. Other studies have used linear probes [24, 48, 53, 57, 64, 67, 69] for the entire study, or for some, switching to use it to study the pleura [56]. The emergence of pocket-sized US machines has been popularized among hospitalist settings over the last 5 years. Pocket-sized ultrasound devices have been comparable to standard devices in screening for ILD in RA patients (e.g., VScan, GE Healthcare, supporting a phased array (1.7–3.8 MHz) transducer) [54]. Similar devices are used in trauma situations, as studied for cases of suspected pneumothorax (e.g., Sonosite 180, 2.4 kg handheld unit, L38 linear array (5–10 MHz) transducer) [36].

Knobology and other controls are similar to what is used for MSUS, but again image optimization in LUS is highly dependent on an understanding of how artifacts, particularly B-lines, develop. Gain, depth, frame rates, and dynamic range are among other equipment-related factors that affect visualization of B-lines. A complete discussion of factors affecting B-line visualization has been described elsewhere [32].

Conclusion

Lung ultrasound is borne out of a better understanding of how artifacts are generated and can be interpreted in the context of pathology. It is mobile, lacks radiation, and is cost- and time-effective as compared to HRCT. LUS has become a clinical tool in the emergency department and ICU settings; however, currently LUS within rheumatology is mostly performed for research purposes. Skills related to rheumatology MSUS are translatable toward LUS, and the knowledge and skills acquired by trainees during medical school and residency training who are entering fellowship training can potentially be built upon to further the use of LUS in rheumatic disease evaluation.

More studies are needed to better define elementary ILD lesions, determine ultrasound's accuracy to assess response to therapy and its relevant impact on overall morbidity and mortality, outline specific indications as to when an ultrasound is warranted, and develop image acquisition and interpretation protocols.

References

1. Volpicelli G. Lung sonography. J Ultrasound Med. 2013;32:165–71.
2. Lichtenstein DA. Ultrasound in the management of thoracic disease. Crit Care Med. 2007;35(5 Suppl):S250–61.
3. Volpicelli G, Elbarbary M, Blaivas M, Lichtenstein D, Mathis G, Kirkpatrick AW, Melniker L, Gargani L, International Liaison Committee on Lung Ultrasound (ILC-LUS) for International Consensus Conference on Lung Ultrasound (ICC-LUS), et al. International evidence-based recommendations for point-of-care lung ultrasound. Intensive Care Med. 2012;38:577–91.
4. Gasho CJ, Torralba KD, Chooljian DM, Cohen A, Dinh VA. Impact of a lung ultrasound course for rheumatology specialists (IMPACT-2). Clin Exp Rheumatol. 2019;37(3):380–4.
5. Picano E, Frassi F, Agricola E, Gligorova S, Gargani L, Mottola G. Ultrasound lung comets: a clinically useful sign of extravascular lung water. J Am Soc Echocardiogr. 2006;19:356–63.
6. American Institute of Ultrasound in Medicine. Ultrasound in Medical Education. https://www.aium.org/communities/usMedEd.aspx. Accessed 22 Sept 2019.
7. Okamoto M, Fujimoto K, Sadohara J, et al. A retrospective cohort study of outcome in systemic sclerosis-associated interstitial lung disease. Respir Investig. 2016;54:445–53.
8. Fischer A, Swigris JJ, Groshong SD, et al. Clinically significant interstitial lung disease in limited scleroderma: histopathology, clinical features, and survival. Chest. 2008;134:601–5.
9. Takei R, Arita M, Kumagai S, Ito Y, Tokioka F, Koyama T, Saito R, Nishimura K, Tokumasu H, Ishi T. Radiographic fibrosis score predicts survival in systemic sclerosis-associated interstitial lung disease. Respirology. 2018;23(4):385–91.

10. Ito Y, Arita M, Kumagai S, Takei R, Noyama M, Tokioka F, Nishimura K, Koyama T, Tachibana H, Ishida T. Radiological fibrosis score is strongly associated with worse survival in rheumatoid arthritis-related interstitial lung disease. Mod Rheumatol. 2019;29(1):98–104.
11. Zamora-Legoff JA, Krause ML, Crowson CS, Ryu JH, Matteson EL. Patterns of interstitial lung disease and mortality in rheumatoid arthritis. Rheumatology (Oxford). 2017;56(3):344–50. https://doi.org/10.1093/rheumatology/kew391.
12. Solomon JJ, Chung JH, Cosgrove GP, Demoruelle MK, Fernandez-Perez ER, Fischer A, Frankel SK, Hobbs SB, Huie TJ, Ketzer J, Mannina A, Olson AL, Russell G, Tsuchiya Y, Yunt ZX, Zelarney PT, Brown KK, Swigris JJ. Predictors of mortality in rheumatoid arthritis-associated interstitial lung disease. Eur Respir J. 2016;47(2):588–96. https://doi.org/10.1183/13993003.00357-2015. Epub 2015 Nov 19.
13. Waseda Y, Johkoh T, Egashira R, et al. Antisynthetase syndrome: pulmonary computed tomography findings of adult patients with antibodies to aminoacyl-tRNA synthetases. Eur J Radiol. 2016;85:1421–6.
14. Parambil J, Myer J, Lindell R. Interstitial lung disease in primary Sjogren syndrome. Chest. 2006;130(5):1489–95.
15. Gunnarsson R, Aaløkken TM, Molberg Ø, et al. Prevalence and severity of interstitial lung disease in mixed connective tissue disease: a nationwide, cross-sectional study. Ann Rheum Dis. 2012;71:1966–72.
16. Bertoli AM, Vila LM, Apte M, et al. Systemic lupus erythematosus in a multiethnic US cohort LUMINA XLVIII: factors predictive of pulmonary damage. Lupus. 2007;16:410–7.
17. Mohammad AJ, et al. Pulmonary involvement in antineutrophil cytoplasmic antibodies. J Rheumatol. 2017;44:10.
18. Alba MA, Flores-Suarez LF, Henderson AG, Xiao H, Hu P, Nachman PH, Falk RJ, Jennette JC. Interstitial lung disease in ANCA vasculitis. Autoimmun Rev. 2017;16(7):722–9.
19. Travis WD, Costabel U, Hansell DM, King TE Jr, Lynch DA, Nicholson AG, Ryerson CJ, Ryu JH, Selman M, Wells AU, Behr J, Bouros D, Brown KK, Colby TV, Collard HR, Cordeiro CR, Cottin V, Crestani B, Drent M, Dudden RF, Egan J, Flaherty K, Hogaboam C, Inoue Y, Johkoh T, Kim DS, Kitaichi M, Loyd J, Martinez FJ, Myers J, Protzko S, Raghu G, Richeldi L, Sverzellati N, Swigris J, Valeyre D, on behalf of the ATS/ERS Committee on Idiopathic Interstitial Pneumonias. An Official American Thoracic Society/European Respiratory Society statement: update of the international multidisciplinary classification of the idiopathic interstitial pneumonias. Am J Respir Crit Care Med. 2013;188(6):733–48.
20. Bryson T, Sundaram B, Khanna D, Kaerooni EA. Connective tissue disease-associated interstitial pneumonia and idiopathic interstitial pneumonia. Semin Ultrasound CT MR. 2014;35:29–38.
21. Fischer A, Antoniou KM, Brown KK, Cadranel J, Corte TJ, du Bois RM, Lee JS, Leslie KO, Lynch DA, Matteson EL, Mosca M, Noth I, Richeldi L, Strek ME, Swigris JJ, Wells AU, Sterling West SG, Collard HR, Cottin V, on behalf of the ERS/ATS Task Force on Undifferentiated Forms of CTD-ILD. An official European Respiratory Society/American Thoracic Society research statement: interstitial pneumonia with autoimmune features. Eur Respir J. 2015;46:976–87.
22. Fischer A, Lee JS, Cottin V. Interstitial lung disease evaluation: detecting connective tissue disease. Respiration. 2015;90:177–84.
23. Oldham JM, Adegunsoye A, Valenzi E, Lee C, Witt L, Chen L, Husain AN, Montner S, Chung JH, Cottin V, Fischer A, Noth I, Vij R, Strek ME. Characterisation of patients with interstitial pneumonia with autoimmune features. Eur Respir J. 2016;47:1767–75.
24. Buda N, Piskunowicz M, Porzezinska M, Kosiak W, Zdrojewski Z. Lung ultrasonography in the evaluation of interstitial lung disease in systemic connective tissue diseases: criteria and severity of pulmonary fibrosis – analysis of 52 patients. Ultraschall Med. 2016;37(4):379–85. https://doi.org/10.1055/s-0041-110590. Epub 2015 Dec 29.
25. Warrick JH, Bhalla M, Schabel SI, Silver RM. High resolution computed tomography in early scleroderma disease. J Rheumatol. 1991;18(10):1520–8.

26. Vizioli L, Ciccarese F, Forti P, Chiesi AM, Giovagnoli M, Mughetti M, Zompatori M, Zoli M. Integrated use of lung ultrasound and chest x-ray in the detection of interstitial lung disease. Respiration. 2017;93:15–22.
27. US Food and Drug Administration. https://www.fda.gov/news-events/press-announcements/fda-approves-first-treatment-patients-rare-type-lung-disease. Last Accessed 27 Sept 2019.
28. Distler O, Highland KB, Gahlemann M, Azuma A, Fischer A, Mayes MD, Raghu G, Sauter W, Girard M, Alves M, Clerisme-Beaty E, Stowasser S, Tetzlaff K, Kuwana M, Maher TM, SENSCIS Trial Investigators. Nintedanib for systemic sclerosis-associated interstitial lung disease. N Engl J Med. 2019;380(26):2518–28. https://doi.org/10.1056/NEJMoa1903076. Epub 2019 May 20. PMID: 31112379.
29. Flaherty KR, Wells AU, Cottin V, Devaraj A, Wawlsh SLF, Inoue Y, Richeldi L, Kolb M, Tetzlaff K, Stowasser S, Coeck C, Clerisme-Beaty E, Rosenstock B, Quaresma M, Haeufel T, Goeldner RG, Schlenker-Herceg R, Brown KK, INBUILD Trial Investigators. Nintedanib in progressive fibrosing interstitial lung diseases. N Engl J Med. 2019;381(18):1718–27.
30. Gargani L, Volpicelli G. How I do it: lung ultrasound. Cardiovasc Ultrasound. 2014;12:25.
31. Lichtenstein DA. Lung ultrasound in the critically ill. Ann Intensive Care. 2014;4(1):1. https://doi.org/10.1186/2110-5820-4-1.
32. Dietrich CF, Mathis G, Cui XW, Ignee A, Hocke M, Hirche TO. Ultrasound of the pleurae and lungs. Ultrasound Med Biol. 2015;41(2):351–65.
33. Lichtenstein DA, Menu Y. A bedside ultrasound is ruling out pneumothorax in the critically ill: lung sliding. Chest. 1995;108:1345–8.
34. Lichtenstein D, Meziere G, Biderman P, et al. The "lung point": an ultrasound sign specific to pneumothorax. Intensive Care Med. 2000;26:1434–40.
35. Lichtenstein DA. Current misconceptions in lung ultrasound: a short guide for experts. Chest. 2019;156(1):21–5. https://doi.org/10.1016/j.chest.2019.02.332. Epub 2019 Mar 11.
36. Kirkpatrick AW, Sirois M, Laupland KB, Liu D, Rowan K, Ball CG, Hameed SM, Brown R, Simons R, Dulchavsky SA, Hamilton DR, Nicolaou S. Hand-held thoracic sonography for detecting post-traumatic pneumothoraces. The extended focused assessment sonography for trauma (EFAST). J Trauma. 2004;57:288–95.
37. Volpicelli G, Melniker LA, Cardinale L, Lamorte A, Frascisco MF. Lung ultrasound in diagnosing and monitoring pulmonary interstitial fluid. Radiol Med. 2013;118:196–205.
38. Volpicelli G, Mussa A, Garofalo G, et al. Bedside lung ultrasound in the assessment of alveolar-interstitial syndrome. Am J Emerg Med. 2006;24:689–96.
39. Dietrich CF, Mathis G, Blaivas M, Volpicelli G, Seibel A, Wastl D, Atkinson NSS, Cui SW, Fan M, Yi D. Lung B-line artefacts and their use. J Thorac Dis. 2016;8(6):1356–65.
40. Lichtenstein D, Meziere G, Biderman P, et al. The comet-tail artifact: an ultrasound sign of alveolar-interstitial syndrome. Am J Respir Crit Care Med. 1997;156:1640–6.
41. Soldati G, Copetti R, Sher S. Sonographic interstitial syndrome: the sound of lung water. J Ultrasound Med. 2009;28:163–74.
42. Wang Y, Gargani L, Barskova T, Furst DE, Cerinic MM. Usefulness of lung ultrasound B-lines in connective tissue disease-associated interstitial lung disease: a literature review. Arthritis Res Ther. 2017;19(1):206. https://doi.org/10.1186/s13075-017-1409-7.
43. Moazedi-Fuerst FC, Kielhauser SM, Scheidl S, Tripolt NJ, Lutfi A, Yazdani-Biuki B, Dejaco C, Graninger WB. Ultrasound screening for interstitial lung disease in rheumatoid arthritis. Clin Exp Rheumatol. 2014;32:199–203.
44. Williamson JP, Grainge C, Parameswaran A, Twaddell SH. Curr Pulmonol Rep. 2017;6:39–47.
45. Cercle des echogarphistes D'Urgence et de Reanimation Fracophones. http://www.ceurf.net/en/index.htm. Last Accessed 22 Sept 2019.
46. Ferro F, Delle Sedie A. The use of ultrasound for assessing interstitial lung involvement in connective tissue diseases. Clin Exp Rheumatol. 2018;36(Suppl. 114):S165–70; image reprinted with permission from the publisher.
47. Delle Sedie A, Terslev L, Bruyn GAW, Cazenave T, Chrysidis S, Diaz M, Di Carlo M, Frigato M, Gargani L, Gutierrez M, Hocevar A, Iagnocco A, Juche A, Mandl P, Naredo E, Mortada M, Pineda C, Porta F, Ravagnani V, Scire C, Serban T, Smith K, Stoenoiu M, Tardella M, Torralba

K, Wakefield R, D'Agostino MA, on behalf of OMERACT US Task Force on Lung US in Rheumatology. Definition and standardization of interstitial lung disease (ILD) assessment by ultrasound: results from a Delphi process and web-reliability exercise by the OMERACT Ultrasound Working Group (WG). Ann Rheum Dis. 2019;78(Suppl. 2):S834.

48. Tardella M, Gutierrez M, Salaffi F, Carotti M, Ariani A, Bertolazzi C, Filippucci E, Grassi W. Ultrasound in the assessment of pulmonary fibrosis in connective tissue disorders: correlation with high-resolution computed tomography. J Rheumatol. 2015;39(8):1641–7.
49. Song GG, Bae SC, Lee YH. Diagnostic accuracy of lung ultrasound for interstitial lung disease in patients with connective tissue diseases: a meta-analysis. Clin Exp Rheumatol. 2016;34(1):11–6. Epub 2016 Jan 20. Review.
50. Gutierrez M, Tardella M, Rodriguez L, Mendoza J, Clavijo-Cornejo D, Garcia A, Bertolazzi C. Ultrasound as a potential tool for the assessment of interstitial lung disease in rheumatic patients. Where are we now? Radiol Med. 2019;124(10):989–99. https://doi.org/10.1007/s11547-019-01053-5. [Epub ahead of print].
51. Sperandeo M, Varriale A, Speerandeo G, Filabozzi P, Piatteli ML, Carnevale V, Duzzi M, Vendemiale G. Transthoracic ultrasound in the evaluation of pulmonary fibrosis: our experience. Ultrasound Med Biol. 2009;35(5):723–9. https://doi.org/10.1016/j.ultrasmedbio.2008.10.009. Epub 2008 Dec 27.
52. Gutierrez M, Salaffi F, Carotti M, Tardella M, Pineda C, Bertolazzi C, Bichisecchi E, Filippucci E, Grassi W. Utility of a simplified ultrasound assessment to assess interstitial pulmonary fibrosis in connective tissue disorders – preliminary results. Arthritis Res Ther. 2011;13:R134.
53. Aghdashi M, Broofeh B, Mohammadi A. Diagnostic performances of high resolution transthoracic lung ultrasonography in pulmonary alveoli-interstitial involvement of rheumatoid lung disease. Int J Clin Exp Med. 2013;6(7):562–6.
54. Cogliati C, Antivalle M, Torzillo D, Birocchi S, Norsa A, Blanco R, Costantino G, Ditto MC, Battelino M, Puttini PCS, Montano N. Standard and pocket-size lung ultrasound devices can detect interstitial lung disease in rheumatoid arthritis patients. Rheumatology. 2014;53:1497–503.
55. Hasan AA, Makhlouf HA. B-lines: transthoracic chest ultrasound signs useful in assessment of interstitial lung diseases. Ann Thorac Med. 2014;9:99–103. https://doi.org/10.4103/1817-1737.128856.
56. Moazedi Fuerst F, Kielhauser S, Brickmann K, Tripolt N, Meilinger M, Lutfi A, Graninger W. Sonographic assessment of interstitial lung disease in patients with rheumatoid arthritis, systemic sclerosis and systemic lupus erythematosus. Clin Exp Rheumatol. 2015;33(4 Suppl 91):S87–91. Epub 2015 Jan 29
57. Pinal-Fernandez I, Pallisa-Nunez E, Selva-O'Callaghan A, Castella-Fierro E, Simeon-Aznar CP, Fonollosa-Pla V, Vilardell-Tarres M. Pleural irregularity, a new ultrasound sign for the study of interstitial lung disease in systemic sclerosis and antisynthetase syndrome. Clin Exp Rheumatol. 2015;33(Suppl 91):S136–41.
58. Vasco PG, de Luna Cardenal G, Garrido IM, et al. Assessment of interstitial lung disease in Sjögren's syndrome by lung ultrasound: a pilot study of correlation with high-resolution chest tomography. Intern Emerg Med. 2017;12:327–31.
59. Buda N, Masiak A, Zdrojewski Z. Utility of lung ultrasound in ANCA-associated vasculitis with lung involvement. PLoS One. 2019;14(9):e0222189. https://doi.org/10.1371/journal.pone.0222189. eCollection 2019.
60. Steen V. Predictors of end stage lung disease in systemic sclerosis. Ann Rheum Dis. 2003;62(2):97–9.
61. Tyndall AJ, Bannert B, Vonk M, Airo P, Cozzi F, Carreira PE, Bancel DF, Allanore Y, Muller-Ladner U, Distler O, et al. Causes and risk factors for death in systemic sclerosis: a study from the EULAR Scleroderma Trials and Research (EUSTAR) database. Ann Rheum Dis. 2010;69(10):1809–15.
62. Doveri M, Frassi F, Consensi A, Vesprini E, Gargani L, Tafuri M, Picano E, Della Rossa A, Delle Sedie A, d'Ascanio A, Giacomelli C, Bazzichi L, Bombardieri S. Ultrasound lung comets: new echographic sign of lung interstitial fibrosis in systemic sclerosis. Reumatismo. 2008;60(3):180–4.

63. Gargani L, Doveri M, D'Errico L, Frassi F, Bazzichi ML, Delle Sedie A, Scali MC, Monti S, Mondillo S, Bombardieri S, Caramella D, Picano E. Ultrasound lung comets in systemic sclerosis: a chest sonography hallmark of pulmonary interstitial fibrosis. Rheumatology. 2009;48(11):1382–7.
64. Delle Sedie A, Doveri M, Frassi F, Gargani L, D'Errico G, Pepe P, Bazzichi L, Riente L, Caramella D, Bombardieri S. Ultrasound lung comets in systemic sclerosis: a useful tool to detect lung interstitial fibrosis. Clin Exp Rheumatol. 2010;28(5 Suppl 62):S54. Epub 2010 Nov 3.
65. Moazedi-Fuerst FC, Zechner PM, Tripolt NJ, Kielhauser SM, Brickmann K, Scheidl S, Lutfi A, Graninger WG. Pulmonary echography in systemic sclerosis. Clin Rheumatol. 2012;31(11):1621–5. https://doi.org/10.1007/s10067-012-2055-8. Epub 2012 Aug 18.
66. Barskova T, Gargani L, Guiducci S, Randone SB, Bruni C, Carnesecchi G, Conforti ML, Porta F, Pignone A, Caramella D, Picano E, Cerinic MM. Lung ultrasound for the screening of interstitial lung disease in very early systemic sclerosis. Ann Rheum Dis. 2013;72(3):390–5. https://doi.org/10.1136/annrheumdis-2011-201072. Epub 2012 May 15.
67. Mohammadi A, Oshnoei S, Ghasemi-rad M. Comparison of a new, modified lung ultrasonography technique with high-resolution CT in the diagnosis of the alveolo-interstitial syndrome of systemic scleroderma. Med Ultrason. 2014;16(1):27–31.
68. Sperandeo M, De Cata A, Molinaro F, Trovato FM, Catalano D, Simeone A, Varriale A, Martines GF, Trovato G. Ultrasound signs of pulmonary fibrosis in systemic sclerosis as timely indicators for chest computed tomography. Scand J Rheumatol. 2015;44:389–98.
69. Cakir Edis E, Hatipoglu ON, Pamuk ON, Mutlucan Eraslan R, Aktoz M, Tuncel SA. Effectiveness of thoracic ultrasonography in the evaluation of the severity of pulmonary involvement in patients with systemic sclerosis. Arch Rheumatol. 2016;31(4):364–70.
70. Gigante A, Fanelli FR, Lucci S, Barilaro G, Quarta S, Barbano B, Biovannetti A, Amoroso A, Rosato E. Lung ultrasound in systemic sclerosis: correlation with high-resolution computed tomography, pulmonary function tests and clinical variables of disease. Intern Emerg Med. 2016;11:213–7.
71. Tardella M, Di Carlo M, Carotti M, Filippucci E, Grassi W, Salaffi F. Ultrasound B-lines in the evaluation of interstitial lung disease in patients with systemic sclerosis. Medicine. 2018;97:18.
72. Hassan RI, Lubertino LI, Barth MA, et al. Lung ultrasound as a screening method for interstitial lung disease in patients with systemic sclerosis. J Clin Rheumatol. 2018;25(7):304–7. https://doi.org/10.1097/RHU.0000000000000860.
73. Gasperini ML, Gigante A, Iacolare A, Pellicano C, Lucci S, Rosato E. The predictive role of lung ultrasound in progression of scleroderma interstitial lung disease. Clin Rheumatol. 2020;39(1):119–23. https://doi.org/10.1007/s10067-019-04686-z. [Epub ahead of print].
74. Reyes-Long S, Gutierrez M, Clavijo-Cornejo D, Alfaro-Rodríguez A, González-Sámano K, Cortes-Altamirano JL, Muñoz-Louis R, Cruz-Arenas E, Camargo K, Gonzalez F, Bertolazzi C. Subclinical interstitial lung disease in patients with systemic sclerosis. A pilot study on the role of ultrasound. Reumatol Clin. 2021;17(3):144–9. https://doi.org/10.1016/j.reuma.2019.05.004. [Epub ahead of print].
75. Goh NS, Desai SR, Veeraraghavan S, et al. Interstitial lung disease in systemic sclerosis: a simple staging system. Am J Respir Crit Care Med. 2008;177:1248–54.
76. Jambrik Z, Monti S, Coppola V, Agricola E, Mottola G, Miniati M, Picano E. Usefulness of ultrasound lung comets as a nonradiologic sign of extravascular lung watter. Am J Cardiol. 2004;93:1265–70.
77. Xie HQ, Zhang WW, Sun S, Chen XM, Yuan SF, Gong ZH, Liu L. A simplified lung ultrasound for the diagnosis of interstitial lung disease in connective tissue disease: a meta-analysis. Arthritis Res Ther. 2019;21(1):93. https://doi.org/10.1186/s13075-019-1888-9.
78. Fairchild R, Chung M, Yang D, Sharpless L, Li S, Chung L. Development and preliminary validation of a novel lung ultrasound interpretation criteria for the detection of interstitial lung disease in patients with systemic sclerosis. Arthritis Care Res (Hoboken). 2020 May 31. https://doi.org/10.1002/acr.24338

Advanced Ultrasound Applications: Elastography and Contrast-Enhanced Ultrasound

19

Paul J. DeMarco

Introduction to Elastography

Ultrasound elastography (EUS) is an imaging technique that capitalizes on the ability of sound to move differently through tissues of different compressibility or stiffness. The technique, first described in the 1990s, was applied to liver disease in the setting of liver fibrosis and portal hypertension [1]. Rapid application to breast, thyroid, prostate, kidney, and lymph node imaging by oncologic radiologists was driven by the observations that tissue infiltration by malignancy changes the stiffness of various soft tissue organ sites. Since any soft tissue has the potential to have its "stiffness" altered by a pathologic state, it would seem reasonable to look outside the oncologic world for applications of elastography. Early work in the musculoskeletal system started with the evaluation of muscle and tendon biomechanics [1, 2]. Elastography applications have become more widely available on smaller, more portable units in the twenty-first century; therefore, elastography is likely to capture the imagination of ultrasonographers in all fields of study.

EUS, using strain elastography, is the most common technique that allows real-time visualization of the elastographic map on the ultrasound screen. There is increasing evidence that EUS can be used to measure the mechanical properties of musculoskeletal tissue in clinical practice with the future potential for early diagnosis to both guide and monitor therapy. Rheumatic conditions that are affected by inflammatory as well as fibrotic processes may be of interest to apply EUS. A summary of disease states identified in the literature is summarized in Table 19.1. The unique information that EUS can provide could add to our understanding of tissue properties in a selected site of interest.

P. J. DeMarco (✉)
Arthritis & Rheumatism Associates PC, Center for Rheumatology and Bone Research, Wheaton, MD, USA
e-mail: pdemarco@arapc.com

M. J. Kohler (ed.), *Musculoskeletal Ultrasound in Rheumatology Review*,
https://doi.org/10.1007/978-3-030-73555-5_19

Table 19.1 Elastography in rheumatic diseases

Achilles tendinopathy [14–18]	Ankylosing spondylitis [17]
Lateral epicondylitis [24–27]	Rheumatoid nodules [43]
Plantar fasciitis [28]	Gouty arthritis [42–44]
Rotator cuff tendinopathy [21–23]	Sarcoidosis [52, 53]
Carpal tunnel syndrome [48–51]	Sjogren's syndrome [13, 29–33]
Myofascial pain [45–47]	Benign hypermobility syndrome [39]
	Psoriasis [19, 20]
Dupuytren's contracture [40, 41]	Scleroderma [34–36]

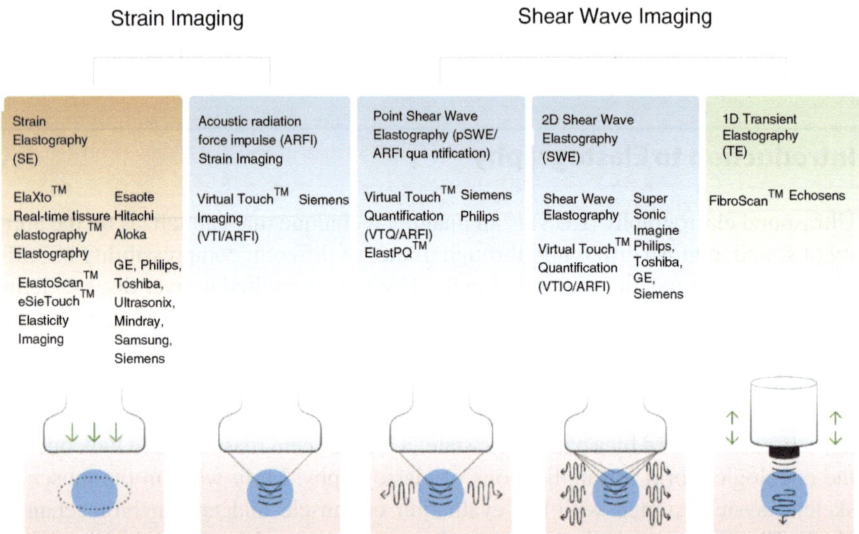

Fig. 19.1 Strain wave imaging versus shear wave imaging. Overview of the grouping of terms and ultrasound machines where these modalities are employed. (Taken from Sigrist et al. [1]. Used with permission)

General Principles

Current applications of EUS include two broad categories: strain elastography (SE) and shear wave elastography (SWE) [1, 3–5]. A summary of the different available technologies by platform/manufacturer type is provided (Fig. 19.1). The two modalities have advantages and disadvantages in musculoskeletal imaging, requiring separate consideration, and are summarized in Table 19.2. Currently, there is considerably more study and more availability of strain elastography (SE) than shear wave elastography (SWE), but both may have a role in the potential evaluation and management of rheumatic disease. Both techniques capitalize on the concept that tissue density is related to tissue compressibility or stiffness. If a tissue is

Table 19.2 Strain wave versus shear wave elastography

Strain elastography (SE)	Shear wave elastography (SWE)
Pros	Pros
Superficial assessment	Relative operator independent due to ARFI
Real time, rapid response	Deep assessment
Broad ROI	Quantitative assessment
Density independent	Cons
Qualitative assessment	Narrow ROI
Cons	Requires serial assessments
Operator dependency	Does not allow real-time response (delay in image acquisition)
Requires subjective scale for grading and following responses	Velocity measurements can be density dependent
	Shear waves do not propagate through fluid (may be important in rheumatologic applications)

deformed or pressured in some way, its relative deformation or compression will depend on its characteristics as well as the characteristics of the surrounding tissue. A soft item will change more dramatically in response to a compressive or sound stimulus, while a firmer or harder item will change less dramatically, nearly retaining its form in response to the stress or remaining unaltered. Further, sound motion and speed through different tissue densities can be readily detected and rapidly classified using the applied physics of the elastic modulus; sound travels faster through a more solid or firmer medium.

Strain Elastography (SE) [Also Known as Real-Time Elastography RTE)]

The overall conceptualization of SE is depicted in Fig. 19.2. This technique operates in a two-dimensional field, where some force is applied from the scanning surface into the tissues deep to the probe [1, 3–5]. Before any elastography imaging begins, the area is assessed by gray scale, and a region of interest (ROI) is chosen by the operator or scanner. Once this area is identified, a vertical compression of the tissue is generated by the operator or the ultrasound probe. One method relies on the ultrasonographer to apply a mechanical, repetitive force in a vertical plane (up and down) onto the surface of the area in question. The force needs to be fairly constant and reproducible for the ultrasound unit to interpret the result of the compression. Most units have a quality assessment tool or "strain indicator" on the image field, which will confirm the adequacy and consistency of compression and assist in selecting the image most representative of the available elastography data. This may differ by ultrasound unit or manufacturer; color bar coding is used in some systems, whereas compression and relaxation curse are used in other units to show the optimal strain at the area of interest. While some units will operate on a manual

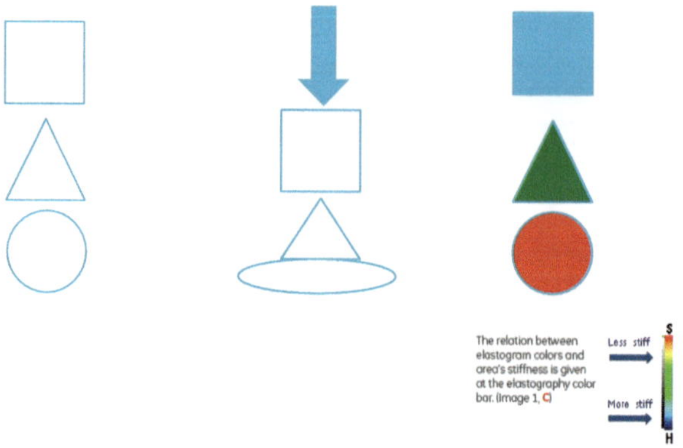

Fig. 19.2 Strain elastography overview. A vertical force (arrow) is applied to the objects of interest, which deform in different degrees. The ultrasound unit codes the objects according to the associated grid, from less stiff, or red hue, to least stiff or most hard, blue hue. The resulting color assignment creates the elastogram

compression, there are other strain wave ultrasound units that will operate with a sound pulse to generate a uniform vertical wave for interpretation of compressibility. The probe generates an acoustic radiation force impulse (ARFI) in the vertical plane to assess the tissue elastography or vertical compressibility [1, 3–5]. Both manual compression units and ARFI units employ the physics involved in the calculation by Young's modulus to distinguish the relative compression of tissues in the field of view, generating a strain wave elastogram [1].

Some tissues are likely to be more easily compressed, such as normal skin (which is not inflamed or infiltrated), and other objects are more likely to retain the shape, size, and contour, such as normal tendon (not mechanically altered by tear or affected by inflammation). The ultrasound unit collects the pattern of geometric alterations and applies a set of assumptions (constant force) through the Young's modulus (see Appendix A), comparing stress and strain to assess elasticity. The resulting image is a color-coded elastogram, which must be interpreted using the color-coding scale provided with each individual ultrasound machine. Many units use a spectrum of a blue hue as the firmest, least compressible tissue type and a red hue as the softest, most compressible tissue; however, it can be reversed on other units. This text will favor using blue as the least elastic and red as the most elastic tissues.

In Fig. 19.3, an egg phantom illustrates the technique of SE by showing that the egg white region, bluer in hue or firm by this machine type, stands in contrast by the yolk type. The soft yolk demonstrates regions of red within them, while the hard yolk is fairly uniformly blue in its elastographic presentation. In an anatomical assessment (Fig. 19.4), the normal Achilles tendon yields a uniform green-blue hue throughout the tendon with regions of red in the soft tissues, outside the grayscale equivalent region, a typical finding for this anatomical region. In contrast, the Achilles tendinitis model, showing areas of tissue stress, notes a red region

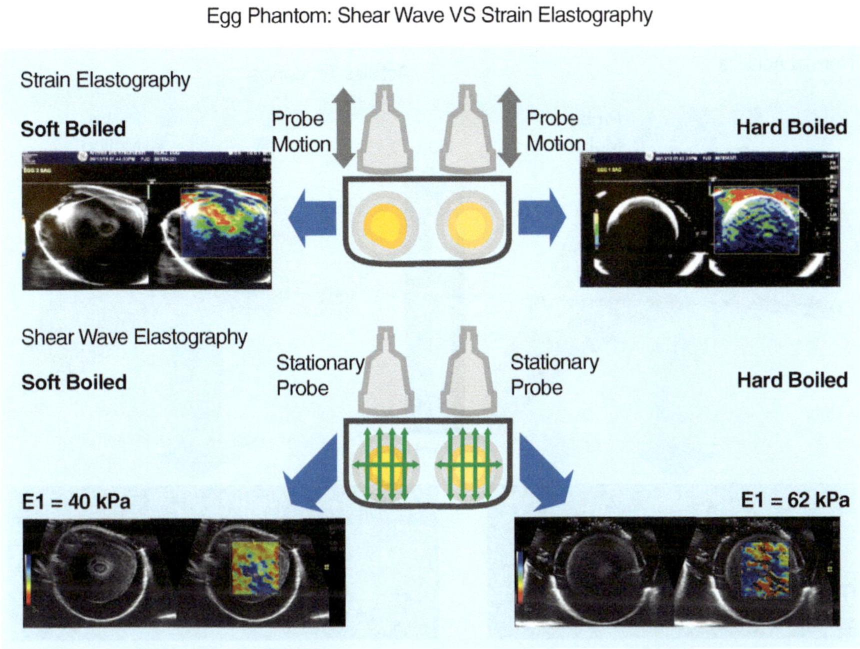

Fig. 19.3 Soft- and hard-boiled egg phantom demonstrating strain wave versus shear wave elastography. Upper series of strain elastography, with soft-boiled egg on the upper left, demonstrates a red hue corresponding to the region of the soft yolk, while the upper right demonstrates a primarily blue hue corresponding to the region of the hard yolk. Lower series of shear wave elastography, with the soft-boiled egg on the lower left, demonstrates a red hue corresponding to the region of the soft yolk, and the shear wave unit assigns a reading of 40 kPa; the lower right demonstrates a primarily blue hue to the region of the hard yolk, and the shear wave unit assigns a reading of 62 kPa, allowing quantitative measure of the difference between the two assessments

throughout the most superficial region of the tendon as well as some red regions in the middle of the Achilles tendon, representing areas of damage or softening. Note that the grayscale region shows some modest widening in the superficial to deep assessment of the tendon, but the elastographic response covers a wider area, suggesting a more broadly affected area.

The resulting elastogram will yield an array of color to allow for qualitative evaluation of the relative softness or firmness/hardness of a tissue type or group. There is inherent difficulty to both reporting an elastographic finding and following a response with such a qualitative measure. To overcome this issue, several authors have evolved scales to facilitate grading of an elastographic finding. For example, in evaluation of lymphadenopathy during an assessment of malignancy [6], an elasticity score of “1” will represent absence of a very small blue area. An elasticity score of “2” will represent a small, scattered blue area that represents 45% but showing green regions. An elasticity score of “4” will represent a blue area with or without a

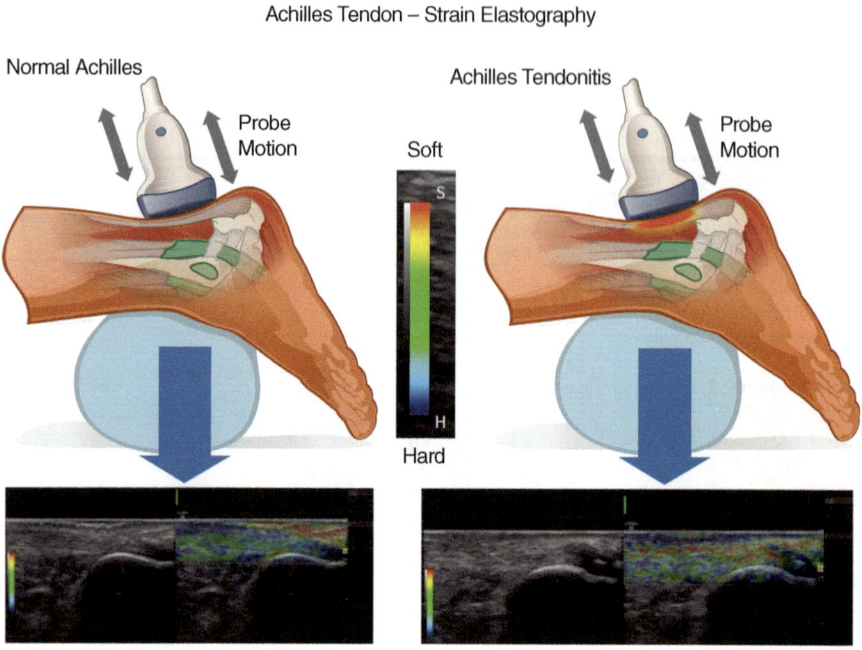

Fig. 19.4 Strain elastography of the Achilles tendon. Lower left elastogram with primarily blue and green in the region of the normal tendon; note the soft tissue above the enthesis is primarily red or soft. Lower right elastogram with streaks of red in the substance of the Achilles tendon, leading up to the insertion, while the soft tissue of the Achilles region sustains it red hue or region of softness

green rim only. An adaptation of this approach for tendon assessment is demonstrated in Fig. 19.5.

Several musculoskeletal articles apply the scale used for grading thyroid nodules [7] which can be either a four-point or a five-point scale. In a five-point strain elastographic score by Rago et al. [8], a score of 1 indicates even elasticity in the whole nodule, a score of 2 indicates elasticity in a large part of the nodule, a score of 3 indicates elasticity only at the peripheral part of the nodule, a score of 4 indicates no elasticity in the nodule, and a score of 5 indicates no elasticity in the nodule or in the area showing posterior shadowing. More in keeping with lymph node scoring, strain elastographic scores by Asteria et al. [9] defined a score of 1 as elasticity in the entire examined area, a score of 2 as elasticity in a large part of the examined area, a score of 3 as stiffness in a large part of the examined area, and a score of 4 as a nodule without elasticity. Other ultrasound units can assign a random score to an ROI and will calculate a comparison to other sites. Investigators of the utility of SE have capitalized on this technique to create a strain ratio (Fig. 19.6); an ROI within a tissue type of interest could be compared to subcutaneous tissue in the same field. The relative compressive response in the tissue of interest (such as a tendon) to the subcutaneous tissue would be labeled as a strain ratio. Strain ratio will increase as

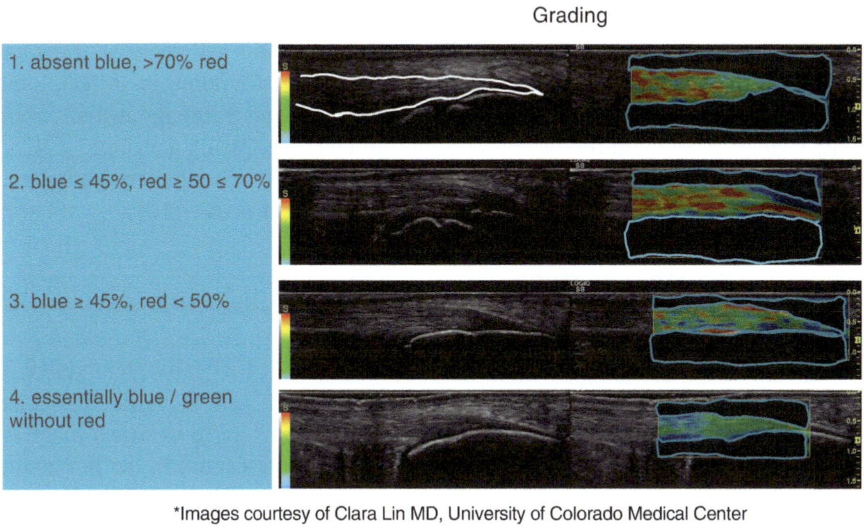

Fig. 19.5 Example of grading tendon elastograms. (Images courtesy of Clara Lin MD, University of Colorado Medical Center). To assist the reader, the non-tendon regions are blackened out to allow the viewer to concentrate on the tendon elastogram

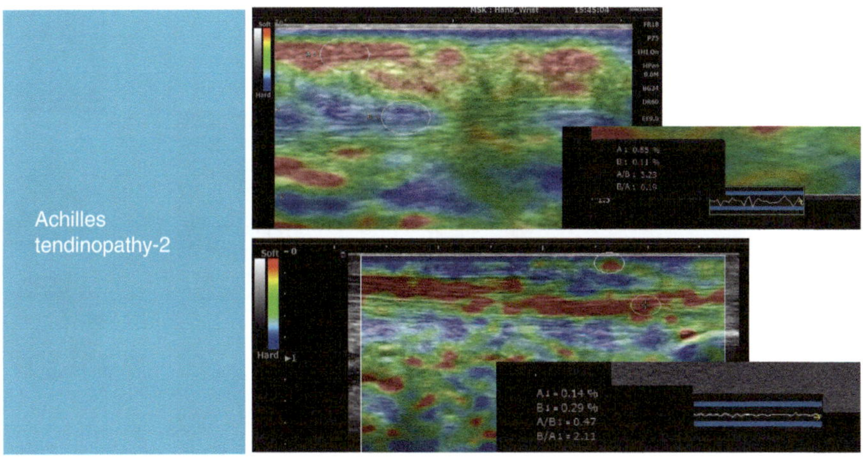

Fig. 19.6 Achilles tendon elastogram demonstrating a tendon strain ratio. Upper Achilles tendon with red hue soft tissue and blue-green hue tendon to create a strain ratio of 5.23. Lower Achilles tendon with red hue soft tissue and regions of red hue within the substance of the Achilles tendon, a sign of tendinopathy, to create a strain ratio of 0.47

tissue increases in stiffness, when the numerator of the tissue of interest, like normal tendon, is harder than the subcutaneous tissue; a strain ratio will decrease if the tissue of interest, like inflamed or mechanically damaged tendon, is softer. Some investigators have noted that elastographic measurements throughout a structure may change in different regions of the same structure. Assessing a change or effect in any one structure over time may benefit from both orthogonal interrogation and measurement at proximal and distal points on the same structure [10].

Shear Wave Elastography (SWE)

The overall conceptualization of SWE is depicted in Fig. 19.7. This technique will interpret sound motion not only in the vertical plane but also in the horizontal plane [11, 12]. The probe-generated ARFI is assessed not only in the vertical plane of motion but also in the speed and tissue deformation that occurs in the horizontal plane: this is the shear wave. The SWE stands in strong contrast to SE where the physical compression or strain ARFI are only interpreted in the vertical plane; in SWE, sound wave propagation also assesses horizontal tissue deformation and horizontal wave speed, or shear wave force. The stationary probe is activated after an

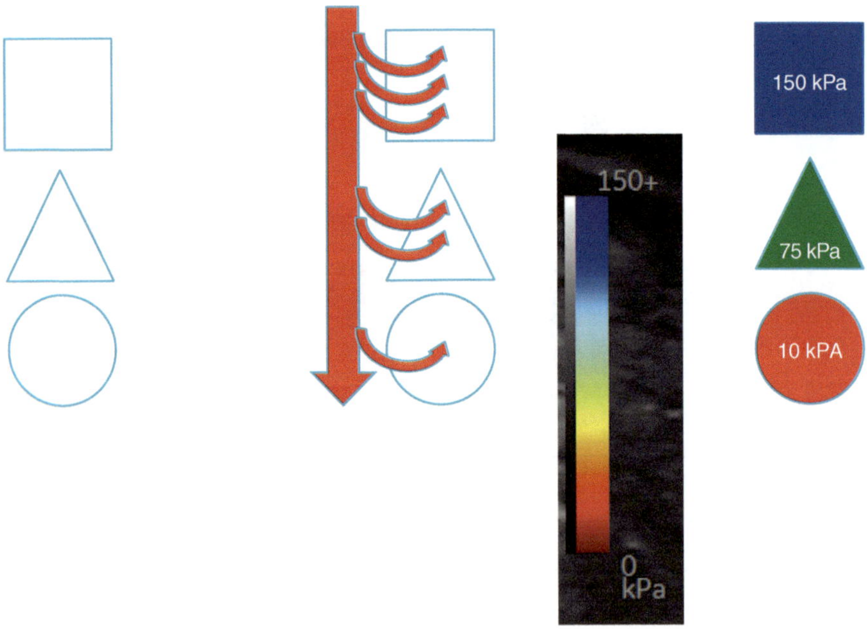

Fig. 19.7 Shear wave elastography overview. The application of a vertical and horizontal force results in a variable speed of wave propagation through the three objects. The deformation and speed of the wave can be calculated and color coded to confirm that the blue hue object conducts force of 150 kPa, the green hue object conducts a force of 75 kPa, and the softest, red hue, object conducts a force of 10 kPa

ROI is chosen; frequently, the ROI is considerably of smaller area in SWE than in SE [11, 12]. This is in large part to the extensive data collected by the probe. The ultrasound system will use a shear modulus calculation to determine the resulting elastic response of the tissue interrogated. The speed of wave propagation through tissue is measured in m/s and/or can be measured in stress force, in units of kilopascal (kPa). Many ultrasound units will allow the operator to evaluate using one method or another but frequently can calculate both.

Basic Physics Measurements in Shear Wave EUS

A review basic physic terms may be useful for understanding the EUS measurement.

- *kPa*: A unit of pressure and stress according to the International System of Units (SI); used for evaluation of sound activity. The kPa equals 1000 Pascals (1000 Pa).
- *Pa*: Pascals is equivalent to one Newton/m^2, a force applied over a designated area.
- *N*: A Newton is the force unit, measuring (kg)(m)/(sec^2), a measurement of weight over a specific acceleration; implicit in this measurement in the ability to define velocity in m/sec, which is part of the reason the elastography units can provide both a kPa reading and a velocity reading in m/sec
- *psi*: Pressure in pounds per square inch (e.g., measurement used in the air in the tires of an automobile)

To make this a more tangible concept, recognize that a normal tire pressure for a car is 220 kPa = 32 psi; further, 1 atmosphere = 101.325 kPa = 14.70 psi. Most elastography ultrasound units use a scale from softest to hardest of 50–150 kPa, roughly half of atmospheric pressure to 1.5× atmospheric pressure.

In the interpretation of SWE, it is important to note that sound will travel more slowly through a softer object and will have a lower kPa response. Conversely, sound will travel faster through a harder object and will have a higher kPa response. Figure 19.3 illustrates this point using a phantom. Note that the yolk region of the soft-boiled egg has an elastographic response of 40 kPa, while the hard-boiled yolk has an elastographic response of 62 kPa. In an anatomical assessment (Fig. 19.8), the normal Achilles tendon yields a uniform green-blue hue throughout the tendon with regions of red in the soft tissues, outside the grayscale equivalent region, a typical finding for this anatomical region. In the shear wave assessment, the normal Achilles tendon is assessed in two regions, closest to the insertion and slightly further away from the insertion. The tendon yields a 169.52 kPa response where the tendon is largely dark blue (E1), and the mixed light-blue and dark-blue region yields a 118.25 kPa response. In contrast, in the Achilles tendinitis assessment, there are scattered red regions in the ROI (the ROI is considerably smaller than a strain wave assessment) which represent areas of damage or softening. In this example, the ROI demonstrating the region of softening, while including some blue hued region, has a lower elastographic measurement, 92.77 kPa in E1, particularly when

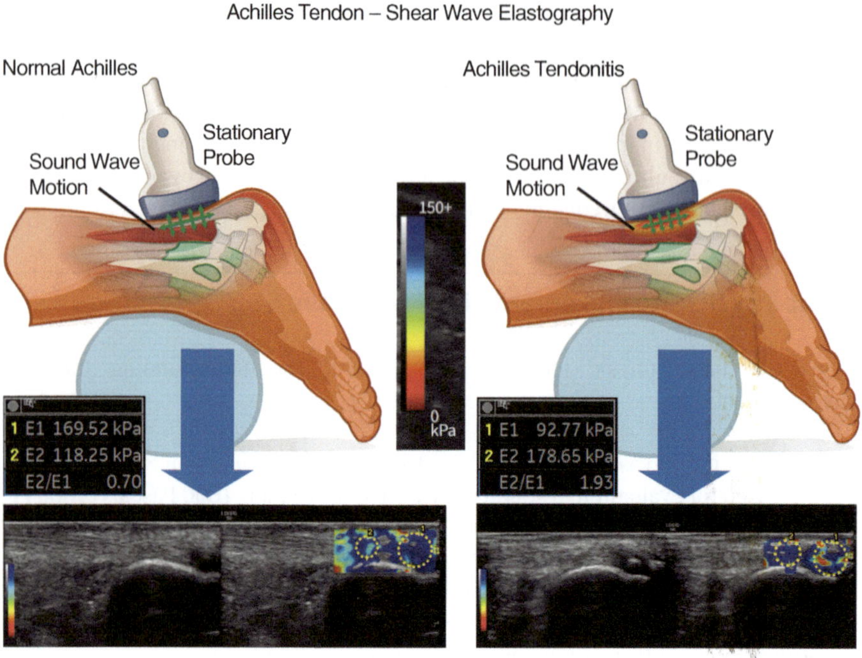

Fig. 19.8 Shear wave elastography of the Achilles tendon. Lower left elastogram of a normal Achilles tendon with uniform tendon elastogram and two elastographic regions that are essentially the same; the ratio is expressed as 0.70. Lower right elastogram of Achilles tendinopathy with a region of softening showing a significantly lower reading of 92.77 kPa while the adjacent uninvolved tendon shows an essentially normal elastographic reading of 178.65 kPa; the ratio of normal to abnormal tendon is expressed as 1.93. Note this ratio of normal to abnormal tendon differs from the ratio of skin to tendon in the prior example

compared to a more uniform blue hue region, E2, yielding an elastographic response closer to that seen in the normal tendon, 178.65 kPa. In the Achilles tendinitis example, SWE can quantitate the ROI representing the region of injury to demonstrate it is considerably different than what would be considered a normal tendon response.

Other important terminology in the understanding of SWE includes:

- *Virtual Touch Imaging (VTI)*: This tracks the ARFI to detect the degree of compression and also tends to require a subjective grading scale. A typical grading scale would assign a "1" to a homogenous spread of white or light-gray pattern; "2" would represent an intermediate, partially mottled gray pattern; and "3" would represent a patchy mixed image with mostly darker gray and black pattern.
- *Virtual Touch Quantification (VTQ)* or *Virtual Touch Imaging Quantification (VTIQ)*: This tracks the ARFI to measure the shear wave velocity within the region of interest and generates that value, usually in meters per second (m/s). The VTQ uses a grayscale display, while the VTIQ uses a color grid display, allowing for distinction of more discreet regions [13].

Achilles/Patellar Tendinopathy

The Achilles tendon, followed by the patellar tendon, is perhaps the most studied site for musculoskeletal elastography [14]. Achilles tendinopathy in SE evaluation has primarily been shown to demonstrate interval softening of the tendon. One study using a lower-frequency probe than traditionally applied in MSK US (i.e., 10–6 MHz vs. traditional 14–6 MHz probe) suggested the opposite effect. This can also occur with positioning as most authorities suggest the foot placed in a neutral, non-tense position as the optimal placement for elastography assessments. There is a concern that the patellar tendon, being in fact a ligament or an attachment between two bones, may behave differently since there is no muscle effect on this site. Studies vary on this interpretation. In addition, Achilles tendon appears to stiffen with age [15], as well as with cigarette smoking [16]. SE appears to perform well in the Achilles tendon, with diagnostic accuracy estimated at 97%–100%: sensitivity (94–97.5%) and specificity (94.5–99%). SWE studies suggest good specificity (68.2–91.5%) and modest sensitivity (35.3–66.7%) [14]. See Table 19.2 for the pros and cons of SE against SWE. The superficial nature of the Achilles tendon may make it more suitable for SE over SWE assessment. In assessing the patellar "tendon" for pathology, the accuracy for diagnosis by SE is 62.9% with sensitivity of 70% and specificity of 53.3% and less than B-mode or Doppler assessment; similar findings were suggested by SWE for patellar tendinopathy (sensitivity 35.3–76.5%, specificity 82.1–92.9%) [14].

There are few studies comparing inflammatory and noninflammatory regions with EUS and none excluding subjects with defined autoinflammatory disorders from the presumed injury cohort. An investigation into the utility of elastography in ankylosing spondylitis (AS) [17] was conducted with 82 Achilles tendons (41 subjects) with AS and 62 Achilles controls (32 unaffected, asymptomatic subjects). Conventional SE performed on the Achilles tendon were characterized as normal when containing blue or green signal, moderately softened when yellow, and severely softened when containing red signal. The distal Achilles was affected in 21/82 subjects, compared to 3/64 healthy subjects, and pain correlated with a softening (yellow or red) response ($P = 0.001$). Lesions in the middle Achilles region were more likely in the asymptomatic controls ($p = 0.053$). Softening also correlated with tendon enlargement and calcaneal erosion. Although there are no histological or alternative imaging correlates, this study suggests there may be a role in the evaluation of inflammatory tendon disorders [17].

The possibility that the response of tendinopathy to therapeutic modalities can be evaluated by SWE was raised by Dirrichs et al. [18]. SWE to assess improvement of the Achilles tendon, patellar tendon, and common flexor/extensor tendons before and after treatment with physiotherapy and a sclerosing agent (polidocanol) performed better than B-mode or Doppler, and SWE correlated better with clinical improvement. Specifically, baseline SWE score of symptomatic tendons was 42 ± 15 kPa and at 6 months after treatment improved to 106 ± 27 kPa ($p < 0.01$). Dirrichs et al. suggest elastography may prove useful in assessment of tendinopathy response to an intervention.

Psoriasis

Psoriasis under elastography demonstrates a diffuse hardening of the dermis (Fig. 19.9). Response of plaque psoriasis to topical corticosteroid application was assessed by ultrasound using SE and computing strain ratio [19]. The strain ratio included an assessment of the dermis and adjacent hypodermis. The focus of this study was to compare 20 MHz to 40 MHz as well as to determine if real-time elastography (SE) can detect steroid-induced skin atrophy in treated plaque psoriasis. The ability to detect change in skin/plaque thickness with the 40 MHz system was superior to the 20 MHz system, and treatment did not appear to influence dermal elasticity (1.61 ± 0.75; follow-up: 1.60 ± 0.60; $P = 0.96$). In a comparison of response of psoriatic plaque to biologic therapy versus DMARD therapy versus topical corticosteroid therapy, Dattola et al. performed EUS with a standard frequency (5–12 MHz) linear probe and equipment-calculated strain ratio of the hypodermis compared to the musculature before and after therapy [20]. Lesional strain ratio was also compared to normal skin. The baseline strain ratio was higher in plaque psoriasis compared with normal skin at baseline (2.8 vs. 0.5). In comparing treatment at baseline to one month, improvement was noted in subjects on biologic therapy (2.9 changing to 0.6) as well as subjects on DMARD therapy (2.8 changing to 1.6). These changes are statistically significantly better ($p < 0.05$) than subjects on topical therapy (2.7 changing to 2.5). This would suggest that SE can serve as a treatment outcome measure for early response to pharmacologic intervention in psoriasis.

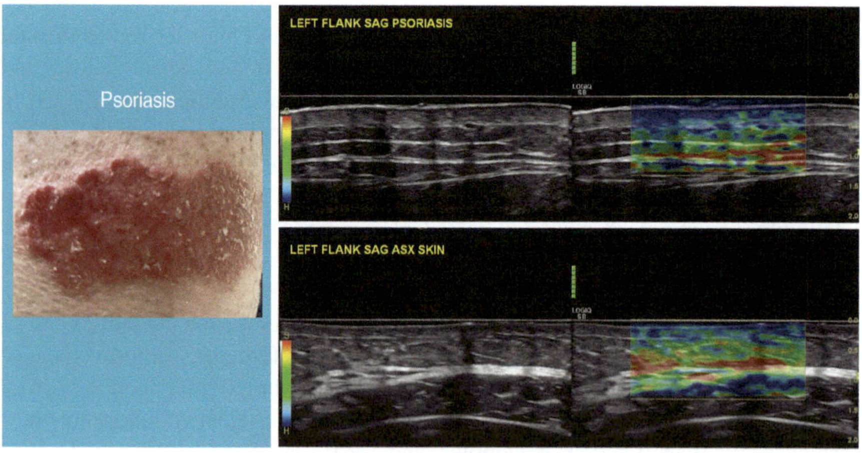

Fig. 19.9 Elastography of plaque psoriasis. Upper image of plaque psoriasis with dark-blue hue in the epidermis but showing more green hue by the dermal layer. Lower image of normal adjacent skin, demonstrating the contrast of green hue in the epidermis

Rotator Cuff Tendinopathy

Investigations into measuring rotator cuff tendon strain with SE have been conducted on a porcine model of 12 fresh porcine shoulders using a probe fitted with an acoustic coupler to compute strain ratios in various settings [21]. Reproducible strain ratio studies were accomplished against reference tissue when the tendon depth was less than 22 mm, suggesting that the correct setting would facilitate accurate reading by SE. A review of the available literature demonstrates three studies with SE of the rotator cuff for tendinopathy with or without tears, as well as assessments of the associated muscles; there are seven in vivo and clinical studies with SWE [22]. The review suggests significant variability in the ability for elastography to correlate rotator cuff pathology with other imaging modalities. Tatta et al. suggest that the conventional limitations of SE make it considerably less attractive than SWE based on the inherent quantification of SWE and stable probe positioning, which may favor correct identification of pathology visualized on B-mode evaluation [21]. None of the available studies correlate with arthroscopic findings and could benefit from histological correlation. SWE demonstrates tendon softening in rotator cuff disease but appears to be better at assessing the proximal tendons in symptomatic subjects [23]. The 55 subjects with an asymptomatic proximal supraspinatus tendon demonstrated an SWV 7.87 ± 1.77 m/s, while the 21 symptomatic proximal supraspinatus tendon demonstrated an SWV of 6.98 ±2.49 ($p = 0.049$); the asymptomatic distal supraspinatus tendon demonstrated an SWV of 8.49 ±2.41,while the symptomatic distal supraspinatus tendon demonstrated an SWV of 7.90 ±2.95 ($p = 0.389$). An incidental, unexpected softening of the deltoid muscle was noted in symptomatic shoulders that the investigators felt bore further investigation.

Lateral Epicondylitis

EUS measurements for lateral epicondylitis/epicondylosis behave in a similar manner as the Achilles tendon (Fig. 19.10). Arslan et al. compared the extensor tendons in 25 normal subjects by B-mode, strain elastography, color Doppler imaging, power Doppler imaging, and Superb Microvascular Imaging (SMI) to 44 subjects with a clinical diagnosis of lateral epicondylosis [24]. B-mode-identified regions of hypoechoic change became the ROI for SE, and with a subcutaneous reference site, a software-generated strain ratio was derived. The mean strain ratio in lateral epicondylosis (2.85 ± 1.99) indicated that the symptomatic tendons were softer than the healthy controls (7.41 ± 2.24; $p > 0.001$); the cutoff strain ratio value between the two groups was 3.94. This yields a sensitivity of 78%, specificity of 92%, PPV of 90.7%, NPV of 80.7%, and accuracy rate of 85.0% [24]. Ahn et al. found that the mean strain ratios were 1.45 ± 0.45 for symptomatic tendons and 2.07 ± 0.70 for asymptomatic tendons [25]. The mean strain ratio was significantly lower for the symptomatic tendons than the asymptomatic tendons. In another study conducted

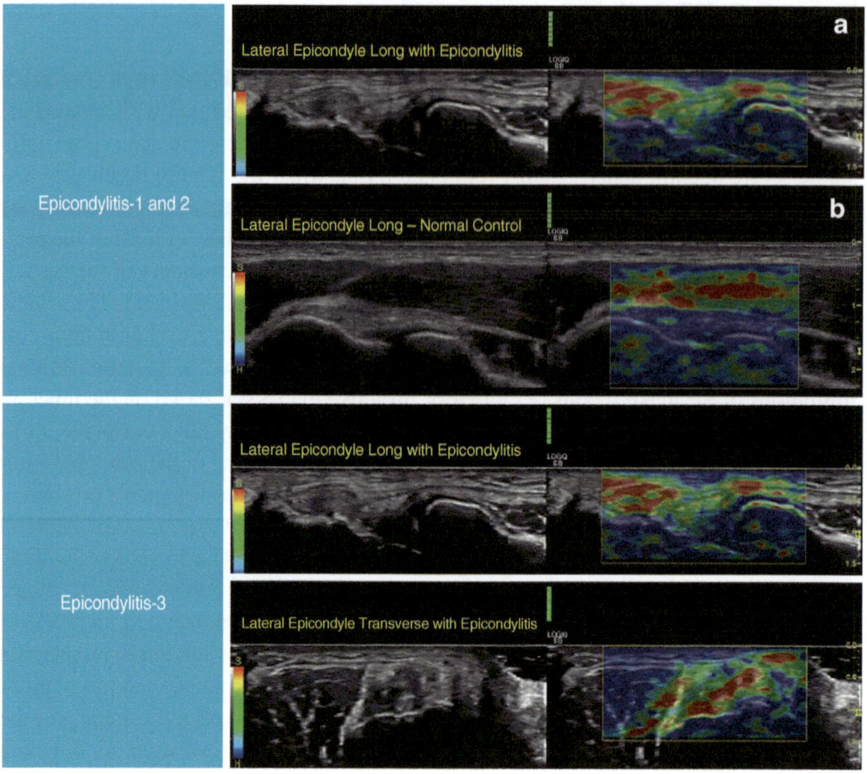

Fig. 19.10 Elastography of epicondylitis. In Epicondylitis-1 and 2, upper image, (**a**) demonstrates grayscale bowing of the tendon with hypoechoic region of damage corresponding to the red hue of softening in the hypoechoic area, which represents tendon damage. By comparison, the lower image, (**b**) is a normal lateral epicondyle, where the tendon is essentially uniformly of blue hue, demonstrating a firm tendon by elastogram. In Epicondylitis-3, upper image is long view of an affected tendon and its corresponding orthogonal view, demonstrating the distribution of the tendon damage in the transverse plane

by De Zordo et al. in patients with lateral epicondylosis, SE gave a sensitivity of 100%, specificity of 89%, and accuracy of 94% [26]. Kocygit et al. studied 17 subjects with clinical evidence of unilateral epicondylosis, using the uninvolved side as the control, with B-mode, Doppler, and SE [27]. A comparison SE of the ROI in the tendon was compared to an ROI in the subcutaneous tissue to create a strain ratio. The tendon was divided by region (medial, middle, and lateral portions) and demonstrated that the strain ratios in these regions of epicondylitis (0.45 ± 0.12, 0.44 ± 0.8, 0.47 ± 0.19) were statistically significantly different than matched "healthy elbows" (0.18 ± 0.13, 0.21 ± 0.13, 0.20 ± 0.14, with $p = 0.001$), indicating that the tendon softening of lateral epicondylitis is detectable by this technique. Strain ratios at the medial portion of the epicondyle correlated with symptom duration and nocturnal pain.

Plantar Fasciitis

Lee et al. used conventional SE to evaluate plantar fasciitis in 18 plantar fasciitis subjects and 18 control subjects [28]. A standardized interpretation of blue regions comprising >50% of the fascia represented normal stiffness; blue regions comprising <50% of the plantar fascia was deemed suggestive of plantar fascial softening or plantar fasciitis. Overall inter-observer agreement was excellent (ICC 0.942) with 89% (16/18) symptomatic subjects versus 50% (9/18) subjects demonstrating softening ($p = 0.027$).

Sjögren's Syndrome

The first attempt to apply EUS to the diagnosis of Sjögren's syndrome by Dejaco et al. used SE to identify primary Sjögren's syndrome (pSS) subjects and discern if this modality could identify impaired salivary gland function [29]. The assessment included B-mode and SE imaging in a cohort of 45 pSS subjects, as defined by American-European Consensus Group (AECG). B-mode grading on 0–48-point scale was compared to a standardized subjective grading scale of SE, range 0–4 applied to right and left parotid and submandibular glands (score 0–16). The score was based on the firm or blue regions: "0" = no hardened (blue) areas; "1" = ≤25%, "2" = 26%–50%, "3" = 51%–75%, and "4" = > 75% of the salivary gland covered by hardened areas. While B-mode ultrasonography identified pSS from control subjects, some inconclusive B-mode images were noted; in these cases, SE scores of ≥6 improved sensitivity and specificity in identifying pSS subjects. Further, SE scoring had a stronger correlation than B-mode US with measures of salivary dysfunction. This group concluded that SE may have a role in the diagnosis and assessment of salivary gland function in Sjögren's syndrome.

In a smaller sample of 15 subjects with ACR 2012 classification of pSS, Samier-Guérin et al. assessed the ability of SWE to distinguish this population from 10 healthy controls [30]. The resulting sampling demonstrated SWE are greater in the pSS parotid glands (2.335 ± 0.315 m/s vs. 1.785 ± 0.384 m/s, $p = 0.001$) but not in the pSS submandibular glands (1.812 ± 0.308 m/s vs. 1.766 ± 0.187 m/s, $p = 0.892$).

Some investigators have suggested that different elastography modalities may yield varying results and sensitivity to diagnosis. Zhang et al. used VTQ and VTIQ in 21 subjects with pSS versus 11 healthy controls and demonstrated that only pSS parotid VTQ values were statistically significantly different than controls (1.33 ± 0.22 m/s vs. 1.18 ± 0.04 m/s, respectively, $p < 0.01$); however, VTIQ in pSS parotid and submandibular glands were both statistically significantly different than controls [31].

In another study comparing EUS modalities in fifty [48] pSS subjects as defined by AECG versus fifty [48] subjects with sicca who did not fulfill criteria for pSS, a comparison of B-mode to RTE to VTI to VTIQ was performed [13]. Standard subjective grading scales for B-mode (grading scale of 1–4), RTE (grading scale of

1–3), and VTI (grading scale of 1–3) were applied, but VTIQ was assessed as an SWV in m/s. In these two subject groups, the analysis of the four modalities suggested only SWV as determined by VTIQ was shown to be statistically significantly different in the pSS salivary glands compared to other sicca subjects, with a parotid gland SWV of 2.99 ± 0.96 m/s and submandibular gland SWV of 2.54 ± 0.76 m/s compared to sicca control parotid gland SWV of 2.16 ± 0.71 m/s and submandibular gland SWV of 2.04 ± 0.40 m/s (for parotid glands, $p < 0.001$ and for submandibular gland, $p = 0.008$).

Using SE with either a 1–4 scoring scale or a strain ratio, Cindil et al. [32] compared the parotid and submandibular glands fifty-eight [56] primary Sjögren's syndrome (pSS) subjects defined by AECG to the salivary glands of 25 healthy controls, generating B-mode and elastography images [32]. Elastography scores and strain wave ratios were statistically significantly different in the pSS group than healthy controls. The average pSS parotid strain ratio of 3.54 was compared to the health control parotid strain ratio of 2.17 ($p < 0.001$) and the average submandibular gland pSS strain ratio 2.21 was compared to the health control submandibular strain ratio of 1.31 ($p < 0.001$). Duration of illness and severity of symptoms increased with increasing strain ratio.

Using shear wave elastography and calculating the SWV, Turnaoglu et al. assessed the submandibular and salivary glands of twenty-five [25] pSS subjects as defined by ACR 2016 criteria and compared the SWV to the salivary glands of twenty-five [25] healthy controls [33]. The resulting observations demonstrated that SWV in the pSS right submandibular gland at 2.20 ± 0.28 m/s, left submandibular gland at 2.39 ± 0.39 m/s, right parotid gland at 2.57 ± 0.48 m/s, and left parotid gland at 2.80 ± 0.44 m/s were statistically significantly higher than the SWV in healthy control right submandibular gland at 1.80 ± 0.14 m/s, left submandibular gland at 1.81 ± 0.14 m/s, right parotid gland at 1.78 ± 0.15 m/s, and left parotid gland at 1.79 ± 0.13 m/s. Further, a cutoff SWV for the pSS submandibular gland of 1.98 and pSS parotid gland of 1.93 yields a favorable sensitivity and specificity.

Taken all together, these six investigations suggest there is a role for the diagnosis, evaluation, and potential management of pSS with elastography, and it may be an adjunct to grayscale B-mode imaging (Fig. 19.11).

Systemic Sclerosis

The first attempt to apply EUS to systemic sclerosis (SSc) was performed with 18 consecutive subjects, comparing the strain wave elastogram on the forearm and fingers on the dominant hand to the same sites on 15 normal controls [34]. Stiffness as manifested by a diffuse blue hue is noted in the tested sites in scleroderma and was significantly different than stiffness measured in controls. The difference in SSc tissue was attributed to the loss of elasticity of the skin with associated dermal fibrosis. This observation was continued in the dermal thickness of the digit, with 22 SSc subjects to determine if the borders of the dermis as defined by a strain wave elastogram would provide better intra-reliability than the same measurement by B-mode ultrasound

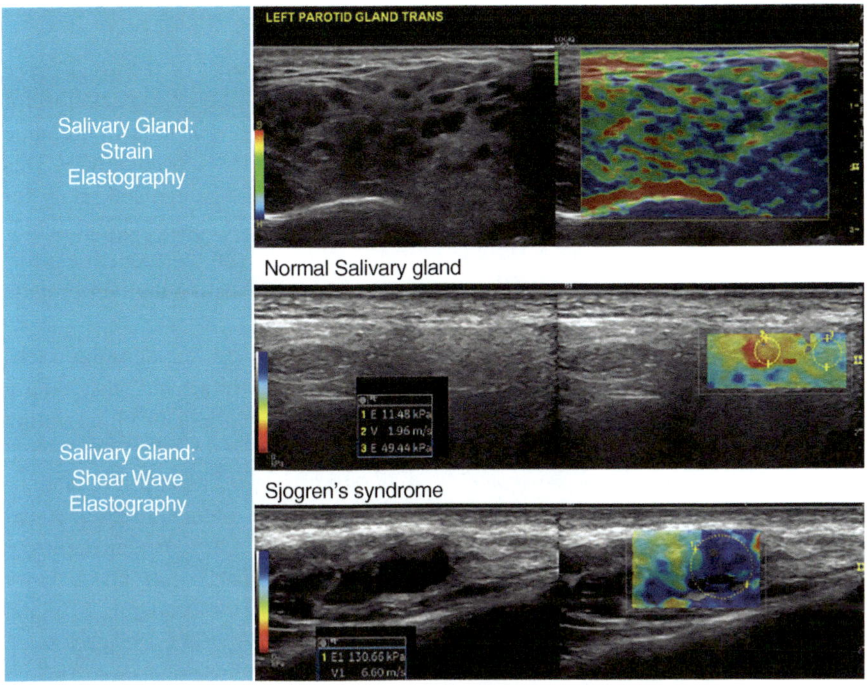

Fig. 19.11 Elastography of salivary glands. Strain wave elastography of the parotid gland with broad area of evaluation to demonstrate the anechoic regions on gray scale is blue hue or firmer regions on the corresponding elastogram. Shear wave elastography with a normal parotid gland demonstrating an elastographic reading of 11.48 kPa and SWV of 1.96 m/s while the lower image shows a limited view of an anechoic region in the parotid gland with an elastographic region of 130.66 kPa and SWV of 6.6 m/s confirming a relative firmness when compared to normal

alone [35]. The intra-class correlation coefficient for the intra-observer and inter-observer agreement was 0.904 and 0.726 for the B-mode measurement but was increased to 0.979 and 0.881 for the elastography-guided measurement. The authors concluded that the reliability of the sonographic measurement is improved with the use of elastography. Additional studies with SE were conducted on the perioral region of six SSc subjects versus six healthy controls, evaluating designated regions in the parasagittal left, parasagittal right, upper axial, and lower axial regions of the mouth [36]. Harder areas identified with largely a blue hue were seen in the SSc subjects, whereas the perioral region in healthy controls was largely flexible or red.

Some preliminary studies of SWE demonstrate the ability to quantitate sclerodermatous skin changes. Hou et al. studied 15 SSc subjects and 15 age-matched controls at 17 sites that are typically the sites of modified Rodnan skin score (mRSS) [37]; there were statistically significantly higher SWV noted in the sclerodermatous skin versus the healthy control skin at the right-hand dorsum (1.912 vs. 1.308 m/s), right forearm (2.703 vs. 1.727 m/s), left-hand dorsum (2.280 vs. 1.193 m/s), left forearm (2.790 vs. 1.728 m/s), right foot dorsum (2.340 vs. 1.432 m/s), and left foot dorsum (1.630 vs. 1.400 m/s) and demonstrated strong intra- and inter-observer reliability. In

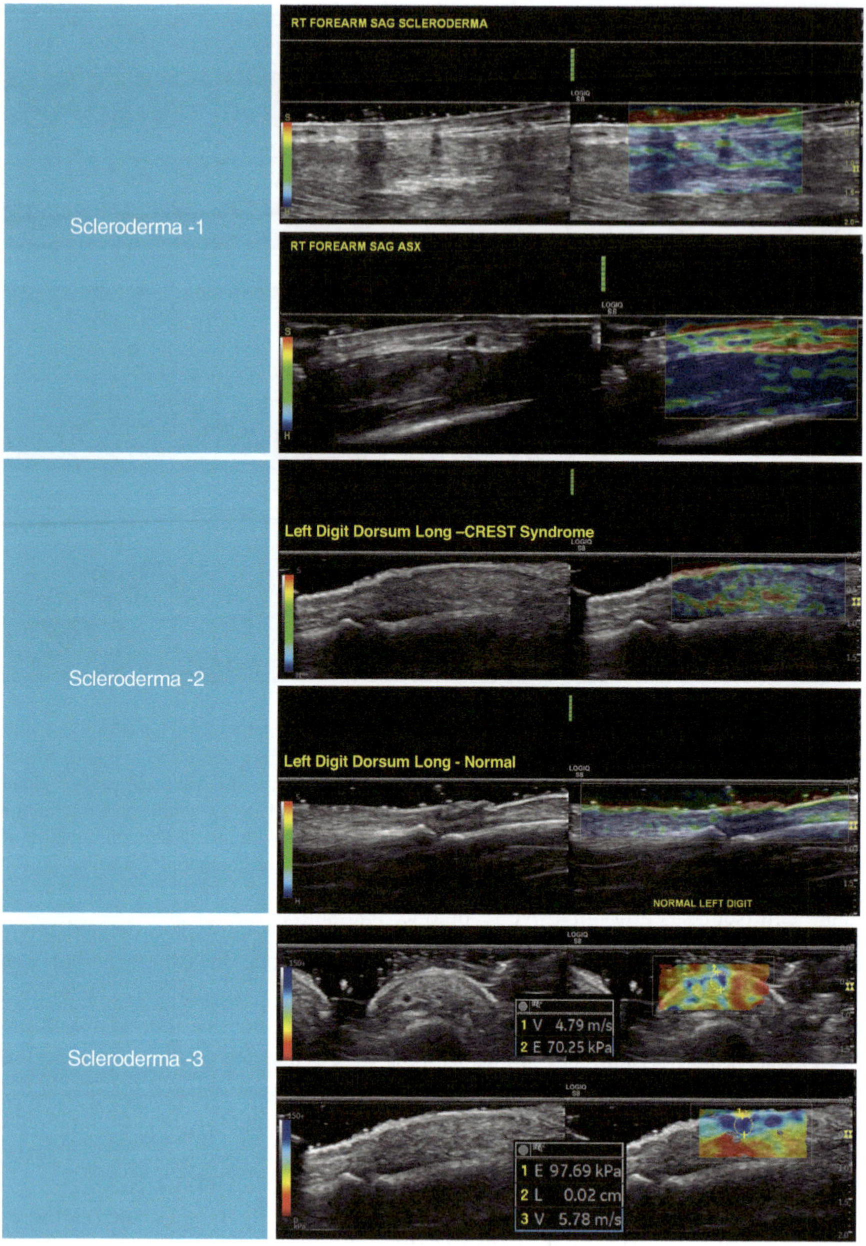

Fig. 19.12 Elastography of scleroderma. Scleroderma-1: Upper image of sclerodermatous involvement of the forearm where the diffuse firmness of the skin with it enhanced blue hue by strain elastography can be contrasted to the lower image of an asymptomatic individual. Scleroderma-2: Upper image of sclerodermatous involvement of the digit where the firmness of the digit skin with its increased thickness and blue hue by strain wave elastography can be contrasted to the green hue of the normal digit skin, in association with the blue hue of the tendon. Scleroderma-3: Upper image of sclerodermatous involvement of the digit, transverse image, by shear wave, with elastography of 70 kPa and SWV of 4.7 m/s as well as sclerodermatous involvement of the digit, long view, with elastography of 97 kPa and SWV of 5.78 m/s

the 9th annual Supplement on Systemic Sclerosis, Santiago et al. reported similar findings [3]. Further pursuits in this area correlated with skin changes by mRSS to isoechoic versus hypoechoic versus hyperechoic skin changes as well as to SWV [38] suggest that skin thickness increases as echogenicity changes (from iso- to hypo- to hyperechoic) and SWV changes from normal, isoechoic skin at 1.83 m/s to hypoechoic skin at 2.16 m/s to 2.55 m/s, but statistically significant change was noted only between the two extremes, isoechoic and hyperechoic skin. The results of these SWE studies showing the ability to quantitate elasticity of skin with shear wave elastography suggest this may be a promising avenue for study in systemic sclerosis (Fig. 19.12).

Hypermobility Spectrum Disorders

SE is used to assess the elastogram of the deltoid, biceps brachii, brachioradialis, rectus femoris, and gastrocnemius muscle as well as the patellar and Achilles tendons in two comparator groups [39]. The 21 subjects with hypermobility spectrum disorder (HSD) were defined with a Beighton Score of ≥4/9 as well as chronic self-reported polyarthralgia for >3 months; these subjects were compared to 22 control subjects. The percentages of "red" areas were graded in the two groups as evidence of elasticity. A strain index was created comparing the elasticity of the muscle or tendon to the subject's skin, and a color pixel analysis of the regions sampled was generated. The strain index identified increased softening in the HSD group with the brachioradialis muscle, patellar tendon, and Achilles tendon reaching statistical significance ($p \leq 0.01$). The color pixel analysis yielded a higher percentage of red (elastic) regions in the HSD group, but only the biceps brachii and the Achilles tendon achieved statistical significance ($p \leq 0.01$); a reduction in blue (stiffer) regions in the HSD was also observed but only achieved statistical significance in the biceps brachii, brachioradialis, and the Achilles tendon ($p \leq 0.01$). The group surmised that SE may evolve as a tool for diagnosis, and monitoring this disorder, including the ability to assess physiotherapy and possibly any pharmacologic intervention that may evolve for this disorder.

Dupuytren's Contracture

While the Dupuytren's cord can primarily appear hypoechoic [40], it has been shown to have a characteristic hardness in strain elastography, localized to the palmar aponeurosis of the hand [41]. When treated with collagenase Clostridium histolyticum, the cord will change its elastogram to a generalized softness when assessed prior to the manual reduction of the contracture (see Fig. 19.13).

Gouty Arthritis

A study of gouty arthritis was undertaken to assess the role of ultrasound in the acute phase versus the intercritical phase of gouty arthritis [42]. All study participants met the 2015 ACR/EULAR Gout Classification Criteria. The first MTP was

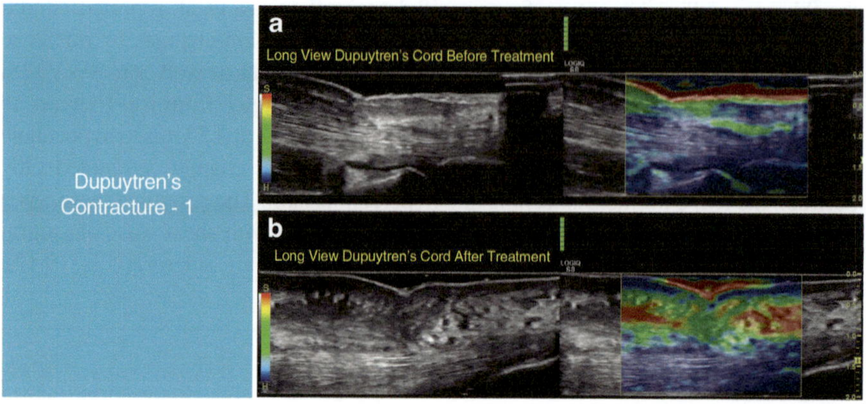

Fig. 19.13 Dupuytren's contracture before and after treatment with collagenase Clostridium histolyticum. Dupuytren's contracture-1: Upper image is a long view before treatment with large superficial region of blue hue demonstrating the firmness of the cord, and lower image is 24 hours later with predominant red hue in the superficial region, corresponding to softening from the enzyme exposure. Dupuytren's contracture-2: Upper image is a transverse view before treatment with circular superficial region of blue hue demonstrating the firmness of the cord in transverse view, above the tendon; the lower image is 24 hours later with circular red-green hue in the superficial region, corresponding to softening from the enzyme exposure, while the lower tendon preserves its blue hue, demonstrating it was not affected by introduction of the enzyme in the superficial tissues

assessed by ultrasound using gray scale, Doppler, and SWE in 57 gout patients. Grayscale changes of synovial thickening, echogenic foci, double contour sign, bone erosion, effusion, and tophus were no different between the two groups. Power Doppler signal grade (0–3 scale) was higher in the acute versus the intercritical phase, but the B-mode characteristics of the regions were not felt to be different between the two groups. SWE targeted the synovium as the ROI and determined the maximal elastic modulus (E_{max}) and mean elastic modulus (E_{mean}) of the two groups. The acute phase E_{max} = 240.4 kPa ± 133.7 (range 70.7–451.9 kPa), and E_{mean} was 101.4 kPa ± 53.0 (range 29.5–235.4 kPa), whereas in the intercritical phase group, E_{max} was 419.7 kPa ± 69.3 (range 285.7–540 kPa), and E_{mean} was 190.0 kPa ± 54.5 (range 109.8–318.3 kPa). The E_{max} and the E_{mean} in the acute phase were lower than the E_{max} and the E_{mean} in the intercritical phase; the synovium is undergoing a "softening" during the acute phase or inflammatory phase of gouty arthritis and then changes to a "harder" phase during the intercritical phase. Comparing the modalities further, the area under the receiver operating characteristic curves (AUROCs) were 0.494–0.553 for B-mode US, 0.735 for CDUS, 0.887 for E_{max}, and 0.882 for E_{mean}; SWE demonstrated the strongest diagnostic performance across the data sets. There may be a role for elastography for determining whether a patient has transitioned to the intercritical period and can begin urate-lowering therapy with a potentially lower risk of flare.

A comparison of eight subcutaneous nodules was performed by blinded readers using SE and identifying the main or prevailing color of the nodule [43], where 1 = blue, 2 = light blue, 3 = green, 4 = yellow, and 5 = red. Rheumatoid nodules were

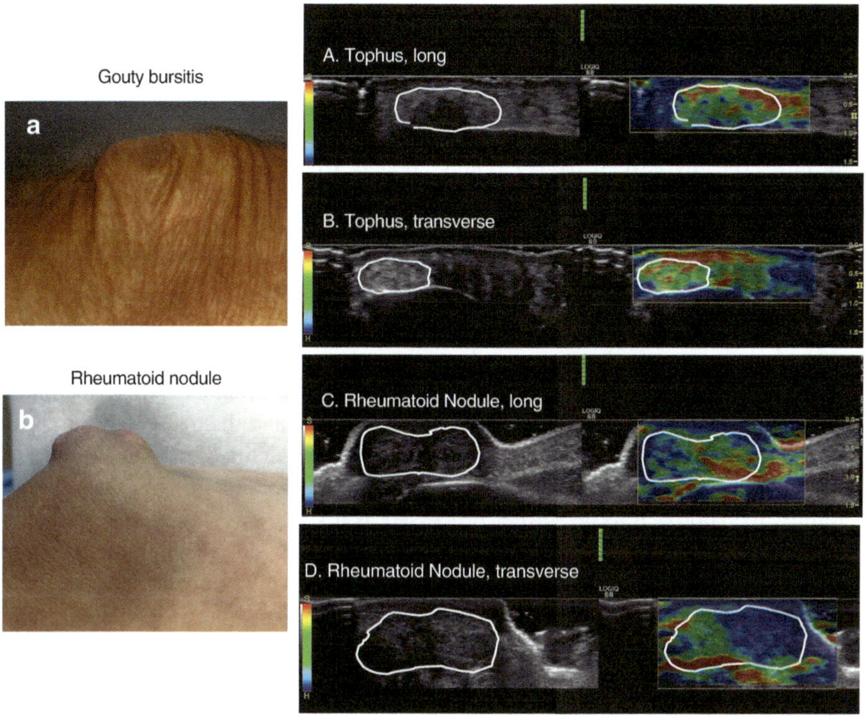

Fig. 19.14 Gouty tophus versus rheumatoid nodule. A and B, tophus long and short, with a white circle placed about the region of the tophus, to demonstrate the relative softness, as described by Sconfienza et al. [43]. where 1 = blue, 2 = light blue, 3 = green, 4 = yellow, and 5 = red. By this group's scale, the gouty tophus is predominantly yellow-red, or 4.5, particularly in the transverse view. The rheumatoid nodule in the transverse plane is predominantly blue or "1"

deemed to be statistically significantly harder than tophi as the median value of the main color was blue or 1 (range 1–3) for rheumatoid nodules and red or 5 (range 3–5) for tophi ($p = 0.024$). While a small sample size, it suggests a role for SE in making a distinction between a rheumatoid nodule and tophus (Fig. 19.14). Other authors have identified that a tophus before treatment is significantly "stiffer" than while under treatment; softening that results during treatment may be an outcome measure for determining pharmacologic response to therapy [44].

Myofascial Pain

Ballyns et al. studied 13 subjects with upper trapezius pain with vibrational elastography with calculated SWE to document stiffer tissue in the symptomatic individuals, 3.5 kPa and viscosity value of 10 Pa/s vice nine pain-free controls with shear modulus of 3.38 kPa and viscosity value of 6.09 Pa/s, to conclude that elastography detects myofascial trigger points [45].

Turo et al. performed an evaluation of myofascial trigger points in trapezius muscle with vibration elastography after three dry needling treatments [46]. The investigators wished to assess the reduction of the involved sites by quantifying the area of involvement, recognizing that the areas of stiffness represented the myofascial trigger points. This technique requires both the elastography and an external vibrating unit. The myofascial trigger points created a heterogenous signal within the elastogram whose area then can be quantified, and reduction of the area of involved tissue corresponded to reduced pain response in those who responded to dry needling.

Jafari et al. also studied SWE in 29 subjects with myofascial trigger points in the sternocleidomastoid muscle [47]. With B-mode ultrasound, his group first identified hypoechoic regions within the muscle as these are previously described representing ultrasound changes in pathologic sites. Applying a mechanical stress, the investigators measured the excursion of muscle in B-mode and then assessed the tissue change. The change in tissue excursion against the calculated applied force was processed by computer software to create an elastic modulus; this is essentially a strain wave approach to be further processed as a shear wave event. The resulting evaluation demonstrated that trigger points have an elastic modulus of 13379.57 ± 1069.75 Pa (13 kPa) and that normal muscle has an elastic modulus of 7078.24 ± 482.92 Pa (7 kPa) and suggested trigger points are in fact stiffer than unaffected muscle.

Median Nerve and Carpal Tunnel Syndrome

Carpal tunnel syndrome, or median nerve entrapment, suggests a system under pressure, and therefore, many investigators have sought the potential role in diagnosis and management of carpal tunnel syndrome. Kantarci et al. [48] evaluated 60 wrist (37 subjects) confirmed with carpal tunnel syndrome (CTS) against 36 control wrists (18 healthy subjects) with SWE to demonstrate that a 40.4 kPa cutoff for diagnosis yielded a specificity of 93.3%, sensitivity of 88.9%, PPV of 93.3%, NPV of 88.9%, and accuracy of 91.7% compared to a gold standard of EMG/NCV measurements [48]. The average mean nerve stiffness in controls was 32.0 ± 8.4 kPa versus 66.7 ± 26.5 kPa ($p < 0.001$) in subjects with CTS. Moreover, moderate to severe CTS demonstrated SWE response of 101.4 ± 26.7 kPa, and mild to moderate CTS demonstrated an SWE response of 55.1 ± 12.9 kPa. Inter-observer variability was superior for SWE interpretation over measurements of CSA.

The kinematics of the carpal tunnel in dynamic motion has also been assessed by elastography [49]. There is evidence to suggest that the standard deviation of cumulative shear strain of the flexor retinaculum is lower in subjects with CTS than normal control, and the axial strain on the median nerve is lower in subjects with CTS than normal controls.

Another study of median nerve stiffness compared cross-sectional area in 222 control hands (111 subjects) versus 402 hands (201 subjects) with rheumatoid arthritis by SE [50]. Despite difference in stiffness in RA patients, all subjects did not display clinical evidence of CTS. Anno et al. demonstrated that there is an increase in nerve stiffness in subjects with rheumatoid arthritis that is not seen in controls, but the cross-sectional area remains unaffected [50]. Distal and proximal cross-sectional area (CSA) is approximately 7.7–10.3 mm^2 in both groups; the rheumatoid arthritis carpal tunnel inlet strain ratio was 2.6 ± 1.4 (right hand) and 2.7 ± 1.3 (left hand), but the control carpal tunnel inlet strain ratio was 2.1 ± 0.9 (right hand) and 2.1 ± 0.8 (left hand). This may be clinically relevant as traditional measurements of carpal tunnel syndrome have been suggested in some studies to be discordant in subjects with rheumatoid arthritis. This group raises the issue of inflammation causing nerve fibrosis as an independent event to nerve widening.

Tezcan et al. used grayscale B-mode ultrasound and SE to assess 17 subjects with untreated carpal tunnel syndrome (CTS) against 17 subjects with CTS before and after treatment with low-level laser [51]. Strain ratio between the cross-sectional area of the medial nerve and adjacent soft tissue at the same depth was calculated by imbedded software. Strain ratio in pretreatment CTS of 0.98 ± 0.21 improved to 0.63 ± 0.24 ($p < 0.001$), whereas strain ratio in control pretreatment subjects remained essentially constant through the study, 0.94 ± 0.44, and posttreatment 0.81 ± 0.43 ($p = 0.081$). Cross-sectional area (CSA) improved in the treatment arm from 13.0 ± 2.9 to 10.9 ± 2.4 ($p < 0.001$) but remained constant in the control group, from 14.4 ± 4.06 to 13.5 ± 3.7 ($p = 0.12$). This investigation suggests that elastography, but specifically strain wave ratio, may have a role in following the clinical response of interventions for carpal tunnel syndrome.

Selected Topics in Pediatric Rheumatology

Elastography in the pediatric population has gained some attention but much more so in the evaluation of solid tumor pathology than the musculoskeletal system [52]. There are many more investigations into the role of SE and SWE in evaluation of liver, kidney, brain, pancreas, lymph nodes, thyroid, and testes. However, some preliminary evaluations of myositis and myopathy have been performed with mixed results. There may be a role in the assessment of muscle stiffness associated with cerebral palsy and torticollis.

Contrast-Enhanced Ultrasound (CEUS)

Contrast-enhanced ultrasound has captured the attention of radiologists and cardiologists for some time. While ultrasound contrast agents are available throughout the world, they are only licensed for use in the United States for cardiology imaging; however, off-label use in tumor imaging has been reported [53]. Most studies to date focus on identifying liver lesions both benign and metastatic, as well as breast, kidney, pulmonary, and cardiac imaging of activity, perfusion, and function. Contrast-enhanced ultrasound may also have a role in procedural ultrasound to assist in identifying sites for biopsy or defer an intervention based on the resulting vascular pattern [54].

Ultrasound contrast agents are essentially microbubbles, which reflect sound during transit through small blood vessels over the time of injection and are rapidly cleared by the body, usually by the lungs. The microbubbles are smaller than a red blood cell, 1–10 um in diameter, and arrive at the site of interest in the arterial phase of circulation approximately 10–20 seconds after injection, lasting in the arterial phase approximately 25 to 30 seconds and then starting a venous phase of flow several seconds later [55]. Therefore, the ultrasonographer has to identify the target area in which the contrast will be sought for image acquisition and follow the region for the contrast transit in order to capture the necessary information. The agents can be divided into soft- and hard-shell bubbles, which are internally filled with different gases. See Table 19.3 for a summary of products. Hard-shell bubbles are mechanically stiffer than soft-shell bubbles, changing the ultrasonic properties and use. Hard-shell bubbles can use natural polymers, gelatin, synthetic polymers, and proteins, such as albumin, and allow the contrast to circulate for up to 10 minutes but can "burst" under high-intensity ultrasound imaging. Soft-shelled microbubbles are composed of phospholipids or stabilized surfactant and, with an improved compliance, can shrink or divide into smaller bubbles.

Use of CEUS in clinical settings remains limited based on labelling restrictions, reimbursement issues, and a recent black box warning. Since 2007, two US-based products, Definity and Opison, have an FDA-mandated black box warning, which reads "serious cardiopulmonary reactions, including fatalities, have occurred uncommonly during or following perflutren-containing microsphere administration. Most serious reactions occur within 30 minutes of administration [56]. This is actively being appealed by the International Contrast Ultrasound Society (ICUS), American Institute of Ultrasound in Medicine, the World Federation of Ultrasound in Medicine and Biology, the Society of Radiologists in Ultrasound, the Society of Diagnostic Medical Sonography, the Society for Pediatric Radiology, the American Society of Echocardiography, and the Liver Imaging Reporting and Data System contrast-enhanced ultrasound working group at the time of publication of this text [57].

Use of CEUS has been advocated in pediatric imaging, citing use in liver, kidney, spleen, trauma, bowel, lung/pleura, and transplantation imaging [58]. An analysis of available case series and case reports allowed Rosado and Riccabona to review the use of CEUS in 502 pediatric subjects with 540 cases of off-label contrast exposure [59]. Most were treated with the sulfur hexafluoride contrast agent. Only 2% has an adverse event with contrast administration; one case of anaphylactic shock was noted while nine cases of a mild transitory event were reported. While most treatment was focused on the liver, it demonstrated that IV use of US contrast is safe and diagnostically useful in the pediatric population. The ability for CEUS to assist in the diagnosis of juvenile inflammatory arthritis of the knee has been established by Doria et al. [60].

Studies applying CEUS in inflammatory states, in a desire to accurately establish early inflammatory arthritis, have been pursued to evaluate both diagnosis and

Table 19.3 Ultrasound contrast agent that have/had been clinically approved

Name	First approved for clinical use	Shell material	Gas	Application (examples)	Producer/distributor	Countries
Sonazoid	2007	Phospholipid	Perfluorobutane	Myocardial perfusion, liver imaging	GE Healthcare, Buckinghamshire, UK/Daiichi Saniko, Tokyo, JP	Japan, South Korea
Imagent/ Imavist	2002, withdrawn	Phospholipid	Perfluorohexane, nitrogen	Echocardiography, heart perfusion, tumor or blood flow anomalies	Schering AG, Berlin, Germany	USA
Lumason/ SonoVue	2001/2014	Phospholipid	Sulphurhexafluoride	Left ventricular opacification, microvascular enhancement (liver and breast lesion detection)	Braceo Diagnostics, Milano, Italy	USA, Europe, China
Definity/ luminity	2001/2006	Phospholipid	Octafluoropropane	Echocardiography, liver and kidney imaging (Canada)	Lantheus Medical Imaging, North Billerica, MA	North America, Europe (approval filed)
Optison	1998	Cross-linked serum albumin	Octafluoropropane	Left ventricular opacification	GE Healthcare, Buckinghamshire, UK	USA, Europe
Levoist	1995, withdrawn	Galactose microparticles	Air	Whole heart imaging, Doppler imaging	Schering AG, Berlin, Germany	Canada, Europe, China, Japan
Albunex	1993, withdrawn	Sonicated serum albumin	Air	Transpulmonary imaging	Molecular Biosystems Inc, San Dieqo, CA	Japan, USA
Echovist	1991, withdrawn	Galactose microparticles	Air	Right heart imaging	Schering AG, Berlin, Germany	Germany, UK

From: Hunt and Romero [53]

monitoring of response of inflammatory arthropathies [61, 62]. This includes studies in rheumatoid arthritis, psoriatic arthritis, and ankylosing spondylitis. Studies of the small joints of the hands are not as prominent in this literature as studies of the large joints, particularly the knee. These studies have documented that early diagnosis and detection of inflammation can be assisted by CEUS [62]. Comparisons to MRI findings suggest that inflammatory synovium detected by CEUS is comparable to other imaging findings. This is particularly impressive in a study by Song et al. [63] where 41 subjects with painful Kellgren-Lawrence grades 2 and 3 osteoarthritis of the knee were assessed with CEUS in comparison to MRI; CEUS was more sensitive for painful knee OA than B-mode or power Doppler ultrasound findings The CEUS findings were comparable to contrast-enhanced MRI studies of the same knee. In psoriatic knee arthropathy, neovasculature identified by CEUS correlated to the presence of CD31+ synovial tissue [64]. Conventional DMARDs, anti-TNF agents, and intra-articular glucocorticoids have been demonstrated to decrease vascular flow when monitored with CEUS. There is a suggestion that CEUS may assist in the diagnosis of vasculitis, based on the principle that neovascularization occurs in the small vessels of the inflamed arterial wall, but experience is limited and bears further study [65].

There are also studies in noninflammatory musculoskeletal disorders where enhanced vascular flow may be an integral part of the pathophysiologic state under investigation. A study of 24 subjects undergoing CEUS for the FDA-approved echocardiogram indication was recruited to have imaging of the median nerve using standard musculoskeletal protocols and demonstrated that detection of the median nerve microvasculature was possible during contrast enhancement. This US-based study was conducted under IRB supervision since CEUS for musculoskeletal indications is not approved in the United States; however, it raises an important issue of CEUS to detect microvascular intraneural inflammation as vascular pattern was detected in the carpal tunnel after administration for the echocardiogram [66]. Further study of CEUS in the carpal tunnel was performed by Motomiya et al. [67]. Blood flow by CEUS was lower preoperatively in the median nerve and then increased at months 1, 2, and 3, while blood flow in the subsynovial space was lower preoperatively and then increased at months 1 and 2 followed by a diminution in blood flow by month 3. All CEUS blood flow values, preoperative and postoperative, were higher than in health controls. Increase of flow to the median nerve with the associated changes in blood flow in the subsynovial tissue may represent the healing phase and recovery after carpal tunnel release.

Conclusion

As advances in technology continue to provide novel techniques for ultrasound, this chapter highlights how these techniques can potentially be clinically applied and further contribute to our understanding of the musculoskeletal system and how tissue change can occur in various disease states.

Review Questions:

Questions:

1. Which of the following techniques uses a strain wave imaging technique?
   (a) Virtual Touch ™ Quantification
   (b) Fibroscan ™
   (c) Real-Time Tissue Elastography ™
   (d) ElastPQ ™
   (e) All of the above
2. Which of the following is a true statement about strain wave image interpretation?
   (a) Tissues will change from "soft" to "hard" when comparing normal to pathologic states
   (b) Tissues will change from blue to red if changing from a "hard" state to a "soft" state
   (c) Strain wave images provide an absolute scale of softness to firmness
   (d) Stain wave images can be graded on a relative scale from soft to firm
   (e) Tissue softening is a sign of healing
3. Shear wave elastography only interprets the sound motion in the vertical plane.
   (a) True
   (b) False
4. Which of the following units is NOT used to measure shear waves?
   (a) kPa
   (b) Newton/m^2
   (c) Grade 2
   (d) m/sec
5. The concept of region of interest (ROI) distinguishes shear wave from strain wave elastography.
   (a) True
   (b) False
6. Which of the following is true regarding elastography of the Achilles tendon?
   (a) It remains constant over a person's lifetime.
   (b) It is independent of smoking status.
   (c) Achilles tendinopathy of ankylosing spondylitis has a distinct elastographic pattern to injury of the Achilles tendon.
   (d) Achilles softening is independent of enlargement or calcaneal erosion.
   (e) The elastography pattern of Achilles tendinopathy may improve in response to treatment.
7. Which is true regarding the assessment of skin by elastography?
   (a) Psoriatic plaque has decreased stiffness compared to normal skin.
   (b) Psoriatic plaque has increased stiffness compared to skin that has been treated for psoriasis.
   (c) Scleroderma has decreased stiffness compared to psoriatic plaque.
   (d) Scleroderma has decreased stiffness compared to normal skin.
   (e) Elastography at Rodnan skin scoring sites correlates to the Rodnan skin score at that site.

8. Which is true regarding elastography of the salivary glands in Sjögren's syndrome?
   (a) Parotid gland elastography correlated with submandibular gland elastography.
   (b) Salivary gland elastography correlates with salivary gland dysfunction.
   (c) Salivary gland elastography correlates with grayscale B-mode grading systems of glandular involvement and severity of anatomical change.
   (d) Salivary gland elastography is used to diagnose Sjögren's syndrome.
   (e) Salivary gland VTQ behaves the same as salivary gland VTIQ.
9. Median nerve stiffness by shear wave elastography correlates with EMG/NCV detection of carpal tunnel syndrome, suggesting the potential for elastography to augment the ultrasound imaging diagnosis of carpal tunnel syndrome.
   (a) True
   (b) False
10. Which of the following substances has not been employed as an agent for contrast-enhanced ultrasound (CEUS)?
   (a) Nitrogen gas
   (b) Phospholipid
   (c) Synthetic polymers
   (d) Gelatin
   (e) Stabilized surfactant

Answers

1. (c) Only Real-Time Tissue Elastography uses strain wave imaging; the other modalities use shear wave imaging techniques to create images.
2. (d) Some tissues have a high baseline tensile strength ("hard") such as tendon, and other have a low baseline tensile strength ("soft") such as skin. Elastography can detect a change in that baseline. Color change depends on the machine assignment of color to firmness, so it is necessary to always look at the scale when interpreting an image. Shear wave provides an absolute scale, not strain wave. Strain wave can be graded on a relative scale. Tissue softening can represent healing or damage.
3. (b) False. Shear wave elastography interprets sound motion in the vertical as well as the horizontal plain.
4. (c) kPa, which is essentially Newton/m^2, and m/sec are used to measure shear wave propagation, while grading scales can be applied to strain wave imaging.
5. (b) False. While all shear wave units will rely on an ROI, some strain wave units will use an ROI to compare two areas of strain wave imaging to create a ratio.
6. (e) Tendon stiffening increases with age as well as smoking status. Elastography has yet to distinguish injury from autoinflammatory states. Achilles softening correlates with tendon enlargement and calcaneal erosion. At least one clinical trial has suggested that elastography of the Achilles tendon improves with treatment.
7. (b) Psoriatic skin and sclerodermatous skin, both infiltrative processes, show increased stiffness and have not be compared directly. Psoriatic skin shows increased stiffness when compared to treatment with TNF inhibitors or corticosteroids. Only certain Rodnan sites correlate with the changes seen on elastography.

8. (b) Elastography measures of infiltration have been associated with salivary gland dysfunction, but other observations of salivary gland elastography have yielded varying results suggesting that study of these modalities is important to correlate by measurement and site of involvement.
9. (a) True
10. (a) Hard-shell bubbles can use natural polymers, gelatin, synthetic polymers, and protein such as albumin. Soft-shelled microbubbles can be composed of phospholipid or stabilized surfactant. Nitrogen gas has not been successfully used in CEUS.

Appendix A: Physics of Elastography

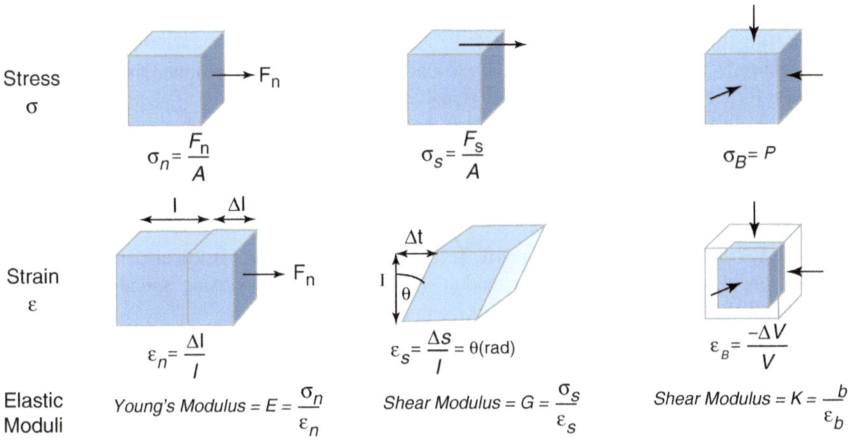

Theranostics
2017; 7(5): 1303-1329. doi: 10.7150/thno.18650

References

1. Sigrist RMS, Liau J, Kaffas AE, Maria Cristina Chammas MC, Juergen K, Willmann JK. Ultrasound elastography: review of techniques and clinical applications. Theranostics. 2017;7(5):1303–29.
2. Levinson SF, Shinagawa M, Sato T. Sonoelastic determination of human skeletal muscle elasticity. J Biomech. 1995;28:1145–54.
3. Martins-Rocha T, Azzolin I, Serban T, Massazza G, Iagnocco AM. New applications in sonoelastography in rheumatology: where are we now? Rheumatology. 2019;58(5):765–9.
4. Barr RG. Elastography in clinical practice. Radiol Clin N Am. 2014;52:1145–62.
5. Drakonaki EE, Allen GM, Wilson DJ. Ultrasound elastography for musculoskeletal applications. Br J Radiol. 2012;85(1019):1435–45.

6. Choi JJ, Kang BJ, Kim SU, et al. Role of sonographic elastography in the differential diagnosis of axillary lymph nodes in breast cancer. J Ultrasound Med. 2011;30:429–36.
7. Kwak JY, Kim E-K. Ultrasound elastography for thyroid nodules: recent advances. Ultrasonography. 2014;33:75–82.
8. Rago T, Santini F, Scutari M, Pinchera A, Vitti P. Elastography: new developments in ultrasound for predicting malignancy in thyroid nodules. J Clin Endocrinol Metab. 2007;92:2917–22.
9. Asteria C, Giovanardi A, Pizzocaro A, Cozzaglio L, Morabito A, Somalvico F, et al. US-elastography in the differential diagnosis of benign and malignant thyroid nodules. Thyroid. 2008;18:523–31.
10. DeMarco A, Bishop M, BassGoldman T, DeMarco PJ. Summative elastography score is superior to single-plane elastography score in Dupuytren's Cord treatment. J Ultrasound Med. 2016;35(suppl):2384881/S15.
11. Ryu JA, Jeong WK. Current status of musculoskeletal application of shear wave elastography. Ultrasonography. 2017;36:185–97.
12. Taljanovic MS, Gimber LH, Becker GW, Latt LD, Klauser AS, Melville DM, Gao L, Witte RS. Shear-wave elastography: basic physics and musculoskeletal applications. Radiographics. 2017;37:855–70.
13. Hofauer B, Mansour N, Heiser C, Gahleitner C, Thuermel K, Bas M, Knopf A. Sonoelastographic modalities in the evaluation of salivary gland characteristics in Sjögren's syndrome. Ultrasound Med Biol. 2016;42(9):2130–9.
14. Washburn N, Onishi K, Wang JH-C. Ultrasound elastography and ultrasound tissue characterization for tendon evaluation. J Orthop Transl. 2018;15:9–20.
15. Turan A, Teber MA, Yakut ZI, Unlu HA, Hekimoglu B. Sonoelastographıc assessment of the age-related changes of the Achilles tendon. Med Ultrason. 2015;17(1):58–61.
16. Ağladıoğlu K, Akkaya N, Güngör HR, Semih Akkaya S, Ök N, Özçakar L. Effects of cigarette smoking on elastographic strain ratio measurements of Patellar and Achilles tendons. J Ultrasound Med. 2016;35:2431–8.
17. Turan A, Tufan A, Mercan R, Teber MA, Tezcan ME, Bitik B, Goker B, Haznedaroğlu S. Real-time sonoelastography of Achilles tendon in patients with ankylosing spondylitis. Skelet Radiol. 2013;42:1113–8.
18. Dirrichs T, Quack V, Gatz M, et al. Shear wave elastography (SWE) for monitoring of treatment of tendinopathies: a double-blinded, longitudinal clinical study. Acad Radiol. 2018;25:265–72.
19. Cucoş M, Crişan M, Lenghel M, Dudea M, Croitoru R, Dudea SM. Conventional ultrasonography and sonoelastography in the assessment of plaque psoriasis under topical corticosteroid treatment –work in progress. Med Ultrasonograph. 2014;16(2):107–13.
20. Dattola A, Altobelli S, Marsico S, et al. Hypodermal adipose tissue sonoelastography for monitoring treatment response in patients with plaque psoriasis. Photomed Laser Surg. 2017;35:484–91.
21. Tatta T, Yamamoto N, Sano H, , Itoi E. In vivo measurement of rotator cuff tendon strain with ultrasound elastography - an investigation using a Porcine model. J Ultrasound Med 2014; 33:1641–1646.
22. Schmalzl J, Fenwick A, Boehm D, Gilbert F. The application of ultrasound elastography in the shoulder. J Shoulder Elbow Surg. 2017;2017(26):2236–46.
23. Hou SW, Merkle AM, Babb JS, McCabe RPT, Gyftopoulos S, Adler RS. Shear wave ultrasound elastographic evaluation of the rotator cuff tendon. J Ultrasound Med. 2017;36:95–106.
24. Arslan S, Karahan AY, Oncu F, Bakdik S, Durmaz MS, Tolu I. Diagnostic performance of superb microvascular imaging and other sonographic modalities in the assessment of lateral epicondylosis. J Ultrasound Med. 2018;37:585–93.
25. Ahn KS, Kang CH, Hong SJ, Jeong WK. Ultrasound elastography of lateral epicondylosis: clinical feasibility of quantitative elastographic measurements. AJR Am J Roentgenol. 2014;202:1094–9.
26. De Zordo T, Lill SR, Fink C, et al. Real-time sonoelastography of lateral epicondylitis: comparison of findings between patients and healthy volunteers. AJR Am J Roentgenol. 2009;193:180–5.
27. Kocyigit F, Kuyucu E, Kocyigit A, Herek DT, Savkin R, Aslan UB, Karabulut N. Association of real-time sonoelastography findings with clinical parameters in lateral epicondylitis. Rheumatol Int. 2016;36:91–100.

28. Lee S-Y, Park HJ, Kwag HJ, Hong H-Y, Park H-W, Lee Y-R, Yoon KJ, Lee Y-T. Ultrasound elastography in the early diagnosis of plantar fasciitis. Clin Imaging. 2014;38:715–8.
29. Dejaco C, De Zordo T, Heber D, Hartung W, Lipp R, Lutfi A, Magyar M, Zauner D, Lackner A, Duftner C, Horwath-Winter J, Graninger WB, Hermann J. Real-time sonoelastography of salivary glands for diagnosis and functional assessment of primary Sjögren's syndrome. Ultrasound Med Biol. 2014;40(12):2759–67.
30. Samier-Guérin A, Saraux A, Gestin S, Cornec D, Marhadour T, Devauchelle-Pensec V, Bressollette L, Nonent M, Jousse-Joulin S. Can ARFI elastometry of the salivary glands contribute to the diagnosis of Sjögren's syndrome? Joint Bone Spine. 2016;83:301–6.
31. Zhang S, Zhu J, Zhang X, He J, Li J. Assessment of the stiffness of major salivary glands in primary Sjögren's syndrome through quantitative acoustic radiation force impulse imaging. Ultrasound Med Biol. 2016;42(3):645–53.
32. Cindil E, Oktar SO, Akkan K, Sendur HN, Mercan R, Tufan A, Ozturk MA. Ultrasound elastography in assessment of salivary glands involvement in primary Sjögren's syndrome. Clin Imaging. 2018;50:229–34.
33. Turnaoglu H, Rahatli FK, Pamukcu M, Haberal KM, Uslu N. Diagnostic value of acoustic radiation force impulse imaging in the assessment of salivary gland involvement in primary Sjögren's syndrome. Med Ultrason. 2018;20(3):313–8.
34. Iagnocco A, Kaloudi O, Perella C, et al. Ultrasound elastography assessment of skin involvement in systemic sclerosis: lights and shadows. J Rheumatol. 2010;37:1688–91.
35. Di Geso L, Filippucci E, Girolimetti R, et al. Reliability of ultrasound measurements of dermal thickness at digits in systemic sclerosis: role of elastosonography. Clin Exp Rheumatol. 2011;29:926–32.
36. Cannao PM, Vinci V, Caviggioli F, et al. Technical feasibility of real-time elastography to assess the peri-oral region in patients affected by systemic sclerosis. J Ultrasound. 2014;17:265–9.
37. Hou Y, Zhu QL, Liu H, et al. A preliminary study of acoustic radiation force impulse quantification for the assessment of skin in diffuse cutaneous systemic sclerosis. J Rheumatol. 2015;42(3):449–55.
38. Liu H, Hou Y, Zhu Q-L, Xu D, Wang L, Li Jc, et al. A preliminary study of skin ultrasound in diffuse cutaneous systemic sclerosis: does skin echogenicity matter? PLoS One. 2017;12(3):e0174481. https://doi.org/10.1371/journal.pone.0174481.
39. Alsiri N, Al-Obaidi S, Asbeutah A, Almandeel M, Palmer S. The impact of hypermobility spectrum disorders on musculoskeletal tissue stiffness: an exploration using strain elastography. Clin Rheumatol. 2019;38:85–95.
40. Morris G, Jacobson JA, Kalume Brigido M, Gaetke-Udager K, Yablon CM, Diong Q. Ultrasound features of palmar fibromatosis or Dupuytren contracture. J Ultrasound Med. 2019;38(2):387–92.
41. DeMarco PJ, Matsumoto A, Thomas N, Bishop M, DeMarco AG, Respicio-Duque G, Beall A, Rosenberg R, Bass-Goldman T, Baraf HSB. Ultrasound imaging with elastography for the medical treatment of Dupuytren's contracture [abstract]. Arthritis Rheumatol. 2015;67(suppl 10)
42. Qiao Wang, Le-Hang Guo, Xiao-Long Li, Chong-Ke Zhao, Ming-Xu Li, Ling Wang, Xin-Ying Liu, Hui-Xiong Xu. Differentiating the acute phase of gout from the intercritical phase with ultrasound and quantitative shear wave elastography. Eur Radiol. 2018;28:5316–27.
43. Sconfienza LM, Silvestri E, Bartonlini B, Garlashi G, Cimmino MA. Sonoelastography may help in the differential diagnosis between rheumatoid nodules and tophi. Clin Exp Rheumatol. 2010;28(1):144–5.
44. DeMarco PJ, Matsumoto AK, Bishop M, DeMarco AG, Thomas NS, Bass-Goldman T, Baraf HSB. Podium Presentation. Elastography as Gouty Arthropathy Outcome (EGO): a pilot study. American Institute of Ultrasound in Medicine Annual Meeting. Hilton Midtown. New York, NY. March 28, 2018.
45. Ballyns JJ, Turo D, Otto P, Shah JL, Hammond J, Gebreab T, Gerber LH, Sikdar S. Office-based elastographic technique for quantifying mechanical properties of skeletal muscl. J Ultrasound Med. 2010;31:1209–19.
46. Turo D, Otto P, Hossain M, Gebreab T, Armstrong K, Rosenberger WF, Shao H, Shah JP, Gerber LH, Sikdar S. Novel use of ultrasound elastography to quantify muscle tissue changes after dry needling of myofascial trigger points in patients with chronic myofascial pain. J Ultrasound Med. 2015;34:2149–61.

47. Jafari M, Bahrpeyma F, Mokhtari-Dizaji M, Nasiri A. Novel method to measure active myofascial trigger point stiffness using ultrasound imaging. J Bodyworks Move Ther. 2018;22:274–378.
48. Kantarci F, Ustabasioglu FE, Delil S, et al. Median nerve stiffness measurement by shear wave elastography: a potential sonographic method in the diagnosis of carpal tunnel syndrome. Eur Radiol. 2014;24:434–40.
49. Liao YY, Lee WN, Lee MR, et al. Carpal tunnel syndrome: US strain imaging for diagnosis. Radiology. 2015;275:205–14.
50. Anno S, Okano T, Mamoto K, Sugioka Y, Takeda S, Hashimoto A, Yamashita E, Morinaka R, Ueda H, Inui K, Koike T, Nakamura H. Comparison of median nerve stiffness with and without rheumatoid arthritis by ultrasound real-time tissue elastography: a propensity score matching study. Mod Rheumatol. 2019; https://doi.org/10.1080/14397595.2019.1602914.
51. Tezcan S, Ozturk FU, Uslu N, Nalbant M, Yemisci OU. Carpal tunnel syndrome: evaluation of the effects of low-level laser therapy with ultrasound strain imaging. J Ultrasound Med. 2019;38:113–22.
52. Thumar V, Squires JH, Spicer PJ, Robinson AL, BSRT, Chan SS. Ultrasound elastography applications in pediatrics. Ultrasound Q. 2018;34:199–205.
53. Hunt D, Romero J. Contrast-enhanced ultrasound. Magn Reson Imaging Clin N Am. 2017;25:725–36.
54. Nolsøe CP, Nolsøe AB, Klubien J, Pommergaard H-C, Rosenberg J, Meloni MF, Lorentzen T. Use of ultrasound contrast agents in relation to percutaneous interventional procedures – a systematic review and pictorial essay. J Ultrasound Med. 2018;37:1305–24.
55. https://www.accessdata.fda.gov/drugsatfda_docs/label/2015/021064s017lbl.pdf.
56. http://www3.gehealthcare.com/~/media/documents/MarketoPDFsnogating/OPT-1H-OSLO_Optison_BK.
57. https://www.radiologybusiness.com/topics/policy/medical-societies-fda-ultrasound-black-box-warning.
58. Rafailidis V, Deganello A, Watson T, Sidhu PS, Sellars ME. Enhancing the role of paediatric ultrasound with microbubbles: a review of intravenous applications. Br J Radiol. 2017;90:20160556.
59. Rosado E, Riccabona M. Off-label use of ultrasound contrast agents for intravenous applications in children - analysis of the existing literature. J Ultrasound Med. 2016;35:487–96.
60. Doria AS, Kiss MH, Lotito AP, et al. Juvenile rheumatoid arthritis of the knee: evaluation with contrast-enhanced color Doppler ultrasound. Pediatr Radiol. 2001;31:524–31.
61. Klauser AS. Value of contrast-enhanced ultrasound in rheumatic disease. Eur Radiol Suppl. 2005;15(Suppl 5):E117–22.
62. Zhao C-Y, Jiang Y-X, Li J-C, Xu Z-H, Zhang Q, Su N, Yang M. Role of contrast-enhanced ultrasound in the evaluation of inflammatory arthritis. Chin Med J. 2017;130(14):1722–30.
63. Song IH, Althoff CE, Hermann KG, Scheel AK, Knetsch T, Schenharting M, et al. Knee osteoarthritis: efficacy of a new method of contrast-enhanced musculoskeletal ultrasonography in detection of synovitis in patients with knee osteoarthritis in comparison with magnetic resonance imaging. Ann Rheum Dis. 2008;67:19–25.
64. Fiocco U, Stramare R, Coran A, Grisan E, Scagliori E, Caso F, et al. Vascular perfusion kinetics by contrast-enhanced ultrasound are related to synovial microvascularity in the joints of psoriatic arthritis. Clin Rheumatol. 2015;34:1903–12.
65. Czihal M, Lottspeich C, Hoffmann U. Ultrasound imaging in the diagnosis of large vessel vasculitis. Vasa. 2017;46(4):241–53.
66. Volz KR, Evans KD, Kanner CD, Dickerson JA. Detection of Intraneural median nerve microvascularity using contrast-enhanced sonography. J Ultrasound Med. 2016;35:1309–16.
67. Motomiya M, Funakoshi T, Ishizaka K, Nishida M, Matsui Y, Iwasaki N. Blood flow changes in subsynovial connective tissue on contrast-enhanced ultrasonography in patients with carpal tunnel syndrome before and after surgical decompression. J Ultrasound Med. 2018;37:1597–604.

Index

M. J. Kohler (ed.), *Musculoskeletal Ultrasound in Rheumatology Review*,
https://doi.org/10.1007/978-3-030-73555-5

T

GPSR Compliance

The European Union's (EU) General Product Safety Regulation (GPSR) is a set of rules that requires consumer products to be safe and our obligations to ensure this.

If you have any concerns about our products, you can contact us on ProductSafety@springernature.com

In case Publisher is established outside the EU, the EU authorized representative is:

Springer Nature Customer Service Center GmbH
Europaplatz 3
69115 Heidelberg, Germany

Batch number: 10732632

Printed by Printforce, the Netherlands